Nutritional Status Assessment

Nutritional Status Assessment

A manual for population studies

Edited by F. Fidanza, MD,
Professor and Director, Institute of Nutrition
and Food Science, University of Perugia, Italy

CHAPMAN & HALL
London · New York · Tokyo · Melbourne · Madras

UK	Chapman & Hall, 2–6 Boundary Row, London SE1 8HN
USA	Van Nostrand Reinhold, 115 5th Avenue, New York NY10003
JAPAN	Chapman & Hall Japan, Thomson Publishing Japan, Hirakawacho Nemoto Building, 7F, 1–7–11 Hirakawa-cho, Chiyoda-ku, Tokyo 102
AUSTRALIA	Chapman & Hall Australia, Thomas Nelson Australia, 102 Dodds Street, South Melbourne, Victoria 3205
INDIA	Chapman & Hall India, R. Seshadri, 32 Second Main Road, CIT East, Madras 600 035

First edition 1991
© 1991 Chapman & Hall
Typeset in 10/12 Ehrhardt by J&L Composition Ltd, Filey, North Yorkshire
Printed in Great Britain by Clays Ltd, St Ives plc

ISBN 0 412 40100 2 (HB) 0 442 31326 8 (USA)

British Library Cataloguing in Publication Data
Nutritional status assessment.
1. Population. Nutrition. Surveillance. Methodology
I. Fidanza, F.
612.3

ISBN 0–412–40100–2

Library of Congress Cataloging-in-Publication Data
Nutritional status assessment: a manual for population studies / edited by F. Fidanza. — 1st ed.
p.   cm.
Based on two workshops held in Perugia in 1984 and 1986.
Includes bibliographical references and index.
ISBN 0–442–31326–8
1. Nutritional—Evaluation—Methodology—Congresses.   I. Fidanza, F. (Flaminio)
[DNLM: 1. Nutrition—congresses.   2. Nutritional Status—congresses.   QU 145 N9785 1984–86]
QP141.N87 1991
613.2'028'7—dc20
DNLM/DLC
for Library of Congress   90–15119
                                                                                                              CIP

Contents

Contributors   xi

Introductory Note   xv

1 **Anthropometric methodology**   1

1.1 Introduction   1

1.2 Stature and supine length   3

1.3 Body mass or weight   6

1.4 Weight/height ratios   12

1.5 Circumferences   16

     Section I   Muscle and fat areas   16

     Section II   Head and chest circumferences   23

     Section III   Waist/hip and waist/thigh ratios   24

1.6 Skinfold thickness   29

1.7 Skeletal diameters   40

Appendix A   The presentation and use of height and weight data for comparing the nutritional status of groups of children under the age of 10 years   44

2 **Body composition methodology**   63

2.1 Introduction   63

2.2 Densitometry   64

2.3 Dilutometry   71

     Section I   Determination of total body water   74

     Section II   Determination of exchangeable potassium   77

     Section III   Determination of total body potassium in a whole-body counter   79

2.4 Advanced methods   83

3 **Physical working capacity and physical fitness methodology**   101

3.1 Introduction   101

3.2 Cardiorespiratory efficiency   102

3.3 Muscle strength   106

3.4 Motor performance   108

3.5 Final comments   112

4 Energy balance methodology   113
4.1 Introduction   113
4.2 Energy intake   115
4.3 Energy expenditure   117

5 Lipid pattern methodology   131
5.1 Introduction   131
5.2 Essential fatty acids by HRGC   131
5.3 Separation and determination of plasma lipids and
    lipoproteins   139
    Section I   Plasma or serum cholesterol determination   140
    Section II   Plasma or serum triglyceride determination   142
    Section III Separation of plasma lipoproteins   144
    Section IV HDL cholesterol determination   148
5.4 The arachidonic acid cascade in the vascular system   153

6 Protein nutriture methodology   165
6.1 Introduction   165
6.2 Indicators of nutritional status: general aspects   167
6.3 Plasma proteins   169
6.4 Urinary creatinine   173
6.5 3–Methyl-histidine   175
6.6 IGF–1 (insulin-like growth factor–1, somatomedin C)   178

7 Vitamin nutriture methodology   185
7.1 Introduction   186
7.2 Vitamin A   191
    Section I   Vitamin A (retinol) in plasma by HPLC   191
    Section II   Vitamin A (retinol) in plasma and serum by
                HPLC-micromethod   195
    Section III β-Carotene in plasma by HPLC   200
7.3 Vitamin D (25-OHD) in serum by competitive
    protein-binding assay   203
7.4 Vitamin E (α-tocopherol)   209
7.5 Vitamin K_1 214
    Section I   Phylloquinone (vitamin K_1) in serum and
                plasma by HPLC   214
    Section II   Trans-vitamin K_1 (phylloquinone) in serum
                by HPLC-micromethod   220
7.6 Thiamin   228
    Section I   Erythrocyte transketolase activity   228
    Section II   Erythrocyte transketolase activity –
                micromethod   233
    Section III Total thiamin in whole blood by HPLC   235

	Section IV	Thiamin in urine	241
7.7	Riboflavin		244
	Section I	Erythrocyte glutathione reductase activity	244
	Section II	Erythrocyte glutathione reductase activity – micromethod	248
	Section III	Flavin adenine dinucleotide (FAD) in whole blood by HPLC	251
	Section IV	Riboflavin in urine by HPLC	256
7.8	Niacin		258
	Section I	Niacin in whole blood by microbiological assay	258
	Section II	Niacin metabolites in urine by HPLC	263
7.9	Vitamin B_6		266
	Section I	Erythrocyte aspartate transaminase	266
	Section II	Pyridoxal 5′-phosphate (PLP) in whole blood by HPLC	271
	Section III	Pyridoxal 5′-phosphate in plasma by radioenzymatic assay using tyrosine decarboxylase apoenzyme	276
	Section IV	4-Pyridoxic acid in urine by HPLC	280
7.10	Folic acid (5–Me–THF) in serum and erythrocytes by radioassay		283
7.11	Vitamin B_{12} (total cobalamins) in serum by competitive protein-binding assay		290
7.12	Biotin		296
	Section I	Biotin in whole blood by microbiological assay	296
	Section II	Biotin in plasma or urine by RIA	300
7.13	Pantothenic acid in whole blood by microbiological assay		304
7.14	Vitamin C		309
	Section I	Vitamin C in plasma and buffy coat layer of blood, by dinitrophenyl hydrazine assay	309
	Section II	Total vitamin C in whole blood and plasma by HPLC-micromethod	315

8	**Essential mineral and trace element nutriture methodology**		331
8.1	Introduction		332
8.2	Sodium		335
8.3	Potassium		341
8.4	Calcium		342
	Section I	Total serum/plasma calcium	344
	Section II	Ionized calcium	345

	Section III	Metacarpal indices	346
	Section IV	Urinary hydroxyproline	348
	Section V	Serum osteocalcin	349
8.5	Phosphorous		350
8.6	Magnesium		353
	Section I	Serum and urinary magnesium	353
	Section II	Serum magnesium by colorimetric method	354
8.7	Iron		355
	Methods for assessing iron deficiency		355
	Section I	Methods for evaluating the risks of iron deficiency (pre-pathogenic period)	356
	Section II	Methods for assessing iron status (pathogenic period)	357
	Section IIA	Indicators for evaluating the size of body iron stores	357
	Section IIB	Indicators of the adequacy of iron supply to the erythroid marrow	362
	Section IIC	Indicators of anaemia	372
	Choice of indicators for assessing iron deficiency in a population		376
	Interpretation of iron status measurements		382
8.8	Zinc		385
	Section I	Zinc in plasma or serum by atomic absorption spectrophotometry	385
	Section II	Plasma or urine zinc	386
	Section III	Serum/plasma zinc – alternative method	387
	Section IV	Zinc in leukocyte and leukocyte subsets	388
	Section V	Hair zinc	391
	Section VI	Alkaline phosphatase	392
8.9	Copper		395
	Section I	Plasma or serum copper by AAS	395
	Section II	Serum/plasma copper by colorimetric method	396
	Section III	Measurement of human serum caeruloplasmin	396
	Section IV	Erythrocyte superoxide dismutase	398
8.10	Selenium		401
	Section I	Blood selenium by spectrophotometry	402
	Section II	Blood selenium by fluorimetric technique	404
	Section III	Glutathione peroxidase activity	406
8.11	Chromium		408
8.12	Manganese		410

9 **Immunocompetence methodology**   425
   9.1 Introduction   425
   9.2 Lymphocyte count   428
   9.3 Delayed cutaneous hypersensitivity   429
   9.4 Complement C3 and factor B   432
   9.5 Secretory IgA   434
   9.6 T-lymphocyte and subset percentage   436
   9.7 Lymphocyte proliferation response   438

10 **Clinical nutriture methodology**   453

11 **Psychometrics and nutrition**   457

   Index   475

Contributors

P.J. Aggett
Department of Child Health, University of Aberdeen, Aberdeen, UK.

J. Arthur
Rowett Research Institute, Bucksburn, Aberdeen, UK.

C. Bates
MRC, Dunn Nutrition Unit, Cambridge, UK.

H. van den Berg
TNO–CIVO Toxicology and Nutrition Institute, Department of Clinical Biochemistry, Zeist, The Netherlands.

R. Bitsch
Ernährungswissenschaft Fakultät, Universität Gesamthochschule, Paderborn, FRG.

I. Bosaeus
Department of Clinical Nutrition, Annedasklinikerna, Sahlgren's Hospital, University of Gothenburg, Gothenburg, Sweden.

P.G. Boshuis
TNO–CIVO Toxicology and Nutrition Institute, Department of Clinical Biochemistry, Zeist, The Netherlands.

N. van Breederode
TNO–CIVO Toxicology and Nutrition Institute, Department of Clinical Biochemistry, Zeist, The Netherlands.

G.B. Brubacher
Institute of Biochemistry, University of Basel, Switzerland.

A.L. Catapano
Istituto di Scienze Farmacologiche, Università di Milano, Italy.

R.K. Chandra
Department of Pediatrics, Memorial University of Newfoundland and Janeway Child Health Centre, St John's, Newfoundland, Canada.

S. Ciappellano
Dipartimento di Scienze e Tecnologie Alimentari e Microbiologiche, Sezione Nutrizione, Università di Milano, Italy.

K.J. Connolly
Department of Psychology, University of Sheffield, UK.

P. Damiani
Istituto di Chimica Bromatologica, Università degli Studi, Perugia, Italy.

A. Dhur
Centre de Recherche sur les Anemies Nutritionnelles, Institute Scientifique et Technique de l'Alimentation, CNAM, Paris, France.

A. Ferro-Luzzi
Instituto Nazionale della Nutrizione, Roma, Italy.

F. Fidanza
Istituto di Scienza dell'Alimentazione, Università degli Studi, Perugia, Italy.

D. Fraser
MRC, Dunn Nutrition Unit, Cambridge, UK.

P. Galan
Centre de Recherche sur les Anemies Nutritionnelles, Institute Scientifique et Technique de l'Alimentation, CNAM, Paris, France.

C. Galli
Istituto di Scienze Farmacologiche, Università di Milano, Italy.

P.M.M. van Haard
Diagnostic Centre SSDZ, Department of Special Analysis, Delft, The Netherlands.

M. Hages
Institute of Nutrition, Department of Pathophysiology of Human Nutrition, University of Bonn, FRG.

S. Hercberg
Centre de Recherche sur les Anemies Nutritionnelles, Institute Scientifique et Technique de l'Alimentation, CNAM, Paris, France.

H. Heseker
Institute of Nutrition, Justus-Liebig University, Giessen, FRG.

S.B. Heymsfield
Columbia University, College of Physicians and Surgeons, New York, USA.

B. Isaksson
Department of Clinical Nutrition, Annedalsklinikerna, Sahlgren's Hospital, University of Gothenburg, Gothenburg, Sweden.

W.P.T. James
Rowett Research Institute, Bucksburn, Aberdeen, UK.

H.E. Keller
Department of Vitamin and Nutrition Research, F. Hoffman-La Roche & Co. Ltd, Basel, Switzerland.

W. Keller
Nutrition, World Health Organization, Geneva, Switzerland.

D.J. Millward
Nutrition Research Unit, London School of Hygiene and Tropical Medicine,
London, UK.

H.A.J. Mocking
TNO–CIVO Toxicology and Nutrition Institute, Department of Clinical
Biochemistry, Zeist, The Netherlands.

N.G. Norgan
Department of Human Sciences, University of Technology, Loughborough,
UK.

J. Pǎrízková
Research Institute of Physical Education, Charles University, Prague,
Czechoslovakia.

G. Pastore
Istituto Nazionale della Nutrizione, Roma, Italy.

A-L.J.M. Pietersma
Reinier de Graaf Gasthuis, Department of Gynecology and Obstetrics, Delft,
The Netherlands.

K. Pietrzik
Institute of Nutrition, Department of Pathophysiology of Human Nutrition,
University of Bonn, FRG.

T. Postma
Diagnostic Centre SSDZ, Department of Special Analysis, Delft, The
Netherlands.

A. Ralph
Rowett Research Institute, Bucksburn, Aberdeen, UK.

D.M. Reid
City Hospital, Aberdeen, UK.

J. Sandhu
MRC, Dunn Nutrition Unit, Cambridge, England.

P. Sarchielli
Istituto di Scienza dell'Alimentazione, Università degli Studi, Perugia, Italy.

J. Schrijver
TNO–CIVO Toxicology and Nutrition Institute, Department of Clinical
Biochemistry, Zeist, The Netherlands.

J.C. Seidell,
Department of Human Nutrition, Agricultural University, Wageningen, The
Netherlands.

M.J. Shearer
Department of Haematology, Guy's Hospital, London, UK.

M.S. Simonetti
Istituto di Scienza dell'Alimentazione, Università degli Studi, Perugia, Italy.

A.J. Speek
TNO–CIVO Toxicology and Nutrition Institute, Department of Clinical Biochemistry, Zeist, The Netherlands.

A. Speitling
Institute of Nutrition, Justus-Liebig University, Giessen, FRG.

G. Testolin
Dipartimento di Scienze e Tecnologie Alimentari e Microbiologiche, Sezione Nutrizione, Università di Milano, Italy.

J.P. Vuilleumier
Formerly at Department of Vitamin and Nutrition Research, F. Hoffmann-La Roche & Co. Ltd, Basel, Switzerland.

Introductory note

Quality control and standardization of methodology in nutritional epidemiology studies are essential items particularly in the comparison of results.

In the past the major reference publication has been that of the Interdepartmental Committee on Nutrition for National Defense [1]. However, methodology has greatly improved in the last few years and consequently the preparation of an updated manual has become necessary. With this intention we organized two Workshops in collaboration with the Group of European Nutritionists [2, 3]. Most of the material presented at these Workshops, together with some changes and many improvements contributed by experts in specific fields, is included in the present Manual.

Other manuals and books on the subject have been published since 1963, but they either cover aspects of the methodology for nutritional status assessment only partially [4–10] or are addressed specifically to clinicians [11, 12].

To avoid a bulky manual, some aspects that can be found in other publications have been omitted. The sampling procedure, for example, which is of basic importance in nutritional epidemiology, can be found in *Practical Human Biology* [13], and also in many Epidemiology textbooks; useful information on this can also be found in the WHO monograph *Cardiovascular Survey Methods* [14]. In this practical publication, the design and planning of cardiovascular surveys covering general aims and types of population studies, the principles of measurement, examination techniques with examples of questionnaires, and the ECG standardized procedure and coding (Minnesota code) are also dealt with.

Details of the carbohydrate tolerance test are included in the above mentioned WHO monograph. Further information and also the definition and classification of diabetes mellitus can be found in the review by Keen and Ng Tang Fui [15].

This is not the place to examine in detail the aims and types of nutritional epidemiological studies. In some of the above publications they are well described. The review by Burr [16] on this topic can also be of some use.

In organizing this Manual we have considered the performance characteristics of most of the methods in detail so as to improve their quality control. Efforts must be made to achieve better comparability and compatibility between laboratory and field results. This is already much improved for anthropometry [17] and laboratory assays [18].

For the standardization of methods (particularly biochemical methods) we need reference material and reference laboratories. As regards reference material, both the National Bureau of Standards (US) and the Community Bureau of Reference of the European Communities Commission can provide this. Requests will be despatched at once. The Netherlands organization for applied scientific research (TNO–CIVO Institutes) in Zeist (The Netherlands) is willing to act as the reference laboratory.

We hope that the above organization will also undertake responsibility for the training of personnel – another important item in epidemiological research.

As editor I have attempted in most cases to render the presentation of each method uniform in this manual, while at the same time leaving the authors some freedom. Uniformity and diversity are sometimes not in conflict and can be interesting; this is a characteristic of the Mediterranean – Latin culture.

F. Fidanza

REFERENCES

1. ICNND. (1963) *Manual for Nutrition Surveys*, Interdepartmental Committee on Nutrition for National Defense, Bethesda.
2. Fidanza, F. (ed.) (1984) *Nutritional Status Assessment of Individuals and Population Groups*, Group of European Nutritionists, Perugia.
3. Fidanza, F. (ed.) (1986) *Nutritional Status Assessment Methodology for Individuals and Population Groups*, Group of European Nutritionists, Perugia.
4. WHO. (1963) *Expert Committee on Medical Assessment of Nutritional Status*, WHO, Geneva. Techn. Rep. Series, No. 258.
5. Jelliffe, D.B. (1966) *The Assessment of the Nutritional Status of the Community*, WHO, Geneva.
6. Weiner, J.S. and Lourie, J.A. (1969) *Human Biology: A Guide to Field Methods*, Blackwell Scientific, Oxford.
7. Sauberlich, H.E., Skala, J.H. and Dowdy, R.P. (1974) *Laboratory Tests for the Assessment of Nutritional Status*, CRC Press, Cleveland (Ohio).
8. Curtius, H.Ch. and Roth, M. (eds) (1974) *Clinical Biochemistry – Principles and Methods. Vol II. Vitamins*, de Gruyter, Berlin, pp. 972–1008.
9. Levenson, S.M. (ed.) (1981) *Nutritional Assessment – Present Status, Future Directions and Prospects*, Ross Laboratories, Columbus (Ohio).
10. Sahn, D.E., Lockwood, R. and Scrimshaw, N.S. (1984) *Methods for the Evaluation of the Impact of Food and Nutrition Programmes*, United Nations University, Tokyo.
11. Jensen, T.G., Englert, D.M. and Dudrick, S.J. (1983) *Nutritional Assessment. A Manual for Practitioners*, Appleton–Century–Crofts, Norwalk (Conn).
12. Wright, R.A., Heymsfield, S. and McManus, C.B. (eds) (1984) *Nutritional Assessment*, Blackwell Scientific, Boston.
13. Weiner, J.S. and Lourie, J.A. (1981) *Practical Human Biology*, Academic Press, London.
14. Rose, G.A. *et al.* (1982) *Cardiovascular Survey Methods*, 2nd edn, WHO, Geneva.
15. Keen, H. and Ng Tang Fui, S. (1982) The definition and classification of diabetes mellitus. *Clin. Endocrinol. Metab.*, **11** (2), 279–305.
16. Burr, M.L. (1985) Nutritional epidemiology. *Prog. Food Nutr. Sci.*, **9**, 149–83.
17. Lohman, T.G., Roche, A.F. and Martorell, R. (eds) (1988) *Anthropometric Standardization Reference Manual*, Human Kinetics Books, Champaign (Illinois).
18. Kallner, A., Bangham, D. and Moss, D. (eds) (1989) Improvement of comparability and compatibility of laboratory assay results in life sciences. *Scand. J. Clin. Lab. Invest.*, **49** [Suppl], 193.

1 Anthropometric methodology

1.1 Introduction *F. Fidanza*	1
1.2 Stature and supine length *F. Fidanza*	3
1.3 Body mass or weight *F. Fidanza and W. Keller*	6
1.4 Weight/height ratios *F. Fidanza*	12
1.5 Circumferences	16
Section I Muscle and fat areas *S.B. Heymsfield*	16
Section II Head and chest circumferences *F. Fidanza*	23
Section III Waist/hip and waist/thigh ratios *J.C. Seidell*	24
1.6 Skinfold thickness *N.G. Norgan, F. Fidanza and P. Sarchielli*	29
1.7 Skeletal diameters *N.G. Norgan*	40
Appendix A	44

1.1 INTRODUCTION

Anthropometric measurements can provide information on gross body size, skeletal form or configuration, and on skeletal and soft-tissue development.

As stated previously in a WHO document [1]

> ... all physical characteristics result from the interaction of heredity and environment. ... Body measurements may not always be used safely for comparing the nutritional status of genetically different populations nor for an assessment of nutritional status by reference to a world standard. They are, however, useful for follow-up of physical state over periods too short for genetic selection to affect the population in a significant way, provided gene flow is negligible.

The number of measurements is very large and the selection depends on the purpose of the study, and the size and age of the sample to be examined. The Committee on Nutritional Anthropometry of the Food and Nutrition Board of the National Research Council (USA) recommended the following items [2]: Body weight, stature, sitting height, iliocristal height, bicristal (biiliac) diameter, biacromial diameter, upper-arm skinfold, and upper-arm circumference. Further measurements for children, according to age, are also included.

The report of the Expert Committee on Medical Assessment of Nutritional Status of the WHO [3] recommended the measurements given in Table 1.1., divided according to age.

Table 1.1   Recommended measurements in nutrition surveys from WHO

Age group (years)	Practical field observations	More detailed observations

0–1	Weight
	Length
		Stem length
		Circumferences:
		  head
		  chest
		Bicristal diameter
		Skinfold:
		  triceps
		  subscapula
		  chest

1–5	Weight
	Length (up to 3 years)
	Height (over 3 years)
	Skinfold over biceps and
	  triceps
	Arm circumference
		Stem length (up to 3 years)
		Sitting height (over 3 years)
		Circumferences:
		  head
		  chest (mid-inspiration)
		Bicristal diameter
		Skinfold:
		  subscapula
		  chest
		Calf circumference
		Posteroanterior X-ray
		  of hand and wrist*

5–20	Weight Height Skinfold over triceps	Sitting height Bicristal diameter Biacromial diameter Skinfold in other sites Posteroanterior X-ray of hand and wrist* Arm and calf circumferences
Over 20	Weight Height Skinfold over triceps	Skinfold in other sites Arm and calf circumferences

* Interpreted by comparison with the Greulich and Pyle atlas [4].

The above report also recommended the publication of a detailed guide describing body measurement techniques and their interpretation. This recommendation was followed by Jelliffe [5], who, in a book on the assessment of the nutritional status of the community, considered nutritional anthropometry in detail. Unfortunately this publication is now out of print.

The group of investigators who met in Geneva in December 1968 proposed the following list as the minimum anthropometric data to be used as criteria for trends of nutritional status in populations: body weight, stature or supine length, sitting height or crown–rump length, upper-arm circumference, triceps skinfold, subscapular skinfold (when practicable), biacromial diameter, and bi-iliocristal diameter.

At about the same time the list of measurements recommended by the International Biological Programme was published [6]. To the basic list of 21 measurements an additional 17 were suggested to achieve a more complete anthropometric examination. This very useful publication has been out of print for years, but much of the material has recently been incorporated in a new publication [7], in which the following anthropometric measurements for assessment of nutritional status are listed: stature, weight, and upper-arm circumference as a minimum; and in addition (if facilities permit) biceps skinfold thickness, triceps skinfold thickness, subscapular skinfold thickness, and calculated muscle circumference.

Another useful and practical publication is that of the Department of Technical Co-operation for Development and Statistical Office of the United Nations for 'Assessing the nutritional status of young children in household surveys' [8]. The procedures for child height or length, weight and mid-upper-arm circumference measurements are fully described and illustrated.

Since methodologies had still not been satisfactorily standardized, a conference was held recently in Arlie (USA) for this purpose. Most of the material was incorporated in an *Anthropometric Standardization Reference Manual* [9]. In this very useful publication most of the measurements not considered in this Chapter can be found described in great detail.

One problem relevant to some measurements is the side on which they should be taken. In the USA the right side is preferred. Most investigators in Europe and the developing countries take measurements on the left side. Although there is a difference between the right and left sides, particularly for some measurements [9], at the moment it seems difficult to reach a consensus. A pragmatic solution is to leave the choice of the side to be measured to the investigator, even if this limits the comparability of the collected data.

1.2 STATURE AND SUPINE LENGTH

1.2.1 Purpose and scope

Stature (standing height) and supine length are considered indicators of general body size and of bone length. In addition to the total height or length, various bony components can be measured for detailed studies of body dimensions.

Assessment of height alone or in association with age may be used as an indicator of the nutritional status of groups and, according to Keller *et al.* [10] it

> ... will estimate past and chronic malnutrition but not necessarily the present nutritional status. It has been shown that the height of African pre-school children was related to the socioeconomic conditions of their families as well as to intakes of energy, protein, and other nutrients. However, the disadvantages of using only height as an indicator are many. The distribution of height is usually narrow; in British pre-school children the third percentile is only 7–8% below the median, a fact that makes grading difficult. Another disadvantage would be the observation made earlier that a deficit in height takes some time to develop; it may not be manifest in infant malnutrition, and when found in infants or young children may be the consequence of small size at birth rather than an indication of postnatal malnutrition.

Genetically determined differences are partly responsible for the differences in height found in any age-group in any population. A preponderance of a genetic trait for large or for small stature in particular ethnic groups has occasionally been shown. In most cases, this will be difficult or impossible to prove, but the possibility of ethnic differences in height cannot be completely discounted.

Weight for height will be examined in detail in the next section. As an indication of the proportion of total height represented by the trunk and legs, the Committee on Nutritional Anthropometry has proposed the measurements of sitting height and cristal height. The relative merit of these variables was not clearly established.

1.2.2 Principle of the method

Using appropriate instruments the stature and supine length of the person in standardized conditions is assessed.

1.2.3 Apparatus

For supine length and crown–rump length there are two main types of instruments: those with a movable footboard and those with movable head and foot contacts. The Harpenden Infant Measuring Table, available from British Indicators Ltd, Sutton Road, St Albans, Herts, UK, is recommended.

Height is measured by a portable measuring rod, in sections ('anthropometer') or by equipment consisting of a board with attached scale ('stadiometer'). The Harpenden Stadiometer (digital read-out wall-mounted with a measurement range of 600–2100 mm to the nearest millimetre) is recommended. For field studies a portable stadiometer (measurement range 840–2060 mm) is available. The digital read-out Harpenden anthropometer with various accessories is also recommended. All the Harpenden instruments can be obtained from British Indicators Ltd (see above). Of course other apparatus are also available. A wall scale employing a suitable steel or plastic tape ruled in centimetres and millimetres is also acceptable. The measuring instrument in this case is a triangular block or an L-shaped bar which makes contact with the wall and the top of the subject's head. The wall must be vertical, the floor horizontal and the position of the tape carefully checked.

An appropriately rigid board should be used for people who cannot stand easily. The board should have a right-angled foot support to bring the feet into position. In this case it should be kept in mind that a person's recumbent length is somewhat greater than his stature.

1.2.4 Procedure

Technique

For supine length (in millimetres) the infant is measured lying supine. One measurer holds the infant's head with the Frankfort plane vertical and applies gentle traction to bring the top of his head into contact with the fixed headboard. A second measurer holds the infant's feet, toes pointing directly upward, and, also applying gentle traction, brings the movable footboard to rest firmly against the infant's heels. When using an instrument with both a movable headboard and footboard, one measurer holds the head with the Frankfort plane vertical with one hand and stabilizes the knees with the other. The second measurer moves the boards firmly against the vertex and feet and reads the value from the scale.

For crown–rump length (in millimetres) the infant lies on his back with the thighs vertical and the knees bent to a right-angle. One measurer holds the infant's head with the Frankfort plane vertical and applies gentle traction to bring it into contact with the fixed headboard. A second measurer supports the infant's legs and brings the movable footboard to rest against his buttocks. When using an instrument with two movable boards, one measurer holds the infant in the correct position as described above and the second measurer moves the boards firmly against the vertex and buttocks and reads the value from the scale.

For stature (in millimetres) the person should stand on a horizontal platform without shoes and socks with the heels together and should stretch upwards to his fullest extent (this may be assured by relaxing the shoulders, taking a deep breath and/or by gentle upward pressure by the measurer on the mastoid processes). The person's back should be as straight as possible. The line of sight, or, more precisely, the Frankfort plane, must be horizontal (this plane is defined by the line joining the left tragion and the lowest point of the inferior margin of the left orbit).

Either the horizontal arm of an anthropometer or the board of a stadiometer is brought down onto the person's head. One measurer should hold the instrument vertically behind the person with the horizontal arm in contact with the subject's head, while another applies gentle upward pressure as above. The subject's heels must be watched to make sure they do not leave the ground.

If stature cannot be measured and the recumbent length is difficult to obtain, arm span can be measured with a wall tape or an anthropometer. With the wall tape, the zero is at the corner of the wall or at a fixed adjustable block. The person stands with his back against the wall and with feet together. Arms are outstretched maximally at the level of the shoulders, with palms facing forwards. The longest finger of the right arm (excluding fingernails) is in contact with the wall or the board. The second measurer takes the reading to the nearest millimetre at the longest finger of the left arm. Of course the tape should be adjusted to the shoulder height of the person. Measurement with a stadiometer is much simpler, particularly if the subject is supine. The stadiometer should pass over the clavicles; therefore two measurers are necessary in this case also.

For segment lengths, measured only for detailed studies, refer to the recent *Anthropometric Standardization Reference Manual* [9].

1.2.5 Performance characteristics

(a) Reproducibility

Using good equipment and well-trained, motivated personnel it is possible to reduce the reading error of the measurement to one millimetre in children.

According to Gordon *et al.* [11] intermeasure mean differences in the Fels Longitudinal Study are: 2.4 mm (SD = 2.1 mm) at 5–10 years; 2.0 mm (SD = 1.9 mm) at 10–15 years; 2.3 mm (SD = 2.4 mm) at 15–20 years; 1.4 mm (SD = 1.5 mm) at 20–55 years and 2.1 mm (SD = 2.1 mm) at 55–85 years.

(b) Validity

Height for age is a direct measure of skeletal growth. Its validity as an indicator of nutrition is questioned because of its association with socioeconomic levels [12]. However, the term nutritional status usually refers only to energy and protein nutrition whereas growth retardation (i.e. low height for age) has been observed as a reaction to dietary deficiency of a large number of vitamins, minerals, and trace elements. Very little is known about the epidemiological importance of most of these specific deficiencies, especially in their milder subclinical stages. Therefore height for age does not have great validity as an indicator.

1.2.6   Reference values

The mean heights, including sitting heights, of children and adults collected under the International Biological Programme are reported in the book of Eveleth and Tanner [13].

In the WHO publication *Measuring Change in Nutritional Status* [14], obtainable on request, tables of length or stature of boys and girls 0–18 years and 49–145 cm in height are reported. Information on standardization procedures and statistical aspects of sampling in studies to assess the nutritional impact of supplementary feeding programmes for vulnerable groups can be found in this publication.

1.2.7   Interpretation

As already pointed out height alone cannot be considered a good indicator of nutritional status of groups of children. The use of height for age, grouping the ages into various classes as suggested by WHO [14], is preferable. The data are then compared with the distribution in a reference population of well-nourished healthy children, as in the tables prepared by WHO [14]. Their use can be found in Waterlow *et al.* (see Appendix A of this chapter (p. 44)). From this comparison it is possible to obtain the percentage of children with the indicator at a low level and the distribution of the indicator within the sampled population in respect to the reference population.

If the age is not available, weight for height can be grouped using height classes as an alternative as suggested by WHO [14]. Further information can be found in a more recent paper by a WHO working group [15].

For adults the weight/height ratios that will be examined in section 1.4 are preferred to actual height. Often tables of height distribution by age are available at national levels. The data have been recorded during national surveys or by societies of actuaries. International tables are not available and in any case their use is limited.

From the sitting height value subtracted from the stature an index called Relative Height of Trunk plus Head can be obtained. It is useful for classifying individuals as regards one aspect of skeletal form, the length of the trunk plus head.

1.3   BODY MASS OR WEIGHT

1.3.1   Purpose and scope

Body mass or body weight are different variables from a physical point of view, but because of the large intraindividual variation and the conditions of the measurement they can be considered biologically synonymous.

Body weight, which measures practically the total body mass, cannot by itself provide any information on body composition, since it does not discriminate whether the mass is partly or mostly composed of muscle, water or fat. Nevertheless repeated measurement of body weight is the most simple, direct, and common assessment of growth in children. According to Keller *et al.* [10]:

... if a single measurement of weight is used to assess the nutritional status, it has to be compared with a reference, the weight of a 'normal' child of the same age. Gomez has introduced weight for age for the classification of malnutrition, and this has been widely used and recommended both for individual patients and for the assessment of the prevalence and severity of malnutrition in communities or populations. The simplest way of classifying a child population is the use of percentages of the reference value as class limits.

A more sophisticated procedure is comparison with the distribution of values in the reference population by using percentiles of the reference population as class limits.

Apart from the general difficulty of defining and finding a 'normal' reference population without overnutrition or undernutrition, the use of weight for age as a measure of nutritional status has two obvious disadvantages. The first is the fact that in severely malnourished children oedema may partly compensate for deficit weight. Such children would thus not be classified as severely malnourished. The second reservation concerns the difference in height or body length that may exist between the population surveyed and the reference population. It is well known that malnutrition in children over some length of time produces a deficit in height as well as in weight, whereas an acute episode of malnutrition, or malnutrition seen in its initial stages, has little effect on skeletal growth. In fact, many malnourished child populations show a weight deficit that increases with age, an observation that often contradicts clinical experience.

An assessment of weight for age will therefore overestimate actual malnutrition by including in the figure children who are unusually small for their age. It will also overestimate overnutrition by the same mechanism.

Keller *et al.* [10] add that

... in order to eliminate the influence of height when comparing weight with a reference standard the weight found at a certain age is often corrected for height by comparing it with the weight of a reference group of the same height rather than of the same age. An indicator of leanness and fatness is thus obtained. Since the commonly used reference standards for weight and height do not give the distribution of weights over height at different ages, weight for height can be expressed as a percentage of the reference median weight for median height at each age. Experience has proved that 80% of the standard is an adequate limit between the malnourished and the adequately nourished.

Moreover, in the only large reference standard containing data on the distribution of weight for height in the United States of America, only 5% of the children of more than 70 cm height are below 87% of the median weight for height and it is possible that less than 1% are below 80% of the standard.

One obvious advantage of using weight for height as an index of nutritional status is its apparent age independence. In the commonly used height and weight standards from well-nourished populations the relationship of the mean or median weights and heights follows (approximately) a straight line and can be adequately expressed by linear equation. By expressing deviations from the standards as a percentage of it, age independence is maintained, i.e., deviation of the weight for height is expressed in proportion to the height.

There are obvious disadvantages and limitations to the use of weight for height. One is the difficulty of measuring body length in young infants, which may make it difficult or sometimes impossible to obtain adequate data in this age-group. Another is inherent in its being a specific expression of leanness–fatness: it gives no information on the duration of malnutrition. For purposes like screening, where the index is applied to individuals, the fact that the errors in measuring height and weight approximately add up to the error of the index weight for height makes the index unreliable in young infants.

For adults the use of relative body weight (percentage of the average weight of individuals of a given height and age as reported in reference tables) was preferred in the past to detect overweight and underweight, and indirectly under- and overnutrition.

But since appropriate reference height–weight tables for adults are not available [16, 17], weight/height ratios are now used, and will be examined in section 1.4.

1.3.2 Principle of the method

Using an appropriate and repeatedly calibrated weighing machine, the body weight of the person in standard conditions is assessed.

1.3.3 Apparatus

For infants a levelled beam balance scale with movable but non-detachable weights is used. The pan should be long enough to support a two-year-old infant. Calibration is carried out with objects of known weights at least every time the scale is moved, making sure that it is positioned on a level plane. When the scale is not in use, the beam is locked and the weights are shifted to zero to reduce wear.

For older children and adults a platform beam scale is used following the above recommendations.

The CMS Weighing Equipment Ltd (18 Camden High Street, London NW1 0JH UK) distributes an all-purpose weighing machine (accurate to ± 50 g up to 160 kg) with extra capacity possibility and a portable Field Survey Scale. Electronic scales are now available (e.g. Seca 770 alpha 0–200 kg × 100 g from Seca Vogel and Halke, Hammer Steindamm 7–25, 2000-Hamburg 76, FRG), which are very accurate, light and easy to transport. Also in this case levelling and calibration are of great importance. A hanging scale (also available from CMS Weighing Equipment Ltd) as well as a beam chair scale can be used in particular conditions.

Spring scales are not recommended because the spring becomes stretched and inaccurate with prolonged use and it is sensitive to hot climates.

1.3.4 Procedure

(a) Technique

Infants should be weighed nude or, if wearing a diaper, the latter's weight should be subtracted. The infant should lie quietly on the pan, with weight distributed evenly on each side of the centre of the pan. Weight is recorded to the nearest 10 g, using the average of three repeated weighings if possible. If the infant or young child is restless the only possibility is to weight it with its mother and then to subtract her weight. This procedure, however, is unreliable because most beam scales measure weight to the nearest 100 g only. This is not the case with an electronic scale. Older children and adults should be weighed nude if possible, or with light underwear or a disposable paper gown.

Shoes and heavy socks should be removed or their weight subtracted later; this may also be necessary in a few cases for ordinary clothing. In general the weight should not be recorded just after a full meal, and sometimes standard conditions are requested.

The individual stands on the centre of the platform, with the body weight evenly distributed on both feet, and without touching anything else. Weight is recorded to the nearest 100 g.

(b) Calculation

In children weight and height for age and weight for height or length are usually transformed into indices. This can be done in two ways, by mathematical relationships between measurements (for example, the Wetzel grid) established for healthy, well-nourished children (the reference populations), or by direct comparison with the measurements of such a reference population. The latter procedure became popular after Gomez *et al.* [18] used it for the classification of malnutrition by weight for age categories; it is the one commonly used at present and internationally recommended [19] for the three indicators: weight for age, height (length) for age and weight for height (length).

Over the years a number of reference data sets on child growth have been prepared and used. The reference population most used at present is the one prepared by the National Center for Health Statistics (NCHS) of the United States of America [20]. The differences between the reference sets from the various affluent countries are not very great and it is perhaps not very important which one is chosen. However, in order to ensure comparability and because of its accessibility the NCHS reference is recommended [19, 21].

The international use of one reference may be criticized. There may be a degree of overnutrition as well as chronic morbidity in the population sample, the secular trend in linear growth may still be continuing or ethnic differences in height between populations may make one reference inappropriate. The last argument has been refuted for many populations [22] but it cannot be completely excluded. It is therefore important to keep in mind the relative nature of even the best reference population and as far as possible to use it as a descriptive reference rather than a standard.

The NCHS reference population has been published as a set of graphs [20] and in tabular form [14]. Computer processing subroutines for mainframe and microcomputers have been prepared by the Centers for Disease Control, Atlanta, USA, and are also available from the World Health Organization. The detailed data sets allow a comparison of distribution rather than means and therefore the estimation of probabilities which is of special importance for screening.

The published graphs and tables gives values for percentiles and means ± 1, 2 and 3 standard deviations of the reference population. This allows for manual classification of each measurement into groups which are more or less wide, sufficient for screening and rough grouping. A more precise calculation of the position of each individual in relation to the distribution of the reference has been described by Waterlow *et al.* (see Appendix A, p. 44) and in a WHO publication [14]. The standard deviation score or Z-score determines the distance of a measurement such as weight from the mean of the reference distribution of weights in the reference population for the given age and sex.

$$Z \text{ score } = \frac{\text{measured value } - \text{ reference mean}}{\text{standard deviation of the reference}}$$

The Z-scores of a sample of measurements can be pooled and their distribution compared with the reference distribution by various statistical and graphic methods. For large sets of observations this is best done with computers.

Another way of processing the data is calculating the proportion of data beyond a cut-off point. Often-used cut-offs are the 5th and 95th percentile or 2 standard deviations above or below the reference means, giving percentage values or prevalences for exceptionally short (stunted), thin (wasted), tall, or 'obese' children.

Because weight for a given height is not completely independent of age, Cole [23] has proposed a method for assessing age-standardized weight for height in children seen cross-sectionally. The standardization has been obtained expressing weight and height as a fraction of the 50th centile for age from a suitable growth standard. A Cole slide-rule calculator, using Tanner–Whitehouse standards for height and weight (0–19 years) is produced by Castelmead Publications, Hertford SG14 1LH, UK.

For adults several regional reference height–weight tables are available, but they have great limitations [16, 17], so instead of presenting relative body weight it is preferred to use weight/height ratios; these will be examined later (section 1.4).

1.3.5 Performance characteristics

(a) Reproducibility

The reliability of the indices and prevalences depends partly on the measurement errors and partly on the variation in both the examined and the reference population due to genetic differences between individuals. With good equipment and well-trained, motivated personnel it is possible to reduce the reading error of the measurement to 100 g or less in weight. Differences remain regarding posture, bowel and bladder contents, and hydration of tissues, which may be larger than the reading or recording errors and may sometimes be unavoidable. In populations without exact birth date records, age determination often presents major difficulties that may make the use of age-dependent indices like height for age or weight for age almost worthless [24].

In a study on 61 children and adults of each sex re-examined within a period of two weeks, Bouchard [25] observed a technical error of 0.4 kg and a coefficient of variation of 0.7 kg for body weight.

Gordon *et al.* [26] reported for the Fels Longitudinal Study a mean intermeasurer difference of 1.2 g (SD = 3.2 g) at 5–10 years, 1.5 g (SD = 3.6 g) at 10–15 years, 1.7 g (SD = 3.8 g) at 15–20 years, and 1.5 g (SD = 3.6 g) for adults. In the Health Examination Survey by the National Center for Health Statistics, the intermeasurer and intrameasurer technical errors were about 1.2 kg within a period of two weeks.

(b) Validity

If the validity of an indicator is the degree to which it measures what is intended then these anthropometric indicators of nutritional status cannot be validated. There is no direct and/or independent measure of nutritional status to compare it with. Validation thus becomes complex and somewhat different for each of the indicators, and includes assumptions about causality.

If weight for height is seen as a measure of the soft body mass and as a measure of the changes of soft body mass in relation to height, its validity must be considered high, since weight is a direct measure of total mass and bone mass is closely related to height. Weight for height is too simple an index to distinguish between body compartments (such as muscle mass and fat content) and changes in their relative size. However, as an indicator of nutritional status and of its changes, weight for height has proved its validity in clinical therapy and rehabilitation.

Although weight for age is a direct measure of body mass and of the changes in it, its validity as an indicator of nutritional status is limited by its simplicity. Without additional information on height a high or low value of this indicator gives no indication of its being due to a large or small skeleton, or to a large or small soft body mass, or to a combination of both. Its validity as an indicator of nutritional status is therefore low. Longitudinally it is often successfully used on growth charts as a simple measure of individual growth velocity.

1.3.6   Reference values

The mean weight and weight for height of children and adults collected under the International Biological Programme are reported in the book of Eveleth and Tanner [13].

The readily available WHO publication *Measuring Change in Nutritional Status* [14] contains tables of reference length, stature and weight by age, length, or stature of boys and girls from 0 to 18 years and 49–145 cm in height based on the NCHS reference population. This publication also gives information on standardization procedures and statistical aspects of sampling in studies to assess the nutritional impact of supplementary feeding programmes for vulnerable groups.

1.3.7   Interpretation

Epidemiologically, many malnourished child populations show a peak in prevalence of low weight for height in the second year of life [27], the age at which a corresponding peak in the incidence of kwashiorkor has been described in many countries [28]. Although minor deviations or changes in weight for height should therefore be interpreted with caution in the absence of other supportive evidence it is the most direct indicator of abnormal or changed nutritional status with regard to energy, since it measures the soft tissue mass that is directly affected by energy imbalances.

Low weight for height and low height for age, or wasted and stunted growth, are probably not due to the same causes. It has been found in many studies that wasting and stunting are associated with different socioeconomic and environmental indicators. This view is supported by the finding that the weight for height and height for age values in a population, expressed as Z-scores, are not correlated [29]. On the other hand weight for age can be reliably predicted from the other two indicators which means that it contains no information in addition to that of weight for height and height for age.

Although by now there is a wealth of information on the low values of these indicators as regards stunting, wasting, and underweight, which has recently been summarized by a working group convened by WHO [15], our experience as to their high values is still limited.

1.4   WEIGHT/HEIGHT RATIOS

1.4.1   Purpose and scope

Weight/height ratios are used to give some indications about body 'build' or shape and about leanness or fatness. Various indices of relative weight have been recommended and applied for many years. The first approach should be the weight per unit height, but using the ratio W/H, raises questions as to why the weight. This is roughly equivalent to a volume, a three-dimensional or cubic unit, and should be standardized in terms of a single linear dimension. If the body had the same form at different heights, weight would tend to be proportional to the third power of the height. This idea was incorporated by Livi in his ponderal index (indice ponderale): the cube root of the body weight divided by the body length or height [30].

Though the body form does not remain constant with increasing length, the ponderal index, or similarly the Rohrer index (W/H^3), has been widely used. Sheldon *et al.* [31] employed an inverted ratio of the ponderal index by dividing the height by the cube root of weight. This 'index of bodily mass' has long been used in attempts at bodily classification.

About 150 years ago, long before the use of any of the above indices, Quetelet [32] explored both W/H^3 and W/H^2 with respect to growth. In recent times there has been a revised interest concerning the W/H^2 index, which was also called 'body mass index' [33]. We have shown [33] that body mass index (W/H^2) in adults is least correlated with height and best correlated with weight and the amount of body fat as obtained with body density measurements. In order that weight be more independent of height, Benn [34] proposed another index (Benn index) which is weight divided by height to the pth power (W/H^p), where p is equal to β, the regression coefficient for weight regressed on height, times the ratio of the mean height to the mean weight (that is, $p = \beta \, (\bar{H}/\bar{W})$.

Besides the fact that the Benn index can only be applied retrospectively, Garn and Pesick [35] have recently shown, from several population surveys, that this index is highly correlated with other body mass measurements and is only fractionally superior to other weight/height ratios. They concluded that the population–specific exponent p in the Benn index adds no material advantage in nutritional assessment.

Because the W/H² has been found to be significantly correlated with height in children, Abdel-Malek *et al.* [36] proposed a new generalized power family index:

$$y = C \frac{W^m}{S^k}$$

where y = % BF, C = constant multiplier, W = weight in kg, S = stature in cm, and m and k = power parameters.

From a sample of the Fels longitudinal Study (*n* = 458; age from 6 to 50 years) they obtained the following formulae:

$$\% \ BF = \frac{W^{1.2}}{S^{3.3}} \cdot 3 \cdot 10^6 \text{ for males}$$

$$\% \ BF = \frac{W^{1.2}}{S^{3.3}} \cdot 4 \cdot 10^6 \text{ for females}$$

A nomogram is available for rapid estimation of % BF.

The mean root squared errors of these estimates of % BF are rather large, as with other direct methods. This obesity index, although significantly correlated with several fat-related measurements, was significantly correlated with S only in adult men.

According to the authors this power model index is preferable to any 'fixed' index as regards generality and flexibility. As for other indices, this index is population or group specific. In order to use it in other populations the direct measures of body composition are needed to compute its C, m, k variables.

A great limitation of the body mass index, as for most of the other weight/height ratios, is that they can be used only for population groups and not for individuals. In fact Durnin *et al.* have shown that individuals with the same weight and height have different percentages of body fat [37].

1.4.2 Principle of the method

With weights and heights collected as previously described, the body mass index can be obtained by dividing the weight by the square of height. Since the other ratios, as discussed above, are not better than the body mass index for adults, they will not be considered here.

1.4.3 Procedure

The procedure is very simple. The body weight and height are collected as described. To obtain the body mass index, weight is divided by the square of height. Thomas *et al.* [38] have produced a nomogram to obtain body mass index (BMI) in kg/m², shown in Fig. 1.1.

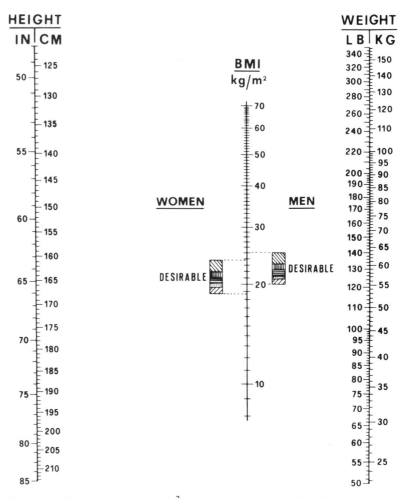

Fig. 1.1 The ratio weight/height^2 is read from central scale. (From 7, with permission.)

1.4.4   Performance characteristics

(a) Reproducibility

Weight/height ratios are derived from basic measurements; thus the reliability of these ratios depends on the reliability of the original measurements.

Womersley and Durnin [39] have computed the standard error of the prediction of W/H^2 in their sample. In men it increases with age, while for women it is high in the age groups 17–19 and 20–29 years, going down in the 30–39 years group and increasing again in the other age groups.

(b) Validity

Validity has been tested only against fatness. Keys *et al.*, in 7426 middle-aged men from nine cohorts of the Seven Countries Study and two groups of Minnesota students and executives, have found that W/H^2 is slightly better correlated than other ratios with the sum of triceps and subscapular skinfolds used as an expression of fatness [33]. Nominal differences were observed with the transformed sum of skinfolds. The situation is the same when these ratios are correlated with body density in Minnesota students and executives only.

Womersley and Durnin [39] found correlation coefficients of 0.49–0.62 between W/H^2 and body fat estimated by densitometry in men aged 17–50 years. For women of the same ages the correlation coefficients ranged from 0.64 to 0.91. Other ratios were less well correlated.

Norgan and Ferro-Luzzi [40] found a correlation coefficient of 0.75 between W/H^2 and percentage of body fat estimated by densitometry. As above, other ratios in this study also showed lower correlations with densitometry in middle-aged Italian shipyard workers.

1.4.5 Reference values

In the nomogram of Thomas *et al.* [38] cut-off points are used to separate desirable, overweight, and underweight values arbitrarily. Garrow [41] has proposed another nomogram indicating a range of desirable weights. Also in this case a frequency or centile distribution from large population samples can be recommended. The cut-off points between physiological and pathological values can be fixed at any point and can be adjusted according to specific criteria (amount of body fat, mortality, etc.).

1.4.6 Interpretation

Weight/height ratios and particularly body mass index have mainly been used as indicators of obesity [33], but, as stated, they have also been used to evaluate leanness in malnourished children in India [42].

In choosing an index of relative weight derived from measures of weight and height, the prime criterion must be the relative independence of the index from height [33]. Lee *et al.* [43] compared the Benn index with the other weight/height ratios in 35 523 individuals of both sexes, aged 18 years and over, and five different ethnic populations in Hawaii. Of the so-called traditional indices, W/H and W/H^2 were highly correlated with weight, but W/H^3 and $W/H^{1/3}$ were only moderately correlated. The ratios W/H^3 and $W/H^{1/3}$ were substantially more biased by height than were W/H and W/H^2. Of the latter two indices, W/H^2 was less biased in males, while W/H was less biased in females. The Benn index (W/H^p) was highly correlated with weight and virtually independent of height in each ethnic–sex-specific population and, more importantly, the same results existed in a mixture of heterogeneous populations. However, the extent of correlation between W/H^p and more direct measures of fatness is still unknown.

In contrast Colliver *et al.* [44] found similarity in measurements obtained with six commonly used weight/height ratios when assessed by correlation and factor analyses performed on data for 951 obese adults participating in a weight-reduction study. Intercorrelations among the indices were found to be very high, with a mean of 0.96. A factor analysis of the six indices resulted in a single factor that accounts for 97% of the aggregate variance in the six indices. The factor analysis performed on the six ratios plus weight and height consistently demonstrated that a two-factor model is sufficient to explain the variability in the eight variables. According to the authors the results indicate that the obesity indices are measuring essentially the same thing, and what they are measuring is independent of height.

In a study of 569 British men and women aged 17–72 years, Womersley and Durnin [39] found that the index $H:W^{0.33}$ is highly correlated with height and therefore is inappropriate as an index of obesity. A marked difference between W/H and body fat obtained by densitometry was also found. 'The measures of obesity which, in their correlation with height, were in best agreement with the assessment of body fat by densitometry, were skinfold thicknesses and the indices W/H^2 and $W/\overline{W}$ (where $\overline{W}$ = reference weight). There was little difference between these three methods'. They also found that '... all the distributions, whatever the method used for estimating body fat, were markedly positively skewed, with a long tail of high values. ... It is evident that in both sexes, compared with the density method, the other four indices all tend to overestimate body fat in individuals whose fat is very small.' In the same study the standard errors for the prediction of body fat from the ratio W/H^2 were calculated, and were found to be from about 3–6% of body weight. With the densitometric method these standard errors were 2–3% of body weight.

The same authors also calculated the linear regression equations for prediction of body fat (as estimated by densitometry) from various weight/height ratios. These should only be used when skinfold measurements are not available.

In a study on 138 Italian shipyard workers aged 22–55 years, Norgan and Ferro-Luzzi [40] computed linear regression equations of % fat from weight–height indices that were rather similar to those of Womersley and Durnin. Because these equations should be regarded as descriptive rather than predictive, prediction equations were drawn up on a validation sample and were cross-validated on another sample. They also presented the % fat at the cut-off points for different degrees of obesity as defined by Garrow from W/H^2 ratios [41]. When age was added as an independent variable the standard errors decreased and the correlation increased. The equation of W/H^2 + age, according to these authors, gives better agreement for people of similar ages when compared with those obtained by other workers.

Garn *et al.* [45] have recently shown some limitations in the use of BMI. Using the data of the first National Health and Nutrition Examination Survey they found that BMI is height dependent, especially in children, and reflects body proportions (ratio of sitting to standing height). Using the data from the Tecumseh study they found that 'BMI reflects *both* the weight of lean tissue and the weight of fat tissue and for some age groups it may at least be a better measure of the amount of lean than of relative fatness'.

1.5 CIRCUMFERENCES SECTION I MUSCLE AND FAT AREAS

1.5.1 Purpose and scope

Muscle and fat area measurements provide information on total body and regional muscle and fat mass [46–48] respectively. Skeletal muscle is the largest component of the fat-free body mass, and thereby this tissue is a major store of total body protein [49]. Hence one major use of muscle area measurements is in the assessment of the amount and rate of change in total body protein. A second application is the use of muscle areas in physical training programmes. A third use of muscle areas, described in another Chapter in this manual, is the evaluation of regional muscle and fat distribution.

Total body fat serves primarily as an energy reserve [49]. Nearly all total body fat is available for oxidation, whereas only about one-half of total body protein is available for this purpose. Hence fat stores are usually equated with total body energy content. Fat is distributed internally around and in the visceral organs and in the subcutaneous space. Fat area measurements are a reflection of subcutaneous fat. Fat area measurements are used for two principal purposes, to provide information on the amount and rate of change in body energy stores and to establish regional fat mass.

1.5.2 Principle of the method

The limbs consist primarily of bone, muscle, and fat. A number of investigators over the years have recognized the relative ease by which these structures can be quantified in living individuals [46–51]. Methods include radiography [52], anthropometry [51], ultrasonography [53], infrared spectroscopy [54], and magnetic resonance imaging [55]. The focus here is on the anthropometric methods of measuring muscle and fat areas.

The basic concept is that the limb resembles a cylinder; measuring limb circumference then provides a means of calculating total limb cross-sectional area. This cross-sectional slice is then the composite of bone, skeletal muscle, and fat. The thickness of the subcutaneous fat layer can next be assessed by measuring fat-fold thickness using a caliper. One-half the measured thickness is then assumed to represent the fat-layer thickness. Equations, described below, can then be formulated to calculate: (1) total limb cross-sectional area, (2) subcutaneous fat area, and (3) muscle plus bone area. Typically these are the three main calculated indices. Estimates of bone area can be used to calculate bone-free muscle area.

The most popular and practical measurement site is the mid-upper arm. The thigh and calf are also used occasionally. The least information is available on forearm areas.

The following recommendations are based upon the Anthropometric Standardization Conference held in Airlie, Virginia, 1985 [9].

SECTION IA CIRCUMFERENCES

1.5.3 Apparatus

Tape-measure. This should be non-extensible, flexible, accurate, easy to use and read, and have a leader before the zero line. Most workers suggest using a narrow (7 mm), flexible, 1–2-metre steel tape. Cloth tapes stretch and are not recommended. Tapes should be periodically calibrated and checked for damage or wear.

Other tapes are available; two examples are the Gulick and Ross tapes. The Gulick tape has a spring-loaded handle in order to maintain constant pressure; this instrument may produce unwanted soft-tissue compression in the obese, in infants, and in the elderly. A non-metallic, flexible tape for measuring arm circumferences was developed by Ross Nutritional Divison for survey and office use. The tape has slots and a reading window. One end of the tape is passed through the slots; this procedure maintains alignment of the reading point.

1.5.4 Procedure

(a) Sites

Arm circumference. (1) With the arm flexed at 90° angle locate the lateral tip of the acromion, make a small mark; (2) drop the tape from this mark and locate the mid-point between the marked acromion and the olecranon. With a felt-tip pen make a mark on the side of the tape; (3) with the arm relaxed and hanging just away from the side of the body the tape is passed around the arm so that it is touching the skin, but not compressing the tissue. The tape should be positioned at a right-angle to the long axis of the arm.

Forearm circumference. The forearm circumference is measured at the maximal circumference of the proximal forearm, no more than 6 cm from the radiale. The arm is extended downward slightly away from the body with the hand supinated and relaxed.

Calf circumference. The subject should either sit on a table so that the leg to be measured is hanging freely off the table, or stand with the feet about 25 cm apart and with weight distributed equally on both feet. A steel tape-measure is positioned around the calf and held snugly against the skin. The tape is then moved up and down the calf to locate the maximum circumference in a plane perpendicular to the long axis of the calf. The maximum circumference is recorded to the nearest millimetre, and replicate measurements should not differ by more than 2.0 mm.

Thigh circumference. For measurements of the middle thigh circumference, the circumference that passes over the site of the thigh skinfold measurement is used: one-half the distance between the inguinal crease and the proximal border of the patella. The proximal border of the patella is located and marked while the subject is standing. To locate the mid-point of the inguinal crease the investigator must first locate the most medial aspect of the superior anterior iliac spine. When the hip is flexed, as when the subject puts one foot on a stool, the anterior superior iliac spine lies just above the mid-point of the inguinal crease. Thus, the mid-point of the inguinal crease can be easily located. Once the proximal border of the patella and the mid-point of the inguinal crease are located the distance from these two points is measured while the subject has one foot raised upon a stool. The halfway mark of this measurement is the point where the mid-thigh circumference is taken.

(b) Technique

The main features of measuring circumferences are the following: (1) The tape should make contact with the skin and follow the contour of the segment, but should not compress to underlying soft tissues; (2) the tape should be placed perpendicular to the long axis of the limb segment; and (3) the tape should be read to the nearest millimetre, although some suggest the last completed millimetre. It is sometimes recommended that the subject stand sideways to the technician for the measurement of upper and lower extremity circumferences.

SECTION IB   SKINFOLDS

Information and recommendations on apparatus, sites and technique for measurement of triceps, biceps, forearm, thigh, and calf skinfolds are provided in the section on Skinfold thickness (section 1.6).

Calculation

The equations for calculating muscle and fat areas are presented in Tables 1.2 and 1.3.

Table 1.2   Equations for calculating limb fat areas[*]

Extremity	Equation	Comment
1. Upper arm	Arm fat area (cm^2) = $$\frac{MAC \cdot TSF}{2} - \frac{\pi \cdot (TSF)^2}{4}$$	This general equation assumes a circular limb and muscle compartment, and a symmetrically distributed fat rim. The accuracy of this equation in predicting mid-upper-arm fat area is unknown. TSF = triceps skinfold (cm); MAC = mid-arm circumference (cm).
2. Thigh	Thigh fat area (cm^2) = $$\frac{MTC \cdot THSF}{2} - \frac{\pi \cdot (THSF)^2}{4}$$	THSF = thigh skinfold (cm); MTC = mid-thigh circumference (cm).
3. Calf	Calf fat area (cm^2) = $$\frac{MCC \cdot CSF}{2} - \frac{\pi \cdot (CSF)^2}{4}$$	CSF = calf skinfold (cm); MCC = mid-calf circumference (cm).

[*] Forearm fat area is calculated using the same general approach. Some workers include the average of the biceps and triceps skinfold thicknesses in equation 1.

1.5.5   Performance characteristics

(a) General considerations

The principle of the method described above must of necessity depend upon a number of assumptions. These assumptions are the following:

The cross-section of the limb can be described by a circle; fat is symmetrically distributed around the muscle bundle; muscle is circular in cross-section; and bone represents an inappreciable component of muscle area.

The evaluation of these assumptions was greatly simplified with the introduction of computerized axial tomography in the 1970s [46]. As might be expected each assumption was found in error to some degree. For example, mid-arm muscle area was overestimated by the standard equation. This was caused by the non-circularity of muscle in cross-section and the inclusion of neurovascular tissue and bone in muscle area. Suggested equations for

Table 1.3 Anthropometric equations for calculating muscle mass [56]*

Equation	Comment
1. Calf muscle area (cm²) = $$\frac{[\text{MCC} - \pi \cdot \text{CSF}]^2}{4\pi}$$	Includes bone area; assumes a circular limb and muscle compartment, and symmetrically distributed fat rim.
2. Thigh muscle area (cm²) = $$\frac{[\text{MTC} - \pi \cdot \text{THSF}]^2}{4\pi}$$	Bone corrections are available
3. Arm muscle circumference (cm) = $$\text{MAC} - \pi \cdot \text{TSF}$$	Same assumption as for equations 1 and 2; includes bone. Note that as muscle loses mass or volume in protein–energy, circumferential measurements will change proportionately less than area measurements. The latter therefore more realistically depicts severity of muscle atrophy.
4. Arm muscle area (cm²) = $$\frac{[\text{MAC} - \pi \cdot \text{TSF}]^2}{4\pi}$$	Same assumption as equations 1 and 2; includes bone. Equation overestimates actual muscle area; by expressing absolute value as % of standard, the error is corrected
5. Arm muscle area (cm²) = (a) Men $$\frac{[\text{MAC} - \pi \cdot \text{TSF}]^2}{4\pi} - 10$$ (b) Women $$\frac{[\text{MAC} - \pi \cdot \text{TSF}]^2}{4\pi} - 6.5$$	Same basic assumptions as equations 1 and 2; the overestimate in equation 4 is corrected and the average value for bone area is also subtracted. Resulting value is therefore bone-free arm muscle area. As for all muscle derivatives on this chart, the resulting value remains an approximation ($\pm$ 8%) of actual muscle area
6. Available arm muscle area = equation 5 (a) or (b) $- 9 \text{ cm}^2$	Subtracts approximate minimal value of arm muscle area compatible with survival. Values at or less than zero are associated with life-threatening protein–energy malnutrition. Values between 2 and 5 cm indicate very severe protein–energy malnutrition, and values above 5 cm but below normal range indicate muscle atrophy.

* Biceps skinfold thickness is sometimes included in upper-arm muscle areas. Forearm muscle area is calculated as for equations 1, 2 and 4.

correcting these errors were developed (Table 1.3), but these are also based on 'average' coefficients, which in the individual subject may lead to error.

Hence, recognizing the limited accuracy of muscle and fat areas is essential in their clinical ap lication. This deficiency must be balanced against the extreme ease and low cost with which these measurements can be made.

(b) Reproducibility

The reliability of muscle and fat area measurements depends largely on the reliability of skinfold and circumferential measurements. The interobserver and between-day variability in triceps skinfold (TSF), mid-arm circumference (MAC), and arm muscle area (AMA) are presented for two observers in Table 1.4. Reliability can be maximized by (1) training the observer thoroughly, (2) periodically checking interobserver variability, (3) using a single observer for repeated measurements in the same subject, and (4) marking the measurement site in some situations.

Table 1.4 Interobserver and between-day variability in anthropometric measurements (equations for arm muscle area)

| | *Interobserver* | | *Between-day* | | | |
| | | | *Observer CM* | | *Observer JS* | |
	CV (%)	*Range*	*CV (%)*	*Range*	*CV (%)*	*Range*
TSF						
Unmarked arm	26.0	0–8.3 mm	7.3	0–2 mm	12.0	0–3.6 mm
Marked arm	21.0	0.5–7.6 mm	7.0	0–1 mm	14.0	0–5 mm
MAC						
Unmarked arm	1.4	0.1–0.9 cm	1.4	0–1 cm	1.2	0–1 cm
Marked arm	1.0	0–0.4 cm	0.5	0–0.4 cm	1.0	0–0.7 cm
AMA						
Unmarked	9.0	0–14 cm^2	3.2	0.1–4.9 cm^2	4.9	
Marked arm	7.1	0.2–9.6 cm^2	2.4	0–2.5 cm^2	4.3	0–6.4 cm^2

AMA = arm muscle area, MAC = mid-arm circumference, TSF = triceps skinfold. From [46].

(c) Validity

The validity of circumference and area measurements is discussed for specific conditions in section 1.5.7. The validity of reference values is of some concern as the population under study may differ markedly in diet, stature, and ethnicity from local patients. Regional norms should be considered, as their development is relatively easy for anthropometric measurements.

1.5.6 Reference values

Either local reference values or published survey data can be used to establish standards. Local norms based on measurements in the practitioners office or laboratory offer the advantage of a predefined population. Examples of survey norms are presented in reference [51].

1.5.7 Interpretation

Muscle 'circumference' and area measurements, principally of the upper arm, have found widespread application both in the hospital and in the field. A brief summary of the validity of muscle areas is now provided:

1. In healthy subjects arm muscle area and grip strength are highly correlated [57]. In diseased patients this correlation is poor.
2. Mid-upper arm muscle area is highly correlated with ^{40}K measurements of lean body mass and 24-hour urinary creatinine excretion (Fig. 1.2). These correlations hold irrespective of the muscle area equation selected from Table 1.3.

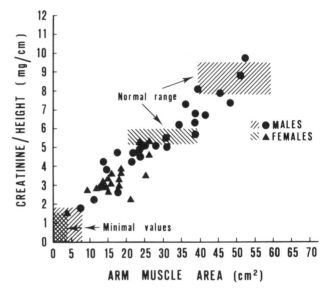

Fig. 1.2 Correlation between muscle indices creatinine/height (ordinate) and arm muscle area (abscissa) in healthy and undernourished subjects. The normal range and minimal values compatible with survival are indicated for males and females.

3. With semi-starvation the upper arm tends to lose muscle tissue more rapidly than the lower extremities [58]. Hence the relative change in any one area may not be directly proportional to the change in total body muscle mass.
4. Short-term changes in nitrogen balance are not readily detected by measuring upper arm muscle area (Fig. 1.3).
5. Upper arm muscle area provides some measure of preoperative surgical risk [59].

   Fat area measurements correlate to a variable degree with total body fat. However recent studies indicate the high frequency of individual 'fat patterning', e.g. [60]. Hence the absolute limb fat area may not be directly proportional to total body fat. Also individual fat areas may change with energy balance at different rates [58]. Therefore the changes in a single fat area may not be directly proportional to changes in total body fat or energy balance.

   Some studies indicate that fat areas provide prognostic information related to patient outcome [59]. However, these associations are considerably weaker than for the muscle areas noted above.
6. In obese subjects precision for circumferences and skinfold measurements are 2% and 11%–24%, respectively [61]. Circumferences may therefore be more reliable than skinfold measurements in obese subjects.

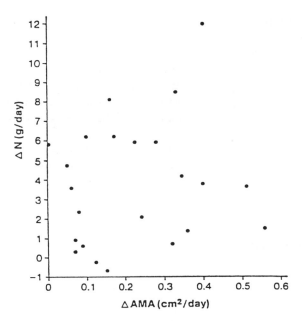

Fig. 1.3 Nitrogen balance (N, ordinate), measured on a metabolic ward, vs change in anthropometric arm muscle area (AMA, abscissa) in subjects undergoing one-week balance studies.

Concern about the interpretation of muscle and fat areas was noted above. Several features of these indices are worthy of mention. Subjects with massive oedema or ascites usually have minimal fluid accumulation in the upper extremities. Thus the fat and muscle areas of the upper arm provide an excellent measure of total body fat, lean body mass, and dry weight. The same applies to the subject with a massive intra-abdominal tumour, in whom body weight is a poor guide to energy–protein status.

A current area requiring additional study is the pattern of muscle and fat area change with ageing. Additional standard values are needed for the elderly.

SECTION II HEAD AND CHEST CIRCUMFERENCES

1.5.8 Purpose and scope

In preschool children head circumference is considered an index of brain growth and its ratio to the chest circumference is reckoned as an indirect measure of nutritional status [62]. In children and adults chest circumference can be used as an index of frame size [62]. The abdominal circumference relative to that of the expanded chest was used by the Medico–Actuarial Mortality Investigation as a mortality classification [63].

1.5.9 Principle of the methods

With an appropriate tape the circumferences at specified places of the head and chest are measured.

1.5.10 Apparatus

The apparatus is detailed in the section on muscle and fat areas circumferences (section 1.5.3).

1.5.11　Procedure

(a) Head circumference

In an infant the measurement is taken with the subject seated, and for older ages with the subject standing. The operator is recommended to stay on the subject's left side [62]. The maximum circumference of the head is measured just above the brow ridges, compressing and excluding the maximum amount of cranial hair. The measurement is recorded to the nearest millimetre.

(b) Chest circumference

With the subject standing erect the tape is passed under the slightly abducted arms. The arms are then lowered to their natural position and the measurement taken at the 3rd and 4th sternebrae, in a horizontal plane at the end of a normal expiration.

For further details of both measurements see Callaway *et al.* [62].

1.5.12　Performance characteristics

Reproducibility

According to Roche *et al.* [64] in the Fels Longitudinal Study the intermeasurer differences for head circumference were small, with a technical error of 0.09 mm and a coefficient of variation of 0.02. Intermeasurer and intertrial reliability coefficients for chest circumference are well within the acceptable range [62].

1.5.13　Reference values

For reference values of head circumference see Meredith [65] and Callaway *et al.* [62]. Data on chest circumference collected under the International Biological Programme are reported in the book by Eveleth and Tanner [13].

SECTION III　WAIST/HIP AND WAIST/THIGH RATIOS

1.5.14　Purpose and scope

Beside measuring body fatness the distribution of fat in the body provides important additional information as regards the risks for morbidity and metabolic aberrations. Although fat distribution can be assessed by other techniques such as skinfolds (subcutaneous fat patterning) and computed tomography (which allows precise quantification of all fat deposits, including the visceral adipose tissue) it seems that in routine clinical investigation and epidemiological studies indices based on simple body circumferences are the most satisfactory.

In the 1960s circumferences were successfully used to derive equations for estimating body fatness [66, 67]. In that period fat distribution was assessed using the complex index constructed by Vague *et al.* [68]: the brachiofemoral adipomuscular ratio (BFAMR) or the index of masculine differentiation (IMD) which, in addition to the BFAMR, used the ratio of nape to sacrum skinfold [60]. The BFAMR was based on skinfolds and circumferences of the arm and thigh and did not include fat deposits on the trunk. As reviewed elsewhere [69] subcutaneous fat patterns measured by skinfolds or combinations of skinfolds and body somatotypes were found to be associated with metabolic risk factors and disease. This review will concentrate on the use of body circumferences for assessing body fat distribution.

In 1980, at three different scientific congresses, several investigators from Wisconsin USA presented data on the relationship between the waist/hip circumference ratio and the prevalence of diabetes [70] and metabolic risk factors [71, 72]. At a congress in 1982 Swedish investigators also showed that the waist/hip ratio was related to metabolic profiles in obese men and women [73]. Since then many studies have been published confirming that the waist/ hip ratio and the waist/thigh ratio are significant indicators of morbidity and metabolic aberrations. In particular, prospective studies showed that waist/hip ratio is a predictor of cardiovascular disease, stroke, diabetes mellitus, total mortality, and some hormone-dependent female carcinomas [74]. Other diseases probably associated with a high waist/hip ratio are menstrual abnormalities and gout. The only condition currently known to be associated with a low waist/hip ratio is varicose veins [69].

Although circumference measurements are very easy to perform it appears that the level for measurement reported in the literature varies considerably. Table 1.5 shows some of these reported levels.

Table 1.5 Reported levels for measurement of circumferences with the purpose of describing fat distribution

Circumference level		*References*
Waist	Umbilicus	Anderson *et al.* [75]
		Andersson *et al.* [76]*
		Haffner *et al.* [77]
		Larsson *et al.* [78]
		Stefanik *et al.* [79]
	Minimal	Evans *et al.* [80]
		Kissebah *et al.* [72]
		Peiris *et al.* [81]
	Minimal between rib cage and iliac crest	Ashwell *et al.* [82]
	Minimal between xiphoid and umbilicus	Lev-Ran and Hill [83]
	Lower border of 10th rib	Johnston *et al.* [84]
	Midway between lower rib margin (or 12th rib) and iliac crest	Lapidus *et al.* [85] Jones *et al.* [86]
	One-third of the distance between xiphoid process and umbilicus	Krotkiewski *et al.* [73]
	Midway between xiphoid process and umbilicus	Krotkiewski and Björntorp [87]
	Maximal circumference	Lanska *et al.* [88]
Hip	Iliac crest	Larsson *et al.* [78] Johnston *et al.* [84]
	Maximal or widest over buttocks or trochanter region	All others
Thigh	Highest (gluteal fold)	Seidell *et al.* [69, 89]
	One-third distance between superior anterior iliac spine and patella	Krotkiewski *et al.* [73]
	Mid-point of thigh	Johnston *et al.* [84]

* Supine position. All other circumferences measured in the standing position.

For the hip circumference there seems to be general agreement in measuring the widest circumference over the buttocks or trochanters. Hip measurements over the iliac crest are not advisable since circumferences at that level may easily include part of the abdominal fat deposits. For the waist many more alternatives have been used. The exact level for measuring the waist circumference has important consequences as regards the average and distribution of the waist/hip values in a given population. A study on about 450 European women in which waist circumferences were measured at different levels illustrates this (Table 1.6).

Table 1.6 Average waist/hip ratios (and SEM) in 450 European women selected from five different centres. Waist circumferences were measured at four different levels,* and hip at the widest circumference in the trochanter region. The percentage of women with a waist/hip ratio greater than 0.8 ('abdominal obesity') is also shown. (Based on Ref. [89].)

Ratio	Sweden		Poland		Netherlands		Verona		Naples	
	mean (SEM)	%	mean (SEM)	%	mean (SEM)	%	mean (SEM)	%	mean (SEM)	%
Waist 1	0.79 (0.006)	37.3	0.79 (0.004)	38.2	0.79 (0.005)	46.4	0.78 (0.006)	32.9	0.89 (0.006)	93.2
Waist 2	0.81 (0.006)	50.6	0.80 (0.005)	44.9	0.79 (0.005)	35.7	0.78 (0.007)	32.9	0.82 (0.004)	70.5
Waist 3	0.77 (0.006)	22.9	0.77 (0.004)	16.9	0.75 (0.005)	11.9	0.74 (0.007)	12.9	0.82 (0.005)	69.8
Waist 4	0.86 (0.006)	89.0	0.84 (0.005)	78.7	0.87 (0.005)	95.2	0.85 (0.007)	77.6	0.94 (0.006)	100.0

* Waist was measured in standing subjects at the following levels:
  waist 1 = midway between the xiphoid process and lower rib margin;
  waist 2 = midway between the lower rib margin and iliac crest;
  waist 3 = minimal circumference between lower rib margin and iliac crest;
  waist 4 = maximal circumference between the lower rib margin and iliac crest.

Details of the study are presented elsewhere [89]. It is clear that to compare studies and classify subjects by this method a waist/hip standardization is essential. Decisions on this will be based on a somewhat arbitrary basis.

Instructions for waist measurements based on easily recognized points of the body such as 'umbilicus', 'minimal', or 'maximal' are convenient for practical purposes such as instructions for self-measurement by patients. However with subjects varying widely in age and degree of obesity such points may also vary widely. Levels that refer to the skeleton are fixed and thus less subject to interobserver variation. In severe obesity, however, the skeleton is not always easily palpable. Some official recommendations [90] have decided on waist measurements based on skeletal reference points. These suggested levels have also been recently included in the list of anthropometric measurements for measuring obesity in the paper entitled *Measuring Obesity* published by the European regional office of WHO. These recommendations are given in section 1.5.16.

It should be noted that there are some dissenting recommendations. At an anthropometric standardization conference at Airlie, Virginia (USA) [91] the waist was defined as the minimum circumference of the mid-section of the body at the level where the waist narrows, seen from the front, and the abdomen circumference defined as the maximum circumference of the mid-section, taken at the level of maximum extension of the stomach in front. Especially in obese men with large bellies there is no narrowing of the waist and it is difficult to decide where to measure the waist as defined by the USA recommendations.

1.5.15 Principle of the method

From measurements at specific sites of the waist, hip and thigh circumferences the waist/hip and waist/thigh circumference ratios can easily be calculated.

1.5.16 Procedure

Recommended sites for measuring body circumferences:

Waist: midway between the lower rib margin (costal margin) and the superior anterior iliac spine (iliac crest);
Hip: widest over the greater trochanters;
Thigh: highest point at the level of the gluteal fold.

Some investigators have proposed taking circumference measurements with subjects in the supine position [76], presumably to get better agreement with CT scan data and have the abdominal fat mass more evenly distributed. In practice this suggestion has not been followed and virtually all investigators have taken measurements in standing subjects. Further research into improvement in precision and reproducibility by measuring circumferences in the supine position is warranted. Since such information is currently lacking I propose to adopt the general agreement for measuring circumferences in standing subjects with their weight equally distributed on both legs. The subjects should breathe lightly and the waist be measured at the end of gentle expiration. All circumferences should be measured horizontally with a flexible tape-measure. Flexible steel as well as plastic tape-measures are appropriate.

On the basis of currently available evidence it is not possible to conclude that either of these ratios is preferable to the other. In several studies the waist measurement alone is as strongly correlated to metabolic variables as the circumference ratios [69, 89].

1.5.17 Performance characteristics

(a) General considerations

Circumference measurements are currently widely used as indicators of fat distribution, but they have also been used to assess body composition and weight loss in the obese [61, 66, 67]. Waist/hip ratio is generally dependent on both age and degree of obesity (BMI). In some populations, such as the relatively short and stout women of Southern Italy, we observed no relationship between BMI and waist/hip ratio [89]. The age of onset of obesity may also be a determinant of fat distribution. In general, subjects with a high waist/hip ratio are older and fatter compared with subjects with a low waist/hip ratio and probably have gained more weight in adult life [74, 86, 92]. Such potentially confounding factors must be controlled in the analysis and interpretation of the data. One of the important characteristics associated with waist/hip ratio is the accumulation of intra-abdominal fat.

Intra-abdominal fat is highly lipolytic and drains into the portal vein. Increased concentrations of FFA may be one of the factors leading to hyperinsulinaemia, insulin resistance, hypertriglyceridaemia and reduced HDL-cholesterol levels frequently observed in people with a high waist/hip ratio [93].

Another characteristic associated with a high waist/hip ratio is a low level of sex hormone binding globulin (SHBG) and elevated levels of unbound androgens [80].

It has been proposed that a high waist/hip ratio is an aggravating symptom of an underlying endocrine abnormality, i.e. elevated production of androgens [80] and/or glucocorticosteroids [94]. Other symptoms of these underlying endocrine factors include a shift towards a higher proportion of type IIb muscle fibres and hypertrophy of muscle fibres [87, 95]. These muscle characteristics could play a role in insulin resistance. All these characteristics associated with waist/hip ratio (endocrine factors, intra-abdominal fat accumulation, and muscle-fibre characteristics) may contribute to metabolic aberrations and clinical disorders [96, 97]. Whatever the waist/hip ratio is really measuring and whatever the underlying mechanisms may be, the fact remains that the waist/hip ratio is a strong risk indicator in both epidemiological and clinical research. It is important to note that waist/hip ratio is a risk factor throughout the range of BMI, which means that the use of this ratio is not confined to the subgrouping of obese subjects into groups with a high and a low waist/hip ratio.

(b) Reproducibility

Bray *et al.* [61] investigated intra-observer variability of skinfold and circumference measurements in obese subjects. The variability was about 2% for circumferences and between 11 and 24% for skinfold measurements. The authors concluded that in the evaluation of obese subjects circumferences are much more reliable than skinfold measurements.

(c) Validity

The validity of waist/hip ratio is difficult to assess, since at present there is uncertainty as to which standard should be employed. If we assume that the volume of intra-abdominal fat deposit is the characteristic we are really measuring with the circumference ratios, then a validity test would be comparison with intra-abdominal fat volumes calculated by computed tomography.

1.5.18 Interpretation

Waist/hip ratio was shown to be correlated with the area of intra-abdominal (or visceral) fat in both women [98] and men [99] as assessed on abdominal computed tomography scans. Waist alone, however, is more strongly related to the intra-abdominal fat deposit. As discussed above the waist/hip ratio seems to be associated with a cluster of other relevant characteristics (endocrine, metabolic, and morphologic). Interpreting waist/hip ratio data is not an easy task. The values depend largely on the level of measurement, and the associated risk with a certain level of waist/hip ratio depends on the disease or abnormality under study and the degree of obesity [100], and probably the age of the subjects as well. To define single cut-off points for waist/hip ratio on the basis of currently available evidence would be to oversimplify and might lead to serious misclassification. 'Normal' values for waist/hip and waist/thigh ratios are still lacking. We therefore recommend presenting percentile and/or frequency distributions of circumference ratios of populations according to sex, age, and degree of obesity (Body mass index).

1.6 SKINFOLD THICKNESS

1.6.1 Purpose and scope

The majority of nutritional problems in the world are problems of energy nutrition, of excess and insufficiency. This applies to the developed and the developing areas of the world. Energy nutritional status is often affected by other nutritional states, e.g. the wasting accompanying inadequate nutrient intakes, and in turn influences the initiation or maintenance of metabolic and endocrine abnormalities leading to a plethora of degenerative diseases. The simplest objective assessment of nutritional status, the measurement of weight and stature, is assessing, in the first instance, energy nutritional status and with this, health. Therefore, measurements of energy nutritional status are key measures in nutritional assessment. A common, simple, inexpensive measurement can be made by measuring skinfold thickness.

Measurements of skinfold thickness play a role in another area of energy nutritional health. It is becoming apparent that in addition to the amount of fat in the body the site of deposition is a separate and additive factor. Skinfold thicknesses allow a description of the distribution or patterning of adipose tissue depots over the body surface. Although the main interest is currently centred on intra-abdominal fat, an area that cannot be assessed from skinfold thicknesses, several consistent and recognizable configurations of subcutaneous fat deposition have been described from measurements of skinfold thicknesses, and associated with mortality and morbidity or with risk factors of the degenerative diseases. Therefore, a consideration of skinfold thicknesses as measures of both fatness and fat location is required.

Energy is stored as fat in adipose tissue located throughout the body, over the abdomen, the hips, buttocks and thighs, between the scapulae and in the abdominal cavity. A measurement of a skinfold thickness is a direct measurement of the subcutaneous adipose tissue thickness (SCAT). (It includes the thickness of the dermis but this can be ignored.) Measurements at a number of sites characterize the total layer of SCAT over the body surface. These by themselves provide sufficient information to make judgements on the energy nutritional status of the populations, and perhaps too the individual, but commonly comparisons are made with reference values from other populations. This latter procedure is common in children, in particular for stature and weight. Often, however, information on the total body fat (fat mass, FM, kg) or fatness (% F) may be required. There are many estimation procedures for calculating FM and % F from skinfold thicknesses. Most of these have not been validated and are specific to the population on which they were formulated [101]. There are, however, equations that have been drawn up with attention to the factors likely to cause specificity [101–103] and that have been cross-validated on other populations [104, 105]. These, although not always more accurate, may perform better at the ends of the range and should be chosen in preference to apparently more accurate but unvalidated equations.

The profiles of adipose tissue deposition have been called fat distribution or fat patterning. Although there is no consensus on the use of these terms, there is much to be said for adopting the suggestion of Bailey and colleagues [106] that fat distribution is used for binary and trinary comparisons of anatomically distinct regions and that fat patterning is reserved for recognizable configurations of a large array of standardized fat thicknesses. The most common indices of fat distribution are ratios of skinfold thicknesses on the limbs (anterior thigh, medial calf, triceps) to those of the trunk (abdominal, suprailiac, subscapular, thorax), allowing the extremity–trunk distribution of fat to be described [107, 108]. Centripetality of fat, a male characteristic, appears a greater risk factor than peripheral fat distribution. However, small numbers of skinfolds may not adequately describe a location and the use of ratios can be confusing [109]. An array of skinfolds overcomes these difficulties and statistical techniques such as principal component analysis identify stable patterns of limb–trunk patterning in all populations and upper–lower body patterning in many others [110–114].

Fat distribution and patterning may be absolute: what is seen and measured; or relative: what appears after differences due to the amount of fat at each site have been removed statistically. The absolute fat pattern is obviously linked to energy nutritional status. The relative fat pattern, being independent of the level of fatness, may be more determined by genetic factors. As the two patterns may pose separate risks to health both types should be assessed.

Skinfold thicknesses illustrate the external fat distribution or pattern. They do not provide information of the internal–external distribution. Attempts to investigate this using skinfolds to estimate external fat, body density, total fat, and by difference, internal fat have not proved fruitful owing to the assumptions involved in the methods [115].

1.6.2 Principle of the method

Using a suitable caliper, the skinfolds are measured at the appropriate sites by a highly standardized technique.

1.6.3 Apparatus

Skinfold thicknesses are measured by skinfold calipers. There are many types but the commonly accepted models have a constant 10 g/mm^2 pressure at all openings and can be read to 0.1 mm. The Harpenden caliper [116], available from British Indicators Ltd, 46 Dumfries St, Luton, UK, has face areas of 90 mm^2 and opens to 40 mm. The Holtain caliper [117], available from Holtain Ltd, Crosswell, Crymmych, Dyfed, UK, is a development of the Harpenden caliper, being lighter with a more easily read dial up to 40 mm. Jaw area is 78 mm^2. The Lange caliper [118], available from Cambridge Scientific Instruments, Inc, 18 Poplar Street, Cambridge, Md, USA, has much smaller jaws, 30 mm^2, designed to remain parallel with the fold up to 60 mm. There is little to choose between these three [119–121].

A further possible model is the inexpensive, lightweight, plastic McGaw caliper, available from McGaw Laboratories, Irvine, California, USA, but this seems to underrecord [122]. Few of the other models have been tested sufficiently.

Calipers may be tested and calibrated using machined metal blocks to check the reading. The jaw pressure can be checked by determining the force required to open the jaws of a clamped caliper. A suitable force can be generated by adding weights to a pan or water to a plastic bottle suspended from the jaw surface until the jaws open completely. From the weight of bottle plus water and jaw surface area, the opening force and hence jaw pressure can be calculated.

Steps towards the automation of recording have begun [117, 123].

1.6.4 Procedures

(a) Technique

The method of taking a skinfold is best described as a sweep rather than a pinch. The skinfold is formed by the thumb and index or middle finger being placed in the skin about 4–8 cm apart and brought together in the defined axis about 1 cm above the marked site. The caliper jaws are applied at the mid-point of the fold where the sides are parallel. The calipers are read after about two seconds, by which time the first component of the decay in reading due to compression is usually over and the second, slow component begun. Such a sharp distinction may not occur with larger folds or those of older subjects, particularly in the abdominal region. However, it is recommended that the same convention be adopted. The fold is held and maintained by the observer during the measurement. The fold is released and swept up again and remeasured. A difference of more than 0.5 mm requires further measurement after a pause to prevent sustained compression of the tissue.

In children it is helpful to demonstrate the measurement by applying the caliper to the back of the measurer's hand. In the obese, a two-handed fold has been used [124] which gives high readings that cannot be compared with reference data.

(b) Sites

Anthropometrists have been unable to reach a consensus on which side of the body to measure [125]. Apart from measurements on the arm, the choice does not make much difference and even on the arm the effect on skinfold values in the general population is negligible.

Location of the correct site is extremely important as small variations may move away from a fat depot. Sites should be marked with dermographic markers. Several good sources of detailed site descriptions are available [7, 117, 126]. The latest manual [9] is clearly illustrated with useful data on reliability and sources of reference data, and can be recommended. The location of sites often varies in different manuals and the description of the sites measured, or a reference, should be given in any publication.

Triceps. The mid-point of the back of the upper arm between the tips of the olecranon and acromial processes is determined by measurement with the arm flexed at 90°. With the arm hanging freely at the side, the calipers are applied vertically above the olecranon at the marked level.

Biceps. The fold is picked up over the belly of the biceps muscle at the same level as the triceps, with the arm hanging freely and the palm facing outwards.

Subscapular. This fold is picked up just below the inferior angle of the scapula at 45° to the vertical along the natural cleavage lines of the skin. Some workers take a vertical fold.

Suprailiac. This measurement is taken just above the iliac crest, in the mid-axillary line with the arm slightly abducted. Again there is variation at this site. Harrison *et al.* [127] recommend following the natural cleavage lines,

Table 1.7   Log transformation of skinfold measurements (Transformation = 100 log 10 (reading in 0.1 mm − 18)

mm	*0.0*	*0.1*	*0.2*	*0.3*	*0.4*	*0.5*	*0.6*	*0.7*	*0.8*	*0.9*
2	30	48	60	70	78	85	90	95	100	104
3	108	111	115	118	120	123	126	128	130	132
4	134	136	138	140	141	143	145	146	148	149
5	151	152	153	154	156	157	158	159	160	161
6	162	163	164	165	166	167	168	169	170	171
7	172	173	174	175	176	176	177	177	178	179
8	179	180	181	181	182	183	183	184	185	185
9	186	186	187	188	188	189	189	190	190	191
10	191	192	192	193	193	194	194	195	195	196
11	196	197	197	198	198	199	199	200	200	200
12	201	201	202	202	203	203	203	204	204	205
13	205	205	206	206	206	207	207	208	208	208
14	209	209	209	210	210	210	211	211	211	212
15	212	212	213	213	213	214	214	214	215	215
16	215	216	216	216	216	217	217	217	218	218
17	218	218	219	219	219	220	220	220	220	221
18	221	221	221	222	222	222	223	223	223	223
19	224	224	224	224	225	225	225	225	226	226
20	226	226	226	227	227	227	227	228	228	228
21	228	229	229	229	229	229	230	230	230	230
22	231	231	231	231	231	232	232	232	232	232
23	233	233	233	233	233	234	234	234	234	234
24	235	235	235	235	235	236	236	236	236	236
25	237	237	237	237	237	238	238	238	238	238
26	238	239	239	239	239	239	239	240	240	240
27	240	240	240	241	241	41	241	241	241	242
28	242	242	242	242	243	243	243	243	243	243
29	243	244	244	244	244	244	244	245	245	245
30	245	245	245	245	246	246	246	246	246	246
31	247	247	247	247	247	247	247	248	248	248
32	248	248	248	249	249	249	249	249	249	249
33	249	250	250	250	250	250	250	250	251	251
34	251	251	251	251	251	251	252	252	252	252
35	252	252	252	253	253	253	253	253	253	253
36	253	254	254	254	254	254	254	254	254	255
37	255	255	255	255	255	255	255	256	256	256
38	256	256	256	256	256	256	257	257	257	257
39	257	257	257	257	258	258	258	258	258	258

inferomedially at 45° to the horizontal. Durnin and Womersley [128] take a vertical fold, but the IBP recommendations [7] are at a site 1 cm above and 2 cm medial to the anterior superior iliac spine.

Abdomen. A horizontal fold 5 cm to the left of the umbilicus is the common site. This skinfold presents great variability, and standardization is essential. Harrison *et al.* [127] propose a site 3 cm lateral and 1 cm inferior to the mid-point of the umbilicus.

Mid-axillary. This site is the most variable of all. A horizontal fold in the mid-axillary line at the level of the xiphoid process can be recommended.

Thigh. This is located in the mid-sagittal plane on the anterior aspect of the thigh, halfway between the inguinal crease and the proximal border of the patella. The subject stands with the knee slightly flexed and the weight on the other leg. The inguinal crease can be evoked by flexing the hip slightly to identify the intersection with the long axis of the thigh. A vertical fold is taken.

Medial calf. With the subject seated and the knee at 90°, a vertical fold on the medial aspect of the calf is picked up at the level of the maximum circumference. This measurement is very tiring if performed repeatedly. The measurer can be seated if the subject is on a raised box or platform.

(c) Calculations

The frequency distributions of most skinfolds are positively skewed. There are various approaches to normalization but in the area of auxology the following transformations are common: transformed skinfold = 100 log 10 (reading in 0.1 mm − 18). This can be applied to all sites in all ages and sexes. The table of transformed values of Edwards *et al.* [116] is given in Table 1.7. Garn *et al.* [129] reported recently that log 10 transformations do not correct skewness but reduce it and change the direction. They recommend normalized Z-scores. Transformation is unnecessary if skinfolds are compared to reference percentiles or analysed by regression or correlation techniques as opposed to parametric tests such as t-tests.

If % F and FM are to be estimated, the validated equations shown in Table 1.8 have much to recommend them. The same authors have given other estimation equations for other combinations of skinfolds, some in different methods of expression.

1.6.5 Performance characteristics

(a) General considerations

Skinfold calipers measure a compressed double fold of dermis plus SCAT, not a single layer of SCAT. Taking a fold of SCAT is probably a time-honoured clinical procedure of estimating nutritional status. However, it was not until 1890 when Richer introduced a caliper that the measurement became objective and repeatable. This first caliper exerted increasing pressure at wider jaw openings, a limitation not overcome until Correnti [131] introduced a constant-loading micrometer with adjustable pressure. The earlier

Table 1.8   Validated equations for the estimation of body density (kg/m^3)

1.   Adults: age (years)

Men

17–19	$D = 1162.0 - 63.0 \log (X_1)$
20–29	$D = 1163.1 - 63.2 \log (X_1)$
30–39	$D = 1142.2 - 54.4 \log (X_1)$
40–49	$D = 1162.0 - 70.0 \log (X_1)$
50+	$D = 1171.5 - 77.9 \log (X_1)$
17–72	$D = 1176.5 - 74.4 \log (X_1)$

Women

16–19	$D = 1154.9 - 67.8 \log (X_1)$
20–29	$D = 1159.9 - 71.7 \log (X_1)$
30–39	$D = 1142.3 - 63.2 \log (X_1)$
40–49	$D = 1133.3 - 61.2 \log (X_1)$
50+	$D = 1133.9 - 64.5 \log (X_1)$
16–68	$D = 1156.7 - 71.7 \log (X_1)$

where X_1 = sum of biceps, triceps, subscapular, and suprailiac skinfold.
(Durnin and Womersley [128])

Men aged 18–61 years
$$D = 1112.0 - 0.435 (X_2) + 0.00055 (X_2)^2 - 0.29 \text{ (age)}$$
$$D = 1213.9 - 31.0 \log_e (X_2) - 0.29 \text{ (age)}$$
$$D = 1109.4 - 0.827 (X_3) + 0.00160 (X_3)^2 - 0.257 \text{ (age)}$$
$$D = 1188.6 - 30.5 \log_e (X_3) - 0.27 \text{ (age)}$$

where X_2 = sum of chest, axilla, triceps, subscapular, abdomen, suprailiac, and thigh
skinfolds.
  X_3 = sum of chest, abdomen and thigh skinfolds.
(Jackson and Pollock [104])

Women aged 18–55 years
$$D = 1097.0 - 0.470 (X_4) + 0.00056 (X_4)^2 - 0.13 \text{ (age)}$$
$$D = 1231.7 - 38.4 \log_e (X_4) - 0.15 \text{ (age)}$$
$$D = 1096.1 - 0.695 (X_5) + 0.0011 (X_5)^2 - 0.07 \text{ (age)}$$
$$D = 1219.9 - 39.4 \log_e (X_5) - 0.11 \text{ (age)}$$
$$D = 1099.5 - 0.993 (X_6) + 0.0023 (X_6)^2 - 0.14 \text{ (age)}$$
$$D = 1213.9 - 40.6 \log_e (X_6) - 0.16 \text{ (age)}$$
where X_4 = sum of chest, axilla, triceps, subscapular, abdomen, suprailiac, thigh.
  X_5 = sum of triceps, suprailiac, abdomen and thigh.
  X_6 = sum of triceps, suprailiac and thigh.
(Jackson *et al.* [105])

2. Children and youths (8–17 years)

Males
$$\% F = 0.735 (X_7) + 1.0$$
$$\% F = 1.21 (X_8) - 0.008 (X_8)^2 - a$$
for $X_8 > 35$ mm, use $\% F = 0.783 (X_8) + 1.6$

Females
$$\% F = 0.61 (X_7) + 5.1$$
$$\% F = 1.33 (X_8) - 0.013 (X_8)^2 - 2.5$$

for $X_8 > 35$ mm, use % $F = 0.546$ $(X_8) + 9.7$

where $X_7 =$ sum of triceps + medial calf skinfold
$\quad\quad\; X_8 =$ sum of triceps + subscapular skinfold

intercept term, a, varies with maturational level and social group:
White males: pre-pubescent, -1.7; pubescent, -3.4; post-pubescent, -5.5;
Black males: pre-pubescent, -3.5; pubescent, -5.2; post-pubescent, -6.8.

(Slaughter *et al.* [130])

---

spring-loaded Franzen caliper [132] gave reproducible pressures at a given opening, but this varied according to jaw opening. The systematic investigations of Brozek and colleagues [133] led to recommendations for caliper design to give a jaw pressure of 10 g/mm^2 and jaw area 20–40 mm^2. The problem with compression is, however, that compressibility varies within and between sites and subjects and reduces the validity of skinfolds for the purpose of estimating energy nutritional status.

The sites measured to estimate subcutaneous fatness by comparison with reference values are the triceps and subscapular. To estimate body density (D) and hence FM and % F, experience has shown that triceps, subscapular and thigh plus abdomen and calf are most favoured [134]. To describe fat distribution and patterning, these sites plus one or more on the lower leg plus suprailiac and mid-axillary are adequate (111). Roche *et al.* [135] have summarized the criteria that determine choice of skinfolds according to the purpose of the investigation. These are shown in Figure 1.4.

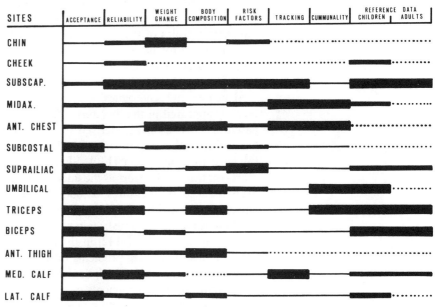

Fig. 1.4 Roche's diagrammatic representation of selected skinfold sites graded as good (▬▬▬), fair (———), and poor (———) with regard to different criteria. Missing data are represented by (– – – –). Reproduced with permission from Roche *et al.* [135].

The estimation of % F and FM from a regression equation with one or more skinfolds in various forms as the independent variables is an extremely common way of interpreting skinfolds in the assessment of nutritional status. There are over a hundred of these equations and the choice may appear perplexing, particularly as most are specific to the populations from which they are derived. However, it is now clear that equations that have been validated on other samples are the equations of choice. Several comprehensive critical reviews have appeared in the last decade [101–103, 136]. Equations tend to be specific to the populations on which they have been drawn up owing to technical, statistical, and biological factors [101]. Attention to these factors and cross validation of the equations should result in a more accurate estimation in other groups. This can be established by measuring % F by a criteria method such as density and comparing the results with those from the skinfold estimation procedure under consideration on a sample of the group.

Validation may have been incorporated in the study that established the relationship or may have come about by the repeated use of the equation and observation of its applicability to a variety of groups. Examples of these are the equations of Jackson and colleagues [104, 105, 137] and those of Durnin and Womersley [128] respectively. These are given in Table 1.8 along with validated equations for children and youths.

The equations are either logarithmic or quadratic to reflect the non-linear relationship between D and skinfolds. Durnin and Womersley's equations cover an age range of 16–72 years but equations for the individual 10-year age groups with lower standard errors of estimate (SEE) and for other combinations of skinfolds are given in their paper. Jackson and Pollock have also produced equations with other combinations of skinfolds.

These SEE cannot be taken as the error of estimate of fatness. They refer to the characteristics of the data of the equation. A second data set will have a greater total error of estimation, as estimation is rarely at the same level for second and subsequent samples and the conversion of density to % F has a further uncertainty as described below.

Slaughter and colleagues' equations for children and youth have only recently appeared in the literature. The advantages of these are that they are based on % F estimates derived from measurements of density, water, and bone mineral, they require only two common skinfolds and have been externally validated to some extent [130]. SEE vary between 3.6 and 3.9% F, which represent truer % F errors as the uncertainty in the conversion of D to % F has been reduced by measures of body water and bone mineral. The earlier equations of Parizkova [138] and Brook [139] were not validated in this way.

There is growing dissatisfaction with body density as a 'gold standard' and a criterion of fatness [140–142] in the individual and in age groups other than young adults. There are problems in the two-component (fat and fat-free or adipose tissue and lean) description of body composition caused by variations in composition of the components as a result of age, sex, habitual activity, and plane of nutrition. These can be reduced by multicomponent descriptions but this is outside the scope of this chapter. In the meantime, in young and middle-aged men, in women, and possibly in youths too, density, % F, and FM can be estimated with an acceptable error of estimate from quadratic or logarithmic equations of the sum of three or more skinfolds [136]. In infants, children, the elderly, and other groups it is inadvisable to estimate fat and fatness from skinfolds or W/H^n ratios. Instead, skinfolds should be compared with reference values. The question of whether to use observed or estimated variables has been addressed recently [143].

(b) Reproducibility

Reliability has two components of variance: imprecision or measurement error determined by re-measuring after a short time, and independability or physiological variation over hours or days [144]. It is imprecision that is usually measured by investigators assessing their reliability. All publications should contain details of the reliability of the measurements. From the information reviewed by Harrison *et al.* [127], reliability varies between sites. Common findings are, for triceps, intrameasurer errors of 0.4–0.8 mm and intermeasurer errors of 0.8–1.9; and for subscapular 0.9–1.6 and 0.9–1.5 respectively. Test–retest correlations invariably exceed 0.9. Measurement errors are shown in Table 1.9 and reliability in Table 1.10. In many cases ranges are given to reflect the results from different surveys and that measurement error increases in a linear manner with increasing skinfold.

Table 1.9 Technical error of the skinfold measurements (mm)

	Intrameasurer	References	Intermeasurer	References
Skinfolds:				
Triceps	0.4–0.8	[145–147]	0.8–1.89	[145,148]
	1.2	[25]		
Biceps	1.0	[25]		
	0.2–0.6	[149,150]		
Subscapular	1.4	[25]	0.88–1.53	[151,152]
	0.88–1.6	[134,153]		
Suprailiac	2.1	[25]	1.53 (children)	[145]
	0.3–1.0	[149,154,155]	1.7 (adults)	[156]
Thigh	0.5–0.7	[149,150]		
Medial Calf	1.9	[25]		
Abdomen	2.0	[25]		
	0.89	[155]		
Mid-axillary			0.95	[155]

(c) Validity

Are infinitely accurate measurements of skinfold thicknesses valid measures (i.e. truly reflecting the aspect one would ideally like to measure) of fat and fatness (and energy nutritional status)? There are several assumptions implicit in the use of skinfolds to represent body fat, as shown in Fig. 1.5. Martin *et al.* [164] regard compressibility as presenting the major problem as it is large and difficult to predict. The dermis thickness is not a constant fraction of the skinfold but the significance of this is unclear. Fat patterning may cause the sites measured to be unrepresentative of average SCAT thickness. However, skinfolds are highly intercorrelated and including more than three in the estimation of fatness does not reduce the error of estimate. The range of fat content of adipose tissue in biopsy material is high, 60–90%, varying according

Table 1.10   Reliability of skinfold measurements

	Intrameasurer reliability				Intermeasurer reliability			
	Intraclass coefficient	*[Ref]*	*Standard error of meas. (mm)*	*[Ref]*	*Interclass coefficient*	*[Ref]*	*Standard error of meas. (mm)*	*[Ref]*
Skinfolds								
Triceps	0.98	[25]						
Biceps	0.96	[25]						
Subscapular	0.98	[25]						
Suprailiac	0.96	[25]						
	0.97	[153]						
Thigh	0.91–0.98	[153,157,158]	1–2	[153,157,158]	>0.90	[159]	3–4	[159]
	0.98	[160]	1.4	[160]	0.97	[160]	2.1	[160]
					0.97	[104]	2.4	[104]
Suprapatellar	>0.90	[153,161]						
Medial calf	0.94	[25]						
	0.98	[162]						
	0.94–0.99	[163]						
Abdomen	0.98	[25]						
	0.97	[153]						
Pectoral (chest)	0.91–0.97	[157,161]	1–2	[157,161]	>0.90	[159]	3–5	[159]
	0.96	[160]	1.45	[160]	0.93	[160]	1.7	[160]
					0.98	[104]	2.1	[104]

to weight and fat status and probably age and sex. Similarly, the internal–external distribution of fat can be expected to vary, although detailed data are lacking.

The effect of these variations is to decrease the reliability, accuracy, and validity of skinfold thicknesses as indicators of body fat and fatness. This is a more serious problem for assessment of individuals than groups and for the estimation of body density and fatness than the practice of comparing skinfolds with reference values.

Skinfolds are used to describe fat distribution and patterning so naturally enough they are affected by it. Robson *et al.* [165] noted that triceps skinfolds of African children fell on much lower percentiles of standard values than subscapular skinfolds. Use of the former would lead to a description of less favourable growth and nutritional status. These ethnic differences seem to arise from European populations varying from others in the world rather than there being considerable inter-ethnic variation. However, within any group, individual variation will confound the use of skinfolds to describe nutritional status. This is less a problem for the population than the individual, and for the latter longitudinal measurements can overcome this difficulty.

1.6.6   Reference values

Reference values for triceps and subscapular skinfolds are given by Tanner and Whitehouse [166], Johnston *et al.* [145, 151], Durnin and Womersley [128] and Frisancho [51]. Much of the early data on triceps and subscapular thicknesses

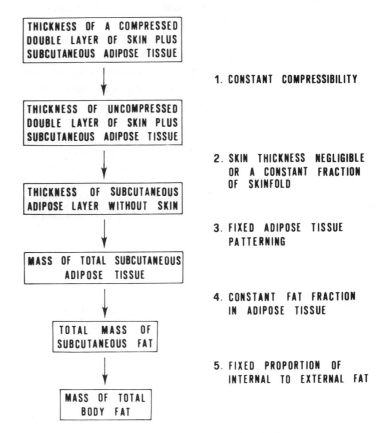

Fig. 1.5 The relations and assumptions between skinfold thickness measurements and body fatness. Reproduced with permission from Martin *et al.* [164].

in populations throughout the world has been collated by Eveleth and Tanner [13]. As with height and weight, there is much to be said for comparing the skinfolds of individuals or groups as percentiles or standard deviation scores rather than as percentages of the mean or median, particularly in children. Sources of reference data for body density are described in Chapter 2 (p. 70).

The assessment of fat distribution and fat patterning is a newer area of use of skinfold thicknesses, and systematic study of population values have not been undertaken to any significant degree. More is known of the fat distribution indices. The multivariate approaches, such as principal component analysis, although able to identify common patterns, do not provide comparable results.

1.6.7 Interpretation

How appropriate are fat and fatness data as indices of energy nutritional status? Ferro-Luzzi [167] has considered energy nutritional status to be a dynamic condition that might be described as the extent to which improvements can be made in terms of functions and capacities (such as work capacity and performance, reproductive competence, disease response, social and be-havioural functions, growth performance, etc.) by changes in energy balance, its components, or the rate of energy flux. This reflects a need to move away from anthropometry to a more functional approach to energy nutritional status. The purpose of nutritional status assessment is to ascertain if an individual or a population is optimally nourished with a view to formulating and implementing appropriate action where necessary to improve or restore the level of nutritional health. To this end it may only be necessary to describe the individual as adequately nourished – no action required; marginally nourished – monitor further; or poorly nourished – institute remedial action. The cut-off points of these categories are at the present time subjective and depend on the size of the problem and the resources available for action. The cut-off points for skinfold thicknesses, their specificity and sensitivity are not well-established. However, there is much data linking weight and overweight to morbidity and mortality, and more prospective studies are including measures of fatness and fat patterning. Roche *et al.* [168] recommend that both fatness and fat content be graded, as they may have separate associations with disease, social effects, and performance.

1.7 SKELETAL DIAMETERS

1.7.1 Purpose and scope

Measurements of skeletal diameters (body breadths) are uncommon in an armoury for the assessment of nutritional status, although they do have an important role in the assessment of frame size. Stature is the usual indicator of body size, but a second dimension to size is reflected by these measurements. Skeletal diameter measurement is an integral part of most procedures of describing body types, as in somatotyping and in clothes sizing. They have also been used in conjunction with circumferences and skinfolds to estimate body composition, particularly the lean or fat-free body mass [169]. Skeletal diameters may provide an indicator of potential weight gain in the anorexic and may substitute for stature when this cannot be measured accurately, e.g. with kyphosis in the elderly, although this is commonly attempted with arm span.

In the assessment of body weight it is recognized that weight varies with stature and with age. It is also recognized that body weight is influenced by muscularity and, more pertinently, by body proportions, particularly width, and bone size. In contrast to stature and age, these cannot be measured with precision, accuracy, or validity. The concept of frame size, a description of build and physique independent of stature and length, helps fill this gap. Frame size is usually described by skeletal diameters, although there is no common agreement on which measures are most appropriate. Frame size description is used to attempt to determine the extent to which body weight at whatever level is influenced by the size of the lean or fat-free mass and its separate components or the size of the fat mass. Considering overweight it is important to distinguish whether this arises from a high fat-free mass or a high fat mass. The selection of frame size variables may be based on a high correlation with weight but low correlation with skinfold thickness. A more useful approach would be one that explains variance unaccounted for by weight or stature. Significant partial correlations of breadths, with fat-free mass controlling for stature, have been shown [170].

As there is no agreement on what constitutes frame size and how it is measured, a variety of skeletal diameters have appeared in the nutrition literature. These include trunk measurements: biacromial (shoulder), biiliac (pelvic), bitrochanteric (hip), bony chest; and limb sites: bicondylar humerus (elbow), bistyloid (wrist), bicondylar femur (knee), and bimalleolar (ankle) diameters. The breadths most commonly used in assessing frame size are wrist, elbow, shoulder, and hip. These are described below.

1.7.2 Principle of the method

Using appropriate instruments, the skeletal diameters are measured by standardized techniques for the reasons described above.

1.7.3 Apparatus

Shoulder and hip breadths are measured by anthropometers such as the Holtain anthropometer (Holtain Ltd, Crosswell, Crymmych, Dyfed, UK). It consists of a rod with one fixed and one movable blade with a digital display to 1 mm. The minimum display is 47 mm. Digital readout anthropometers should be calibrated each day as the gear mechanism and blades can be damaged easily. The minimum and maximum readings should remain constant. For elbow and wrist breadth, sliding calipers, similar to the anthropometer in having one fixed and one movable blade but usually with a flat bar and scale engraved in centimetres and millimetres. Calipers should be cleaned frequently and lubricated with graphite to prevent sticking.

1.7.4 Procedures

The landmarks of the skeletal breadths are typically bony protuberances. The anthropometer is held by the blades with the bar resting on the wrists or hands. The tops of the blades are held by the thumb and middle finger while the index finger is used to palpate the landmark. The non-movable blade is placed on the landmark and the movable blade brought onto the opposite landmark. As the measurement is of the skeleton, firm pressure should be used to reduce the influence of subcutaneous adipose tissue. Once a stable reading has been obtained, the blades should be removed, reapplied and a duplicate reading taken. Duplicates should agree to within 2 mm. The measurements described are taken with the observer behind the subject, except where stated.

Biacromial breadth This is measured from behind the subject, with the shoulders bared. The shoulders are relaxed with the arms at the side. The lateral borders of the acromial processes are palpated and the blade pushed firmly onto them. The measurement is not recommended for individuals less than two years of age.

Bitrochanteric breadth The subject stands with arms folded and the feet 50 mm apart and at a 15° angle. The trochanters are palpated from behind. The blades are applied firmly if the intention is to achieve a skeletal measurement at this site as there may be considerable amounts of soft tissue.

Biiliac breadth This is more commonly measured than the bitrochanteric breadth but is measured in the same way with the anthropometer blade applied to the iliac crests at the maximum diameter. Firm pressure may be required.

Bicondylar humerus breadth The arm is raised and the elbow flexed at 90°, with the palm of the hand towards the individual. From the front of the subject, the epicondyles of the humerus are palpated and the blades of the sliding caliper applied. An angle of 45° to bisect the elbow angle is recommended [171] and, as the medial epicondyle is lower than the lateral epicondyle, the calipers are at a slight angle to the arm.

Bistyloid breadth Measure from the front of the subject who stands with the upper arm by his or her side, the elbow flexed at 90°, and the hand held out, palm down. Holding the blades of spreading or sliding calipers, palpate the outer aspects ulnar and radial styloids. Bring the blades onto these landmarks firmly.

Earlier descriptions of measurement procedures have been given by Behnke and Wilmore [172], Weiner and Lourie [7], Cameron [173], and Lohman *et al.* [9].

1.7.5 Performance characteristics

(a) General considerations

Early uses of skeletal diameters in the assessment of nutritional status were the ratio of the sum of the biacromial and bicristal diameters to height, the laterality–linearity index, and the ratio of biacromial to bicristal (biiliac), a masculinity index. Both were recommended for the assessment of nutritional status [2] and were applied in cardiovascular epidemiology [174].

An early use of frame size to improve the description of body weights associated with lowest mortality was the Metropolitan Life Insurance Company [175] ideal weights at each height in three frame-size categories. However, frame sizes are based on self-reports, which are unreliable [176] and no definitions were provided. In the 1983 tables [177], three frame size categories were formulated based on the 25th and the 75th percentiles of American data (NHANES I) for elbow breadth collected between 1971 and 1974. But frame size was not measured in those used to assess subsequent mortality. Frisancho and Flegal [178] suggested elbow breadth to be a suitable measure of frame size based on a low correlation with log-transformed skinfolds and age in over 16 000 adults from NHANES I. Subsequently, Frisancho [179] published tables of weight, triceps and subscapular skinfolds, and bone-free arm muscle area percentiles in sex, height, and three frame-size categories based on elbow breadth in over 21 000 adults in NHANES I and II. Frame sizes corresponded to below, between, and above the 15th and 85th percentiles in the separate age and sex groups. At about the same time Katch and Freedson [180] produced a bivariate frame-size model based on stature and the sum of biacromial and bitrochanteric diameters, called ΣAT, of 300 young adults. The cut-off points for small, medium, and large frames were perpendiculars 1 SD above and below the mean stature on the regression line of ΣAT on stature.

In the estimation of body composition, skeletal breadths are important estimators of fat-free mass [169, 181]. Roche [182] has reviewed the studies that have related frame size to body composition measures. In brief, in the estimation of body density and hence fatness and leanness, frame size may not be useful in boys; biacromial diameter has been useful in girls and young women, chest, knee, and elbow widths are useful in women, and biiliac diameter and ankle and chest circumferences in young men.

(b) Reproducibility

Reliability of skeletal diameters depends on the age and sex of the individual and possibly the level of fatness too. The published information has recently been collected together [171]. Behnke and Wilmore [172] state that biacromial, bitrochanteric and biiliac are highly reproducible if the soft tissues are compressed. Test and retest correlations invariably exceed 0.95 and technical errors of measurement of 1–3 mm are reported in children and young adults. The ratio of the technical error of measurement to the variability of the data is low and thus these measurements are highly reproducible provided the standard protocol is rigorously adhered to, e.g. if the shoulders are not relaxed but are pulled back, the biacromial diameters may decrease 20–30 mm. For the elbow and wrist, technical error of measurement are similarly low but the population data are less variable. However, these are very reproducible too, with good technique.

(c) Validity

If frame size is to be useful in the interpretation of body weight, differences in body weight in the different size categories should be associated with only one of the components of body composition. In the small sample of males of Katch and Freedson [180], differences in body weight between frame size groups was primarily due to differences in lean body weight. However, in females there was a small but statistically significant increase in fat weight but not in lean body weight when frame size was allowed for by dividing lean weight by frame size. Garn *et al.* [183] also found differences in weight but not in fatness as evinced by skinfolds in frame size groups based on bony chest breadth (BCB) in 2200 middle-aged men. However, weight/BCB was interpreted as an indication of relative fatness and bony chest breadth of lean body mass. Similarly, Himes and Frisancho [184] found small but significant correlations between body breadths and per cent fat or fat weight controlling for fat-free mass, in both men and women. Thus, our measures of frame size are independently related to fatness and leaness.

1.7.6 Reference values

Good reference data are available for elbow breadth [178]. Other suitable reference data have been listed recently [171] and data on groups throughout the world identified [13].

1.7.7 Interpretation

Evidence that frame size improves the identification of those at increased risk of morbidity and mortality is lacking. Bony chest breadth and weight/BCB were positively associated with 16 years cardiovascular mortality in middle-aged Scots [183], but Himes and Frisancho [184] point out that it is unclear whether BCB is indeed superior to weight alone or weight for stature. There are no data linking frame size adjusted weight or fatness to morbidity. Despite the paucity of supporting data it is still widely accepted that frame size will influence the body weight with lowest morbidity and mortality.

Appendix A

The presentation and use of height and weight data for comparing the nutritional status of groups of children under the age of 10 years

J. C. WATERLOW,[1] R. BUZINA,[2] W. KELLER,[3] J. M. LANE,[4] M. Z. NICHAMAN,[5] & J. M. TANNER [6]

This paper presents recommendations for the analysis and presentation of height and weight data from surveillance or surveys involving nutrition and anthropometry in young children up to the age of 10 years. These recommendations are only for the analysis of data collected on a cross-sectional basis. The basic indices recommended are height for age and weight for height, each considered either in terms of centiles or in a cross-classification scheme using standard deviation scores. It is hoped that these methods of analysis and presentation will prove widely acceptable, so that international comparisons will be made easier.

In the past, the nutritional status of groups of children has been most frequently assessed by using a classification based on a deficit in weight for age, originally proposed by Gomez and modified by Jelliffe (*1, 2, 3*). The Eighth Joint FAO/WHO Expert Committee on Nutrition (*4*) emphasized the importance of distinguishing between acute and chronic, or present and past, malnutrition. Several authors have suggested methods for the classification of nutritional status, based on measurements of height and weight, which take into account this distinction (*5, 6, 7*). Recently, an FAO/UNICEF/WHO Expert Committee on Nutritional Surveil-lance (*8*) recommended the use of height for age and weight for height as primary indicators of nutritional status in children.

The results of surveys made in different regions, or in the same region at different times, should be analysed and reported in such a way that comparisons are facilitated. This paper suggests methods of classification that we hope will be widely acceptable and thus make international comparisons possible. The classifications are intended for use in analysing data from cross-sectional surveys made as part of nutritional monitoring or surveillance programmes. In the context of this paper, nutritional monitoring includes the cross-sectional collection of measurements of height and weight on a continuous basis as part of regular health care services (surveillance) as well as the making of periodic studies of population samples (surveys).

These recommendations, although specifically for use in the analysis of cross-sectional data from groups of children, do not conflict in any way with the use of weight and height for following the progress of individual children in clinics. The reader should recognize, however, that there are specific problems related to the evaluation of growth of an individual child that are not discussed in this paper.

[1] Head, Department of Human Nutrition, London School of Hygiene and Tropical Medicine, Keppel Street (Gower Street), London WC1, England.

[2] Head, Department of Nutrition, Institute of Public Health of Croatia, Rockefellerova 7, Zagreb, Yugoslavia.

[3] Medical Officer, Nutrition, WHO, Geneva, Switzerland.

[4] Director, BSE, Preventable Diseases and Nutrition, Center for Disease Control, Public Health Service, Department of Health, Education, and Welfare, Atlanta, GA, USA.

[5] Chief, Nutrition Section, BSE, Preventable Diseases and Nutrition, Center for Disease Control, Public Health Service, Department of Health, Education, and Welfare, Atlanta, GA, USA.

[6] Professor of Child Health and Growth, Department of Growth and Development, Institute of Child Health, University of London, London, England.

THE REFERENCE POPULATION

It is frequently convenient to compare measurements made in different places, or in the same place at different times, by relating them to a single reference population. The anthropometric data to be used in the development of such a reference population should fulfil the following criteria.

1. Measurements should relate to a well-nourished population.

2. The sample should include at least 200 individuals in each age and sex group.

3. The sample should be cross-sectional, since the comparisons that will be made are of a cross-sectional nature.

4. Sampling procedures should be defined and reproducible.

5. Measurements should be carefully made and recorded by observers trained in anthropometric techniques, using equipment of well tested design and calibrated at frequent intervals.

6. The measurements made on the sample should include all the anthropometric variables that will be used in the evaluation of nutritional status.

7. The data from which reference graphs and tables are prepared should be available for anyone wishing to use them, and the procedures used for smoothing curves and preparing tables should be adequately described and documented.

At present, there are three bodies of data that may be considered for use as an international reference. These are: the measurements of Dutch children reported by van Wieringen (*9*); those of US National Academy of Sciences (*10*); and those of British children reported by Tanner et al. (*11*).

Although none of these sets of measurements meets all the criteria listed above, we suggest that the data recommended by the US National Academy of Sciences are, on balance, most suitable for use as an international reference. These data are drawn from a defined sample of American children which contains between 300 and 1600 children in each yearly age group. In addition to height and weight, other anthropometric variables are available including measurements of skinfold thickness, limb circumference, and head circumference. A detailed analysis and description of the reference population and the sampling procedures is obtainable from the US

National Center for Health Statistics and will be published as a monograph of that agency. The data from this reference population are available for both sexes as centile curves of weight for age and height for age up to 18 years, and of weight for length or height up to the age of puberty (*12*). The data are also available as tabulations of centiles and mean $\pm$ SD of height and weight for each month of age up to the age of 18 years, and of weight for height for each 0.5 cm height interval up to 145 cm for boys and 137 cm for girls. These tabulations are available from the Chief Medical Officer, Nutrition, World Health Organization, who will also offer facilities for consultation on the computer analysis of results for presentation in the ways recommended below.

Anthropometric measurements are being made, or are in the process of being analysed, on large groups of children in other countries, e.g., Cuba and United Kingdom (*13, 14*). When these analyses are complete, a detailed comparison of all the results should be undertaken to determine how far the reference data that we are recommending are representative of well-nourished children in different countries.

When the reference population data are being used, a distinction must be made between the concept of a reference and that of a standard or target. The question of whether all child populations throughout the world have the same genetic potential for growth in size is still unresolved (*15, 16*). Clearly, if there were differences dependent on different gene distributions, then the target for one population would not be the same as the target for another. This does not, however, affect the use of the reference data for comparisons between populations.

We suggest that there are in effect two stages in the analysis of data from cross-sectional surveys. The first stage is recording and grouping the observations in such a way that they are internationally intelligible and comparable. It is for this purpose that a reference base is needed, and it is immaterial from what population that base is drawn, provided that it is large enough for proper statistical definition.

Because the reference population cannot be used as a universal target, the question of what is a realistic goal in any particular situation does become important. If it is felt that the growth of children in an industrialized country is not a realistic target in another country in which the population has a different genetic and environmental background, two courses are possible: the first is to construct a local standard, although this may present considerable difficulties; the second is to make an arbitrary and perhaps temporary adjustment in the cut-off points derived from the reference population that are used for grouping the data and making value judgements about them (see below). For example, if it is felt that in a particular population even well-nourished children are shorter in stature than the children of the North American reference population, then it might be reasonable to set the target for height as 95% of the reference height rather than 100%. Decisions of this kind have to be taken locally, and it is not possible to make international recommendations about them.

ANALYSIS AND PRESENTATION OF DATA

Indicators

We recommend that for the assessment of nutritional status in cross-sectional studies, primary reliance should be placed on weight for height as an indicator of the present state of nutrition and on height for age as an indicator of past nutrition. Although weight for age has for many years been a mainstay in the evaluation of nutritional status, it has the disadvantage that it does not distinguish between acute and chronic malnutrition. On the other hand, weight for age as well as height for age are useful indices when serial measurements are made, as in clinics for children under 5 years of age. Weight for age is particularly useful in children under 1 year old and, if length measurements are not performed accurately, weight for age may be the most valid index.

Both the Dutch data of van Wieringen and the American data show that in these populations weight for height is nearly independent of age between 1.0 and 10.0 years. This means that, at a given height, both median weight and range of weight are independent of the age of the children concerned. Weight for height is probably also relatively independent of ethnic group, particularly in the age groups between 1 and 5 years (*15, 17, 18*). At ages of less than 1 year, at a given height (or length) the older child tends to be heavier. This source of error, which in any case is not very great (*19*), is minimized if in the first year of life children are classified in fairly narrow age ranges, as recommended below. Neither weight for age nor height for age can be determined when ages are unknown, and in these situations the use of weight for height for the assessment of nutritional status is particularly advantageous.

Age groups

In many contexts, children up to the age of 5 years are considered to be a homogeneous group and are referred to under the heading of preschool children. This leads to errors because the pattern of malnutrition tends to change as children grow older (*6*). At 1–2 years of age the deficit in weight for height is often very marked; by 3–4 years this deficit may be made up, but the child remains with a deficit in height for age and weight for age. For this reason it is recommended that data be presented in the age groups shown in Table 1. If the numbers of children are large enough (at least 100 in each age group) we strongly recommend the groupings in column A. In many situations the age groups shown in column B will be the most useful. The wider groupings in column C should be used only when numbers are small; we believe that such data will have limited value.

Table 1. Recommended age groups for the presentation of anthropometric data

A Highly recommended	B Recommended	C Permissible
0 – 2.99 months		
3.0 – 5.99 months	0 – 5.99 months	
6.0 – 8.99 months		
9.0 – 11.99 months	6.0 – 11.99 months	0 – 11.99 months
1.0 – 1.99 years	1.0 – 1.99 years	1.0 – 1.99 years
2.0 – 2.99 years		
3.0 – 3.99 years	2.0 – 3.99 years	
4.0 – 4.99 years		
5.0 – 5.99 years	4.0 – 5.99 years	2.0 – 5.99 years
6.0 – 6.99 years		
7.0 – 7.99 years	6.0 – 7.99 years	
8.0 – 8.99 years		
9.0 – 9.99 years	8.0 – 9.99 years	6.0 – 9.99 years

Analysis and presentation of results for each age and sex group

In all cases an accurate description of the population from which the results were obtained, including the numbers of children, should be provided in tabular or graphic form. Suppose, then, that measurements have been made on a number of children of one sex between the ages of 1 and 2 years; this forms a specific age and sex group. The set of measurements from this group can be analysed in two ways: by centiles, or by standard deviations from the mean (SD score).

Centiles

Data for an individual child (sex, age, height, and weight) are used to place the child in the appropriate centile of weight for height (or length), height for age, and weight for age. Under the age of 1 year, weight for age centiles are particularly useful. The specific centile into which a child falls can be determined by calculation; alternatively, the range within which each child lies can be obtained from graphs such as the examples (based on the National Center for Health Statistics/CDC reference population) shown in Fig. 1–6 or from appropriate tables. In these graphs and tables the weight for height, height for age, and weight for age centiles of the reference population are shown at selected intervals, including the third, fifth, ninety-fifth, and ninety-seventh centiles, which are presented so that the extremes can be better characterized.

Height and weight data for a group of children can be summarized in a table or a figure. Examples

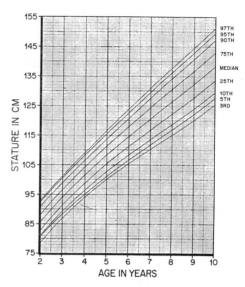

Fig. 2. Girls, 2–10 years, stature by age, percentiles (reference population).

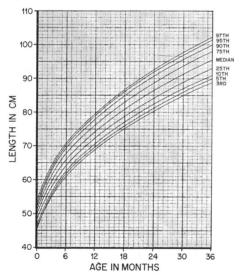

Fig. 1. Girls, 0–36 months, supine length by age, percentiles (reference population).

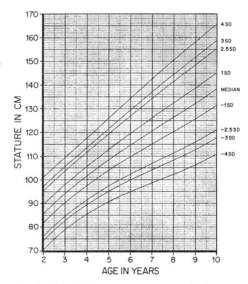

Fig. 3. Girls, 0–36 months, supine length by age, standard deviations (reference population).

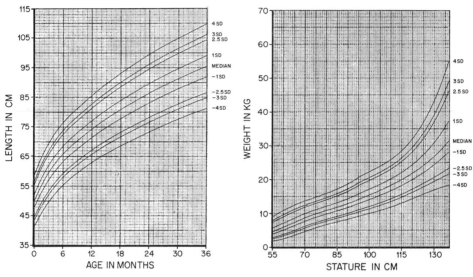

Fig. 4. Girls, 2–10 years, stature by age, standard deviations (reference population).

Fig. 6. Girls, weight by stature, standard deviations (reference population).

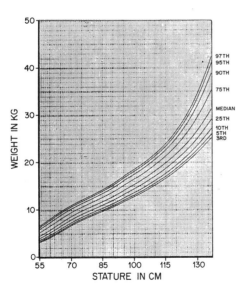

Fig. 5. Girls, weight by stature, percentiles (reference population).

of the presentation of height for age are shown in Table 2 and Fig. 7; similar presentations are appropriate for weight for height and weight for age. Fig. 7 shows that the sample contains an excess of children whose height for age lies in the lower centile ranges of the reference population. The advantage of relating results to centiles is that no error arises from the fact that weight for height in the reference population, and probably in all populations, has a skewed distribution. This skewness makes direct calculation of standard deviations inappropriate. The disadvantage of the method is that extremes of variation are less easy to characterize than in the standard deviation method. There are many populations in less developed countries where large numbers of children are so far outside the range of the reference population that they cannot be accurately classified by centiles.

Standard deviation score

In populations where many children lie outside the extreme centiles of the reference population, classification has usually been based on percentage deviation from the median of the reference population (*2, 6, 19*). In such classifications it has been usual to

Table 2. Example of presentation of the centile distribution of height for age in a sample group of children (aged between 1 and 2 years) as compared to the reference population

Centile		Male	Female	Total
00.0 – 02.9	n	15	23	38
	%	2.4	3.4	2.9
00.0 – 04.9	n	86	59	145
	%	13.9	8.7	11.2
00.0 – 09.9	n	211	208	419
	%	34.0	30.6	32.3
10.0 – 19.9	n	77	107	184
	%	12.4	15.8	14.2
20.0 – 29.9	n	81	100	181
	%	13.1	14.7	13.9
30.0 – 39.9	n	67	54	121
	%	10.8	8.0	9.3
40.0 – 49.9	n	48	46	94
	%	7.7	6.8	7.2
50.0 – 59.0	n	45	47	92
	%	7.3	6.9	7.1
60.0 – 69.9	n	26	41	67
	%	4.2	6.0	5.2
70.0 – 79.9	n	25	29	54
	%	4.2	6.0	5.2
80.0 – 89.9	n	18	23	41
	%	2.9	3.4	3.2
90.0 – 99.9	n	22	24	46
	%	3.5	3.5	3.5
95.0 – 100.0	n	10	9	19
	%	1.6	1.3	1.5
97.0 – 100.0	n	2	4	6
	%	0.3	0.6	0.5

distinguish grades of deficit (mild, moderate, and severe) by establishing arbitrary cut-off points.

Waterlow and others (*5, 6, 19, 20*) have pointed out the additional usefulness of looking at the deficit in weight for height (wasting) and the deficit in height for age (stunting) together. The cut-off points proposed in this system, which were based on percentage deviations from the median, were chosen because they were assumed to correspond approximately to 1, 2, and 3 standard deviations of height for age and weight for height. Fig. 8 and Tables 3 and 4 show, however, that this is only an approximate relationship. As an example, at a height of 65 cm (girls) 90% of median weight for height is equal to 1.00 SD below the median (—1 SD) whereas at 85 cm, it is equal to 1.30 SD below the median (the 17th and 10th centiles respectively). The relative proportions of children diagnosed as malnourished by using a cut-off of 80% of median weight for height as compared to using a cut-off of —2 SD changes somewhat with increasing age and size of children. For this reason it is recommended that in those populations where large numbers of children fall above the upper or below the lower centiles, their weight for height and height for age should be expressed as multiples of the standard deviation of the reference population rather than as percentages of the median.

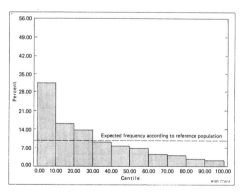

Fig. 7. Height for age distribution of a sample population in centiles as compared to the reference population; **total number in sample = 4780.**

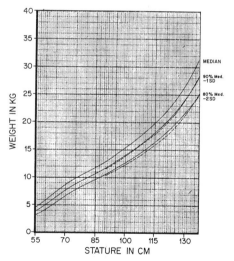

Fig. 8. Girls, weight by stature, standard deviations and percentages of median curves (reference population).

Table 3. Relationship of selected levels of percentage of median to SD scores and centiles for weight for height at various heights (girls)

Height (cm)	Weight for height (girls)					
	120% of median		90% of median		80% of median	
	SD score	centile	SD score	centile	SD score	centile
65	+ 1.9	97th	− 1.0	17th	− 2.0	3rd
85	+ 2.5	99th	− 1.3	10th	− 2.5	0.6th
95	+ 1.7	96th	− 1.1	13th	− 2.3	1st
105	+ 1.9	97th	− 1.1	13th	− 2.3	1st
115	+ 1.9	97th	− 1.2	12th	− 2.3	1st

Table 4. Relationship of selected levels of percentage of median to SD scores and centiles for height for age at various ages (boys)

Age (months)	Height for age (boys)					
	95% of median		90% of median		85% of median	
	SD score	centile	SD score	centile	SD score	centile
6	− 1.3	10th	− 2.5	0.6th	− 3.8	0.008th
12	− 1.4	8th	− 2.8	0.2nd	− 4.2	0.002th
24	− 1.3	10th	− 2.6	0.5th	− 3.9	0.005th
48	− 1.2	12th	− 2.4	0.8th	− 3.6	0.02nd
72	− 1.2	12th	− 2.4	0.9th	− 3.6	0.02nd

Table 5. Examples of calculation of standard deviation scores

Height of subject (boys) (cm)	Weight of subject (kg)	Median weight ± 1.00 SD for height (kg)	(kg)	Subjects' SD score
60	5.1	5.8	− 0.643	− 1.1
70	9.3	8.5	+ 0.841	+ 1.0
90	15.1	13.0	+ 1.069	+ 2.0
110	15.3	18.7	− 1.610	− 2.1

Formula for calculation of the SD score of subjects with a weight below the median weight for the subject's height:

$$\text{SD score of subject} = \frac{\text{median weight for height} - \text{weight of subject}}{1.00 \text{ SD lower}}$$

Formula for calculation of the SD score of subjects with a weight above the median weight for the subject's height:

$$\text{SD score of subject} = \frac{\text{weight of subject} - \text{median weight for height}}{1.00 \text{ SD upper}}$$

Because the weight for age and weight for height distributions were highly skewed at the upper centiles, different estimates of the standard deviation for values above and below the median were made for these variables. This was done by fitting empirical centiles of each half distribution with half of a Gaussian curve. In the case of height for age, which is normally distributed, standard deviations were calculated in the normal fashion.

Charts showing selected multiples of the standard deviation in the reference population are reproduced in Fig. 3, 4, and 6. Since in many situations there are obese as well as undernourished children, provision should be made for excess weight for height as well as for deficits. The determination for each child of the appropriate standard deviation score for weight for height, height for age, and weight for age can be done by calculation or by comparison with these graphs. The formulae for calculating the standard deviation score for a child, as well as a number of examples using weight for height, are shown in Table 5. Similar calculations to determine the standard deviation score for height or weight for age can be made by substituting the age of the subject, the height or weight of the subject, the median height or weight for age, and the appropriate ±1.00 SD value as required. It is then a simple matter to summarize the results by giving, for each age and sex group, the number and proportion of children in specified standard deviation ranges. However, as each child may in varying degrees be both under weight for height (acutely malnourished) and under height for age (chronically malnourished), it is an advantage to get a more complete picture of the various combinations. For this purpose a 4×4 table was originally introduced (6, 19). If account is to be taken of children who are overweight and of more than average height, the number of cells in the table should be increased.

Applications

In presenting height and weight data to describe the nutritional status of children from relatively well-nourished populations, centile distributions of height for age and weight for height are the most appropriate (see Table 2 and Fig. 7). In relatively undernourished populations the cross-tabulation of height for age against weight for height is recommended using standard deviation scores instead of percentage deviations from the median. The approximate relation-

Table 6. Example of cross tabulation in SD scores of weight for height and height for age, in a developing country, of children aged between 1 and 5 years (number in sample = 6482)

SD score of weight for height	SD score of height for age (percentage of population)				
	More than − 2.00	− 2.00 to − 2.99	− 3.00 to − 3.99	− 4.00 or less	Total
More than − 2.00	24.3	24.8	21.3	15.1	85.5
− 2.00 to − 2.49	2.3	2.6	2.3	1.7	8.9
− 2.50 to − 2.99	0.8	1.2	1.1	0.7	3.7
− 3.00 or less	0.4	0.5	0.5	0.4	1.8
Total	28.0	29.0	25.1	17.9	100.0

Table 7. Example of cross tabulation in SD scores of weight for height and height for age, in a developed country, of children aged between 1 and 5 years (number in sample = 9448)

SD score of weight for height	SD score of height for age (percentage of population)				
	More than − 1.50	− 1.50 to − 1.99	− 2.00 to − 2.99	− 3.00 or less	Total
+ 2.00 or more	5.3	0.4	0.5	0.5	6.7
1.99 to + 1.00	13.4	0.9	0.8	0.4	15.5
+ 0.99 to − 1.99	66.6	5.0	3.8	0.9	76.3
− 2.00 or less	1.3	0.1	0.0	0.0	1.4
Total	86.6	6.4	5.2	1.8	100.0

ships between SD scores, deviations from the median and centiles for weight for height (girls) and height for age (boys) are shown in Tables 3 and 4. With such information, appropriate classification limits and numbers of cells can be chosen.

Previous use of this system has shown that 80% of median weight for height and 90% of median height for age in undernourished populations are useful classification limits for identifying significantly malnourished groups of children. In deciding on appropriate classification limits in both undernourished and overnourished populations, the following principles should be observed.

1. It is desirable to include ±2.0 SD units for both height for age and weight for height in the classification scheme.

2. In undernourished populations, −2.0 SD weight for height corresponds approximately to 80% of the median weight for height and 90% of the median height for age. If further extension below −2.0 SD units is desired, it should be done in units of 0.5 or 1.0 SD, and the classification points at −3.0 SD, −4.0 SD units, respectively, should be maintained.

3. In populations where overnutrition is a problem, the same principle should be applied in extending upwards or downwards from +2.0 SD units for weight for height particularly. It should be noted from Table 3 that +1.0 SD corresponds approximately to 110% of median weight for height and +2.0 SD corresponds approximately to 120% median weight for height.

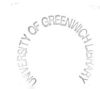

4. In practice this will usually mean analysing the population data in 0.5 SD units and later grouping these data into appropriate SD groups. It is recommended that in most cases classification points at —2.0 SD or +2.0 SD units be included, depending on whether the population is basically undernourished or overnourished. When data are put together using these principles, it will usually not be necessary to have more than a 4 × 4 cross-tabulation.

Examples showing the appropriate use of these principles in populations of developing and developed countries are given in Tables 6 and 7. The systems of analysis and presentation so far discussed have dealt with the distribution of height for age and weight for height (length) in population groups. It may sometimes be useful to present a single figure to describe the extent to which a population differs from the reference population. For this purpose, the average of the standard deviation scores for children in specific age and sex groups can be calculated. Such averages can be used for comparing the overall position of different groups.

ACKNOWLEDGEMENTS

The authors are grateful to James B. Goldsby, mathematical statistician at the Center for Disease Control, Atlanta, GA, USA, who made the statistical calculations and graphs on which the paper is based.

RÉSUMÉ

PRÉSENTATION ET UTILISATION DES DONNÉES RELATIVES À LA TAILLE ET AU POIDS POUR LA COMPARAISON DE L'ÉTAT NUTRITIONNEL DE GROUPES D'ENFANTS DE MOINS DE 10 ANS

Dans le présent article sont formulées des recommandations pour l'analyse et la présentation des données relatives à la taille et au poids fournies par la surveillance ou des enquêtes nutritionnelles et anthropométriques chez des enfants jusqu'à l'âge de 10 ans. Ces recommandations sont destinées uniquement à l'analyse des données recueillies sur une base transversale. Les indicateurs fondamentaux recommandés sont la taille pour l'âge et le poids pour la taille, chacun étant présenté soit en centiles soit sous une forme de classement à plusieurs entrées utilisant les valeurs des écarts-types. On espère que ces méthodes d'analyse et de présentation pourront être largement acceptables et rendront ainsi plus faciles les comparaisons sur le plan international.

REFERENCES

1. BENGOA, J. M. The problem of malnutrition. *WHO Chronicle*, **28**: 3-7 (1974).
2. GOMEZ, F. ET AL. Mortality in second and third degree malnutrition. *Journal of tropical pediatrics and African child health*, **2**: 77 (1956).
3. JELLIFFE, D. B. The assessment of the nutritional status of the community. Geneva, World Health Organization, 1966 (WHO Monograph Series No. 53).
4. WHO Technical Report Series, No. 477, 1971 (Joint FAO/WHO Expert Committee on Nutrition. *Eighth report*).
5. SEOANE, N. & LATHAM, M. C. Nutritional anthropometry in the identification of malnutrition in childhood. *Journal of tropical pediatrics and African child health*, **17**: 98-104 (1971).
6. WATERLOW, J. C. & RUTISHAUSER, I. H. E. Malnutrition in man. In: *Early malnutrition and mental development*. Symposia of the Swedish Nutrition Foundation XII, p. 13-26. Uppsala, Almqvist and Wiksell, 1974.
7. MCLAREN, D. S. & READ, W. W. C. Classification of nutritional status in early childhood. *Lancet*, **2**: 146-148 (1972).
8. WHO Technical Report Series No. 593, 1976 (*Methodology of nutritional surveillance*).
9. VAN WIERINGEN, J. C. Secular changes of growth. 1964-1966 height and weight surveys in the Netherlands. Leiden, Netherlands Institute for Preventive Medicine, TNO, 1972.
10. US FOOD AND NUTRITION BOARD. Committee on Nutrition Advisory to CDC. Comparison of body weights and body heights of groups of children. US Department of Health, Education and Welfare, Public Health Service. Center for Disease Control, Atlanta, Georgia, 1974.

11. TANNER, J. M. ET AL. Standards from birth to maturity for height, weight, height velocity and weight velocity: British children 1965. *Archives o, disease in childhood*, **41**: 454, 613 (1966).

12. NATIONAL CENTER FOR HEALTH STATISTICS. Growth Charts. US Department of Health, Education and Welfare, Public Health Service, Health Resources Administration, Rockville, MD., 1976. (HRA76 - 1120, **25**, 3).

13. JORDAN, J. ET AL. The 1972 Cuban national child growth study as an example of population health monitoring, design and methods. *Annals of human biology*, **2**: 153-171 (1975).

14. RONA, R. & ALTMAN, D. G. Standards of attained height, weight and triceps skinfold in English children from 5-11 years old. *Annals of human biology* (in press).

15. HABICHT, J.-P. ET AL. Height and weight standards for preschool children: Are there really ethnic differences in growth potential? *Lancet*, **1**: 611-615 (1974).

16. EVELETH, P. B. & TANNER, J. M. World-wide variation in human growth. London, Cambridge University Press, 1976.

17. KPEDEKPO, G. M. K. Preschool children in Ghana—the use of prior information. *Journal of the Royal Statistical Society*, *A*, **134**: 372-373 (1971).

18. WRAY, J. D. Child Care in the Peoples' Republic of China—1973, Part II. *Pediatrics*, **55**: 723 (1975).

19. WATERLOW, J. C. Note on the assessment and classification of protein energy malnutrition in children. *Lancet*, **1**: 87-89 (1973).

20. WATERLOW, J. C. Classification and definition of protein calorie malnutrition. *British medical journal*, **3**: 566-569 (1972).

We acknowledge the World Health Organization for permission for reproduction of this paper published in Bulletin of the World Health Organization 1977; 55 489–98.

REFERENCES

1. WHO. (1970) *Nutritional status of populations – A manual on anthropometric appraisal of trends*, WHO, Geneva. Doc. No. Nutr/70.129.
2. Committee on Nutritional Anthropometry. Food and Nutrition Board, National Research Council. (1956) Recommendations concerning body measurements for the characterization of nutritional status. *Hum. Biol.*, **28**, 111–23.
3. WHO. (1963) *Expert Committee on Medical Assessment of Nutritional Status – Report*, WHO, Geneva. Techn. Rep. Series No. 258.
4. Greulich, W.W. and Pyle, H.I. (1950) *Radiographic Atlas of Skeletal Development of the Hand and Wrist*, Stanford University Press, Stanford (California).
5. Jelliffe, D.B. (1966) *The Assessment of the Nutritional Status of the Community*, WHO, Geneva.
6. Weiner, J.S. and Lourie, J.A. (1969) *Human Biology: A Guide to Field Methods*, Blackwell Scientific, Oxford.
7. Weiner, J.S. and Lourie, J.A. (1981) *Practical Human Biology*, Academic Press, London.
8. United Nations – National Household Survey Capability Programme. (1986) *How to Weigh and Measure Children*, New York. United Nations – Department of Technical Co-operation for Development, and Statistical Office.
9. Lohman, T.G., Roche, A.F. and Martorell, R. (eds) (1988) *Anthropometric Standardization Reference Manual*, Human Kinetics Books, Champaign (Illinois).
10. Keller, W., Donoso, G. and DeMaeyer, E.M. (1976) Anthropometry in nutritional surveillance: A review based on results of the WHO collaborative study on nutritional anthropometry. *Nutr. Abstr. Rev.*, **46**, 591–609.
11. Gordon, C.C., Chumlea, W.C. and Roche, A.F. (1988) Stature, recumbent length, and weight, in *Anthropometric Standardization Reference Manual* (eds T.G. Lohman, A.F. Roche and R. Martorell), Human Kinetics Books, Champaign (Illinois), pp. 3–26.
12. Keller, W. (1983) Choice of indicators of nutritional status, in *Evaluation of Nutrition Education in Third World Communities* (ed. B. Schürch), Hans Huber, Bern, pp. 101–13.
13. Eveleth, P.B. and Tanner, J.M. (1976) *Worldwide Variation in Human Growth*, Cambridge University Press, Cambridge.
14. WHO. (1983) *Measuring Change in Nutritional Status*, WHO, Geneva.
15. WHO Working Group. (1986) Use and interpretation of anthropometric indicators of nutritional status. *Bull. WHO*, **64**, pp. 929–41.
16. Keys, A. (1980) Overweight, obesity, coronary heart disease and mortality. *Nutr. Rev.*, **38**, 297–307.
17. Geissler, C.A. and Miller, D.S. (1985) Problems with the use of 'weight for height' tables. *J. Nutr.*, **115**, 1546–9.
18. Gomez, F., Galvan, R.R., Cravioto, J. and Frenk, S. (1955) Malnutrition in infancy and childhood with special reference to kwashiorkor, in *Advances in Pediatrics*, Vol. VII (ed. S. Levine), Yearbook Publishers, Chicago.
19. WHO. (1981) *Development of Indicators for Monitoring Progress Towards Health for All by the Year 2000*, WHO, Geneva.
20. National Center for Health Statistics. (1976) *Growth Charts*, US Department of Health, Education and Welfare, Washington (DC).
21. Waterlow, J.C., Buzina, R., Keller, W. *et al.* (1977) The presentation and use of height and weight data for comparing the nutritional status of groups of children under the age of 10 years. *Bull. WHO.*, **55**, 489–98.
22. Habicht, J.P., Martorell, R., Yarbrough, C. *et al.* (1974) Height and weight standards for preschool children: How relevant are ethnic differences in growth potential? *Lancet*, **i**, 611–15.

23. Cole, T.J. (1979) A method for assessing age-standardized weight-for-height in children seen cross-sectionally. *Ann. Hum. Biol.,* **3**, 249–68.

24. El Lozy, M. (1976) Computer simulation of the effects of errors in birth registration on age-dependent anthropometric methods. *Am. J. Clin. Nutr.,* **29**, 585–90.

25. Bouchard, C. (1985) Reproducibility of body composition and adipose tissue measurements in humans, in *Body Composition Assessment in Youths and Adults* (ed. A.F. Roche), Ross Laboratories, Columbus (Ohio), pp. 9–13.

26. Gordon, C.C., Chumlea, W.C. and Roche, A.F. (1988) Stature, recumbent length, and weight, in *Anthropometric Standardization Reference Manual* (eds T.G. Lohman, A.F. Roche and R. Martorell), Human Kinetics Books, Champaign (Illinois), pp. 3–8.

27. Keller, W. and Fillmore, C.M. (1983) The prevalence of malnutrition. *World Health Stat. Q.,* **36**, 129–67.

28. Waterlow, J.C. and Vergara, A. (1956) La malnutrition prothéique au Brésil. *Bull. Org. Mond. Santé,* **15**, 165–201.

29. Keller, W. (1983) Choice of indicators of nutritional status, in *Evaluation of Nutrition Education in Third World Communities* (ed. B. Schürch), Hans Huber, Bern, pp. 101–4.

30. Livi, R. (1897) L'indice ponderale o il rapporto tra la statura e il peso. *Atti Soc. Romana Antrop.,* **5**, 125–53.

31. Sheldon, W.H., Stephen, S.S. and Tucker, C.B. (1940) *The Varieties of Human Physique. An Introduction to Constitutional Psychology,* Harper, New York.

32. Quetelet, A. (1836) *Sur l'Homme et le Developpement des Facultés,* Hauman, Brussels.

33. Keys, A., Fidanza, F., Karvonen, M.J. *et al.* (1972) Indices of relative weight and obesity. *J. Chron. Dis.,* **25**, 329–43.

34. Benn, R.T. (1971) Some mathematical properties of weight-for-height indices used as measures of adiposity. *Br. J. Prev. Soc. Med.,* **25**, 42–50.

35. Garn, S.M. and Pesick, S.D. (1982) Comparison of the Benn index and other body mass indices in nutritional assessment. *Am. J. Clin. Nutr.,* **36**, 573–5.

36. Abdel-Malek, A.K., Mukherijee, D. and Roche, A.F. (1985) A method for constructing an index of obesity. *Hum. Biol.,* **57**, 415–30.

37. Durnin, J.V.G.A., McKay, F.C. and Webster, C.I. (1985) *A New Method of Assessing Fatness and Desirable Weight, for Use in the Armed Services,* Ministry of Defence, London.

38. Thomas, A.E., McCay, D.A. and Cutlip, B.M. (1976) A nomograph method for assessing body weight. *Am. J. Clin. Nutr.,* **29**, 302–4.

39. Womersley, J. and Durnin, J.V.G.A. (1977) A comparison of the skinfold method with extent of 'overweight' and various weight–height relationships in the assessment of obesity. *Br. J. Nutr.,* **38**, 271–84.

40. Norgan, N.G. and Ferro-Luzzi, A. (1982) Weight–height indices as estimators of fatness in men. *Hum. Nutr. Clin. Nutr.,* **36C**, 363–72.

41. Garrow, J.S. (1981) *Treat Obesity Seriously. A Clinical Manual,* Churchill Livingstone, Edinburgh.

42. Visweswara Roa, K. and Singh, D. (1970) An evaluation between nutritional status and anthropometric measurements. *Am. J. Clin. Nutr.,* **23**, 83–93.

43. Lee, J., Kolonel, L.N. and Hinds, M.W. (1981) Relative merits of the weight-corrected-for-height indices. *Am. J. Clin. Nutr.,* **34**, 2521–9.

44. Colliver, J.A., Frank, S. and Frank, A. (1983) Similarity of obesity indices in clinical studies of obese adults: a factor analytic study. *Am. J. Clin. Nutr.,* **38**, 640–7.

45. Garn, S.M., Leonard, W.R. and Hawthorne, V.M. (1986) Three limitations of the body mass index. *Am. J. Clin. Nutr.,* **44**, 996–7.

46. Heymsfield, S.B., McManus, C., Smith, J. *et al.* (1982) Anthropometric measurement

of muscle mass: revised equations for calculating bone-free arm muscle area. *Am. J. Clin. Nutr.*, **36**, 680–90.

47. Bistrian, B.F., Blackburn, C.L., Vitale, J. *et al.* (1976) Prevalence of malnutrition in general medical patients. *JAMA*, **235**, 1567–70.

48. Jelliffe, E.F.P. and Jelliffe, D.B. (1969) The arm circumference as a public health index of protein–calorie malnutrition of early childhood. *J. Trop. Pediatr.*, **15**, 179–92.

49. Garrow, J.S., Stalley, S., Diethelm, R. *et al.* (1979) A new method for measuring the body density of obese adults. *Br. J. Nutr.*, **42**, 173–83.

50. Gurney, J.M. and Jelliffe, D.B. (1973) Arm anthropometry in nutritional assessment: nomogram for rapid calculation of muscle circumference and cross-sectional muscle and fat mass. *Am. J. Clin. Nutr.*, **26**, 912–15.

51. Frisancho, A.R. (1981) New norms of upper limb fat and muscle areas for assessment of nutritional status. *Am. J. Clin. Nutr.*, **34**, 2540–5.

52. Heymsfield, S.B., Olafson, R.P., Kutner, M.H. *et al.* (1979) A radiographic method of quantifying protein–calorie undernutrition. *Am. J. Clin. Nutr.*, **32**, 693–702.

53. Bullen, B.A., Quade, F., Olesen, E. and Lund, S.A. (1965) Ultrasonic reflections used for measuring subcutaneous fat in humans. *Hum. Biol.*, **37**, 375–84.

54. Conway, J.M., Norris, K.H. and Bodwell, C.E. (1984) A new approach for the estimation of body composition: infrared interactance. *Am. J. Clin. Nutr.*, **40**, 1123–30.

55. Heymsfield, S.B., Rolandelli, R., Casper, K. *et al.* (1987) Application of electromagnetic and sound waves in nutritional assessment. *JPEN*, **11** [Suppl 5], 64S–69S.

56. Heymsfield, S.D. McManus, C., Stevens, V. and Smith, J. (1982) Muscle mass: reliable indicators of protein–energy malnutrition severity and outcome. *Am. J. Clin. Nutr.*, **35**, 1192–9.

57. Heymsfield, S.B. and Casper, K. Anthropometric assessment of the adult hospitalized patient. *JPEN*, **11** [Suppl 5], 36S–41S.

58. Garrow, J.S. (1974) *Energy stores: Their Composition, Measurement and Control. Energy Balance and Obesity in Man*, North Holland, Amsterdam, pp. 177–224.

59. Busby, G.P. and Mullen, J.L. (1984) Analysis of nutritional assessment indices – prognostic equations and cluster analysis, in *Nutritional Assessment* (eds R.A. Wright, S. Heymsfield and C.B. McManus III), Blackwell Scientific Publications, Boston, pp. 141–55.

60. Vague, J. (1956) The degree of masculine differentiation of obesities: a factor determining predisposition to diabetes, atherosclerosis, gout, and uric calculous disease. *Am. J. Clin. Nutr.*, **4**, 20–34.

61. Bray, G.A., Greenway, F.L., Nolitch, M.E. *et al.* (1978) Use of anthropometric measures to assess weight loss. *Am. J. Clin. Nutr.*, **31**, 769–73.

62. Callaway, C.W., Chumlea, W.C., Bouchard, C. *et al.* (1988) Circumferences, in *Anthropometric Standardization Reference Manual* (eds T.G. Lohman, A.F. Roche and R. Martorell), Human Kinetics Books, Champaign (Illinois), pp. 39–54.

63. Medico-Actuarial Mortality Investigation. (1914) The Association of Life Insurance Medical Directors and The Actuarial Society of America, New York. Vol IV Part I, pp. 19–23.

64. Roche, A.F., Mukherie, D., Guo, S. and Moore, W.M. (1987) Head circumference reference data: Birth to 18 years. *Pediatrics*, **79**, 706–12.

65. Meredith, V.H. (1971) Human head circumferences from birth to early adulthood: racial, regional and sex comparisons. *Growth*, **35**, 233–51.

66. Behnke, A.R. (1963) Anthropometric evaluation of body composition throughout life. *Ann. N.Y. Acad. Sci.*, **110**, 450–61.

67. Steinkamp, R.C., Cohen, N.L., Gaffey, W.R. *et al.* (1965) Measures of body fat and

related factors in normal adults – II – a simple clinical method to estimate body fat and lean body mass. *J. Chron. Dis.*, **18**, 1291–8.

68. Vague, J., Boyer, J., Jubelin, J. *et al.* (1969) Adipomuscular ratio in human subjects, in *Physiopathology of Adipose Tissue* (ed. J. Vague), Excerpta Medica, Amsterdam, pp. 360–86.

69. Seidell, J.C., Deurenberg, P. and Hautvast, J.G.A.J. (1987) Obesity and fat distribution in relation to health – current insights and recommendations. *World Rev. Nutr. Diet.*, **50**, 57–91.

70. Hartz, A.J., Rupley, D.C., Kalkhoff, R.D. and Rimm, A.A. (1983) Relationships of obesity to diabetes: influence of obesity level and body fat distribution. *Prev. Med.*, **12**, 351–7.

71. Kalkhoff, R.K., Hartz, A.J., Rupley, D. *et al.* (1983) Relationship of body fat distribution to blood pressure, carbohydrate tolerance, and plasma lipids in healthy obese women. *J. Lab. Clin. Med.*, **102**, 621–7.

72. Kissebah, A.H., Vydelingum, M., Murray, R. *et al.* (1982) Relation of body fat distribution to metabolic complications of obesity. *J. Clin. Endocrinol. Metab.*, **54**, 254–60.

73. Krotkiewski, M., Björntorp, P., Sjöström, L. and Smith, U. (1983) Impact of obesity on metabolism in men and women – importance of regional adipose tissue distribution. *J. Clin. Invest.*, **721**, 1150–62.

74. Björntorp, P. (1986) Adipose tissue distribution and morbidity, in *Recent Advances in Obesity Research, V* (eds S.M. Berry *et al.*) Libbey, London, pp. 60–5.

75. Anderson, A.J., Sobocinski, K.A., Freedman, D.S. *et al.* (1988) Body fat distribution, plasma lipids and lipoproteins. *Arteriosclerosis*, **8**, 88–94.

76. Andersson, B., Terning, K. and Björntorp, P. (1987) Dietary treatment of obesity localized in different regions – the effect of dietary fibre on relapse. *Int. J. Obesity*, **11**, [Suppl 1], 79–85.

77. Haffner, S.M., Stern, M.P., Hazuda, H.P. *et al.* (1987) Do upper-body and centralized obesity measure different aspects of regional body fat distribution? *Diabetes*, **36**, 43–51.

78. Larsson, B., Svärdsudd, K., Welin, L. *et al.* (1984) Abdominal adipose tissue distribution obesity, and risk of cardiovascular disease. *Br. Med. J.*, **288**, 1401–4.

79. Stefanik, M.L., Williams, P.T., Krauss, R.M. *et al.* (1987) Relationship of plasma estradiol, testosterone, and sex hormone binding globulin with lipoproteins, apolipoproteins, and high density lipoprotein subfractions in men. *J. Clin. Endocrinol. Metab.*, **64**, 723–9.

80. Evans, D.J., Hoffman, R.G., Kalkhoff, R.K. and Kissebah, A.H. (1983) Relationship of androgenic activity to body fat topography, fat cell morphology, and metabolic aberrations in premenopausal women. *J. Clin. Endocrinol. Metab.*, **57**, 304–10.

81. Peiris, A.N., Mueller, R.A., Smith, G.A. *et al.* (1986) Splanchnic insulin metabolism in obestiy – influence of body fat distribution. *J. Clin. Invest.*, **78**, 1648–57.

82. Ashwell, M., Chinn, S., Stalley, S. and Garrow, J.S. (1982) Female fat distribution – a simple classification based on two circumference measurements. *Int. J. Obesity*, **6**, 143–52.

83. Lev-Ran, A. and Hill, L.R. (1987) Different body fat distribution in IDDM and NIDDM. *Diabetes Care*, **10**, 491–4.

84. Johnston, F.E., Wadden, T.A. and Stunkard, A.J. (1988) Body fat deposition in adult obese women. I. Patterns of fat distribution. *Am. J. Clin. Nutr.*, **47**, 225–8.

85. Lapidus, L., Bengtsson, C., Larsson, B. *et al.* (1984) Distribution of adipose tissue and risk of cardiovascular disease and death: a 12-year follow-up of participants in the population study of women in Gothenburg. *Br. Med. J.*, **289**, 1261–3.

86. Jones, P.R.M., Hunt, M.J., Brown, T.P. and Norgan, N.G. (1986) Waist/hip

circumference ratio and its relation to age and overweight in British men. *Hum. Nutr. Clin. Nutr.*, **40C**, 239–47.

87. Krotkiewski, M. and Björntorp, P. (1986) Muscle tissue in obesity with different distribution of adipose tissue-effects of physical training. *Int. J. Obesity*, **10**, 331–41.

88. Lanska, D.J., Lanska, M.J., Hartz, A.J. *et al.* (1985) A prospective study of body fat distribution and weight loss. *Int. J. Obesity*, **9**, 241–6.

89. Seidell, J.C., Cigolini, M., Charzewska, J. *et al.* (1988) Regional obesity and serum lipids in European women born in 1948 – a multicenter study. *Acta Med. Scand.*, [Suppl 723], 189–97.

90. Apfelbaum, M., James, W.P.T., Björntorp, P. *et al.* (1988) Statement on reporting of obesity treatment programmes. *Int. J. Obesity*, **12**, 93.

91. Mueller, W.H. (1985) The biology of human fat patterning, in *Human Body Composition and Fat Distribution* (ed. N.G. Norgan), EURO-NUT rep. 8, pp. 159–74.

92. Lanska, D.J., Lanska, M.J., Hartz, A.J. and Rimm, A.A. (1985) Factors influencing the anatomic location of fat tissue in 52953 women. *Int. J. Obesity*, **9**, 29–38.

93. Björntorp, P. (1987) Adipose tissue distribution, plasma insulin, and cardiovascular disease. *Diabete et Metab.*, **13**, 381–5.

94. Hiramatsu, R., Yoshida, K. and Sato, T. (1983) A body measurement to evaluate the pattern of fat distribution in central obesity – a screening and monitoring technique for Cushing's syndrome. *JAMA*, **250**, 3174–8.

95. Lillioja, S., Young, A.A., Culter, C.L. *et al.* (1987) Skeletal muscle capillary density and fibre type are possible determinants of in vivo insulin resistance in man. *J. Clin. Invest.*, **80**, 415–24.

96. Kissebah, A.H., Evans, D.J., Peiris, A. and Wilson, C.R. (1985) Endocrine characteristics in human obesities: role of sex steroids, in *Metabolic Complications of Human Obesities* (eds J. Vague *et al.*), Elsevier, Amsterdam, pp. 115–30.

97. Kissebah, A.H., Peiris, A. and Evans, D.J. (1986) Mechanisms associating body fat distribution with the abnormal metabolic profiles in obesity, in *Recent Advances in Obesity Research* (eds S.M. Berry *et al.*), Libbey, London, pp. 54–9.

98. Ashwell, M., Cole, T.J. and Dixon, A.K. (1985) Obesity: new insight into anthropometric classification of fat distribution shown by computed tomography. *Br. Med. J.*, **a90**, 1692–4.

99. Seidell, J.C., Oosterlee, A., Thijssen, M.A.O. *et al.* (1987) Assessment of intra-abdominal and subcutaneous abdominal fat – relation between athropometry and computed tomography. *Am. J. Clin. Nutr.*, **45**, 7–13.

100. Rimm, A.A., Hartz, A.J. and Fisher, M.E. (1988) A weight shape index for assessing risk of disease in 44820 women. *J. Clin. Epidemiol.*, **44**, 459–65.

101. Norgan, N.G. and Ferro-Luzzi, A. (1985) The estimation of body density in men: are general equations general? *Ann. Hum. Biol.*, **12**, 1–15.

102. Katch, F.I. and Katch, V.L. (1980) Measurement and prediction errors in body composition assessment and the search for the perfect prediction equation. *Res. Q.* **51**, 249–60.

103. Katch, V. (1987) Assessment of body composition: comments on prediction, in *Human Body Composition and Fat Distribution* (ed. N.G. Norgan), EURO–NUT Rep. 8, Wageningen, 15–30.

104. Jackson, A.S. and Pollock, M.L. (1978) Generalised equations for predicting body density of men. *Br. J. Nutr.*, **40**, 497–504.

105. Jackson, A.S., Pollock, M.L. and Ward, A. (1980) Generalised equations for predicting body density of women. *Med. Sci. Sports Exerc.*, **12**, 175–82.

106. Bailey, S.M., Garn, S.M., Katch, V.L. and Guire, K.E. (1982) Taxonomic identification of human fat patterns. *Am. J. Phys. Anthropol.*, **59**, 361–6.

107. Mueller, W.H. and Stallones, L. (1981) Anatomical distribution of subcutaneous fat: skinfold site choice and construction of indices. *Hum. Biol.*, **53**, 321–35.

108. Kaplowitz, H.J., Mueller, W.H., Selwyn, B.J. *et al.* (1987) Sensitivities, specificities and positive predictive values of simple indices of body fat distribution. *Hum. Biol.*, **59**, 809–25.

109. Norgan, N.G. and Ferro-Luzzi, A. (1986) Simple indices of subcutaneous fat patterning. *Ecol. Food Nutr.*, **18**, 117–23.

110. Mueller, W.H. and Reid, R.M. (1979) A multivariate analysis of fatness and relative fat patterning. *Am. J. Phys. Anthropol.*, **50**, 199–208.

111. Mueller, W.H. and Wohlleb, J.C. (1981) Anatomical distribution of subcutaneous fat and its description by multivariate methods: how valid are principal components? *Am. J. Phys. Anthrop.*, **54**, 25–35.

112. Norgan, N.G. and Ferro-Luzzi, A. (1985) Principal components as indicators of body fatness and subcutaneous fat patterning. *Hum. Nutr. Clin. Nutr.*, **39C**, 45–53.

113. Mueller, W.H., Deutsch, M.I., Malina, R.M. *et al.* (1986) Subcutaneous fat topography: Age changes and relationship to cardiovascular fitness in Canadians. *Hum. Biol.*, **58**, 90–8.

114. Baumgartner, R.N., Roche, A.F., Guo, S. *et al.* (1986) Adipose tissue distribution: the stability of principal components by sex, ethnicity and maturation stage. *Hum. Biol.*, **58**, 719–36.

115. Davies, P.S.W., Jones, P.R.M. and Norgan, N.G. (1986) The distribution of subcutaneous and internal fat in man. *Ann. Hum. Biol.*, **13**, 189–92.

116. Edwards, D.A.W., Hammond, W.H., Healy, M.J.R. *et al.* (1955) Design and accuracy of calipers for measuring subcutaneous tissue thickness. *Br. J. Nutr.*, **9**, 133–43.

117. Cameron, N. (1984) *The Measurement of Human Growth*, Croom Helm, London, pp. 87–93.

118. Lange, K.O. and Brozek, J. (1961) A new model of skinfold caliper. *Am. J. Phys. Anthropol.*, **19**, 98–106.

119. Imbimbo, B., Fidanza, A.A., Caputo, V. and Moro, C.O. (1968) Valutazione comparativa di tre differenti plicometri. *Quad. Nutr.*, **28**, 332–40.

120. Parizkova, J. and Goldstein, H. (1970) A comparison of skinfold measurements using the Best and Harpenden calipers. *Hum. Biol.*, **40**, 436–41.

121. Parizkova, J. and Rath, Z. (1972) The assessment of depot fat in children from skinfold thickness measurements by Holtain caliper. *Hum. Biol.*, **44**, 613–18.

122. Burgett, S.L. and Anderson, C.F. (1979) A comparison of triceps skinfold values as measured by the plastic McGaw caliper and the Lange caliper. *Am. J. Clin. Nutr.*, **32**, 1431–533.

123. Jones, P.R.M. and West, G.M. (1983) A microprocessor system, for data recording and analysis for the modified (HERO) skinfold caliper. *Ann. Hum. Biol.*, **10**, 86–7.

124. Damon, A. (1965) Notes on anthropometric technique II. Skinfolds – right and left sides; held by one or two hands. *Am. J. Phys. Anthropol.*, **23**, 305–11.

125. Martorell, R., Mendoza, F., Mueller, W.H. and Pawson, I.G. (1988) Which side to measure: right or left? in *Anthropometric Standardization Reference Manual* (eds T.G. Lohman, A.F. Roche and R. Martorell), Human Kinetics Books, Champaign (Illinois), pp. 87–91.

126. Behnke, A.R. and Wilmore, J.H. (1974) *Evaluation and regulation of body build and composition*, Prentice Hall, New Jersey.

127. Harrison, G.G., Buskirk, E.R., Lindsay Carter, J.E. *et al.* (1988) Skinfold thicknesses and measurement technique, in *Anthropometric Standardization Reference Manual* (eds T.G. Lohman, A.F. Roche and R. Martorell), Human Kinetics Books, Champaign (Illinois), pp. 55–80.

128. Durnin, J.V.G.A. and Womersley, J. (1974) Body fat assessed from total body-density and its estimation from skinfold thickness: measurements on 481 men and women aged from 16 to 72 years. *Br. J. Nutr.*, **32**, 77–97.

129. Garn, S.M., Sullivan, T.V. and Tenhave, T. (1987) Which transformation for normalising skinfold and fatness distributions? *Lancet*, **ii**, 1326–7.

130. Slaughter, M.H., Lohman, T.G., Boileau, C.A. *et al.* (1988) Skinfold equations for estimation of body fatness in children and youth. *Hum. Biol.*, **60**, 709–23.

131. Correnti, V. (1947) Il malachistometro – Nuovo apparecchio per la misura dello spessore delle parti molli. *Riv. Antrop.*, **35**, 439–42.

132. Franzen, R. and Palmer, G.T. (1934) The ACH index of nutritional status. *Child. Health Bull.*, **10**, 26–33.

133. Brozek, J., Brock, J.F., Fidanza, F. *et al.* (1954) Skinfold caliper estimation of body fat and nutritional status. *Fed. Proc.*, **13**, 19.

134. Lohman, T.G. (1981) Skinfolds and body density and their relation to body fatness: A review. *Hum. Biol.*, **53**, 181–255.

135. Roche, A.F., Abdel-Malek, A.K. and Mukherjee, D. (1985) New approaches to clinical assessment of adipose tissue, in *Body Composition Assessment in Youth and Adults* (ed. A.F. Roche), Ross Laboratories, Columbus (Ohio), pp. 14–19.

136. Norgan, N.G. (1991) Anthropometric assessment of body fat and fatness, in *Anthropometric Assessment of Nutritional Status* (ed. J.H. Himes), A.R. Liss, New York, pp. 197–212.

137. Jackson, A.S. and Pollock, M.L. (1984) Practical assessment of body composition. *Phys. Sports Med.*, **13**, 76–82.

138. Parizkova, J. (1961) Total body fat and skinfold thickness in children. *Metabolism*, **10**, 794–807.

139. Brook, C.G.D. (1971) Determination of body composition of children from skinfold measurements. *Arch. Dis. Child.*, **46**, 182–4.

140. Johnston, F.E. (1982) Relationships between body composition and anthropometry. *Hum. Biol.*, **54**, 221–45.

141. Ross, W.D., Eiben, O.G., Ward, R. *et al.* (1986) Alternatives for the conventional methods of human body composition and physique assessment, in *Perspectives in Kinanthropometry* (ed. J.A.P. Day), Human Kinetics Books, Champaign (Illinois), pp. 203–20.

142. Roche, A.F. (1987) Some aspects of the criterion methods for the measurement of body composition. *Hum. Biol.*, **59**, 209–20.

143. Roche, A.F. (1987) Population methods: anthropometry and estimations, in *Human Body Composition and Fat Distribution* (ed. N.G. Norgan), EURO–NUT Rep. 8, Wageningen, pp. 31–47.

144. Mueller, W.H. and Martorell, R. (1988) Reliability and accuracy of measurement, in *Anthropometric Standardization Reference Manual* (eds T.G. Lohman, A.F. Roche and R. Martorell), Human Kinetics Books, Champaign (Illinois), pp. 83–6.

145. Johnston, F.E., Hamill, P.V.V. and Lemeshow, S. (1974) *Skinfold Thickness of Youths 12–17 years, United States, 1966–1970*. National Center for Health Statistics, Rockville (MD). (Vital health statistics series 11, No. 132. Data from the National Health Survey 74 [DHEW publication (HRA) 74–1614]).

146. Malina, R.M. and Buschang, P.H. (1984) Anthropometric asymmetry in normal and mentally retarded males. *Ann. Hum. Biol.*, **11**, 515–31.

147. Martorell, R., Habicht, J.P., Yarbrough, C. *et al.* (1975) The identification and evaluation of measurement variability in the anthropometry of preschool children. *Am. J. Phys. Anthropol*, **43**, 347–52.

148. Johnston, F.E. and Mack, R.W. (1985) Interobserver reliability of skinfold measurements in infants and young children. *Am. J. Phys. Anthropol.*, **67**, 285–90.

149. Melesky, B.W. (1980) *Growth, Maturity, Body Composition and Familiar Characteristics of Competitive Swimmers 8 to 18 years of age.* [Unpublished doctoral dissertation]. University of Texas, Austin (Texas).

150. Zavaleta, A.N. (1976) *Densitometric Estimates of Body Composition in Mexican Americans.* [Unpublished doctoral dissertation]. University of Texas, Austin (Texas).

151. Johnston, F.E., Hamill, P.V.V. and Lemeshow, S. (1972) *Skinfold Thickness of Children 6–11 years, United States 1963–1965.* National Center for Health Statistics, Rockville (MD). (Vital and health statistics series 11, No. 120. Data from the National Health Survey 72 [DHEW publication (HSM) 73–1602]).

152. Sloan, A.W. and Shapiro, M. (1972) A comparison of skinfold measurements with three standard calipers. *Hum. Biol.,* **44**, 29–36.

153. Wilmore, J.H. and Behnke, A.R. (1969) An anthropometric estimation of body density and lean body weight in young men. *J. Appl. Physiol.,* **27**, 25–31.

154. Buschang, P.H. (1980) *Growth Status and Rate in School Children 6 to 13 years of Age in a Rural Zapotec-Speaking Community in the Valley of Oxaca, Mexico.* [Unpublished doctoral dissertation]. University of Texas, Austin (Texas).

155. Zavaleta, A.N. and Malina, R.M. (1982) Growth and body composition of Mexican American boys 9 through 14 years of age. *Am. J. Phys. Anthropol.,* **57**, 261–71.

156. Haas, J.D. and Flegel, K.M. (1981) Anthropometric measurements, in *Progress in Cancer Research. Vol. 17. Nutrition and Cancer Etiology and Treatment* (eds G.R. Newell and N.M. Ellison), Raven Press, New York, pp. 123–40.

157. Pollock, M.L., Hickman, T., Kendrick, Z. *et al.* (1976) Prediction of body density in young and middle-aged men. *J. Appl. Physiol.,* **40**, 300–4.

158. Zuti, W.B. and Golding, L.A. (1973) Equations for estimating percent body fat and body density in active adults. *Med. Sci. Sports Exerc.,* **5**, 262–6.

159. Lohman, T.G., Pollock, M.L., Slaughter, M.H. *et al.* (1984) Methodological factors and the prediction of body fat in female athletes. *Med. Sci. Sports Exerc.,* **16**, 92–6.

160. Pollock, M.L. (1986) Unpublished data. University of Florida, Department of Exercise Science, Gainsville (Florida).

161. Pollock, M.L., Laughridge, E.E., Coleman, B. *et al.* (1975) Prediction of body density in young and middle-aged women. *J. Appl. Physiol.,* **38**, 745–9.

162. Perez, B.M. (1981) *Los Atletas Venezolanos. Su tipo físico.* Universidad Central de Venezuela, Caracas (Venezuela).

163. Carter, J.E.L. (1986) Unpublished data. San Diego State University, Department of Physical Education, San Diego.

164. Martin, A.D., Ross, W.D., Drinkwater, D.T. and Clarys, J.P. (1985) Prediction of body fat by skinfold caliper: assumptions and cadaver evidence. *Hum. Biol.,* **9**, 31–9.

165. Robson, J.R.K., Bazin, M. and Soderstrom, R. (1971) Ethnic differences in skinfold thickness. *Am. J. Clin. Nutr.,* **24**, 864–8.

166. Tanner, J.M. and Whitehouse, R.H. (1975) Revised standards for triceps and subscapular skinfolds in British children. *Arch. Dis. Child.,* **50**, 142–5.

167. Ferro-Luzzi, A. (1988) Marginal malnutrition: some speculation on energy sparing mechanisms, in *Capacity for Work in the Tropics* (eds K.J. Collins and D.F. Robert), Cambridge University Press, Cambridge, pp. 141–64.

168. Roche, A.F., Siervogel, R.M., Chumlea, W.C. and Webb, P. (1981) Grading body fatness from limited anthropometric data. *Am. J. Clin. Nutr.,* **34**, 2831–8.

169. Lohman, T.G. (1988) Anthropometry and body composition, in *Anthropometric Standardization Reference Manual* (eds T.G. Lohman, A.F. Roche and R. Martorell), Human Kinetics Books, Champaign (Illinois), pp. 125–9.

170. Himes, J.H. and Bouchard, C. (1985) Do the new Metropolitan Life Insurance

weight–height tables correctly assess body frame and body fat relationships? *Am. J. Publ. Health*, **75**, 1076–9.

171. Wilmore, J.H., Frisancho, R.A., Gordon, C.C. *et al.* (1988) Body breadth equipment and measurement techniques, in *Anthropometric Standardization Reference Manual* (eds T.G. Lohman, A.F. Roche and R. Martorell), Human Kinetics Books, Champaign (Illinois), pp. 27–38.

172. Behnke, A.R. and Wilmore, J.H. (1974) *Evaluation and Regulation of Body Build and Composition*, Prentice Hall, Englewood Cliffs (New Jersey), pp. 39–43.

173. Cameron, N. (1984) *The Measurement of Human Growth*, Croom Helm, London and Sydney, pp. 75–81.

174. Keys, A. *et al.* (1967) Epidemiological studies related to coronary heart disease: characteristics of men aged 40–59 in seven countries. *Acta Med. Scand.*, **460** [Suppl].

175. Metropolitan Life Insurance Company (1959) New weight standards for men and women. *Stat. Bull.*, **40**, 1–4.

176. Katch, V.L., Freedson, P.S., Katch, F.I. and Smith, L. (1982) Body frame: validity of self-appraisal. *Am. J. Clin. Nutr.*, **36**, 676–9.

177. Metropolitan Life Insurance Company (1983) Metropolitan height and weight tables. *Stat. Bull.*, **64**, 2–9.

178. Frisancho, A.R. and Flegal, P.N. (1983) Elbow breadth as a measure of frame size for U.S. males and females. *Am. J. Clin. Nutr.*, **37**, 311–14.

179. Frisancho, A.R. (1984) New standards of weight and body composition by frame size and height for assessment of nutritional status of adults and the elderly. *Am. J. Clin. Nutr.*, **40**, 808–19.

180. Katch, V.L. and Freedson, P.S. (1982) Body size and shape: derivation of the 'HAT' frame size model. *Am. J. Clin. Nutr.*, **36**, 669–75.

181. Behnke, A.R. (1959) The estimation of lean body weight from skeletal measurements. *Hum. Biol.*, **31**, 295–315.

182. Roche, A.F. (1984) Anthropometric methods: new and old, what they tell us. *Int. J. Obesity*, **8**, 509–23.

183. Garn, S.M., Pesick, B.S. and Hawthorne, V.M. (1983) The bony chest breadth as a frame size standard in nutritional assessment. *Am. J. Clin. Nutr.*, **37**, 315–18.

184. Himes, J.H. and Frisancho, A.R. (1988) Estimating frame size, in *Anthropometric Standardization Reference Manual* (eds T.G. Lohman, A.F. Roche and R. Martorell), Human Kinetics Books, Champaign (Illinois), pp. 121–4.

2 Body composition methodology

2.1 Introduction   *N.G. Norgan*   63
2.2 Densitometry   *N.G. Norgan*   64
2.3 Dilutometry   *I. Bosaeus and B. Isaksson*   71
    Section I   Determination of total body water   74
    Section II   Determination of exchangeable potassium   77
    Section III Determination of total body potassium in a
                 whole-body counter   79
2.4 Advanced methods   *S.B. Heymsfield*   83

2.1 INTRODUCTION

The tissues of the body are acquired from and exchanged with the environment. Nutritional status is an index of the state of this exchange and accretion. One component of this index is the amounts of the constituents of the body that are present at any given time. This is the composition of the body. In addition, during changing plane of nutrition, the amounts of a nutrient/body constituent alter before there is any compromise in the function of the nutrient. For example, a decrease in energy intake may cause a fall in adipose tissue before any of the adaptive phenomena such as reduced physical activity or resting metabolic rate are markedly affected. Thus, measurements of body composition may represent an early indication of changing or unsatisfactory nutritional status. Paramount in this process is a knowledge of the levels associated with

Table 2.1 Some body composition methods and the compartments they estimate

Method	Estimate
Densitometry	Fatness and fat mass
Neutron activation	Muscle mass, total body calcium
24-hour urinary creatinine	Muscle mass
Photon absorption	Total body calcium
Gamma radiometry (^{40}K)	Total body potassium (fat-free mass)
Isotope dilution	Total body water (fat-free mass)
Electrical impedance	Total body water (fat-free mass)
Induced conductivity	Total body water (fat-free mass)
Computed tomography	Various
Magnetic resonance imaging	Various

good health and the boundaries that identify suboptimal states. As with many of the nutrient requirements, there is uncertainty about these levels in many age and sex groups. The study of body composition or analytic somatology as it has been called by Roche [1] incorporates a number of physical and chemical procedures. Some of these relevant to the assessment of nutritional values are listed in Table 2.1. Each is an indirect *in vivo* measurement based on one or more assumptions. To what extent these assumptions are invalidated by severe malnutrition or illness is described in the relevant section.

2.2 DENSITOMETRY

2.2.1 Purposes and scope

Densitometry allows a description of the body as fat mass and fat-free mass. Thus the purposes and scope of the measurement overlaps with those of skinfold thicknesses (see section 1.6) in that they are concerned primarily with the assessment of energy nutritional status. However, it can be expected to be more accurate than the anthropometric approaches in most cases and density has become something of a 'gold standard'. There are, however, doubts about this. Densitometry has been applied to subjects from 6 to 80 years, but except in adolescents, youths, and young adults the proportion of any group willing to give informed consent to participation in the procedure may be small.

2.2.2 Principle of the method

If the density of a body (D) and the density of its two constituents are known then the proportions of the constituents can be calculated. For the assessment of human body composition the body is commonly described as a two-compartment system of fat (F) and fat-free mass (FFM) of constant composition. Hence,

$$\frac{1}{D} = \frac{f}{Df} + \frac{ffm}{Dffm} \tag{1}$$

where:
f   = proportion of fat
ffm = proportion of fat-free mass.

The Df and Dffm have been estimated from animal studies and cadaver analysis, and from study of the individual constituents of FFM.

Body density is given by D = mass/volume, $kg.m^{-3}$

The problem in densitometry is how to measure the volume of an irregularly shaped object, the human body. The solution was realised by Archimedes on lowering himself into a full bath. The volume of water displaced is equal to the volume of the body. This is the principle of one method of densitometry, volumetry. The common and more accurate method, underwater weighing, utilizes Archimedes' principle of buoyancy, that the loss of weight of a body in water compared to air is equal to the weight of water displaced. This weight displaced by the body can easily be converted to a volume of water from volume displaced = loss of weight divided by the density of water. This volume is corrected for the residual air (RV) at BTPS in the lungs. Thus,

D = Mass in air/((Mass in air − mass in water)/density of water) − RV (2)

Dffm is taken to be 1100 and Df 900 kg.m^{-3}. Since the main interest in nutritional status assessment is the proportion or percentage of fat not density per se, equation (1) is rearranged to

$$f = \frac{1}{D} \cdot \frac{(Dffm \cdot Df)}{(Dffm - Df)} - \frac{Df}{(Dffm - Df)} \tag{3}$$

This may be written as a general equation.

$$f = \frac{1}{D} \cdot \frac{(D_2 \cdot D_1)}{(D_2 - D_1)} - \frac{(D1)}{(D_2 - D_1)} \tag{4}$$

Using 1100 and 900 kg.m^{-3} for D_2 and D_1 respectively, the equation simplifies to

$$f = \frac{4950}{D} - 4.5 \tag{5}$$

This is known as Siri's equation [2].

Lung residual volume (RV) is measured by the three-breath nitrogen dilution technique of Rahn *et al.* [3] popularized by Durnin and Rahaman [4]. The principle is that alveolar air is assumed to be 80.00% nitrogen. If the amount of nitrogen can be determined the residual volume can be calculated. The nitrogen is diluted and washed out with a known volume of oxygen, in adults three litres, and the nitrogen in the mixed air (N) determined. The extent of the dilution depends on the residual volume

Then

$$0.80 \, RV = N \, (3.00 + RV) \tag{6}$$

rearranging and using percentages;

$$RV = 3.00 \, (N/(80 - N)) \tag{7}$$

Further corrections are required for the small amounts of nitrogen (n) in the original oxygen, to convert volumes to BTPS, and to correct for the dead space (DS) of a snorkel and three-way tap.

The full formula is:

$$\begin{matrix} RV \\ \text{(litres)} \end{matrix} = 3.00 \cdot \frac{(N - n)}{(80 - N)} \cdot \frac{Bp}{Bp - 47} \cdot \frac{310}{273 + t} - DS \tag{8}$$

Where Bp is barometric pressure, mmHg, 47 is the saturated vapour pressure, mmHg, at 37°C, and t the temperature °C of oxygen in the rebreathing bag.

There are few readily available detailed descriptions of the measurement of body density [5-8] so a detailed description is given here.

2.2.3 Apparatus

The apparatus to measure body density is often custom made but an inexpensive system built up from apparatus found in a well-equipped human biological laboratory has been described by Jones and Norgan [9], which has since been further improved. An advantage of this system is that it can easily be stored and does not require dedicated space. The major drawback is that access is by ladder.

The water tank should be 3.5 m³ or more. Larger volumes reduce the oscillations caused by water movement as the subject changes position. The interior should be treated to prevent corrosion, and PVC fittings used underwater. The tank should be situated on a firm floor near to a single-phase electric supply, water mains, and drains. The tank is fitted with a large-volume charcoal filter and a recirculating pump to keep the water clean. Small-sized tanks require frequent water replacement, i.e. after five to six subjects. Water temperature is maintained at $35 \pm 0.5°C$ by electric heaters connected to 3 mA earth leak trip safety devices. A plastic chair fitted with a foot rail at the front and a dead weight and seat belt for low-density subjects,is suspended by stainless steel rigging from the weighing device. This may be a force transducer connected to a digital voltmeter and calibrated to read to 0.01 kg. Electronic filtering allows weight to be measured to 0.02 kg in co-operative subjects and to 0.05 kg in others. The force transducer is mechanically protected against damage from excess weight arising when the subject is out of water. Alternative weighing devices are dial-reading autopsy scales or underwater floor-mounted force transducers [10]. The transducer is calibrated by suspending from it known weights of 0–4 kg.

A three-litre calibrated syringe is used to deliver medical 100% O_2 to the rebreathing bag. These are standard 4-litre anaesthetic bags fitted with a three-way aluminium tap. The closed end is removed and fitted with tubing through which the bag can be washed out and evacuated with a vacuum pump before filling, and the temperature measured.

The contents of the bag after rebreathing are analysed with electronic analysers for oxygen (e.g. Servomex 570A) and carbon dioxide (e.g. ADC, 0–10% range). These are zeroed and spanned with the appropriate gases and calibrated with a certificated or chemically analysed test gas of about 65–70% O_2, 5% CO_2 and remainder nitrogen. Nitrogen is determined by difference $(100 - (O_2 + CO_2))$. If nitrogen is determined directly it should be remembered that formula (8) for RV is derived for nitrogen by difference which includes the inert gases.

2.2.4   Procedure

(a) Training and preparation

For all but frequent swimmers, underwater weighing is a strange experience. For some they may be undecided if they wish or are able to complete the measurement. Therefore, before a study or measurement begins the procedure should be explained fully, they should be encouraged to visit the laboratory, individually, with friends or in a group and given a comprehensive description of what is involved. This is always required to achieve the necessary written, informed consent of the volunteers, but much can be achieved by spending time with the subjects in a friendly, sympathetic but at all times highly professional atmosphere.

Subjects should refrain from eating before the measurement. On arrival at the laboratory, the bladder should be emptied. The subject should shower and wash the hair, and put on light swimwear. Body weight is recorded to 0.05 kg, then the subject enters the tank, via a footbath.

The underwater weighing measurement involves the subject submerging, expiring maximally through a snorkel and after 5–8 s rebreathing 3 l of oxygen. The procedure should be practised a step at a time, allowing the subject to dictate the pace at which the training proceeds. Firstly, the subject should sit correctly and comfortably in the chair. Ensure that he or she is seated centrally with feet on the bar, and holding the sides of the chair rather than the chair guide-wires. The subject can then be instructed on how to submerge. This is a key movement as too quick or jerky a submersion disturbs the water, introducing oscillations into the measuring system and hence requiring a longer time with the breath held. The subject is fitted with an ordinary snorkel held in place by an adjustable headband and told to breathe normally through the snorkel. A check is made that a good seal is achieved by the lips around the mouthpiece. A tightly fitting nose-clip occludes the nose. The subject leans forward in the chair and lowers the head towards the knees by bending at the waist and elbows.

Instructions can be given about the rate of entry and when the head and shoulders are covered. For those who are very apprehensive about submerging themselves, training may begin with the subject standing up holding the side of the tank and dipping below the surface at will.

The second manoeuvre to rehearse is expiring maximally and maintaining a stationary position. The submerged subject is instructed to continue breathing normally though the snorkel then to make a maximum expiration and to sit very still. On the first occasion, the subject is encouraged to hold his or her breath as long as possible and to breathe when required. This will demonstrate to the observer if a stable reading is obtained and the general disposition of the subject. This is repeated until a stable weight can be obtained, usually 5–8 s after the end of maximal expiration.

The rebreathing sequence is explained to the subject. After maximal expiration and reading of weight, the contents of the rebreathing bag must be inhaled and exhaled through the snorkel in 3 s. The cycle is repeated twice according to the observer's instructions. The subject is shown the bag containing, at this stage during practice, 3 l of room air, and informed that inhalation and exhalation needs to be fairly rapid and deep but that the timed instructions of the observer must be followed. This sequence may be practised on the first occasion with the head out of water so that the subject can see the necessary deflation and inflation of the bag. Most subjects will be able to proceed to rehearsing the procedure underwater straight away. After each trial, the subject should be allowed to rest and recover. The trained subject will perform the three cycles over 9 s, emptying the bag and returning close to 3 l each cycle. The subject should now be able to perform all three manoeuvres satisfactorily in sequence.

(b) Measurement of underwater weight and residual volume

The first of the trials can begin.

Underwater weight Submersion and expiration are carried out as above. As the subject submerges there is a tendency for the chair to move back and then forward and eventually centre again. The observers can dampen these movements by resistance on the guide-wires above the chair, in this way causing movement to cease sooner. The observer checks that neither the subject nor the chair touch the side or bottom of the tank. The subject is instructed to make a maximal expiration; again movement is dampened out and the voltmeter is read. With expiration the underwater weight increases and continues to increase after the end-point of expiration is reached. The reading will then stabilize (to within 0.02 kg) or fluctuate due to water movement, etc. If the fluctuations are within 0.04 kg, a central point can be taken. If they are greater than this, the subject is instructed to surface and the procedure repeated.

Residual volume Immediately after the underwater weight is taken the rebreathing commences as described above. To complete the manoeuvres in the allotted time, the observer must give the instruction 'breathe in' or 'breathe out' before the actual time in order that the subject responds at the right time. A stop-watch or timer is required by the observer. The contents of the bag are analysed for oxygen and carbon dioxide. Measurements can now be made of the tank water temperature, to 0.1°C, and the weight of the unloaded chair. The transducer calibration is checked using a known weight of similar magnitude to the underwater weight. An interval of 10 min between RV determinations is required to allow the composition of alveolar air to return to normal. During this time the body density can be calculated.

The measurement is repeated. Duplicates to within 0.5–1% body weight as fat are acceptable. A third measurement may be required to achieve agreement in some subjects. If four or more trials are necessary equipment malfunction or imperfect rebreathing should be suspected and care applied as to which readings to use.

2.2.5 Performance characteristics

(a) Effect of measurement conditions

The effect of varying the subject condition can be easily calculated. Drinking 1 l of water will decrease the body density by 1.2 $kg.m^{-3}$, which is equivalent to 0.6% fat. The effect is less dramatic than expected because the weight and volume appear in the numerator and the denominator of body density. Dehydration due to induced sweating has been shown to influence body density [11]. Therefore, a normal level of hydration is mandatory. The effects of meals and carbonated drinks were investigated by Durnin and Satwanti [12] and found to be less than 1% body fat on average.

A further importance of food is in relation to intestinal gas. Estimations vary from 0.028 to 1.330 litres with a mean of 0.1 litres proposed as a correction factor [13]. Although this correction causes an increase in density of 1.7 $kg.m^{-3}$, equivalent to 0.8% fat, it gives an unwarranted sense of accuracy to the data. These figures do illustrate, however, how important the accurate measurement of body volume is, of which the measurement of RV is probably the crucial measurement. As a precaution, measurement should be made in the fasting condition, but fluid intake need not be restricted.

RV can be measured by closed-circuit methods with inert tracer or diluent gases such as nitrogen, hydrogen, helium, or as in this case, oxygen, and open-circuit methods where nitrogen is washed out with oxygen. The method described here, originally by Rahn *et al.*[3] is similar to that of Wilmore and colleagues [14] who employed 5–7 breaths. This was found to be reliable ($r = 0.99$) and valid ($r = 0.92$), comparing favourably ($r = 0.89$) with the nitrogen washout technique, involving seven minutes of rebreathing. Rahn *et al* [3] established three breaths in 9 s as the optimal balance between thorough mixing and oxygen uptake (which is to a large extent balanced by carbon dioxide release). The method has been validated against a two-tracer method [15].

There is general agreement that the RV is best determined at the time the underwater weight is taken. This avoids any difference due to varying position or hydrostatic pressure on the thorax that may exist when the measurement is made sitting or standing upright out of water.

Measuring underwater weight at maximum inspiration or at functional residual capacity have been suggested as alternatives to RV. However, these volumes require more lengthy and complex procedures than the simple, rapid measurement of RV.

(b) Reproducibility

The precision of the density method is high. The standard error of repeated measurements is about $2 \, \mathrm{kg.m^{-3}}$, with a product–moment correlation coefficient of 0.95 or more. This is equivalent to an error in per cent fat of 1%, i.e. 5% of an average fat content or 1% of the fat-free mass. However, as discussed below the true error in terms of fat or fat-free mass is greater if the assumptions on which the methods are based are violated. As this cannot be established without considerable further investigation, the accuracy of the method in each individual is unknown.

(c) Comparability

Alternatives to underwater weighing have been proposed. The direct measurement of water displacement has been tried but the rise in a water column for a given volume depends on the area of the column. Narrow containers are most accurate but are claustrophobic. Even so accuracy is limited to about 0.2 l. The test–rest reliability of the volumeter has been shown to be lower (0.96) compared with underwater weighing (0.99) in one laboratory [16]. It gave significantly lower per cent fat, (19.4 vs 20.1) in a group of 67 men.

Plethysmographic methods have been described [17–19]. Here, body volume without the need for residual volume measurement is calculated from the difference between expected and actual pressure changes on introducing a known volume of gas to the closed chamber containing the subject. The method has not been widely adopted.

(d) Validity

The densitometric approach to body composition rests on the assumption that the body consists of two components of known and fixed composition and hence density [20]. It has been known for many years that this is not strictly true. Siri, who put forward the values of $900 \, \mathrm{kg.m^{-3}}$ and $1100 \, \mathrm{kg.m^{-3}}$ for the densities of fat and fat-free mass following the pioneering work of several laboratories [21–23], emphasized the variation in hydration of the fat-free mass (1–3%) and the variation in protein: mineral ratio (2%) in healthy men. The theoretical error of estimating fatness in a population from density was calculated to be 3.8%, a figure confirmed by Lohman [24]. The figures are based on young adult men and women. For other groups less is known of the extent of the variation. In children the composition of the fat-free mass is different and the density of fat-free mass is calculated to be 1080 kg.m^{-3} [25]. During pregnancy the density of the fat-free mass changes and equations relating body density to fatness (equations (3)–(5) on p. 65) can be revised to take this into account [26, 27]. Fat density too is not invariable. Interstitial muscle fat and central nervous system fat have higher density than depot fat. However, as they are usually small in comparison to storage fat they have little effect on the overall density.

Revisions to Siri's equation for differences in the density of FFM with muscular development, obesity, and ageing have been proposed [28]. For young adults alternatives to Siri's equation have appeared [29]. These give results to within 1% fat over density ranges of 1030–1100 kg.m^{-3}.

One course of action that has not received much attention is to use density values themselves as an indication of change in compositional status, rather than converting the density to per cent fat or fat mass. Density is a precise measurement and reference data have been identified [30]. However, in the field of nutritional status assessment, fat and lean are more useful concepts and most workers have been prepared to accept the decreased accuracy when the assessment is of an individual as opposed to the population.

Although body density as an estimate of energy stores is not without criticism, in the assessment of changes in fatness it is more accurate than ^{40}K isotope dilution or skinfold thicknesses [31]. However, to improve the accuracy of body composition estimates, particularly in the young, in women, and the elderly – groups who may be most at risk nutritionally – more than one method should be used. A multi-component method – density, total body water or skeleton mass – has been advocated [25], to take the study and application of body composition forward.

2.2.6 Reference values

Roche [30] has listed sources of reference data for body density for groups that were not selected on the basis of factors known to be associated with body density. The majority of studies were North American. The large series of individuals measured in order to establish density–skinfold relationships (See section 1.6, p. 34) are rarely well described and seem to be composed of University and Research Institute staff or their peers. Measurements of body density in Italian shipyard workers [32] represent some of the few data on European industrial workers. As with body weight, reference data should not be regarded as prescriptive.

2.2.7 Interpretation

There are several two-component descriptions of body composition; these are not interchangeable. Fat mass (a chemical entity) is not equivalent to adipose tissue (an anatomical entity), and fat-free mass differs from lean body mass. Densitometry produces an estimate of leanness as well as fatness, an index that may be of interest in the assessment of nutritional status. However, the application of the method to malnutrition, as opposed to varying levels of fatness, will be compromised by changing composition of the fat-free mass. In patients, the method is not recommended in wasting and oedematous states. Many ill patients could not complete the procedures.

There is as yet little evidence linking fat or fatness, as opposed to over- or underweight, to raised mortality or morbidity, as described in Chapter 1. There may be separate risks to health by fat (fat mass, kg) and fatness (per cent fat) and it is recommended that these be graded separately.

2.3 DILUTOMETRY

2.3.1 Purpose and scope

Dilutometry is a general methodology for estimating the size of certain body compartments such as plasma volume, extracellular volume, cell mass, or fat mass, or certain body constituents such as body water, body potassium, or body sodium.

Such data are of value in studies of various physiological and pathological conditions. They allow estimations of body composition changes with age, pregnancy and lactation, athletic training, etc. They can be used for diagnostic purposes and for evaluation of the effect on body composition of disease or therapy.

The first attempts to estimate body compartments by dilutometry as opposed to elemental analyses of body carcass were made during the first half of this century. A number of chemical substances such as Evans' blue, inulin, sucrose, thiosulphate, urea, etc. were used to quantify plasma volume, extracellular

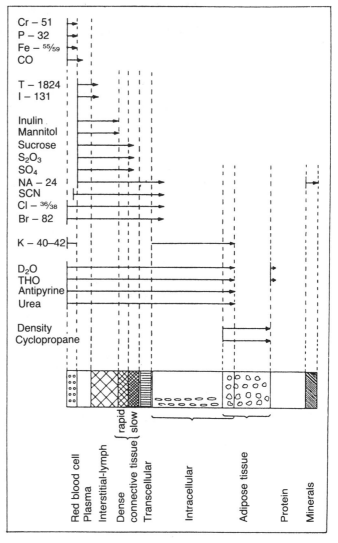

Fig. 2.1 Applications of dilutometry. Determination of various spaces using the principle of dilution.

volume, total body water, etc. A number of these applications are summarized in Fig. 2.1. These methods using chemical substances to measure various 'spaces' were of substantial interest to clinical physiologists during the 1950s–1960s but are seldom used today, as they give different data for some spaces which are often difficult to interpret. In 1935 de Hevesy introduced the use of isotopes to determine certain body constituents, i.e. deuterium-labelled water for total body water determination. In 1950 Francis Moore and his associates applied radioactive isotopes such as ^{42}K, ^{24}Na, ^{35}Cl etc. [33] to measure body compartments as well as constituents. The isotope techniques have found many applications in nutrition research. Both total body water (TBW) and total body potassium (TBK) have been used to calculate lean body mass (LBM). This concept creates some interpretation difficulties.

According to the primary definition by Benedict in 1915 [34], launched again by Behnke in 1942 [20], lean body mass was defined as:

$$Body = LBM + AT$$

where AT stands for adipose tissue. In later literature, however, lean body mass is defined as:

$$Body = LBM + FAT$$

since adipose tissue contains water in a varying and unknown quantity, impossible to determine.

However, lean body mass is not fat-free. It contains structural fat and there may also be some intracellular deposits of fat as well as circulating lipoproteins. Hence, the concept fat-free mass (FFM) has been introduced and defined as follows:

$$Body = FFM + FAT$$

The interest in determining LBM or FFM from TBW and TBK depends to a large extent on the interest in estimating body fat.

Especially in pathological conditions, different components of LBM can be expected to deviate from normal. These considerations have led to the development of a four-compartment model for body composition [35] at present used in our laboratory (Fig. 2.2).

$$Body = FFECS + BCM + ECW + BF$$

where FFECS = Fat-free extracellular solids; BCM = Body cell mass; ECW = Extracellular water; BF = Body fat.

The compartments are estimated from simultaneous determination of TBW and TBK, as will be described in the methods section.

The assumptions made and the sources of error, apart from methodological errors in TBW and TBK discussed below, are as follows:

1. **Fat-free extracellular solids** FFECS is not readily measured by any method presently available to us. The assumption is made that FFECS is 12% of normal (not actual) weight for height. This is based on data from the few carcass analyses made of dry fat-free bone weight [33, 36], and our assumption that this covers 70% of FFECS.

2. **Body cell mass** The factor 8.33 to calculate BCM from TBK is taken from

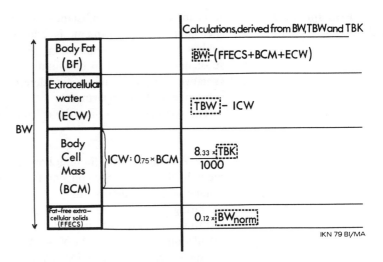

Fig. 2.2 Four-compartment model of body composition determination from TBW and TBK.

Moore [33], who assumed a potassium : nitrogen ratio of 3 mmol/g and a total wet weight equal to the nitrogen content multiplied by 25 for cells. The potassium : nitrogen ratio is supported by analyses of skeletal muscle [37–40]. Recent data from whole-body nitrogen measurements by neutron activation analysis indicate that the total body potassium : total body nitrogen ratio may vary in nitrogen depletion and repletion [41], and this should be kept in mind when studying such patients.

3. Intracellular water The assumptions in sub-section 2 above result in a factor of 0.75 for calculating intracellular water (ICW) from BCM (i.e. from TBK), and an intracellular potassium concentration of 160 mmol/kg water. Moore *et al.* [33] estimated this concentration to be 150 mmol/kg water from isotope dilution studies (with ^{42}K, D_2O and ^{82}Br), but direct measurements strongly support the 160 mmol/kg water figure [37, 42–44].

4. Extracellular water Our calculations will, of course, give figures close to those determined from ^{82}Br space by Moore *et al.* [33], as the coefficients used are based on similar assumptions. Wang and Pierson [45] give much lower figures for ECW/ICW, based on determination of TBW and $^{35}SO_4$ space in only four normals. This would imply an intracellular potassium concentration of 110–130 mmol/kg, which is not in accordance with the studies mentioned above.

5. Body fat BF denotes body lipids and includes lipids in adipose tissue as well as in all other cells. In the four-compartment model BF is calculated by subtracting the sum of the other three compartments from body mass. The error in this calculation is therefore dependent on the assumptions discussed above. The main error source in the calculation is the estimation of FFECS. Imprecision in the determination of TBW will have a larger influence than imprecision in TBK, as can be deduced from Fig. 2.2.

2.3.2 Principle of the methods

A standard dose of a substance or isotope, assumed to diffuse freely into a specific body compartment, is administered orally or intravenously to the subject. After the equilibration period, i.e. the period of time when the substance is expected to distribute equally within the compartment, a representative sample is taken for determination of the concentration of the substance in the compartment.

The volume V (litre) may be calculated from the equation:

$$V = A/c$$

where A is the amount (in mmol or MBq) of the substance or isotope given to the individual, and c the concentration (mmol/l or MBq/l) of the substance or isotope in the compartment.

During the equilibration period a certain amount (B) of the substance may be lost from the body with urine etc., which must be collected and analysed. The calculation of V will thus be $V = (A - B)/c$.

Moreover, part of the substance given may metabolize or diffuse outside the specific body compartment under study. In both instances the volume will be overestimated. Therefore, instead of saying that V is the volume of the compartment, the data is often described as the 'A-space'.

The techniques for determination of total body water and total body potassium are given later. The more modern method for determining total body potassium, i.e. counting the natural isotope ^{40}K in a whole-body counter, will also be described in this chapter, even though it is not a dilutometry method. The gamma radiation from the naturally present radionuclide ^{40}K, which is a constant fraction of all natural potassium, is counted in a whole-body counter in a well-shielded low-activity background laboratory.

SECTION I   DETERMINATION OF TOTAL BODY WATER

2.3.3 Chemicals and apparatus

(a) Chemicals

Tritiated water, e.g. Amersham International, England;
Liquid-scintillation fluid, e.g. Rialuma (LKB Chemicals Sweden).

(b) Solutions

Stock solution of tritiated water;
Test solution prepared by dilution of stock solution to a specific activity of 100 µCi/ml (3.7 MBq/ml);
Standard solution prepared from test solution by two-step dilution of test solution to 1:40 000 (i.e. to a specific activity of 92.5 Bq/ml).

(c) Apparatus

Vacuum sublimation unit with test tube connected to a receiver placed in a Dewar vessel with dry ice;
Liquid scintillation counter, e.g. Packard Tri-Carb model 3320.

2.3.4 Subject preparation

It is preferable to perform determinations in the morning after an overnight fast.

The subjects should not be in a fasted state but the risk of incomplete absorption from the gut due to delayed gastric emptying or extensive fluid losses from the bowel has to be considered.

The subject must also deliver a urine specimen of at least 10 ml before isotope administration (0-urine).

2.3.5 Procedure

(a) Technique

One hundred microcuries (3.7 MBq) ^{3}H water is added to an ordinary drinking glass containing approximately 100 ml tapwater.

The administration of 100 µCi (3.7 MBq) gives a radiation dose of approximately 0.5 milliSievert, comparable to a chest X-ray. The subject has to take this amount and in addition at least two 50 ml portions of tap water used to rinse the glass.

The drinking of the isotope solution and the rinsing water must be closely supervised in order to avoid spilling, and intravenous administration of the isotope solution may be considered in some subjects.

If repeated measurements are required in the same subject it is wise to give only 10–50 µCi on the first occasion, followed by doubled doses at each new measurement, up to the maximum dose allowed by the Ethics committee. A period of at least 14 days between measurements is recommended.

After an equilibration period of at least 2 h a sample of about 10 ml blood is drawn from a cubital vein. After clotting and centrifugation of the blood two samples of 2–3 ml serum and the 0-urine are sublimated in vacuo. Sublimation is preferred to distillation as the latter procedure will not separate volatile substances that may have quenching properties.

Half a millilitre serum water and 0-urine water from each sublimated sample and standards (diluted 1:40 000, see below) are mixed with 4.0 ml scintillation fluid in standard scintillation vials. If a suitable commercial scintillation liquid is not available the mixture of Moss is recommended (200 g naphthalene, 25 g PPO, 100 mg POPOP in 2000 ml dioxane).

Samples and standards are counted for 10 min in the liquid scintillation counter at least twice. In each batch of samples, four standard vials are included, two from the previous run and two freshly prepared. Background activity is counted in vials with tap water and scintillation fluid.

(b) Calculation

Total body water (TBW) is calculated from the equation:

$$\text{TBW} = \frac{\text{Dose} \cdot 40\,000 \cdot (\text{Std count} - \text{Blank count})}{1000 \cdot (\text{Serum count} - \text{Urine count})}$$

where TBW = Total body water (litres); Dose = Amount (in ml) of test solution administered; 40 000 = Standard solution dilution factor; Std count = Activity in standard solution (counts/10 min); Blank count = Background activity (counts/10 min); 1000 = Conversion from ml to litres; Serum count = Activity in serum water (counts/10 min); Urine count = Activity in 0-urine water (counts/10 min).

2.3.6 Performance characteristics

(a) General considerations

An equilibration period of 2 h is sufficient in most cases. However, subjects with oedema, ascites or other forms of fluid retention in tissues may require prolonged equilibration time. If so, the data must be corrected for isotope losses through urine and faeces (measured) during the prolonged period, and insensible losses via skin and expired air (assumed to have a volume of 800 ml/ 24 h). Thus, such data must be interpreted with caution.

Urine samples have been used instead of plasma; however, they have been reported to overestimate the total body water volume, probably due to the presence of unlabelled urine. In our experience this overestimation amounts to a mean of 10% [35].

The usual coefficient for calculation of lean body mass (or fat-free mass) is TBW/0.73. The equation LBM = TBW/0.73 comes from direct analyses in the rabbit [21]. Nevertheless, the water content seems to be similar in other species including man, judged from the few direct analyses available. Calculations made in different populations also give an average figure very close to 0.73, with a small individual variation.

Data from a Gothenburg population are given in Table 2.2.

Table 2.2 Ratio of total body water to lean body mass in a Gothenburg population

Age range	n	TBW/LBM (means ± SD)
Females		
20–29	56	0.721 ± 0.016
30–39	30	0.718 ± 0.019
40–49	50	0.715 ± 0.018
50–59	128	0.709 ± 0.018
60–69	35	0.714 ± 0.017
70 +	56	0.712 ± 0.018
Males		
20–29	24	0.717 ± 0.008
30–49	10	0.712 ± 0.010
50–59	51	0.717 ± 0.014
70+	49	0.729 ± 0.017

Although LBM water content seems to vary little in healthy conditions, during pathological conditions fluid retention or dehydration can result in considerable deviations from the 0.73 value. Calculations as above are based on the assumption that LBM is homogeneous and constant with respect to the variable measured.

(b) Reproducibility

The precision of the measurement is dependent on the accuracy of administration and equilibration as commented on above. The total error has been determined in a group of 20 women measured twice at about a one-month interval, once in the early follicular phase and again in the premenstrual phase. The error was ± 1.03 l.

(c) Validity

At the moment there is no direct measurement method available to test the validity.

2.3.7 Reference values

In a number of publications [33, 35, 46–49] reference values are given for total body water in clinically healthy individuals.

Attempts have been made to describe so-called reference ranges for these variables in relation to body weight, body height, and/or age as well as sex. A number of single and multiple regression equations have been developed. These equations may be sufficiently reliable for the group examined but one must doubt their value when evaluating the data of an individual from another population. Nevertheless, data from clinically healthy individuals may be used for reference if these limitations are kept in mind.

2.3.8 Interpretation

Interpretation is dealt with in section 2.3.13.

SECTION II DETERMINATION OF EXCHANGEABLE POTASSIUM

2.3.9 Chemicals and apparatus

(a) Chemicals

^{42}K, obtained from an isotope-producing factory in the vicinity of the laboratory (due to the short half-life; see Technique below);
KCl, p.a.

(b) Solutions

Stock solution of ^{42}K, about 150 µCi/ml;
Test solution prepared by dilution with 1% KCl of stock solution to a specific activity of 10 µCi/ml;
Standard solution prepared by a two-step dilution of test solution to 1 : 2000– 1 : 5000 with 1% KCl.
1% potassium chloride in distilled water.

(c) Apparatus

10-ml Geiger–Müller liquid counter, e.g. Model M6, 20th Century Electronic Ltd;
Flame photometer, e.g. Eppendorf.

2.3.10 Procedure

(a) Technique

Because of the short half-life (12.4 h) and also its rapid decay, ^{42}K is checked immediately on arrival from the supplier. Test solutions and standards should be prepared without delay.

The isotope ^{42}K has a slow equilibration (up to 40 h) in the body. Both factors strongly influence the procedure. If possible the isotope delivered from the supplier should arrive in the laboratory around noon, and be given in the afternoon in a proper dilution to the subject, who should return in the morning of the second day, about 40 h after the isotope intake.

Add 10.0 ml of the test solution to a drinking glass containing about 100 ml tapwater. Allow the subject to drink this amount and in addition at least two portions of 50 ml water, used to rinse the glass.

Rather high doses of radioactivity should be received from the factory due to the short half-life of the product. The laboratory must be equipped for the proper handling of the radioactive material.

The equilibration period is usually 42 h, during which time all urine has to be collected.

After the equilibration period the subject has to deliver two spot urine samples of at least 20 ml each, at about 2-h interval.

It is essential that all losses of activity during the long equilibration period are collected and determined. Losses through vomiting, diarrhoea, ileostomy, etc. must be measured.

Standard solution, urine collection, and the two spot urine samples are measured in a 10-ml Geiger–Müller liquid counter and corrected for background and decay.

The concentration of potassium in the three urine samples is determined by flame photometry.

(b) Calculation

U_1 = urine collection during equilibration period;
U_2 and U_3 = spot urine samples in equilibrium;
Exchangeable potassium K_e (mmol), calculated from urine sample U_2:

$$K_e = \frac{(5000 \cdot \text{Std} - U_1 \text{ count} \cdot U_1 \text{ vol}/10) \cdot K_{U_2} \cdot 10}{U_2 \text{ count} \cdot 1000}$$

where 5000 = standard dilution factor; Std = activity in standard solution (counts/10 min); U_1 count = activity in 10 ml of urine sample U_1; U_1 vol = total volume of U_1 urine collection; K_{U_2} = potassium concentration in urine sample U_2 (mmol/l); U_2 count = activity in 10 ml U_2 sample (counts/10 min).

K_e is calculated in the same way for urine sample U_3, and the result expressed as the mean.

All counts measured have to be corrected for decay during analysis, i.e. the real-time of counting is noted and corrected to zero time (start of analysis) using the decay curve.

This laborious procedure has been replaced by determination of ^{40}K in a whole-body counter but is useful if the latter equipment is not available.

2.3.11   Performance characteristics

(a) General considerations

At a meeting of the NY Academy of Sciences in 1963 Moore introduced the equation:

$$\text{MAN} = \text{BCM} + \text{EST} + \text{FAT}$$

where BCM = Body cell mass and EST = Extracellular supporting tissue.

The body cell mass is the most variable part of LBM. In addition, it can be estimated quite accurately from TBK, since 98% of TBK resides intracellularly.

(b) Reproducibility

The coefficient of variation in counting radioactivity in the system used in our laboratory was ± 1.1% and the coefficient of variation in the flame photometry determination of potassium was ± 1.5%. Under these conditions, the coefficient of variation of a K_e determination, based on 644 paired measurements, was ± 4.5%.

(c) Validity

No direct method exists to test validity.

2.3.12 Reference values

In a number of publications [33, 35, 46–49] reference values are given for total body potassium in clinically healthy individuals. Attempts have been made to describe so-called reference ranges for these variables in relation to body weight, body height, and/or age as well as sex. A number of single and multiple regression equations have been developed. These equations may be sufficiently reliable for the group examined but one must doubt their value when evaluating the data of an individual from another population. Nevertheless, data from clinically healthy individuals may be used for reference if these limitations are kept in mind.

2.3.13 Interpretation

Use Figs. 2.3 and 2.4 for the interpretation of observed value in relation to predicted value from body height, body weight, sex, and age.

SECTION III   DETERMINATION OF TOTAL BODY POTASSIUM IN A WHOLE-BODY COUNTER

2.3.14 Apparatus

Whole-body counter.

2.3.15 Procedure

(a) Technique

The procedure depends on the performance of the whole-body counter. We use a highly sensitive 3 π whole-body counter containing four plastic scintillators with a total volume of 700 dm³. The shielding consists of a room with 15 cm thick iron walls and ceiling, lined on the inside with 3 mm lead [50].

The counter was calibrated for the 1.46 MeV gamma radiation from ^{40}K by administrating ^{42}K to a group of volunteers. ^{42}K emits 1.5 MeV gamma radiation and is measured by a slight adjustment of the energy window under identical circumstances to those of ^{40}K counting.

Thus, a calibration curve for subjects of various body mass and length can be obtained. In order to reduce the effect of contaminating isotopes such as disintegration products of radon the subjects are asked to bath and wash their hair the day before measurement.

(b) Calculation

Obtained from computer software.

2.3.16 Performance characteristics

(a) General considerations

The usual coefficient for calculation of lean body mass (or fat-free mass) is TBK/68.1. The equation LBM = TBK/68.1 seems to originate from direct

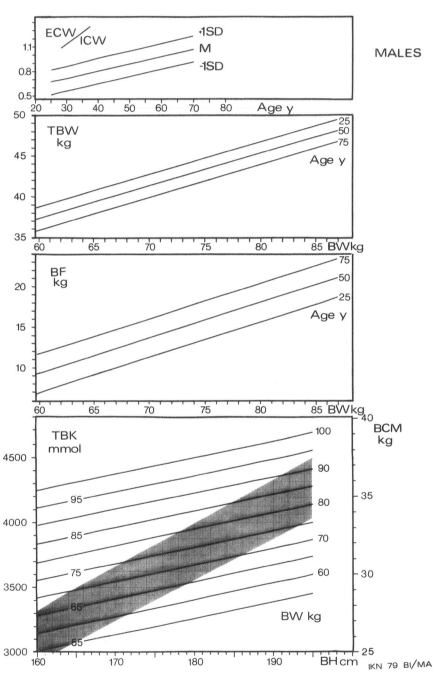

Fig. 2.3   Males. Chart for prediction of normal TBK, body fat, TBW, and ECW/ICW from body height, body weight, sex, and age. Shaded area represents 'normal' weight for height (mean ± 10%).

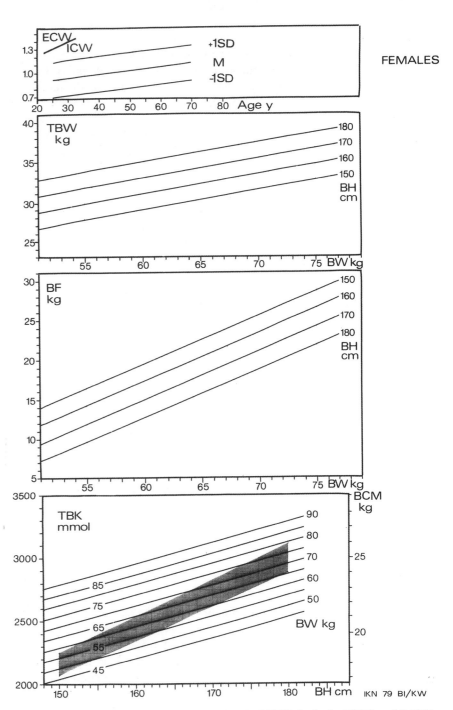

Fig. 2.4 Females. Chart for prediction of normal TBK, body fat, TBW, and ECW/ ICW from body height, body weight, sex and age. Shaded area represents 'normal' weight for height (mean ± 10%).

analysis of four human bodies [51]. It is widely quoted although it seems clear that this relation is not constant but varies with the size of LBM, simply because potassium is an intracellular ion. Data on the apparent variation in a Gothenburg population are presented in Table 2.3 and indicate that the figure 68.1 is relevant to younger males only. These figures were derived from the simultaneous determination of TBW and TBK, using the body composition model described previously. Thus it should be kept in mind that there is no independent determination of LBM.

Table 2.3   Ratio of total body potassium to lean body mass in a Gothenburg population

Age range	n	TBK/LBM (mean ± SD)
Females		
20–29	56	60.3 ± 4.4
30–39	30	59.9 ± 5.5
40–49	50	57.3 ± 5.4
50–59	128	56.0 ± 5.3
60–69	35	53.1 ± 5.2
70+	56	54.1 ± 5.0
Males		
20–29	24	69.1 ± 2.9
30–49	10	68.3 ± 3.7
50–59	51	61.6 ± 4.4
70+	49	56.7 ± 4.4

(b) Reproducibility

The accuracy of the determination depends on the performance of the whole-body counter and the choice of calibration method. In our laboratory, a count duration of 100 s gives a standard deviation in counting statistics of ±50 mmol. The standard deviation of a single potassium determination in adults is approximately ± 80 mmol.

The main error source is the presence of contaminating radionuclides, mainly disintegration products of radon, present in certain stone buildings. Another source of error is the calibration method used in correction for body size and shape.

(c) Validity

At the moment no direct method exists to test validity.

2.3.17   Reference values

In a number of publications [33, 35, 46–49] reference values are given for total body potassium in clinically healthy individuals. Attempts have been made to describe so-called reference ranges for these variables in relation to body weight, body height, and/or age as well as sex. A number of single and multiple regression equations have been developed. These equations may be sufficiently reliable for the group examined but one must doubt their value when evaluating the data of an individual from another population. Nevertheless, data from clinically healthy individuals may be used for reference if these limitations are kept in mind.

2.3.18 Interpretation

Interpretation is dealt with as in section 2.3.13.

2.3.19 General applications

The above methods have been used in samples from epidemiological surveys in the Gothenburg population. From these studies regression equations for the compartments based on sex, age, body weight, and body height have been developed [35]. The equations are given in Table 2.4 and nomograms for them in Fig. 2.3 for males and Fig. 2.4 for females.

Table 2.4 Multiple regression analyses. Dependent variables: Total body potassium (TBK), Total body water (TBW) and Body fat (BF). Independent variables: Body weight (BW), Body height (BH) and Age. The multiple regression equations are also given. SE = standard error of estimates

	Males			*Females*		
	TBK *R*	*TBW* *R*	*BF* *R*	*TBK* *R*	*TBW* *R*	*BF* *R*
BW	0.434	0.731	0.725	0.507	0.706	0.900
BH	0.566	0.345	0.067	0.505	0.473	0.032
BW, BH	0.625	0.740	0.747	0.640	0.769	0.923
BW, BH, Age	0.831	0.755	0.780	0.690	0.773	0.925

TBK = 27.3 BW + 11.5 BH − 21.9 Age + 778
  SE ± 314 mmol

TBW = 0.40 BW + 0.023 BH − 0.056 Age + 12.1
  SE ± 3.5 l

BF = 0.43 BW − 0.044 BH + 0.096 Age − 14
  SE ± 3.8 kg

TBK = 16.7 BW + 16.7 BH − 7.9 Age − 821
  SE ± 275 mmol

TBW = 0.24 BW + 0.20 BH − 0.03 Age − 13.9
  SE ± 2.8 l

BF = 0.61 BW − 0.23 BH + 0.04 Age + 15
  SE ± 3.0 kg

For clinical purposes the method is applied for monitoring body composition changes in the treatment of patients with gross obesity and patients on long-term nutritional support programmes, e.g. short-gut patients and some cancer patients.

In research, most studies on the effects of nutritional therapy include monitoring of body composition by these methods.

2.4 ADVANCED METHODS

2.4.1 Purpose and scope

The purpose of advanced body composition methodology is to provide measures of body fat and fat-free soft-tissue mass. Methodology in this category is generally more costly, less available, but more accurate than anthropometric counterparts. This section reviews advanced techniques in current use at body composition research centres. The material is abstracted from earlier reports [52–54].

2.4.2 Principles of the methods

Computerized axial tomography (CT) Based upon an earlier theoretical framework, G.N. Hounsfield introduced the first operational CT scanner in 1972 [55]. The CT system consists of an X-ray tube and receiver mounted on opposite poles of a circular gantry [56]. The subject rests upon a platform located in the centre of and perpendicular to the gantry. The X-ray beam is rotated about the subject; the attenuated X-rays are recorded, and the information is stored. The scanner computer next applies complex reconstruction algorithms to create the cross-sectional image.

The CT image is assembled from square (1 mm $\times$ 1 mm) picture elements or 'pixels'. As the CT slice has a definable depth, this is referred to as volume element or 'voxel'. The degree of X-ray beam attenuation is reflected in the pixel shading, which is quantified as the CT number in Hounsfield units [53]. The major determinant of X-ray attenuation is tissue physical density. Thus, high image contrast is noted between fat, lean tissues, and bone.

Nuclear magnetic resonance (NMR) NMR was first introduced independently by Bloch and Purcell in 1946 [57, 58]. By the 1970s NMR was widely applied to the *in vitro* analysis of chemical compounds. Referred to as NMR spectroscopy (NMRS), this technique shows promise in the study of human tissue metabolism. More recently techniques became available for creating an image from the NMR signal [59]. This process of NMR imaging is often referred to as magnetic resonance imaging or MRI.

NMR is based upon the principle that nuclei containing an odd number of protons or an odd number of neutrons, or both, have an angular momentum arising from their inherent spin [59]. Examples of these nuclei are ^1H, ^{31}P, ^{13}C and ^{23}Na. The electrical charge and spin of these nuclei generates a magnetic field that creates a dipole. When surrounded by an external magnetic field, these nuclei align themselves in a parallel or anti-parallel orientation relative to the field's line of induction. A 90° shift in the orientation of these nuclei can be induced by a radiofrequency pulse. Discontinuation of the radio signal allows the nuclei to return gradually to the equilibrium state and dissipate the absorbed energy into the surrounding environment. In an NMR scanner the external magnetic field is applied while the sample is surrounded by a coil connected to a source of radiofrequency power. The signal generated when the nuclei return to the parallel orientation is collected in the NMR receiver and then stored in a computer for subsequent analysis. A useful NMR signal is generated when the compounds possessing nuclear spin are in sufficiently high tissue concentration and are relatively mobile.

NMR imaging is currently based upon the high concentration, naturally abundant ^1H nucleus. Measuring the relaxation times (T1 and T2) in different projections provides the information needed to construct an image [59]. Image contrast is a function of proton density, T1, and T2 among neigbouring tissues. Imaging based upon ^{23}Na and ^{31}P is currently in an early phase of development, whereas ^{13}C imaging is not yet feasible.

Whole-body counting and *in vivo* neutron activation analysis (IVNA) Whole-body counting is used in association with some neutron activation analysis systems to quantify elements such as Ca, P, and Na [60]. In addition, ^{40}K whole-body counting is used *per se* to estimate total body potassium [61]. An earlier section (p. 79) reviewed whole-body counting in detail. This chapter presents a brief review of whole-body counting and its combined use with neutron activation analysis.

Intracellular potassium (K) concentration is relatively constant, there is little K outside cells, and K is distributed entirely within the fat-free tissues. Hence, total body K (TBK) can be used as a component in models that aim to provide estimates of intracellular fluid volume, body cell mass, and total fat-free body mass [33]. TBK can be estimated using radioactive ^{42}K, a procedure rarely used today due to the isotope's short half-life (p. 77). The alternative is to quantify TBK by counting the gamma rays emitted during the natural decay of ^{40}K, which constitutes a fixed percentage of potassium *in vivo* [61]. The approach is to first provide an area with sufficient shielding to eliminate or minimize background radiation. The instruments *per se* differ in design and configuration, but most rely on scintillation counters that detect the ^{40}K gamma rays. Appropriate anthropomorphic corrections are required in order to convert raw counts into estimated TBK. Typically such correction algorithms are based on ^{42}K experiments in appropriately selected subjects. Whole-body counting is a safe, non-invasive procedure that involves no radiation exposure to the patient [61].

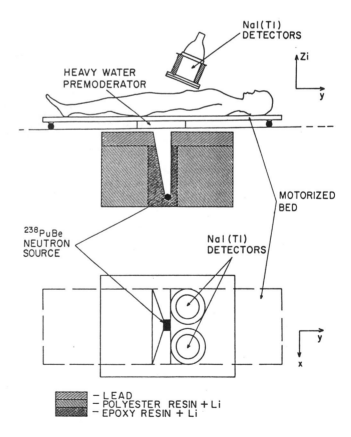

Fig. 2.5 Brookhaven National laboratory PBNA facility for total body nitrogen and hydrogen. Patient is scanned over a collimated neutron beam from 77 Ci of ^{238}Pu and Be. (From [53] with permission.)

The IVNA approach encompasses a broad range of techniques that share in common exposure of the subject to a neutron source followed by counting the activated nuclei as they decay to their stable forms [62]. The following elements can now be measured *in vivo*: H, C, O, N, Ca, P, Na, and Cl. Methods are also available for measuring iron, lead, and other heavy metals. Activation is accomplished by exposure to a neutron source that generates elemental forms which decompose either quickly or slowly. The decomposition products represent a fingerprint of the element, allowing conversion of spectral analysis into elemental content. Rapid decay of activated nuclei requires simultaneous counting, so called prompt-gamma IVNA [63]. Figure 2.5 presents a schematic diagram of the Brookhaven National Laboratory (BNL) prompt-gamma IVNA system used in the measurement of total body N and H. Slower decay can be counted following activation, termed delayed gamma IVNA. At BNL the delayed counting procedure is performed in a whole-body counter located at a distance from the activation unit. The patient is transported between the activation site and counting chamber within minutes of neutron exposure.

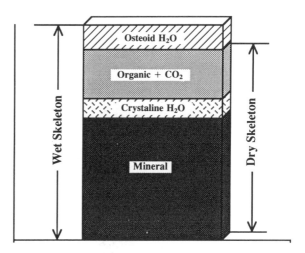

Fig. 2.6 Composition of representative human bone. (From [53] with permission.)

IVNA presents an unparalleled opportunity to study human body composition. The methods are expensive to implement and maintain, limiting their use to research centres. Finally, the radiation exposure is considerable relative to other methods, excluding pregnant women and healthy children from analysis.

Dual photon absorptiometry (DPA) Photons passing through human tissues are attenuated in relation to the substances with which they interact. Soft tissue and the bone mineral fraction of the skeleton (Fig. 2.6) attenuate photons to differing degrees, a property which underlies the dual photon absorptiometry (DPA) method [64]. DPA systems have a source that generates photons at two energy levels, for example, ^{153}Gd in classic DPA and filtered X-rays in newer systems (DEXA) [65]. By solving several simultaneous equations, DPA systems provide estimates of soft-tissue and bone mineral mass (Fig. 2.7). The

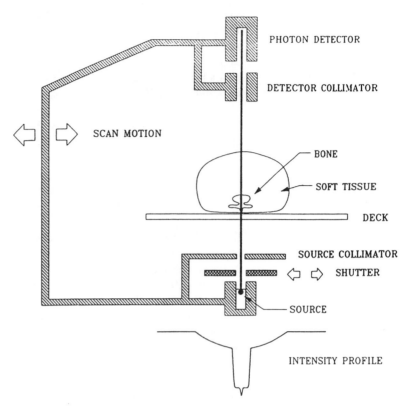

Fig. 2.7 A typical DPA scanner showing essential components. Photon beam intensity for a single line scan is shown at bottom. (From [53] with permission.)

proportion of soft tissue as fat and lean also influences photon attenuation, and this property can be used to estimate the proportion of body weight as fat. Hence DPA systems generate estimates of body fat and bone mineral mass.

Bioimpedance analysis (BIA) The BIA method is based on the principle that a frequency-dependent impedance to the spread of an applied alternating electrical current develops in biological tissues [66]. At frequencies of between 500 and 800 kHz, the current passes through both intra- and extracellular fluids. Due to the high conductivity of fluids, the fat-free tissues have a far greater conductivity than fat. The approach is to fasten electrodes at predefined anatomic sites and then to measure electrical conductance (1/resistance) as an excitation current is introduced into the subject. These results are then used to develop a prediction equation for total body water, fat, or fat-free body mass, which are estimated by other advanced methods [67]. The equations can then be used in clinical practice to calculate body composition based on BIA measurements.

Total body electrical conductivity (TOBEC) The TOBEC technique, as with BIA, is based on the differences in electrical properties of fat and fat-free tissues [68]. The measurement chamber of the TOBEC instrument consists of a large cylindrical coil. An oscillating electrical current is injected into the coil, inducing an electromagnetic field in the space enclosed by the coil. A meter coupled to the system measures the change in coil impedance as the subject passes through the instrument's core. The change in impedance is related to the dielectric and conductive properties of the body, and as for BIA, equations for water, fat, and fat-free body mass can be developed.

2.4.3   Procedure

Computerized axial tomography (CT) The CT scanner usually takes less than 10 s to complete each slice. The number of slices performed depends upon the question under study. A pre-scan 'scout' view allows precise definition of the anatomic location of each slice. Most scanners now have a variety of standard programs that allow reconstruction of the image and processing of specific aspects of the image data. These include:

1. defining the area of a structure of interest by tracing the image directly on the viewing console [69];
2. evaluating the CT number in a defined region of interest [60];
3. plotting the image pixels in the form of a histogram that allows separation of the tissues of differing density [69, 70];
4. reconstruction of complex images from a series of contiguous CT slices, including three-dimensional views that can be rotated and visualized from different angles.

In regard to body composition analysis, the usual approach is to first practice with a series of phantoms of known cross-sectional area, volume, and/or density. This initial step ensures the observer is using a calibrated instrument with proper settings for tracing and recording densities. The information then available from each cross-sectional CT slice includes the area and CT number

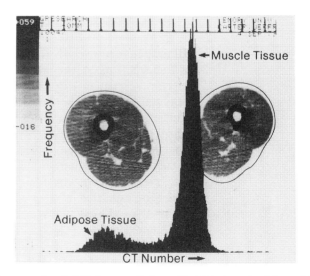

Fig. 2.8 Cross-sectional CT image of the mid-thigh in a healthy subject and a histogram of the image pixels. (From [53] with permission.)

of selected tissues (e.g. muscle, liver, etc.) (Fig. 2.8). A histogram of the slice pixels can also be plotted. By selecting appropriate boundaries, the histogram pixels can be separated into lean and adipose tissues.

Nuclear magnetic resonance (NMR) The NMR image and signal can be processed in a fashion similar to that described earlier for CT. Hence, essentially the same types of body composition analysis are possible.

Whole-body counting and *in vivo* neutron activation analysis (IVNA) The procedure usually requires less than 30 min. Patients are placed within the counter, and rest quietly during the study interval. Usually anthropometric measurements are made before or after whole-body counting, and these results are used in the TBK calculation. Some counters, such as the one at Brookhaven National Laboratory, have built-in methods of adjusting counts for body size (e.g. a cadmium sheet placed beneath the patient). Instruments are calibrated at regular intervals using reference phantoms.

With IVNA patients dress in a light gown, and are then placed in the neutron activation system. Techniques such as prompt-gamma IVNA (nitrogen) and neutron inelastic scattering (carbon) require about one hour for simultaneous neutron exposure and counting. Delayed gamma IVNA requires a 9-min initial exposure, followed by transfer to the whole-body counter. The whole body counting procedure requires about 10–15 min. Calibrations of reference solutions and anthropometric corrections are needed for most IVNA methods.

Dual photon absorptiometry (DPA) The DPA scanner is first calibrated, and patient studies then follow. With ^{153}Gd systems patients rest quietly for 45–55 min for whole-body scans. The newer DEXA method is faster, requiring 10–15 min for whole-body analysis. When studies of fat are of interest, either internal scanner algorithms or beef phantoms can be used in the calculation. The chemically analysed phantoms are scanned before or after the patient, and results are used to calibrate the per cent fat calculation.

Bioimpedance analysis (BIA) The usual approach is to make measurements several hours (about 2) after the last meal and to have the subject void prior to electrode placement. Shoes and socks are removed, and the subject rests quietly in the supine position. The aluminium foil electrodes are then placed on the middle dorsal surfaces of the hands and feet in specific anatomic positions in relation to bony landmarks. The 800-μA 50-kHz current is then introduced into the subject at the distal electrodes of the hands and foot with voltage detection at the proximal electrodes.

Total body electrical conductivity (TOBEC) As with BIA, the preferably fasting subject removes all large pieces of metal (coins, jewellery) and shoes prior to resting supine on the TOBEC platform. The system operator then activates the platform drive, which then moves the patient into and back out of the coil and electrical field. The procedure requires about one minute, after which the patient dresses; results are displayed on the system's computer terminal.

2.4.4 Evaluation

Computerized axial tomography CT represents a major advance in body composition methodology. In particular the novel use of CT in depicting internal or visceral fat and subcutaneous fat is now widely recognized and applied.

A point worth mentioning is that CT pixels derived from an area of adipose tissue represent the complete adipocyte with intracellular triglyceride, rather than the classic 'ether extractable fat'. [71]. Some workers recommend calculating 'fat' from CT adipose tissue by assuming a specific lipid content of the adipocyte. The inverse also applies: the 'lean tissue' as defined by CT also includes a small amount of fat. A final relevant point is that CT provides a measure of tissue volume; conversion to tissue mass requires appropriate adjustment for density. Figure 2.9 demonstrates the subdivision of body weight by CT into adipose tissue and adipose tissue free or lean body mass.

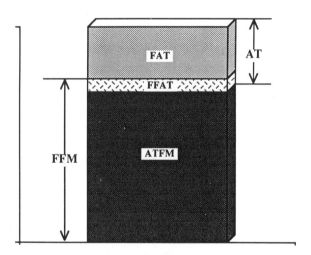

Fig. 2.9 The two components of fat-free body, fat-free adipose tissue (FFAT), and adipose tissue free mass (ATFM). Adipose tissue (AT) = FFAT + FAT, and fat-free body mass (FFM) = FFAT + ATFM. (From [53] with permission.)

Nuclear magnetic resonance A major current limitation of NMR is the difficulty in localizing the signal source and lack of NMR sensitivity of some nuclei. For example, ^{31}P-NMR spectroscopy of a human extremity is now possible using a small-bore superconducting magnet combined with a surface coil draped over the limb. Initial ^{31}P studies are now being reported for human myocardial tissue. A recent study examined the effects of dietary manipulation on the myocardial high-energy phosphorous intermediates in an infant with a severe cardiomyopathy [72]. This study was feasible due to the combined presence of a small body size, a greatly enlarged heart, and a thin chest wall. The advances in this field are of enormous significance to those investigators focusing on the interrelation between body composition and tissue metabolism.

The major advantage of NMR over CT with respect to the study of body composition is that the former produces no ionizing radiation. Thus both children and pregnant women can be evaluated by NMR; repeated studies are also possible. Major NMR installations are currently limited, thus restricting investigator access.

Whole-body counting and *in vivo* neutron activation analysis The raw counts are converted to TBK by use of anthropometric or other internal calibration procedures, and next converted to intracellular water, body cell mass, or fat-free body mass based on human body composition models [33, 61]. These components of body weight are central to the fluid metabolic model of body composition (Fig. 2.10).

With IVNA the raw elemental results are of interest *per se* (Fig. 2.11), but more commonly data is converted into a body compartment based on models, a few examples are as follows: Cl (extracellular fluid) ([73], Fig. 2.10); N (protein) ([73], Fig. 2.10); C (fat) ([74], Figs 2.10, 2.11); and Ca (bone mineral ash) [73]. These compartmental results are then analysed in the usual manner; as for example, patients total body protein vs expected for age, sex, height, and weight. Models are also developed that allow calculation of muscle and non-muscle protein or FFM (Fig. 2.10), and connective and intracellular protein based on ratios of TBK and TBN [74].

Dual photon absorptiometry This procedure provides for the first time a practical method of evaluating human skeletal weight in vivo. The relatively low radiation exposure allows for repeated studies, with the exclusion of children and pregnant females. The fat estimates are also useful, although the accuracy

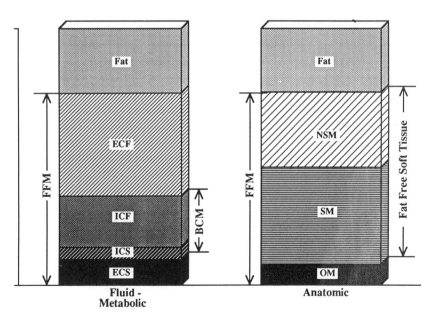

Fig. 2.10 Human body composition models based on fluid–metabolic (left) and anatomic (right) models. Abbreviations: BCM = body cell mass; ECF and ECS = extracellular fluid and solids; FFM = fat-free body mass; ICF and ICS = intracellular fluid and solids; NSM = non-skeletal muscle; OM = osseous mineral; SM = skeletal muscle. (From [53] with permission.)

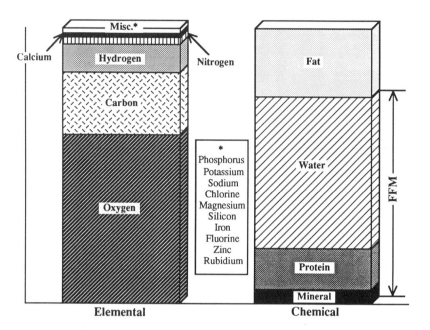

Fig. 2.11 Human body composition models based on elemental (left) or chemical (right) models. (From [53] with permission.)

of this aspect of DPA remains uncertain. The DPA method is a major advance in the study of osteoporosis.

Bioimpedance analysis The BIA instrument measures resistance and reactance at the specified electrical frequency. Resistance is the primary term used by investigators to predict body composition. Typically a prediction equation is developed in which resistance is used in association with such other variables as weight, height, age, and sex. In some cases a geometric model is developed in which resistance is used in association with height squared [75]. The equation is completed by calibrating the impedance and other preselected terms against body composition derived by hydrodensitometry, [40]K whole-body counting, or isotopic water dilution. Hence BIA prediction equations are available for total body water, fat, and fat-free body mass [75].

Total body electrical conductivity As with BIA, the raw signal received by TOBEC is used either alone or with other terms (e.g. weight, height, etc.) to predict body composition. TOBEC thus produces estimates of total body water, fat, and fat-free body mass [76].

(a) Reproducibility

Computerized axial tomography Excellent agreement is observed between CT estimates of phantom limb and organ weights. The CV for repeated per cent fat estimates based on CT is 2–3%. The relatively high radiation exposure of CT limits usefulness to either simple studies or to longitudinal regional evaluations.

Nuclear magnetic resonance No published results are yet available for evaluating NMR CVs.

Whole-body counting and *in vivo* neutron activation analysis The CV for ^{40}K whole-body counting is typically 2–7%, with the better systems in the 2–4% range [33, 61].

There are now cadaver studies that validate IVNA elemental estimates [77]. Moreover, animal and phantom experiments support compartmental estimates based on IVNA. As or all aspects of body composition analysis, additional validation experiments are needed, particularly in abnormal states such as obesity and cancer.

The CVs of elemental analyses vary between 1% (e.g. TBCa) and 3% (TBNa). Multi-compartment models that predict percent fat based on neutron activation give CVs between 1% and 3% [73].

Dual photon absorptiometry The CV for repeated DPA (^{153}Gd) bone mineral studies in humans is 1%. The CV for percent fat estimates is 2.7%. The newer DEXA systems are more reliable, demonstrating improved bone mineral and fat CVs [65]. Hence, longitudinal studies of osteoporosis and its treatment are feasible, based on the high reproducibility of dual photon systems.

Bioimpedance analysis The CV of repeated BIA measurements of fat-free body mass is less than 2% in healthy adults [74].

Total body electrical conductivity As for BIA, the between-day reproducibility of TOBEC in healthy adults is excellent, with between-day CVs of less than 2–3% for estimates of fat-free body mass [75].

(b) Validity

Computerized axial tomography The assumptions of CT involve: (1) conversion of the cross-sectional image to a tissue volume; (2) calculating (in some cases) tissue mass from volume; and (3) integrating the volume or mass of contiguous slices into an organ or tissue volume or mass. The validity of the three steps is relatively easy to recreate in non-living phantoms, such as water-filled balloons, pieces of meat, or whole animal carcasses. These various approaches confirm the validity of CT as a body composition instrument.

In contrast the accuracy of CT in evaluating body composition *in vivo* is more difficult to establish. Technical factors such as patient movement, slice width and interslice distance, and any number of additional considerations are involved. Nevertheless, CT clearly presents a unique opportunity to explore compartments not accessible by other methods except NMR (MRI).

Nuclear magnetic resonance As for CT, NMR can be validated using phantoms. The reservations expressed above for *in vivo* CT also apply for NMR.

Whole-body counting and *in vivo* neutron activation analysis As noted earlier IVNA is now nominally validated in phantoms and human cadavers.

A larger concern relates to the models in which IVNA provides the estimates of compartmental mass. These models are based on assumptions that should be carefully reviewed before final interpretation of results.

Dual photon absorptiometry There are now many validation studies of DPA both *in vitro* and *in vivo*. The most relevant experiments involve the correlation between DPA bone mineral and neutron activation total body calcium ($r = 0.94$–0.96) [78]. The latter is presently considered the benchmark method of evaluating skeletal mineral content *in vivo*. The fat estimates based on DPA correlate well with other conventional techniques. More studies in this area, particularly in malnourished and obese patients, are needed.

Bioimpedance analysis Current BIA instrumentation provides whole-body or regional estimates of resistance and reactance. Extensive between-instrument comparisons indicate extremely good agreement for both resistance and reactance, so validity in this respect is of relatively minor concern.

The next issue involves validity of BIA in estimating total body water. Agreement here also appears relatively good (SEE = 1.8–2.1 l) [68, 75, 79], given a reasonably high confidence interval in the prediction of water *per se*. There is one proviso, however, which is that subjects must be in a relatively stable state under predefined conditions. Acute fluid shifts, a full urinary bladder, and other factors can all contribute to error. In the absence of other techniques for measuring total body water, BIA can provide a reasonable bedside estimate.

The final and most difficult question involves the validity of BIA in providing estimates of fat and fat-free body mass. Here we focus on whole-body estimates, with the assumption that similar conclusions are worthy of mention. First, BIA estimates of fat are inaccurate in patients who have disturbances in fluid or electrolyte balance. Surgical patients and subjects with oedema secondary to chronic lung disease or congestive heart failure are typical examples in which BIA cannot be used with confidence to predict fat or fat-free body mass.

The second concern relates to the BIA instrument's prediction equation. Was it developed for use in patients with severe malnutrition, obesity, or the elderly? These are important considerations as there is now good evidence that prediction equations developed in healthy young adults are inaccurate when applied outside these boundaries.

The third concern relates to the confidence limit of predicted results. Most studies show that BIA improves prediction of body fat over anthropometrics, but the differences are not large in healthy, normal-weight adults (e.g. 2.7% vs 3.9% body fat) [79].

Our expectation is that both BIA technology and clinical BIA testing will improve this method and clarify its uses over the coming years. Until this process evolves the practitioner should be aware of the BIA instrument's limitations as described herein.

Total body electrical conductivity TOBEC provides excellent correlations with total body water, protein, and fat-free body mass in chemically analysed rat carcasses. Similar good results are observed in miniature pigs and in inanimate phantoms. There are considerably fewer human TOBEC instruments and thus a critical examination of the method's validity is not as clear as that for BIA. Almost identical concerns over BIA also pertain to TOBEC. Assuming good instrument calibration and upkeep, estimates of total body water under steady-state conditions are reasonably good. Fat estimates in young healthy, non-obese adults are likewise satisfactory. The concern, however, is with body composition estimates outside of these narrow constraints. As for BIA, additional studies are anticipated as new and improved TOBEC instruments are installed throughout the world.

2.4.5   Interpretation

Computerized axial tomography Baseline results are compared to appropriate published norms (e.g. total body fat) or to locally developed control results. The patients own results are used for comparative purposes in longitudinal studies.

Nuclear magnetic resonance Nuclear magnetic resonance results are interpreted as for CT.

Whole-body counting and *in vivo* neutron activation analysis TBK results are expressed either as absolute TBK or as compartmental masses. Some investigators also use the ratio of TBK to either nitrogen or fat-free body mass to calculate skeletal muscle and non-skeletal muscle protein, or extracellular and intracellular protein [74].

Results of IVNA are typically expressed as compartmental masses (e.g. fat, fat-free body mass, protein, etc.). Standard reference sources are available for comparing patient results to reference standards. Most centres with IVNA facilities develop their own norms.

Dual photon absorptiometry Bone mineral estimates are compared to age and sex adjusted standards. New reference values are needed that also account for body weight and ethnicity. For example, both obese and black subjects have increased mineral relative to lean and white individuals respectively [80]. Bone density measurements, also provided by DPA, can be used to screen for osteoporosis. Fat estimated by DPA is interpreted similar to other approaches to evaluating body fat.

Bioimpedance analysis The three main body composition components provided by BIA are total body water, fat, and fat-free body mass. Published norms are available for all three components based on height, weight, age and sex [81]. We also recommend developing a set of local reference standards based on a clearly defined 'normative' population.

A more difficult question is the interpretation of hydration estimates (e.g. TBW/FFM). In theory a patient's fluid status could be established by BIA, although this approach is not presently sufficiently sensitive for use in seriously ill patients. As mentioned earlier, improvements in data interpretation and instrument design could eventually lead to BIA becoming a useful clinical tool in assessing fluid status.

Total body electrical conductivity Similar normative tables and equations applied to BIA can be used for TOBEC estimates of water, fat, and fat-free body mass. New developments in TOBEC design may also eventually lead to valid estimates of hydration in disease states.

REFERENCES

1. Roche, A.F. (1987) Some aspects of the criterion methods for the measurement of the body composition. *Hum. Biol.*, **59**, 209–20
2. Siri, W.E. (1956) *Body Composition from Fluid Spaces and Density: Analysis of Methods*, UCRL-3349 University of California Radiation Laboratory, Berkeley (California).
3. Rahn, H., Fenn, W.O. and Otis, A.B. (1949) Daily variations of vital capacity, residual air, and expiratory reserve including a study of the residual air method. *J. Appl. Physiol.*, **1**, 725–43.
4. Durnin, J.V.G.A and Rahaman, M.N. (1967) The assessement of the amount of fat in the human body from measurement of skinfold thickness. *Br. J. Nutr.*, **21**, 681–8.
5. Buskirk, E.R. (1961) Underwater weighing and body density: a review of procedures, in *Techniques for Measuring Body Composition* (eds J. Brozek and A. Henschel), National Academy of Sciences – NCR, Washington (DC), pp. 90–106.
6. Goldman, R.F. and Buskirk, E.R. (1961) Body volume measurement by underwater weighing: description of a method, in *Techniques for Measuring Body Composition* (eds J. Brozek and A. Henschel), National Academy of Sciences – NCR. Washington (DC), pp. 78–89.
7. Consolazio, C.F., Johnson, R.E. and Pecora, L.J. (1963). *Physiological measurements of metabolic functions in man*, McGraw-Hill, New York, pp. 288–99.
8. Rich, G.O. and Scherer, G.D. (1980) A description of laboratory hydrostatic weighing methodology and descriptive data for young–middle age adults and athletes, in *Symposium Papers 1980* (eds R.H. Cox and J.K. Nelson), AA HPERD Research Consortium, Washington (DC), pp. 76–92.
9. Jones, P.R.M. and Norgan, N.G. (1974) A simple system for the determination of human body density by underwater weighing. *J. Physiol.*, **239**, 71–3.
10. Akers R. and Buskirk E.R. (1969) An underwater weighing system utilising "force cube" transducers. *J. Appl. Physiol.*, **26**, 649–52.
11. Girandola, R.N., Wiswell, R.A. and Romero, G. (1982) Body composition changes resulting from fluid ingestion and dehydration. *Res. Quart.*, **48**, 299–303.
12. Durnin, J.V.G.A., and Satwanti. (1982) Variations in the assessment of the fat content of the human body to experimental technique in measuring body density. *Ann. Hum. Biol.*, **9**, 221–5.
13. Keys, A. and Brozek, J. (1953) Body fat in adult man. *Physiol. Rev.*, **33**, 245–325.
14. Wilmore, J.H., Vodak, P.A., Parr, R.B. *et al.* (1969) Further simplification of a method for determination of residual lung volume. *Med. Sci. Sports Exerc.*, **12**, 216–18.
15. Nunneley, S.A., Edward, T., Flynn, J.R. and Camporesi, E.M. (1974) Two-tracer method for rapid determination of residual volume. *J. Appl. Physiol.*, **37**, 286–9.
16. Ward, A. Pollock, M.L., Jackson, A.S. *et al.* (1978) A comparison of body fat determined by underwater weighing and volume displacement. *Am. J. Physiol.*, **234**, E94–E96.
17. Garrow, J.S., Stalley, S., Diethielm, R. *et al.* (1979) A new method for measuring the body density of obese adults. *Br. J. Nutr.*, **42**, 173–83.
18. Gundlach, B.L., Nijkrake, H.G.M. and Hautvast, J.G.A.J. (1980) A rapid and simplified plethysmometric method for measuring body volume. *Hum. Biol.*, **52**, 23–33.

19. Gundlach, B.L. and Visscher, G.J.W. (1986) The plethysmometric measurement of total body volume. *Hum. Biol.*, **5**, 783–99.

20. Behnke, A.R., Feen, B.S. and Welham, W.C. (1942) The specific gravity of healthy men; body weight/volume as an index of obesity, *JAMA.*, **118**, 495–8.

21. Pace, N. and Rathbun, E.N. (1945) Studies on body composition, III. The body water and chemically combined nitrogen content in relation to body fat. *J. Biol. Chem.*, **158**, 685–91.

22. Rathbun, E.N. and Pace, N. (1945) Studies on body composition, I. Determinations of body fat by means of specific gravity. *J. Biol. Chem.*, **158**, 667–76.

23. Fidanza, F., Keys, A. and Andersen, J.T. (1953) The density of human body fat. *J. Appl. Physiol.*, **6**, 252–6.

24. Lohman, T.G. (1981) Skinfolds and body density and their relation to body fatness. *Hum. Biol.*, **53**, 181–225.

25. Lohman, T.G. (1986) Applicability of body composition techniques and constants for children and youths. *Exer. Sports Sci. Rev.*, **14**, 325–57.

26. Fidanza, F. (1987) The density of fat-free body mass during pregnancy. *Int. J. Vit. Nutr. Res.*, **57**, 104.

27. Raaij, J.M.A.V., Peek, M.E.M., Vermaat-Miedema, S.H. *et al.* (1988) New equations for estimating body fat mass in pregnancy from body density or total body water. *Am. J. Clin. Nutr.*, **48**, 24–9.

28. Womersley, J., Durnin, J.V.G.A., Boddy, K. and Mahaffy, M. (1976) Influence of muscular development, obesity and age on the fat-free mass of adults. *J. Appl. Physiol.*, **41**, 223–9.

29. Brozek, J., Grande, F., Andersen, J.T. and Keys, A. (1963) Densitometric analysis of body composition: revision of some quantitative assumptions. *Ann. N.Y. Acad. Sci.*, **110**, 113–40.

30. Roche, A.F. (1984) Anthropometric methods: new and old, what they tell us. *Int. J. Obesity*, **8**, 509–23.

31. Garrow, J.S. (1987) Methods for measuring changes in body composition, in *Human Body Composition and Fat Distribution* (ed. N.G. Norgan), EURO-NUT rep 8, Wageningen, pp. 75–80.

32. Norgan, N.G. and Ferro-Luzzi, A. (1985) The estimation of body density in men: are general equations general? *Ann. Hum. Biol.*, **12**, 1–15.

33. Moore, F.D., Olesen, K.H., McMurray, J.D. *et al.* (1963) *The body cell mass and its supporting environment*, W.B. Saunders, Philadelphia, London.

34. Benedict, F.G. (1915) *A study of prolonged fasting*, Carnegie Institution, Washington (DC).

35. Bruce, A., Andersson, M., Arvidsson, B. and Isaksson, B. (1980) Body composition. Prediction of normal body potassium, body water and body fat in adults on the basis of body height, body weight and age. *Scand. J. Clin. Lab. Invest.*, **40**, 461–73.

36. Moore, F.D. (1967) Body composition and its measurement in vivo. *Br. J. Surg.*, **54**, 431–5.

37. Bergstrom, J. (1962) Muscle electrolytes in man. Determination by neutron activation analysis on needle biopsy specimens. *Scand. J. Clin. Lab. Invest.*, **14**, [suppl], 68.

38. Dickerson, J.W.T., and Widdowson, E.M. (1960) Chemical changes in skeletal muscle with development. *J. Biochem.*, **74**, 247–57.

39. Flear, C.T.G., Carpenter, R.G. and Florence, I. (1965) Variability in the water, sodium, potassium, and chloride content of human skeletal muscle. *J. Clin. Pathol.*, **18**, 74–81.

40. Talso, P.J., Miller, C.E., Carballo, A.J. and Vasquez, I. (1960) Exchangeable potassium as a parameter of body composition. *Metabolism*, **9**, 456–71.

41. Russell, D.M. and Jeejeebhoy, K.N. (1984) Radionuclide assessment of nutritional depletion, in *Nutritional assessment* (eds R.A. Wright and S. Heymsfield), Blackwell Scientific, Boston, pp. 83–109.
42. Graham, J.A., Lamb, J.F. and Linton, A.L. (1967) Measurement of body water and intracellular electrolytes by means of muscle biopsy. *Lancet*, **ii**, 1172–6.
43. Litchfield, J.A. and Gaddie, R. (1958) The measurement of the phase distribution of water and electrolytes in skeletal muscle by the analysis of small samples. *Clin. Sci.*, **17**, 483–97.
44. Valentin, N. and Olesen, K.H. (1973) Measurement of muscle tissue water and electrolytes. *Scand. J. Clin. Lab. Invest.*, **32**, 155–60.
45. Wang, J. and Pierson, R.N. (1976) Disparate hydration of adipose and lean tissue require a new model for body water distribution in man. *J. Nutr.*, **116**, 1687–93.
46. Hume, R. and Weyers, E. (1971) Relationship between total body water and surface area in normal and obese subjects. *J. Clin. Pathol.*, **24**, 234–8.
47. Boddy, K., King, P.C., Hume, R. and Weyers, E. (1972) The relation of total body potassium to height, weight, water, and age in normal adults. *J. Clin. Pathol.*, **25**, 512–17.
48. Ellis, K.J., Shukla, K.K. and Cohn, S.H. (1974) A predictor for total body potassium in man based on height, weight, sex and age: application in metabolic disorders. *J. Lab. Clin. Med.*, **83**, 716–27.
49. Pierson, R.N., Lind, D.H.Y. and Phillips, R.A. (1974) Total body potassium in health: The effects of age, sex, height, and fat. *Am. J. Physiol.*, **226**, 206–12.
50. Arvidsson, B., Sköldborn, H. and Isaksson, B. (1972) Clinical application of a high-sensitive whole-body counter, in *The Third International Conference on Medical Physics*, Chalmers University of Technology, Göteborg, **41**, 2.
51. Forbes, G.B., Gallup, J. and Hursh J.B. (1961) Estimation of total body fat from potassium-40 content. *Science*, **133**, 101–2.
52. Heymsfield, S.B. (1987) Human body composition: analysis by computerized axial tomography and nuclear magnetic resonance, in *AIN Symposium Proceedings* (ed. O.A. Levander) American Institute of Nutrition. Bethesda, MD, pp. 92–6.
53. Heymsfield, S.B. *et al.* (Chapter in press) in *Assessment of body composition* (ed. P. Bjorntorp), Lippincot, Philadelphia.
54. Heymsfield, S.B., Rolandelli, R., Casper, K. *et al.* (1987) Application of electromagnetic and sound waves in nutritional assessment. *JPEN*, 11 [Suppl 5], 64S–72S.
55. Hounsfield, G.N. (1973) Computerized transverse axial tomography. *Am. J. Roentgenol.*, **127**, 3–9.
56. Haus, A.G. (1979). *The Physics of Medical Imaging: Recording System Measurements and Techniques*, American Institute of Physics, New York (NY).
57. Purcell, E.M., Torrey, H.C. and Pound, R.V. (1946) Resonance absorption by nuclear magnetic moments in a solid. *Phys. Rev.*, **69**, 37.
58. Gunby, P. (1982) The new wave in medicine: Nuclear magnetic resonance. *JAMA*, **247**, 151.
59. Roth, K. (1984) *NMR-Tomography and Spectroscopy in Medicine: An Introduction*, Springer-Verlag, Heidelberg.
60. Cohn, S.H. (1987) Noninvasive techniques for measuring body elemental composition. *Biol. Trace Elem. Res.*, **13**, 179–84.
61. Pierson, R.N., Lin, D.H.Y. and Phillips, R.A. (1974) Total body potassium in health: effects of age, sex, height, and fat. *Am. J. Physiol.*, **226**(1) 206–12.
62. Whitman, G.J.R., Chance, B., Bode, H. *et al.* (1985) Diagnosis and therapeutic evaluation of a pediatric case of cardiomyopathy using phosphorus-31 nuclear magnetic resonance spectroscopy. *JACC*, **5**(3), 745–9.
63. Vartsky, D. Ellis, K.J. and Cohn S.H. (1963) In vivo quantification of body

nitrogen by neutron capture prompt gamma-ray analysis. *J. Nucl. Med.*, **20**, 1158–65.

64. Mazess, R.B., Peppler, W.W. and Gibbons, M. (1984) Total body composition by dual-photon (153Gd) absorptiometry. *Am. J. Clin. Nutr.*, **40**, 834–9.

65. Heymsfield, S.B., Wang, J., Aulet, M. *et al.* (in press) Dual photon absorptiometry: validation of mineral and fat measurements, in *In Vivo Body Composition Studies* (eds S. Yasumura and J.E. Harrison), IPSM.

66. Lukaski, H.C. (1986) Use of the tetrapolar bioimpedence to assess body composition, in *Human body composition and fat distribution* (ed. N.G. Norgan), EURO-NUT rep 8, Wageningen, pp. 143–58.

67. Segal, K., Gutin, B., Presta, E. *et al.* (1985) Estimation of human body composition by electrical impedance methods: a comparative study. *J. Appl. Physiol.*, **58**, 1565–71.

68. Kushner, R.F., and Schoeller, D.A. (1986) Estimation of total body water by bioelectrical impedance analysis. *Am. J. Clin. Nutr.*, **44**, 417–24.

69. Sjostrom, L., Kvist, H., Cederblad, A. and Tylen, U. (1986) Determination of total adipose tissue and body fat in women by computed tomography, ^{40}K and tritium, *Am. J. Physiol.*, E736–E745.

70. Kvist, H., Chowdhury, B., Grangard, U. *et al.* (1988) Total and visceral adipose tissue volumes derived from measurements with computed tomography in adult men and women: predictive equations. *Am. J. Clin. Nutr.*, **48**, 1351–61.

71. Heymsfield, S.B., Olafson, R.P., Kutner, M.H. *et al.* (1979) A radiographic method of quantifying protein calorie undernutrition. *Am. J. Clin. Nutr.*, **32**, 1734–40.

72. Barrett, E.J., Alger, J.R. and Zaret, B.L. (1985) Nuclear magnetic resonance spectroscopy: its evolving role in the study of myocardial metabolism. *J. Am. Coll. Cardiol.*, **6**, 497–501.

73. Cohn, S.H., Vaswani, A.N., Yasumura, S. *et al.* (1984) Improved models for determination of body fat by in vivo neutron activation. *Am. J. Clin. Nutr.*, **40**, 255–9.

74. Burkinshaw, L., Hill, G.L. and Morgan, D.B. (1979) Assessment of the distribution of protein in the human body by in vivo neutron activation analysis. *IAEA-SM*, **227**(139), 787–98.

75. Lukaski, H. (1987) Methods for the assessment of human body composition: traditional and new. *Am. J. Clin. Nutr.*, **46**, 537–56.

76. Harrison, G.G. and Van Itallie, T.B (1982) Estimation of body composition: A new approach based on electromagnetic principles. *Am. J. Clin. Nutr.*, **32**, 524–6.

77. Knight, G.S., Beddoe, A.H., Streat, S.J. *et al.* (1986) Body composition of two human cadavers by neutron activation and chemical analysis. *Am. J. Physiol.*, **250**, E179–E185.

78. Mazess, R.B. (1971) Estimation of bone and skeletal weight by direct photon absorptiometry. *Invest. Radiol.*, **6**, 52–60.

79. Baumgertner, R.N., Chumlea, W.C. and Roche, A.F. (1988) Bioelectric impedance phase angle and body composition. *Am. J. Clin. Nutr.*, **48**, 16–23.

80. Lohman, T.G. (1984) Research progress in validation of laboratory methods of assessing body composition. *Med. Sci. Sports Exerc.*, **16**(6), 596–603.

81. Report of the Task Group on Reference Man. (1975) *Int. Comm. Radiol. Protection Report No 23*, Pergamon Press, Oxford.

3 Physical working capacity and physical fitness methodology

3.1 Introduction   *J. Pařízková*   101
3.2 Cardiorespiratory efficiency   *J. Pařízková*   102
3.3 Muscle strength   *J. Pařízková*   106
3.4 Motor performance   *J. Pařízková*   108
3.5 Final comments   *J. Pařízková*   112

3.1 INTRODUCTION

Among the measurements of nutritional status and health the evaluation of physical fitness and functional capacity have an important place. They belong to the most important characteristics of the human organism: its level of development, growth, and maturation. Their reduction and deterioration are often the first signs of a certain degree of malnutrition, illness and/or any other pathological state.

By functional capacity we understand first of all the ability to perform physical work, which depends mostly on the efficiency of the cardiovascular, respiratory, and neuromuscular systems as related to the function of all other systems of the human organism. In the type of work that engages large muscle groups (especially when one's body weight is transferred along a distance) the limiting factor is the individual's ability to transport oxygen to the working tissues. From the measurements of functional capacity we can characterize not only so-called 'normality', but also 'positive health' according to the World Health Organization definition. An adequate level of functional capacity and physical fitness are important not only from the point of view of well-being, but also of economic productivity, which especially applies to the developing countries. As often stated, it is more important to be healthy and fit, than to achieve certain bodily dimensions.

Adequate nutrition is necessary for optimal development of physical fitness and functional capacity [1].

Malnutrition, both in a positive and negative sense of energy intake, has a negative impact on the functional characteristics. Obese as well as excessively underweight persons have a low level of physical fitness. However, this deterioration is differentiated according to the character of physical activity and work-load. A very lean person can have very good results as regards dynamic performance (e.g. running), but his gross work output demanding muscle strength may be reduced. On the other hand an obese person has very bad results in dynamic performance, but is frequently strong. The impact of dietary intake and nutritional status is related to the changes of body weight and body composition. Special deficiencies, e.g. that of iron (causing anaemia), or vitamin C (resulting in increased fatiguability, more frequent common colds, etc.), even if slight, may cause a considerable reduction in the level of physical fitness and physical performance. The same applies to a number of other micronutrients, trace elements, and so forth. Studies concerning the relationship between physical fitness and intake of the above-mentioned food components have only been initiated recently.

The impact of malnutrition of specific character manifests both in developing as well as industrially developed countries. As regards the latter, the impact of overeating, usually together with hypokinesia, results in deterioration of cardiorespiratory efficiency that may predispose the subject to diseases of the cardiovascular system. On the other hand the impact of low intakes of energy on gross work output in developing countries is well known.

Similarly, as with other physical traits in humans, there exists a wide variability in physical fitness and functional capacity, which depends both on genetic and/or environmental factors. Adaptation processes can significantly modify the capacity for performing physical work at all ages. The impact of a systematic work-load of a sufficient intensity, but within the adaptation limits of the organism, can markedly increase the work performance. This applies especially during the growing period, when an appropriate stimulation helps to develop an optimal level of all bodily systems, and especially those involved in physical work. This is particularly applicable to the cardiorespiratory system. However, if the growing organism is overburdened, it can significantly interfere not only with normal development but also with the desirable functional capacity currently as well as in later periods.

The evaluation of functional capacity and physical fitness have become an integral part of research, not only in nutritional sciences but also in research in physiology (theoretical and clinical), epidemiology, human biology, and so forth.

The level of functional capacity and physical fitness can be evaluated by a number of methodological approaches that concern cardiovascular, respiratory and neuromuscular systems.

For practical purposes these can be divided into laboratory and/or clinical, half-field, and field methods, according to the aims and circumstances of the study in question.

3.2 CARDIO-RESPIRATORY EFFICIENCY

3.2.1 Purpose and scope

Physical performance, i.e. the ability to perform a physical work-load, depends first of all on the capacity of the cardiovascular and respiratory systems, which are closely interrelated. The limiting factor for performing a physical work-load is the ability to transport oxygen to the working muscles and all the other tissues involved, i.e. the aerobic power, assessed for example by the direct measurement of $\dot{V}O_2$ max. This is quite demanding and requires first-class laboratory conditions and a high level of motivation and co-operation from the subjects tested. Measurements of the O_2 uptake are carried out during a gradually increasing work-load, either on a treadmill, or bicycle ergometer. These may not always be available, especially for field measurements; this also applies to analysers for O_2, CO_2, etc.

The maximal aerobic power can be estimated indirectly, i.e. from the results of the submaximal tests. With the help of extrapolation the 'oxygen ceiling' (i.e. $\dot{V}O_2$ max) can be calculated and gives an idea of the overall level of the organism's functional capacity [2].

As regards working performance, the results of submaximal work load testing (e.g. physical working capacity at 170 heart beats per minute – PWC_{170}) can be interesting as this is closer to the daily activities. These tests are again performed on a treadmill or bicycle ergometer, but the level of performance achieved is lower.

When facilities are limited, a step test may be used as an alternative to the other tests.

3.2.2 Principle of the methods

The ability to perform physical work depends first of all on the capacity of the cardiovascular and respiratory systems, which can be characterized by aerobic power – submaximal and maximal. Like the ability to carry as much oxygen as possible to the working tissues, mostly muscles, the efficiency of the cardio-respiratory fitness can be evaluated by measuring the oxygen uptake during a particular work-load on a treadmill or bicycle ergometer, together with other necessary variables such as heart and ventilation rate, ventilation volume, carbon dioxide output, RQ, etc. Most important are the measurements of the maximal oxygen uptake ($\dot{V}O_2$ max) in absolute and relative values (i.e. per kg body weight and/or lean body mass, or per single heart beat), which gives information on the physical limits of performance. PWC_{170}, however, is also widely used, especially in children and adolescents.

With the step test the heart rate is recorded after stepping on a bench, varying its height and the frequency of stepping according to the age and sex of the subject.

3.2.3 Procedure

Testing procedures are described in various textbooks [2–5]. The use of methods adopted for the International Biological Programme (maximal oxygen uptake during step-wise increasing work-load, and/or PWC_{170}) are highly recommended for an exact and world comparable evaluation of functional capacity.

The PWC_{170} test is performed on a stationary cycle ergometer, the subject being required to pedal continuously for a total of not more than nine minutes, during which the work-load is increased twice (at three and six minutes), making three loads in all. Heart rate is measured during the last 15 s of each load, and the work-load increases are regulated so that the heart rate achieved at the end of the test approaches 170 beats per minute. This procedure was recommended especially for testing children [6].

From our experience we give further information, in particular for the step test. In the original Harvard step test the height of the bench (50 cm or 20 inches) and the stepping frequency (30 steps/min) were selected so that only roughly one-third of the subjects would be able to perform the test for a five-minute period. The heart rate was counted during recovery from the exercise with the subject sitting on the bench (from 1 to 1.5 minutes). Modifications of the Harvard step test have also been used, e.g. the height of the bench was lowered, or the frequency reduced for the subjects with a lower level of physical fitness, children, obese subjects, etc. Procedures for the continuous registration of heart rate (HR) were developed using leads from the chest and continuous registration by computer. Under simple field conditions a stethoscope with a very long rubber tube can serve the same purpose. In such cases the heart rate is registered during three minutes rest, then during five minutes work load (mounting a bench) and per cent minutes of recovery, i.e. for a total of 13 minutes when necessary. From the data the establishment of steady state, the shape of the heart-rate curves, and also the economy of the reaction of the cardiorespiratory system to work-load can be evaluated by various indices [7].

Calculations

The aerobic power is given by two maximal consecutive values of the oxygen uptake during a graded work-load. This value is given in absolute numbers and/or per kg body weight and/or lean body mass.

When testing PWC_{170} it is possible to determine the work-load corresponding to a heart rate of 170 beats per minute by extrapolation or interpolation. The score is made more meaningful if divided by the subject's weight (kg).

From the respiratory variables measured during step-wise maximal work-load the ventilatory anaerobic threshold can also be determined non-invasively from the dependence of pulmonary ventilation on oxygen uptake and/or carbon dioxide output by means of two-part discontinuous linear models. Aerobic power can also be calculated using a nomogram for adult men and women [2]. As regards aerobic power, modifications in the evaluation of HR during the step test are numerous. The step test is evaluated from the values of HR during work-load and recovery in relation to work performed (see Fig. 3.1).

3.2.4 Performance characteristics

(a) Reproducibility

The measurement of maximal oxygen uptake varied from 4.5 to 5.8% in most laboratories when measured repeatedly in the same subjects under the same conditions. The standard error in the estimate of step test measurements was approximately in the same range, i.e. 4–6%. However, when individual motivation, in particular performance, is requested, the homogenization of the experimental conditions may be difficult, and perfect co-operation with the measured subjects is indispensable.

(b) Validity

The values of the aerobic power, both maximal and submaximal, especially when expressed per kg body weight and/or lean body mass, have proved a valid characteristic of the cardiorespiratory efficiency, which has a typical trend of age changes, and varies in individuals adapted to different work loads, diets, and so forth.

No better tests of validity are available at the moment.

STEP TEST	
Name:	Date of birth:
Date of examination:	Hour of the examination:
	Weight:

rest   Work   recovery

(HR/min)

$\bar{x}$ A   B

HR $(\bar{x})$ = mean heart rate per minute at rest
HR$_{WR}$ = sum of heart beats during work (A) and recovery (B)
HR$_P$ = HR$_{WR}$ − 10 · HR $(\bar{x})$
CEI =: $\dfrac{Kpm}{HR_{WR}}$
CEI$_P$ = $\dfrac{Kpm}{HR_P}$
HR$_R$ = B − 5 · HR $(\bar{x})$
Index = = $\dfrac{30000}{\sum 2\ min\ +\ 3rd\ min\ +\ 5th\ min\ B}$

where:
Kpm   = weight of the child · 150 · height of the step (0.25 m)
(150   = 30 mounts during 5 min)
HR$_P$ = heart rate for performance
CEI   = cardiac efficiency index (5)
CEI$_P$ = cardiac efficiency index for performance

Fig. 3.1 Form for step test and relative indices in children.

3.2.5 Reference values

Reference values for different population groups as regards, sex, age, physical activity, etc. are available [2–4, 6, 8, 9]. Nevertheless, more data for reference values on an international scale are needed.

3.2.6 Interpretation

The peak of aerobic power appears around puberty and decreases with ageing. The impact of dietary intake and nutritional status on aerobic power is significant and related to the changes of body weight and body composition. Obese people have low aerobic power which can be improved after weight-reducing therapy. People with marginal malnutrition who are lean and have lower body weight often have higher aerobic power than people with normal body weight and standard body composition. Severe malnutrition with extreme emaciation was never tested, but low aerobic power may be assumed.

Among the methods for cardiorespiratory efficiency is the Ruffier test, which is the simplest of all.

Measurement of lung capacity has not been included because it is fully described in many books as mentioned above [2–10].

The same applies to the results of the step test when the degree of malnutrition is excessive. However, when only marginal malnutrition is present the results of the step and/or Ruffier tests, and maximal oxygen uptake per kg total and lean body weight, may be quite satisfactory and comparable to the values ascertained in well-nourished people with standard body weight.

3.3 MUSCLE STRENGTH

3.3.1 Purpose and scope

Muscle strength depends on the number of motor units activated and the frequency of their contraction. With increasing work-load, recruitment of more units is most important. Muscle strength is usually divided into static (isometric) and dynamic strength. Static strength can be further subdivided into maximum isometric strength and maximum isometric endurance. Maximum isometric strength is the maximal force that can be exerted in an 'attempted' movement; the position during measurement must be fixed and well-defined. Maximal isometric endurance is the maximum time a certain percentage of the maximum isometric strength can be maintained in tension. Maximum dynamic strength can generally be considered as two forms of work, namely concentric or positive work and eccentric or negative work. It can be measured, for example, as the maximum weight that can be lifted (positive work) or lowered (negative work), always during a well-defined movement and with a maximum of one repetition.

As in other functional parameters, muscle strength changes in a characteristic way during the life-span. It increases during growth – the maximum strength is reached between the ages of 20 and 30 years – after which it decreases gradually so that the strength of the 60-year old is approximately 80% of that attained between 20 and 30 years [2]. Males generally have greater muscle strength. Adaptation to exercise, especially static, increases muscle strength in both sexes and at all ages. The impact of nutrition is remarkable: the greatest muscle strength is achieved in people with great lean body mass, especially muscle mass.

3.3.2 Principle of the method

To measure muscle strength many modifications of the spring balance principle have been suggested, substituting the spring balance with mechanical or electrical dynamometers.

3.3.3 Apparatus

The cable tensiometer and/or strain-gauge dynamometer are based on mechanical principles. Manometric dynamometers were much used in the past. Now electric and/or electronic dynamometers are used under laboratory conditions. These apparatuses are sometimes constructed as prototypes for specific research purposes in different laboratories. Certain types are also available from firms (e.g. Hottiger, FRG).

3.3.4 Procedure

The test may be carried out either using the relatively simple technique of cable tensiometry, or strain-gauge dynamometers. Under laboratory conditions, the muscular strength of flexors and extensors is usually assessed by means of an electric dynamometer constructed on the tensiometric principle. The muscle strength measurements at the following positions have been recommended:

1. Backward extension of the trunk;
2. Leg extension;
3. Knee extension;
4. Forward flexion of the trunk;
5. Horizontal push.

In particular studies the impact of environmental conditions, including nutrition, on muscle strength in absolute Newtons (N) and relative values (N . kg^{-1}) in boys and girls was ascertained: trunk extensors, elbow-joint flexors and extensors, knee-joint flexors and extensors, plantar flexors, and hand-grip strength.

Under field conditions, hand-grip strength measurements can be carried out with the help of hand-grip dynamometers. The instrument should be adjusted so that the second joint of the forefinger flexes on the gripping bar of the dynamometer at a right angle. The instrument should be adjusted to a comfortable grip. The scale reading before gripping should be half the distance from the tip of the thumb to the tip of the fingers. The handle must be locked after rotation. The subject is allowed to try the apparatus, and then the best of the three readings is taken with the subject gripping as he flexes the forearm. The test is performed on each arm in turn. A note is made as to which hand is dominant.

Calculation

The values of muscle strength are read in Newtons (N). Both absolute values (N) and/or relative values are given (N . kg^{-1} body weight, or N . kg^{-1} lean body mass), which may be compared with reference values (see below).

3.3.5 Performance characteristics

(a) Reproducibility

The standard error of estimation is approximately 4–6%.

(b) Validity

No validity tests are available at present.

3.3.6 Reference values

Reference values of muscle strength have been given by Hettinger [11], Asmussen and Heeball-Nielsen [12], Dal Monte [13], Collins and Weiner [4] and others. In Table 3.1 the values of hand-grip strength (the most often measured) from 3762 men and women in age categories 12, 15, 18, 25, 35, 45, and 55 years are given. The age tabulation was made by extrapolation and intrapolation from 11 to 21 years at one-year intervals and from 21 to 59 at two-year intervals [8].

Table 3.1   Hand-grip strength: right and left hand (N)

Men		Age	Women	
R	L	(years)	R	L
183	170	11	180	166
234	216	12	206	190
282	259	13	228	209
324	299	14	245	225
361	332	15	258	238
390	360	16	268	247
413	381	17	276	255
431	399	18	282	260
445	413	19	287	264
456	422	20	290	267
464	430	21	293	270
475	441	23	296	273
482	448	25	298	275
486	451	27	299	275
488	453	29	299	275
489	454	31	299	275
489	454	33	298	275
489	453	35	297	274
488	453	37	296	273
487	451	39	295	272
486	450	41	294	271
485	449	43	293	269
484	447	45	292	268
483	446	47	291	267
482	444	49	290	266
479	443	51	288	265
479	441	53	287	263
478	440	55	286	262
477	438	57	285	261
475	436	59	283	259

3.4 MOTOR PERFORMANCE

3.4.1 Purpose and scope

A great variety of simple tests are in use among researchers. Most of these are not specific for testing general working performance, especially in children. Nevertheless, some basic motor abilities (speed, coordination, etc.) are characterized by these tests, and the results are comparable with data from the countries where they have been widely used.

One of the most commonly used battery of motor tests is that of AAHPER (American Association for Health, Physical Education and Recreation), consisting of seven items:

(a) Pull-ups;
(b) Sit-ups;
(c) Shuttle run;
(d) Standing broad jump;
(e) 50-yard dash;
(f) Soft-ball throw for distance;
(g) 600-yard run-walk.

At present in Europe similar items in the framework of Eurofit testing, are used mostly for evaluating physical performance and fitness in children and adolescents.

The International Biological Programme (IBP) [3] suggested the measurement and evaluation of pull-ups (in the original and/or modified form), straddle-chinning, flexed arm hang, sit-ups, shuttle-run, standing broad jump, 50-yard dash, soft-ball throw for distance, etc. Most measurements were done in groups of subjects from 12 to 55 years, especially performance in standing broad jump (characterizing the explosive strength of the lower limbs) and ball throw (2 kg; strength of upper limbs, and coordination).

The distance covered in 12 minutes is also used as a criterion of motor abilities, namely endurance capacity. The results can also be used to calculate oxygen consumption.

The above-mentioned tests characterize mainly gross motor development. There are also tests for fine motorics, i.e. tests for accuracy of movement, tests for coordination of hand movements, and so forth. However, these tests are mainly used by psychologists, work physiologists, researchers involved in studies of child development, etc. Some of the tests may of course also be suitable for checking nutritional status.

3.4.2 Principle of methods and procedures

(a) Pull-ups

The pull-ups test for male subjects is performed hanging from a beam high enough for the feet to be clear of the floor when the arms are fully extended. The overhand grasp is used. The subject raises his body by his arms until his chin is above the bar and then lowers himself to the straight position. No swinging of the body or kicking of the legs is permitted. The exercise is repeated as often as possible without resting, and the score is the number of complete pull-ups achieved.

Modified pull-up. In the modified pull-up for female subjects a horizontal bar, set at about chest level, is grasped with both hands, using an overhand grasp. The subject extends her legs under the bar and extends her arms fully. The arms should form a 90° angle with the straight trunk and the legs should form an angle of 45° with the floor. The heels should be braced (for instance against the scorer's feet) to prevent slipping. From this position, keeping the body straight, the subject raises herself by the arms until the chest touches the bar and then returns to the starting position. No resting is permitted. The score is the number of completed pull-ups to a maximum of 40.

Flexed arm hang. The subject pulls herself up with an overhand grasp on a horizontal bar at her own standing height until her chin is above the level of the bar. The score is the number of seconds that this position can be maintained.

Straddle chinning. This is a second alternative to the modified pull-up for female subjects. The subject lies supine and grasps the hands of a partner standing astride her. Keeping the body straight, she pulls herself up by her arms until her trunk touches the inside of her partner's thighs, in this position the arms should be parallel to the trunk, and then lowers herself to the starting position. The exercise is repeated as often as possible and the score is the number of complete straddle chinnings achieved.

(b) Sit-ups

The sit-up test is performed with the subject lying supine on the floor with the legs extended and feet about 60 cm apart. The hands are placed on the back of the neck with the fingers interlaced and the elbows against the floor. A partner holds the ankles down and acts as scorer. To perform the test, the subject sits up turning the trunk to the left and touching the right elbow to the left knee and returns to the starting position; then sits up turning the trunk to the right and touching the left elbow to the right knee. The exercise is repeated, alternating sides. In scoring, one point is given for each complete movement of touching elbow to knee. No score is counted if the fingertips do not maintain contact behind the head, if the knees are bent when the subject lies on his back, or when he begins to sit, or if he pushes up off the floor with an elbow. The original test specifies a maximum score, but to abolish this arbitrary limit it is recommended that the maximum number of sit-ups achieved in one minute be scored.

(c) Shuttle-run

For the shuttle-run two parallel lines are marked on the floor 9.2 m apart, and two small blocks of wood ($5 \times 5 \times 10$ cm) are placed beyond one of the lines. Starting from behind the other line the subject runs to the blocks, picks one up, runs back to the starting line and places the block behind the line, runs back and picks up the second block and runs back with it across the starting line (Fig. 3.2). At least two scorers should be present with stop-watches so that at least two subjects can run at the same time. Two trials are allowed, with a rest between. The score is the shorter of the two times, to the nearest tenth of a second.

(d) Standing broad jump

For the standing broad jump the subject stands with feet apart and toes just behind the take-off line. To prepare for jumping the subject swings the arms backwards and bends the knees.

The jump is accomplished by simultaneously extending the knees and swinging the arms forward. The jump is measured to the point nearest the take-off lines where the heel or other part of the body touches the floor. Three trials are allowed and the score is the longest of the three jumps measured to the nearest centimetre.

(e) 50-yard dash

This test is performed by two or more subjects at a time, depending on the number of timers with stopwatches available. The starter drops his arm on the

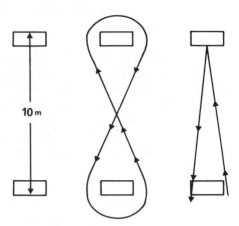

Fig. 3.2 Shuttle-run.

command 'go' to give the timer a visual signal. This test is performed once only and the score is the time taken to run 50 yards (46 m) measured to the nearest tenth of a second.

(f) Soft-ball throw for distance

A standard 30.5 cm circumference soft-ball is used. Starting from a line 2 metres behind the take-off line the subject throws the soft-ball overhand from behind the take-off line as far as possible. The throw is measured from the point of landing to the nearest point on the take-off line. Three throws are allowed, and the score is the furthest of the three throws, measured to the nearest 25 cm.

(g) 600-yard run-walk

The score for this test is the time taken for the subject to cover 600 yards (551 m) measured if possible with a stopwatch to the nearest tenth of a second. The test is performed once only.

3.4.3 Performance characteristics

(a) Reproducibility

The measurements of motor performance may vary according to the actual fitness level, absence or presence of fatigue due to previous physical work-load, level of satiety and so forth. Skill tests may be more easily repeated than longer runs. Characteristic patterns for motor abilities can be found among individuals. Few repeated reliable measurements have been performed up to now under precisely comparable conditions.

(b) Validity

The results of the whole battery of motor tests give valid information on the individual items of motor skills as well as the general level of physical fitness as regards motor abilities.

3.4.4 Reference values

Data from IBP [3, 4] may be used as reference values. More recently AAHPER test results, and Eurofit results have been made available [6].

**3.5 FINAL
COMMENTS**

For all these indicators of physical fitness and work performance some standard values for different population groups with regard to age, sex, physical activity regimens, occupational work-load, etc. have already been established in some industrially developed countries. These standard values are much rarer than those for morphological measurements, such as height and weight. More data for establishing general norms and standards are needed.

With regard to nutritional status, most representative evaluation can be given by a complex of data. Along with basic anthropometric measurements and body composition assessment, tests of functional capacity as characterized by aerobic power, muscle strength, and when possible also by motor performance and skill should be used to complete the nutritional characteristics of the organism.

REFERENCES

1. Pařízková, J. (1982) Nutrition and work performance, in *Critical Reviews in Tropical Medicine*, Vol. 1 (ed. R.K. Chandra), Plenum Press, New York, pp. 307–33.
2. Åstrand, P.O. and Rodahl, K. (1989) *Textbook of work physiology*, 3rd edn, McGraw-Hill Book Company, New York.
3. Weiner, J.S. and Lourie, J.A. (1969) *Human Biology: A Guide to Field Methods*, Blackwell Scientific, Oxford (out of print).
4. Collins, K.J. and Weiner, J.S. (1977) *Human Adaptability. International Biological Programme. A History and Compendium of Research*, Taylor and Francis, London.
5. Shepherd, R.J. (1978) *Human Physiological Work Capacity. International Biological Programme No 15*, Cambridge University Press, Cambridge.
6. Committee of Experts on Sports Research: Eurofit. (1988) *Handbook for the EUROFIT Tests of Physical Fitness*, Rome.
7. Pařízková, J., Adamec, A., Berdychová, J. *et al.* (1984) *Growth, Fitness and Nutrition in Preschool Children*, Charles University, Prague.
8. Seliger, V. and Bartůněk, Z. (eds) (1976) *Mean Values of Various Indices of Physical Fitness in the Investigation of Czechoslovak Population Aged 23–55 Years*, Czechoslovak Association of Physical Culture (ČSTV), Praha.
9. Weiner, J.S. and Lourie, J.A. (1981) *Practical Human Biology*, Academic Press, London.
10. Seliger, V. and Bartůněk, Z. (1977) *Tělesná Zdatnost Obyvatelstva ČSSR ve Věku 12–55r*, Universita Karlova, Praha.
11. Hettinger, T. (1957) *Theorie und Praxis der Körperkultur. Sonderheft 1957*, **6**, 57.
12. Asmussen, E. and Heeball-Nielsen, K. (1961) Isometric muscle strength of adult men and women. *Comm. Dan. Nat. Ass. Infant Paral.*, **11**, 3–43.
13. Dal Monte, A. (1983) *La valutazione funzionale dell'atleta*. Sansoni, Firenze.

4 Energy balance methodology

4.1 Introduction   *A. Ferro-Luzzi and N.G. Norgan*   113
4.2 Energy intake   *A. Ferro-Luzzi and N.G. Norgan*   115
4.3 Energy expenditure   *G. Pastore and A. Ferro-Luzzi*   117

4.1 INTRODUCTION

Energy balance can be described by the energy balance equation:

Energy intake − Energy expenditure = change in energy stores

As energy intake is discontinuous but energy expenditure is continuous, man is constantly alternating between positive and negative energy balance. Thus, energy balance must be expressed over some time period, usually one day. Short-term daily energy balance can be described by energy intake and energy expenditure alone, as fluctuations in energy stores are likely to be small in everyday life. Over longer period of time measurements of energy intake and energy expenditure become problematic and energy balance may be approximated by measures of changing energy stores. However, there is much to recommend simultaneous measurements of the three components of energy balance, as none of them can be assessed with any degree of accuracy and pitfalls exist in attempting to describe energy balance from one or two of its components.

The overall purpose of energy balance assessment is similar to that of other types of nutritional status assessment, i.e. to ascertain if an individual or a group of individuals are optimally nourished, with a view to formulating and implementing appropriate action to improve or restore the level of nutritional health.

As with the nutrients, the scope of energy balance assessment should involve much more than nutritional aspects. The reasons for undernutrition and overnutrition often lie far removed from the questions of the availability of food or the opportunities for exercise and work. For the appropriate remedial action to be implemented these origins must be identified. It is rarely necessary to allocate individuals or groups into more than three categories of nutritional health, such as good, marginal and poor. This should allow three courses of action, namely no action, investigate further or again in the near future, and action required now. However, the methods may need to be accurate and precise to ensure high sensitivity and specificity.

Why measure energy balance in the assessment of nutritional status? Energy nutritional status cannot be described from measurements of energy intake alone. Energy intake can be compared to figures of requirements or, even better, to figures of measured energy expenditure. However, it is advisable to bear in mind that energy balance is only a proxy for functional capacities, which are the real indicators of energy nutritional status.

We propose that the recommended energy balance methodology for free-living subjects following their everyday lives is the conventional seven-day weighed food intake, diary record of activities with measured energy cost of the activities, plus a measure of energy stores. This may characterize individuals well enough for the purpose of grouping subjects into one of the three categories of energy balance and, ultimately, of energy nutritional status. However, there are major reservations about the validity of this methodology:

The method is lengthy and expensive;
The appropriate methodology will depend on the problems being investigated.

We ourselves share these reservations but, whilst investigating alternatives, we do not advocate change until the new is shown to be superior to the familiar. Also, impure data is less of a problem than impure usage: impure data used conservatively can be useful; good data used unscientifically is dangerous.

Regarding the interpretation of energy balance data, a state of balance (energy intake = energy expenditure) is not by itself evidence of energy well-being. It may be found in adaptation to undernutrition and static obesity. Levels of energy stores may not add further useful information: long-distance runners may have very low energy stores yet be capable of sustained heavy work. Therefore, a judgment of a level of energy balance is necessary.

The convention is to measure energy balance over seven days. This may be too short a period for many individuals. The number of days necessary for achieving a desired degree of accuracy in the individual energy balance results, in relation to its specified variability, has been calculated with the formula of Beaton *et al.* [1] and the results for a situation of moderately high and moderately low intraindividual variability are presented in Fig. 4.1. Seasonal variations require repeated measurements.

Any report giving energy balance data should describe fully the methods used, as suggested by Durnin and Ferro-Luzzi [2], in order that the information can be fully appraised.

In view of the reservations about the methods of energy balance that can be applied to free-living subjects, the effort and expense required to collect data and the problems in interpreting energy balance data – caused partly by lack of precision of the methods and the possibility of adaptation to varying planes of nutrition – it is not recommended that measurements of energy balance be included in routine assessment of nutritional status. Levels or changes in energy stores or growth determined anthropometrically will be a much more cost-effective approach. Measurements of energy balance are, however, well-employed in examining nutritional enigmas, e.g. populations with low intakes but without widespread malnutrition [3]. Even here definite answers have not been forthcoming. When applied to normal, healthy subjects, the methodology has posed as many questions as it has answered [4]. There therefore seems little reason to recommend the direct measurement of energy balance in most assessments of nutritional status.

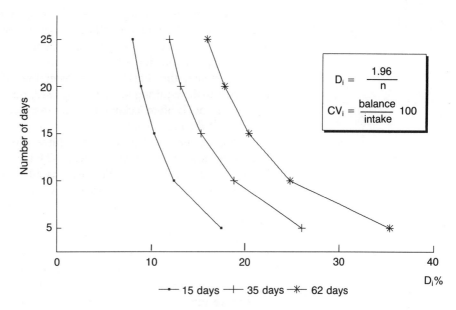

$$D_i = \frac{1.96}{n}$$

$$CV_i = \frac{balance}{intake} 100$$

—•— 15 days —+— 35 days —*— 62 days

Fig. 4.1 Percent deviation of individual observed mean energy balances from true mean (D_i), with increasing number of days of observation, at 95% confidence. (CV_i = coefficient of interindividual variation).

4.2 ENERGY INTAKE

4.2.1 Purpose and scope

Data on energy intake are obtained by means of dietary surveys. Dietary survey methodology is very flexible and versatile; for these reasons it can be utilized for a multiplicity of purposes such as the assessment of current consumption by individuals, or by groups of individuals, or at the household level. It can also serve to provide retrospective information on dietary intakes, etc. In epidemiological studies it may be sufficient to consistently classify subjects according to a specified nutrient intake. The scope of these types of studies would be to correlate groups by the association of specific dietary profiles with the prevalence of a given biochemical or functional disorder on a group basis.

4.2.2 Generalities

Three basic recent publications are at the moment available. The first one is a EURO-NUT report on *The diet factor in epidemiological research* [5]; the second is a review of S.A. Bingham on *The dietary assessment of individuals: methods, accuracy, new techniques and recommendations* [6]; and the third is a Handbook from the IUNS Committee on Food Consumption Surveys [7]. We refer the reader to the above publications for any further information.

It will suffice here to emphasize that the dietary survey should be regarded as a scientific tool, and as such should be handled with skill and care: it needs to be tested over all its components to verify its working conditions; it must be calibrated to avoid bias in the results; it must be standardized to allow the comparability of the data, etc. The apparent simplicity of the survey methods masks inherent multiple difficulties that stem from the rather large subjective component of the technique, from the risk of introducing undesirable and unrecognized behavioural modifications, and from the limited precision of the various components of the technique (tables of food composition, sampling techniques, intraindividual variance, etc.).

Furthermore, the dietary survey technique, if properly carried out, is an expensive tool, requiring skilled manpower, time, organization, etc. Recognition of this fact is often lacking. In order to reduce the costs and to alleviate the pressure of the high degree of co-operation required from the subjects by the more precise methodology of dietary intake, a number of simplified versions have been developed and used, such as 24-hour recall techniques, the dietary history, questionnaires, etc. The main problem with these simplified versions based on interviews is their high subjective component, and the resultant loss of reliability. The respondents being mostly untrained in nutrition, their replies inevitably reflect their subjective ability to recall, to average through time, to estimate and quantify exact portion sizes, etc. This ability is not a fixed characteristic and varies with age, sex, culture, ethnicity, time-span covered, environment, existence of a defined eating pattern, and the interviewer's ability to probe the subjects deep enough without eliciting the phenomenon of retroactive interference. Forgetting curves are different and identity between responses in original and interpolated activities yields facilitation while differences between responses yield interference of forgetting [8]. The effect of the interviewer may also differ in relation to his or her training, background,

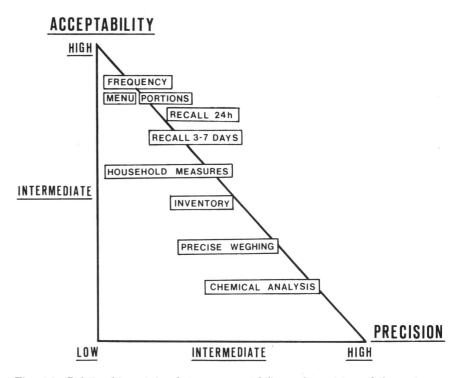

Fig. 4.2 Relationship existing between acceptability and precision of the various methods for assessing individual dietary intakes.

personality, etc. [9, 10]. This creates problems of comparability when different interviewers are used in the same survey, or in different surveys [9].

As a general introductory statement it can be reasonably said that the precision and validity of the results of a survey technique are in inverse relation to the acceptability of the survey by the subjects, (Fig. 4.2 [11]).

Although the precise weighing methodology for assessing individual dietary intake is a putative gold standard and is considered as a valuable reference and check for less reliable techniques, it is far from being immune from faults, limitations, and imprecision. The factors that can affect the reliability of the results of a dietary survey can be grouped under three major headings:

1. The first is related to the ability to assess correctly and precisely the energy that is actually consumed during the observation period (measurement error).
2. The second factor relates to the actual representativity of the observation period in relation to the time frame to which the data are extrapolated (weeks, months, seasons, etc.) and are influenced by the intraindividual variability ('construct validity') [12].
3. The third factor relates to the changes brought about in the habitual dietary habits by 'observational interference'. This would be a special case of 'construct validity'.

Double-labelled water, recently shown as an accurate method for measuring energy expenditure, can be used to validate energy intake assessed by any dietary record methods, as indicated by Bingham [6, 13]. Recent improvements to diet record methods have been suggested to correct for the large daily variation usually present [14]. More complex statistical analysis, taking into account the ratio of between-individual and within-individual variance, have been suggested.

4.3 ENERGY EXPENDITURE

4.3.1 Purpose and scope

Energy expenditure measurements are needed for the definition of the energy requirement of an individual or a community, as set out in the 1985 FAO/WHO/UNU Expert Consultation recommendations [15]. Energy expenditure assessments may also be useful when monitoring the dynamic evolution of the energy nutritional status of both individuals and groups.

Metabolically useful energy is 'produced' through the oxidation of nutrients and is used to perform chemical work (biosynthesis), osmotic work (generating ion gradients), and mechanical work (muscular contraction). Heat released during oxidation and work maintains body temperature in man. The total energy expenditure of an individual is composed of several parts:

1. Basal metabolic rate (BMR), which includes the cost of tissue maintenance and the internal work of the body.
2. Energy expended to perform physical work.

3. Diet-induced thermogenesis, namely the increase in the rate of resting energy expenditure in response to feeding.
4. Energy needed for the synthesis of tissues, during growth, pregnancy, lactation, and any deposition of muscular and/or adipose tissue.
5. Cold-induced thermogenesis, namely any extra energy for maintaining body temperature in extreme environmental conditions.

The largest proportion of the total energy expended by man is associated with BMR. In an average 70-kg man, BMR may represent 60–75% of total energy output [16]. The highest energy turnover per gram of tissue is found in the liver, brain, heart and kidneys. Under resting conditions these organs utilize between 60% and 70% of the total energy expenditure while accounting for only 6% of the body weight [17].

Physical activity contributes under normal conditions about 15–30% of total daily expenditure [16]. Obviously, this proportion is highly variable and depends upon the activity pattern (i.e. the intensity, type, and duration of the work), the muscle masses involved in the activity, and the weight of the subject.

Dietary-induced thermogenesis accounts for about 10% of total energy expenditure [16]. The highest increase in energy expenditure associated with food is that found in response to the ingestion of protein or aminoacids (10–35% of the ingested food energy) [17]; much lower values follow the intake of carbohydrates and fats (2–5%).

4.3.2 Approaches to energy expenditure assessment

The methods can be grouped into three major classes: direct measurement of the heat released by the body (direct calorimetry), indirect measure of heat by monitoring the oxygen used to oxidize the nutrients (indirect calorimetry), and non-calorimetric methods. The first two approaches rely on the first law of thermodynamics, which states that when the chemical energy content of a system changes, the sum of all the forms of energy given off or absorbed by the system will be equal to the magnitude of the change.

(a) Direct calorimetry

Direct calorimetry is based on the principle that all energy used by the body for both external or internal work is ultimately liberated as heat. The measurement of the sum of radiant heat losses and of convective, conductive, and evaporative heat transfer is thus the fundamental measure of energy expenditure.

(b) Indirect calorimetry

It can safely be assumed that all the oxygen consumed by the body is used to oxidize degradable fuels and produces carbon dioxide. The total amount of energy 'produced' is assessed from the total oxygen consumption and/or the carbon dioxide production. The body has only a very small oxygen storage capacity, so oxygen consumption rises immediately in response to the demand for extra internal or external work.

(c) Non-calorimetric methods

This third approach relies on predicting the relationship between various physiological phenomena, e.g. heart rate or pulmonary ventilation, and the oxygen consumed by the body.

In this chapter only indirect calorimetry will be considered, since the others are of limited practical interest in the present context, which is the assessment of total energy output in free-living populations.

4.3.3 Principles of indirect calorimetry

The two approaches include the traditional measurement of oxygen uptake, and the new 'doubly labelled water method' (DLW), based on estimating carbon dioxide production.

The DLW method is based upon the instantaneous equilibrium reached between oxygen in the body's bicarbonate pool and body water. This means that by labelling body water with both deuterium and oxygen 18 it is possible to estimate the total carbon dioxide produced in the body. The turnover in the body of oxygen 18 exceeds that of deuterium, since the labelled oxygen in body water will be diluted by unlabelled CO_2 production and water intake, whereas the deuterium label will be diluted only by the inflow of unlabelled water. Thus the difference between the two turnovers reflects CO_2 production.

The advantages of the $D_2^{18}O$ method are significant: it allows an unrestricted pattern of behaviour of subjects and it is totally non-invasive, since the stable isotopes are given orally and small urine samples are used to monitor body water labelling. Increasing evidence suggests that the technique – using standardized protocols, measurement techniques, and specific assumptions on isotopic fractionation – can be applied validly to infants, sick patients, and other groups who are difficult to study by other methods.

The principal drawbacks of the $D_2^{18}O$ method are the high costs of the labelled oxygen (isotope 18) and of the analytical equipment (mass spectrometer). Furthermore, highly skilled personnel are needed to perform the analyses. Other problems relating to the assumptions about isotopic loss from the body continue to be investigated.

The traditional indirect calorimetry methods monitor oxygen consumption. They may be grouped into long-, middle- and short-term calorimetry.

Long- and middle-term calorimetry are those using either calorimetric chambers or ventilated hoods. A stream of air is directed over the subject thereby mixing with the expired air; a sample of the mixed air is then collected. In the ventilated hood the sample is collected from a transparent Perspex hood placed over the subject's head, whereas in calorimetric chambers the air is sampled either in the chamber or from the chamber outflow. The rate of energy expenditure can then be calculated by determining the flow rate of air through the hood or chamber and the oxygen and carbon dioxide concentrations of the incoming and outgoing air.

Short-term calorimetry differs from the above because the undiluted expired air is directly sampled and analysed for its O_2 and CO_2 content. Douglas bags are used with a mouthpiece and nose-clip attached to a respiratory gas valve for collecting expired air. The Kofranyi–Michaelis (KM) meter may be used for collecting expired breaths while subjects move about. The KM meter takes a precise proportion of the expired air for analysis and thereby avoids the need to collect large volumes of air.

Calorimetric chambers and ventilated hoods are more comfortable because subjects are able to breathe naturally without having to use a mask or a mouthpiece. If a mask is used leakage is also a potential source of error, and when mouthpiece and nose-clip are used the subject may experience various discomforts [18]. On the other hand the ventilated hood can be used only for static activities (e.g. monitoring basal, resting, or sleeping metabolic rates). Calorimetric chambers only simulate real-life activities of free-living individuals. An accurate description of the calorimetric chambers or ventilated hoods may be found elsewhere [19–21].

In this chapter only the short-term calorimetry method by Douglas bags or by Kofranyi–Michaelis respiration gas meter will be considered, and the so-called factorial method will be described so that the reader can apply the method to free-living subjects.

4.3.4 Assessment of daily energy expenditure in free-living individuals

The most popular method for assessing daily energy expenditure is the so-called factorial method. This method relies on the accurate description and timing of activities over each hour of the day, and on the measurements of the energy cost of each activity. Thus the daily total energy expenditure (TEE) of an individual is the sum of the products of the duration of each activity multiplied by its energy cost.

Estimation of the daily energy expenditure is performed in three stages. Firstly, an accurate account of all the time spent on each and every activity by the subject is required. Several days, e.g. a week, may be needed if representative habitual activity pattern is to be assessed. Changes at weekends and with season must also be considered. Secondly, the energy cost of each activity needs to be measured by means of reliable short-term calorimetry. (When the energy cost of activities cannot be assessed directly it is possible to derive approximate values from the literature [22].) Finally, the integration of the data on time allocation with those of their energy cost have to be performed for each individual.

The next section will describe in some detail the apparatus, procedures, and calculation required for applying the factorial method.

(a) Time and motion assessment

A timed record of activities is normally made by using a specially designed diary. Only a watch and a diary are needed. Activities are recorded minute by minute. A shorthand notation for activities can be developed, and simple code letters are often employed for the most usual activities of the day (Fig. 4.3).

Whenever possible the subject should be continuously observed in order to record data more reliably. This technique, although expensive, constraining, and complex yields data of high accuracy and reliability.

When an observer cannot be used subjects may be asked to keep a record of their own activities. Their diaries should be checked daily by skilled personnel, first to verify that all the 1440 minutes of the day have been accounted for, and secondly to settle any difficulties in classifying activities.

An even simpler method involves an interview that examines the previous day(s)' activities. In this case the recall of the time devoted to each activity can be assisted by subdividing the day into short intervals of time. This method requires that the subject has a reliable memory and that the interviewer is highly skilled. The method is cheaper than the recorded time–motion technique, since one observer may follow a large number of individuals simultaneously. It has also the advantage that the subject is not influenced by the continued presence of an observer and will not tend to modify his or her activity pattern.

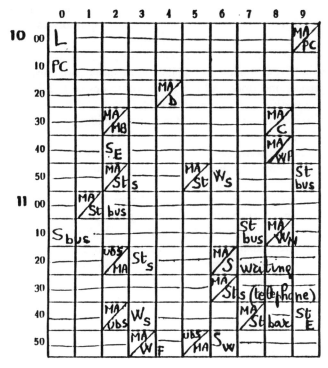

Fig. 4.3 Page from an activity diary.

(b) Energy cost of activities

The energy cost of the various activities can be measured by means either of Douglas bag technique (for static activities) or of the Kofranyi–Michaelis respiration gas meter. For both procedures the technique consists of two stages, the first one during which expired air is measured (KM) or collected (Douglas bag), and the second stage during which expired air is analysed for its gas concentration.

4.3.5 Apparatus

Douglas bags of leakproof PVC, fitted with an inlet (1 inch diameter) and a sampling tube (0.5 cm diameter), capacity from 50 to 200 litres. Douglas bags are convenient for the collection and temporary storage of expired air during static activities.

Kofranyi–Michaelis respiration gas meter (KM). The use of a KM meter is particularly indicated when the activities to be measured involve displacement of the body, as it allows considerable freedom of movements. It is a lightweight backpack, with an inbuilt gas-meter for the measure of the volume of exhaled air. An enclosed thermometer measures the temperature of the expired air. A sampling device automatically samples 0.3% or 0.6% of each breath and stores it in a bag for later analysis. The instrument needs to be regularly calibrated. For this procedure see Consolazio *et al.* [19] and/or Durnin and Brockway [23]. The KM weighs about 3 kg and is worn on the back using shoulder harnesses. More detailed description may be found elsewhere [19, 22, 23].

Three-way stopcocks with low dead-space, of light metal, connected to the Douglas bag's inlet on one side and to the tubing and respiratory valve on another side. The third arm is open to the atmosphere.

Two-way respiratory valves, low dead-space, low flow resistance, low weight. There are several different models in commerce, of various weights, flow resistance, dead-space, and price. All are fitted with a device to allow for unidirectional air flow. (For description see [19].)

Several segments of 1-inch diameter corrugated rubber tubing.

Mouthpiece, nose-clips, stopwatch, clamps.

Sampling bags, 2–3 litres capacity, rubber or, preferably, PVC.

Gas meter, wet or dry, regularly calibrated, with dial or digital reading of 0.05 litres, and a capacity of at least 50 litres/minute.

Barometer, either mercury or aneroid, sensitive to 0.5 mmHg.

Oxygen analyser. Oxygen concentration of expired gases can be measured either with paramagnetic or polarographic analysers of high sensitivity and stability. The paramagnetic analysers are based upon the magnetic susceptibility of oxygen. Polarographic oxygen detectors consist essentially of an electrochemical transducer that responds to changes in the partial pressure of the oxygen.

Carbon dioxide analyser. CO_2 concentration is normally determined by non-dispersive infra-red absorption technique. This is based on the property of polyatomic non-elemental gases to absorb radiations in the middle infra-red region of the spectrum.

Calibration gas cylinders of certified concentration. Pure nitrogen, carbon dioxide in nitrogen, and oxygen in nitrogen are required; the composition of these mixtures must be defined according to the recommendation of the analysers' manuals.

4.3.6 Procedure

Respiratory gases must be collected in a rigorously leak-free manner. Errors can easily occur either as contamination of the sample with atmospheric air, or as undetected leaks to the atmosphere.

(a) The Douglas bag technique

After having emptied the Douglas bag completely, either manually or by a vacuum pump, the subject is connected to it by means of a three-way tap, a length of corrugated tubing, and a respiratory valve. The subject's nose is closed with a nose-clip. The absence of leaks either from the nostrils or the mouth is accurately checked. The three-way tap is open to the atmosphere. Allow enough time for the subject to equilibrate and reach a steady state. During this time the tubing and connection will be washed out with expired air. The steady state has been reached when there is a balance between the oxygen requirement and the oxygen supply; under these condition O_2 consumption, CO_2 production, body temperature, pulse rate and respiration rate are kept at a fairly constant level.

Start the measure by turning the three-way-stopcock to connect the subject to the Douglas bag, and simultaneously note the time to the nearest second.

The collection of expired air should last either about 10 minutes, or until there are at least 50 litres of expired air in the bag.

Heart rate and respiratory rate may be re⌐
measure to provide an indication of the steady

At the end of the measure, close the th⌐
record the duration of the collection to the near⌐
subject. To improve the accuracy of the measure, the who⌐
repeated twice or thrice at brief intervals.

Mix the Douglas bag's contents by kneading vigorously a few ⌐
remove a measured aliquot (1.5 litres) for gas analysis. Care must be exer⌐
not to contaminate the aliquot with atmospheric gases. (For details see [19].)

The volume of the air in the Douglas bag is measured by passing the whole bag's content through a calibrated gas meter at a constant steady rate. The volume of the expired air must be read to the nearest 0.05 litres.

Gas temperature, measured at the outlet of the gas-meter, should be recorded to the nearest 0.5°C. Record the barometric pressure to the nearest 0.5 mmHg.

(b) KM technique

This portable instrument can be used to measure the energy costs of activities requiring that freedom of movement of the subject is unhampered. It is not advisable to use the KM for measuring static, low-energy-cost activities, because of the unreliable reproducibility of the instrument at low ventilation rates.

The KM is strapped on the back of the subject by two shoulder harnesses. After closing the nose with a nose-clip and fitting a mouthpiece to the subject, leaks from the respiratory valve, mouth, and nose are checked. An empty sampling bag is attached and clamped at the proper outlet of the KM. The selection of aliquot of each breath to be sampled should be set (0.3% or 0.6%) according to the expected ventilation rate.

Initial meter reading and initial temperature are recorded: the subject is invited to start performing the selected task. Allow enough time to reach the steady state (1–3 minutes, according to the intensity of the activity), and to flush all tubing of the KM with expired air.

To begin the measure, the sample bag is unclamped, the watch started and, simultaneously, the meter engaged by turning the appropriate switch. The duration of the measure will depend on the ventilation rate and should allow at least 50–100 litres to be passed through the gas meter.

At the end of the measure the meter is switched off and the time simultaneously recorded at the nearest second. The sampling bag is clamped and the temperature and volume of expired air ar noted.

The content of the sampling bag should be analysed immediately in order to minimize gas diffusion through the rubber walls. To limit such diffusion the use of PVC sampling bags is preferable.

(c) Calculations

Each component is considered separately for simplicity.

Pulmonary ventilation. The pulmonary ventilation ($\dot{V}$) is the mass movement of gas in and out of the lungs. In adults the resting $\dot{V}$ may range between 4 and 6 litres per minute; it can reach 80–150 l/min during physical activities of various intensity, and during very hard work and on trained subjects can reach as much as 180–220 l/min.

The $\dot{V}$ is calculated according to the following equation:

$$\dot{V} = \frac{(V2 - V1) + VS}{Time} \cdot \text{gas meter factor} \cdot \text{STPD factor}.$$

where:
$\dot{V}$ = litres/minute of expired air, STPD (0°C, 760 mmHg, dry); V1 = Initial reading of the gas meter (litres); V2 = Final reading of the gas meter (litres); VS = Volume of the sample taken for the analysis (litres); Time = Time of gas collection (minutes); gas meter factor = Value for correcting constant errors (if any) of the gas meter; STPD factor = Value for reducing the volume of the gas to that at 0°C and 760 mmHg, in a dry state (Table 4.1).

Table 4.1 Equation to transform a given volume of gas to STPD

STPD factor = $[1-(PW/P)] \, (P/760) \, [273/(273+t)]$	
STPD factor	= Value for reducing a given volume of gas to that at 0°C and 760 mmHg, in a dry state
PW	= Water Pressure
P	= Atmospheric pressure
t	= Temperature (°C)

True oxygen of expired air. The true oxygen represents the millilitres of oxygen consumed for every 100 ml of expired air; it is the quantity of O_2 removed from the inhaled air.

$$\text{True oxygen} = FE \, N_2 \cdot (FI \, O_2 / FI \, N_2) - FE \, O_2$$
$$\text{True oxygen} = [100 - (FE \, O_2 + FE \, CO_2)] \cdot 0.265 - FE \, O_2$$

where:
$FE \, N_2$ = nitrogen concentration in expired air (%); $FE \, O_2$ = oxygen concentration in expired air (%); $FE \, CO_2$ = carbon dioxide concentration in expired air (%); $FI \, O_2$ = oxygen concentration in inspired air (%); $FI \, N_2$ = nitrogen concentration in inspired air (%).

True carbon dioxide of expired air. The true carbon dioxide represents the millilitres of CO_2 produced for every 100 ml of expired air.

$$\text{True carbon dioxide} = FE \, CO_2 - FI \, CO_2$$

where:
$FE \, CO_2$ = carbon dioxide concentration in expired air; $FI \, CO_2$ = carbon dioxide concentration in inspired air (0.03 for outdoor air).

Respiratory quotient (RQ).

$$RQ = \frac{\text{True carbon dioxide}}{\text{True oxygen}}$$

RQ is the ratio of CO_2 produced to O_2 consumed.

In normal resting condition RQ is on average 0.82 [19]; after 12–18 h fast most energy is derived from fatty acids, so the RQ tends towards 0.7. After a light meal RQ approaches the value of 1.0 (Table 4.2). There are a number of physiological conditions that may spuriously modify the RQ. The production of lactic acid during heavy exercise provokes the liberation of extra CO_2 from the bicarbonate pool and raises the RQ up to values as high as 1.5. After exercise the reverse process occurs, causing CO_2 to be trapped as bicarbonate and lowering RQ even below 0.7. Hyperventilation can cause washing out of CO_2 in excess of the amount produced in the oxidation of substrates, resulting in an RQ greater than 1.0; hypoventilation can reduce the RQ to values below 0.7.

Table 4.2 O_2 consumption, CO_2 production, value of RQ, and energy output for the oxidation of different organic substrata

	O_2 cons. (ml/g)	CO_2 prod. (ml/g)	RQ	Energy (kcal/g)
Starch	829	829	1.000	4.183
Animal fat	2019	1427	0.707	9.461
Protein	966	782	0.809	4.442

Moreover, lipogenesis gluconeogenesis and ketone-body metabolism may also potentially modify the RQ value. More details about these metabolic processes and their relation with the RQ value have been described elsewhere [24].

Oxygen consumption and carbon dioxide production.

$$\text{Oxygen consumption} = \text{True oxygen} \cdot \dot{V}$$
$$\text{Carbon dioxide production} = \text{True } CO_2 \cdot \dot{V}$$

Oxygen consumption (in millilitres of O_2 consumed per minute) is strictly dependent on the work-load. A healthy adult has an O_2 consumption ranging between 0.2 and 0.5 l/min at rest and 5–6 l/min during physically demanding activities.

Energy cost of activities and daily total energy expenditure (TEE). The energy cost of each individual activity is given by the energy equivalence of the volumes of oxygen consumed over the period of measurements at the given RQ (Table 4.3). The latter should in principle be corrected for the amount of energy lost in the incompletely oxidized nitrogenous compounds lost through the kidneys over the same period.

The different equations proposed to compute the energy expenditure from oxygen consumption (Table 4.4) have been reviewed elsewhere [29, 31]. Weir [25] and subsequently Consolazio [19] pointed out that these equations are unnecessarily cumbersome. In practice it is adequate for many purposes to calculate energy expenditure from equations that omit the protein correction

Table 4.3 Equation to calculate the energy equivalent of expired air for a given RQ value

Energy equivalent of 1 litre expired air $= [a + (RQ - x) \cdot (b - a)/(y - x)]$

RQ = RQ of expired air
a   = Constant, representing the energy equivalent of 1 litre oxygen consumed in the metabolism of fat
b   = Constant, representing the energy equivalent of 1 litre oxygen consumed in the metabolism of carbohydrates
x   = RQ of fat
y   = RQ of carbohydrates

(Source [29])

and do not require the measurement of carbon dioxide concentration in the expired air. Weir [25] proposed the following simplified equation:

$$\text{Energy cost (kcal/min)} = \dot{V} \cdot c \cdot \Delta O_2$$

where $\dot{V}$ is the STP ventilation rate; c is a constant $= 0.0504$ [25]; and ΔO_2 is the difference in oxygen concentration between inspired and expired air.

Table 4.4 Proposed reference formula for calculation of energy expenditure

Energy expenditure (kcal/min) $= VO_2 + y\ VCO_2 - z\ N$				
Authors		*x*	*y*	*z*	Ref.
Weir	(1949)	3.941	1.106	2.1	[25]
Consolatio *et al.*	(1963)	3.78	1.16	2.98	[19]
Brower	(1965)	3.866	1.20	1.43	[26]
Frayn	(1983)	3.76	1.18	0.88	[27]
Passmore and Eastwood	(1986)	3.77	1.16	2.87	[28]
Brockway	(1987)	3.96	1.08	1.41	[29]
Garlick	(1987)	3.76	1.16	1.78	[30]
Jequier and Faber	(1987)	3.84	1.09	0.61	[31]

The error in neglecting to correct for urinary nitrogen would be only about $\pm 1.0\%$ for each 12.3% of the total calories arising from proteins [25]. On the other hand it has been stated that the above formula, which neglects to correct for both urinary nitrogen and carbon dioxide production, can be used with an accuracy of better than $\pm 3\%$ [29], or at the most $\pm 4\%$ [32].

Daily TEE can be calculated factorially, once the cost of each activity performed over the 24 hours is known. The duration of each activity has only to be multiplied by its energy cost and summed up.

$$\text{TEE} = (t_1 \cdot \text{AEE}_1) + (t_2 \cdot \text{AEE}_2) + (t_3 \cdot \text{AEE}_3) + (t_n \cdot \text{AEE}_n)$$

where t_1, t_2, t_n = Time (min) devoted to each activity; $\text{AEE}_1, \text{AEE}_2, \text{AEE}_n$ = Activity energy expenditure.

4.3.7 Performance characteristics

(a) Technical reproducibility

The reliability of a method can be assessed on the basis of its technical performance.

The recording of the duration of activities requires considerable effort on the part of the observer and/or the subject. It is difficult to check that this is performed accurately, routinely, or consistently. Alternative data logging systems have not yet been proved to be of sufficient merit.

Volume recording apparatus has an accuracy of greater than 99% but this may decrease in the hands of an inexperienced observer using poorly maintained or badly calibrated equipment. Apparatus must be calibrated correctly [23] and routinely serviced and maintained. Experience shows that the manufacturer's calibration factors should be checked. Sampling systems may cause more problems than the volume-recording parts of the apparatus.

Error analysis of the KM method using a well-calibrated KM suggest a maximum range of error of -14 to $+1\%$ [19]. There is no reason to suppose that other methods will be any more precise.

(b) Biological reproducibility

Replicated measurements of energy expenditure usually show good agreement although there may be 5–10% fluctuation from one 15-min period to another [33]. However, variation during the day and between days may exceed 5%. The origin of such variations in individuals under standard conditions is not precisely known. Exercise, temperature, plane of nutrition, and type of diet may contribute to further intraindividual variation [34]. The inability to quantify this variation without interfering with the subject's way of life is probably the largest single error in the factorial method of measuring daily energy expenditure. Attempts to get over this should include taking as many measurements as possible of the activities pursued for long periods, ensuring that the measurement period is long enough [33] and that the activities are adequately described in the recording.

(c) Validity

The factorial method is usually taken as the reference method for daily energy expenditure in free-living subjects. It has been described as 'the most commonly used and probably the best available for measuring 24 hour energy expenditure' [35]. However, its accuracy is unknown or uncertain, although it is thought to be some 10% [36].

The validity of the method is affected by:

1. errors in the recording of the duration of the separate activities;
2. failure to define the activity accurately;
3. failure of the subjects to behave in a typical fashion while the energy cost of an activity is being measured;
4. errors in the technique of measuring the metabolic cost of an activity [23].

To these can be added disturbance of the subject's normal routine because of the study.

There are several studies comparing daily energy expenditure determined by direct and indirect calorimetry in farm animals and in men which have shown good but not invariable agreement in the methods [36]. However, the full factorial method has not often been compared with other methods. Self-recording of activities produces records not significantly different from those of independent observers, over two days [36] or two weeks [37]. Over a two-hour period, continuous measurements of energy expenditure and the factorial method have given results not significantly different [38].

Energy expenditure determined by the factorial method has been compared with that estimated from long-term energy intake and energy stores changes. In a study over several months it has been found that factorial energy expenditure was 6% greater than energy expenditure from energy intake and energy stores [39]. In 7 of 12 subjects the methods produced results to within 10%. Borel *et al.* [40] found a better agreement in 12 subjects over 5 weeks, 2% in men, 5% in women. In these studies, group means agree well but individual data are much more variable.

The field measurements of the energy costs of tasks is very time consuming. The estimation of energy expenditure using literature values would represent a considerable saving in effort and resources. With regards to this, Durnin and Passmore [22] state 'Far more important than taking large numbers of measurements by indirect calorimetry is the accurate recording of the time spent in each activity'. Moreover it has been found [39] that there was no significant difference in daily energy expenditure estimated by using measured energy costs or taking values from literature. This appears as surprising considering Garrow's analysis of related and random intra- and inter-individual variation of the energy costs of tasks [35].

REFERENCES

1. Beaton, G.H., Milner, J., Corey, P. *et al.* (1979) Sources of variance in 24-hour dietary recall data: Implications for nutrition study design and interpretation. *Am. J. Clin. Nutr.*, **32**, 2546–59.
2. Durnin, J.V.G.A. and Ferro-Luzzi, A. (1982) Conducting and reporting studies on human energy intake and output: Suggested standards. *Am. J. Clin. Nutr.*, **35**, 624–6.
3. Norgan, N.G., Ferro-Luzzi, A. and Durnin, J.V.G.A. (1974) The energy and nutrient intake and the energy expenditure of 204 New-Guinean adults. *Philos. Trans. R. Soc. Lond. [Biol.]*, **268**, 309–48.
4. Durnin, J.V.G.A. (1984) Some problems in assessing the role of physical activity in the maintenance of energy balance, in *Energy Intake and Activity* (eds E. Pollit and P. Amante), Alan Liss, New York, pp. 101–13.
5. Hautvast, J.G.A. and Klaver, W. (eds) (1982) *The Diet Factor in Epidemiological Research*, EURO-NUT rep. 1, Wageningen.
6. Bingham, S.A. (1987) The dietary assessment of individuals; methods, accuracy, new techniques and recommendations. *Nutr. Abstracts Rev. (Series A)*, **57**, 705–42.
7. Cameron, E.D. and van Staveren, W. (eds) (1988) *Manual on Methodology for Food Consumption Studies*, Oxford Medical Publications, Oxford.
8. Osgood, C.E. (1953) *Method and Theory in Experimental Psychology*, Oxford University Press, New York.
9. Church, H.N., Clayton, M.M., Young, C.M. and Foster, W.D. (1954) Can different interviewers obtain comparable dietary surveys data? *J. Am. Diet. Assoc.*, **30**, 777–9.

10. Eagles, J.A., Grant Whiting, M. and Olson, E.E. (1966) Dietary appraisal. Problems in processing dietary data. *Am. J. Clin. Nutr.*, **19**, 1–9.

11. Ferro-Luzzi, A. (1982) Meaning and constraints of energy-intake studies in free-living populations, in *Energy and Effort* (ed. G.A. Harrison), Taylor and Francis, London, pp. 115–37.

12. Burk, M.C. and Pao, E.M. (1976) *Methodology for Large Scale Surveys of Households and Individual Diets*, USDS Home Economics Research Rep. No. 40, Washington (DC).

13. Prentice, A.M. (1988) Applications of the doubly-labelled water method in free-living adults. *Proc. Nutr. Soc.*, **47**, 258–68.

14. Borrelli, R., Cole, T.J., Di Biase, G. and Contoldo, F. (1989) Some statistical considerations on dietary assessment methods. *Eur. J. Clin. Nutr.*, **43**, 451–60.

15. FAO/WHO/UNU (1985) *Expert Consultation. Energy and Protein Requirement*, WHO, Geneva.

16. Woo, R., Daniels-Kush, R. and Horton E.S. (1985) Regulation of energy balance. *Ann. Rev. Nutr.*, **5**, 411–33.

17. Bursztein, S., Elwyn, D.H., Askanazi, J. and Kinney, S.M. (1989) *Energy Metabolism, Indirect Calorimetry and Nutrition*, William and Wilkins, Baltimore (USA).

18. Segal, K.R. (1987) Comparison of indirect calorimetry measurements of resting energy expenditure with a ventilated hood, face mask and mouthpiece. *Am. J. Clin. Nutr.*, **45**, 1420–3.

19. Consolazio, C.F., Johnson, R.E. and Pecora, L.J. (1963) *Physiological Measurements of Metabolic Functions in Man*, McGraw-Hill, New York.

20. Dauncey, M.J., Murgatroyd, P.R. and Cole, T.J. (1978) A human calorimeter for the direct and indirect measurement of 24 h energy expenditure. *Br. J. Nutr.*, **39**, 557–66.

21. Shetty, P.S., Sheela, M.L., Murgatroyd, P.R. and Kurpad, A.V. (1987) An open circuit indirect whole body calorimeter for the continuous measurement of energy expenditure of man in the tropics. *Indian J. Med. Res.*, **85**, 453–60.

22. Durnin, J.V.G.A. and Passmore, R. (1967) *Energy, Work and Leisure*, Heinemann Educational, London.

23. Durnin, J.V.G.A. and Brockway, J.T. (1959) Determination of the total daily energy expenditure in man by indirect calorimetry: Assessment of the accuracy of a modern technique. *Br. J. Nutr.*, **13**, 41–53.

24. Ferrannini, E. (1988) The theoretical basis of indirect calorimetry: a review. *Metabolism*, **37** (3), 287–301.

25. Weir, J.B. de V. (1949) New methods of calculating metabolic rate, with special reference to protein metabolism. *J. Physiol.*, **109**, 1–9.

26. Brower, E. (1965) Report of sub-committee on constant and factors, in *3rd Symposium on Energy Metabolism* (ed. K.L. Blaxter), European Association for Animal Production. Publ. No. 11. Academic Press, London, pp. 441–3.

27. Frayn, K.N. (1983) Calculation of substrate oxidation rates in-vivo from gaseous exchange. *J. Appl. Physiol.*, **55**, 628–34.

28. Passmore, R. and Eastwood, M.A. (1986) *Davidson and Passmore, Human Nutrition and Dietetics*. 8th edn, Churchill Livingstone, Edinburgh, pp. 18–19.

29. Brockway, J.M. (1987) Derivation of formulae used to calculate energy expenditure in man. *Hum. Nutr. Clin. Nutr.*, **41**C, 463–71.

30. Garlick, P.J. (1987) Evaluation of the formulae for calculating nutrient utilisation rates from respiratory gas measurements in fed subjects. *Hum. Nutr. Clin. Nutr.*, **41**C, 165–76.

31. Jequier, E. and Felber, J.P. (1987) Indirect calorimetry. *Clin. Endocrinol. Metab.*, **1**(4), 911–35.

32. McArdle, W.D., Katch, F.I. and Katch, V.L. (1986) *Exercise Physiology. Energy, Nutrition and Human Performance*, Lea and Febiger, Philadelphia.

33. Garrow, J.S. and Haves, S.F. (1972) The role of amino acid oxidation in causing 'specific dynamic action' in man. *Br. J. Nutr.*, **27**, 211–19.

34. Garrow, J.S. and Webster, J.D. (1984) Thermogenesis to small stimuli, in *Human Energy Metabolism: Physical Activity and Energy Expenditure Measurements in Epidemiological Research Based Upon Direct and Indirect Calorimetry* (ed. A.J.H. Van Es), EURO-NUT rep. 5, Wageningen, pp. 215–24.

35. Garrow, J.S. (1974) *Energy Balance and Obesity in Man*, North Holland, Amsterdam.

36. Durnin, J.V.G.A. (1978) Indirect calorimetry in man: a critique of practical problems. *Proc. Nutr. Soc.*, **37**, 5–12.

37. Brockett, J.E., Konishi, F., Brophy, E.M. *et al.* (1957) *The Energy Expenditure of Men in a Training Company*, USA Medical Research and Nutrition Laboratory Rep. No. 212 (cited in Ref. [23]).

38. Rankin, A.D., Konishi, F., Insull, W. and Marcinek, J. (1956) US Army Medical Nutrition Laboratory Rep. No. 188 (cited in Ref. [23]).

39. Acheson, K.J., Campbell, I.T., Edholm, O.G. and Miller, D.S. (1980) The measurement of daily energy expenditure – an evaluation of some techniques. *Am. J. Clin. Nutr.*, **33**, 1155–64.

40. Borel, M.J., Riley, R.E. and Snook, J.T. (1984) Estimation of energy expenditure and maintenance energy requirements of college age men and women. *Am. J. Clin. Nutr.*, **40**, 1264–72.

5 Lipid pattern methodology

5.1 Introduction *F. Fidanza*   131
5.2 Essential fatty acids by HRGC *M.S. Simonetti, P. Damiani
    and F. Fidanza*   131
5.3 Separation and determination of plasma lipids and
    lipoproteins *A.L. Catapano*   139
      Section I   Plasma or serum cholesterol determination   140
      Section II   Plasma or serum triglyceride determination   142
      Section III Separation of plasma lipoproteins   144
      Section IV   HDL cholesterol determination   148
5.4 The arachidonic acid cascade in the vascular system *C. Galli* 153

5.1 INTRODUCTION

Fatty acid composition of lipids in tissues and body fluids is correlated with the fatty acid composition of dietary fats.

As signs of deficiency of essential fatty acids are well documented, in this chapter we present first the method for assessment of nutritional status in these fatty acids. Because the separation and determination of plasma lipids and lipoproteins is needed in some epidemiological studies, their assessment is described in the next section (p. 139).

In recent years the problem of eicosanoids has become·very important, and we examine the arachidonic cascade in the vascular system from a general point of view. This is an area of very rapid development and consequently the complete methods cannot be reported in detail as yet. Researchers interested in any specific problems can contact the Authors, who have considerable experience in this field.

5.2 ESSENTIAL FATTY ACIDS BY HRGC

5.2.1 Purpose and scope

Coronary heart disease and a number of other diseases are thought to be related aetiologically to the intake and composition of dietary fats. Assessment of the fatty acid composition of lipids in tissues and body fluids, e.g. plasma, erythrocyte membranes, phospholipids, adipose tissue, and cheek cell phospholipids, is correlated with the fatty acid composition of dietary fats, and its measurement is thought to provide a valid index of nutritional status [1–7].

A decrease in the polyunsaturated fatty acids (PUFA) of the n-6 and n-3 families and an increase in the polyunsaturated fatty acid of the n-9 family are the most prominent findings. Diversity of unsaturation and of the balance of chain length in the fatty acids contributes to the stability of the cell membrane; therefore the profound changes in fatty acid composition induced by essential fatty acid (EFA) deficiency may alter the integrity and function of the membrane structure.

The experience of Holman *et al.* [1] indicates that the fatty acid pattern of serum phospholipids (PL) most clearly reflects essential fatty acid status. Analyses of total lipids (TL) also indicate EFA status but the long-chain PUFAs, which are the best indicators of EFA status, are found in the highest proportion in the PLs; in the TLs they are diluted by the presence of high proportions of 16 and 18 carbon acids that are abundantly present in triglycerides and cholesteryl esters and in free fatty acids, which occur in variable proportion in TLs.

5.2.2 Principle of the method

The plasma phospholipids are separated from other lipid classes by thin-layer chromatography after extraction with chloroform-methanol (2:1 v/v). The fatty acid methyl esters of phospholipids are prepared by transesterification with a large excess of anhydrous methanol in the presence of an acidic catalyst (H_2SO_4). The methyl esters are then separated and quantified by HRGC procedure. The methyl esters are identified by comparison with relative retention times of standard mixtures analysed under the same conditions.

5.2.3 Chemicals and apparatus

(a) Chemicals

Fatty acid methyl esters, e.g. Sigma, Supelco, Alltech Associates
Methanol (CH_3OH) p.a.
Chloroform ($CHCl_3$) p.a.
Deionized and double-distilled water
2, 6-Di-tert-butyl-p-cresol (butylated hydroxy toluene, BHT) ($C_{15}H_{24}O$) p.a.
Acetic acid (CH_3COOH) p.a.
Petroleum ether, 30°–50° p.a.
Diethylether (($C_2H_5)_2O$) p.a.
2′, 7′-dichlorofluorescein ($C_{20}H_{10}Cl_2O_5$) p.a.
Ethanol (C_2H_5OH) p.a.
Sulphuric acid, 95–97% (H_2SO_4) p.a.
Sodium bicarbonate ($NaHCO_3$) p.a.
Anhydrous sodium sulphate (Na_2SO_4) p.a.
Silica gel plates, 20 × 20 cm, 250 μm in thickness.

(b) Solutions

Chloroform-methanol, 2:1 (v/v)
Petroleum ether-diethylether-acetic acid, 70:30:1 (v/v)
0.1% BHT: 1 g BHT dissolved in chloroform to make 1000 ml
0.2% 2′,7′-dichlorofluorescein (2 g 2′,7′-dichlorofluorescein dissolved in ethanol to make 1000 ml)

4% (v/v) H_2SO_4 in methanol (41.67 ml 95–97% H_2SO_4 made up to 1000 ml with methanol)

Saturated solution of sodium bicarbonate in water

Fatty acids methyl esters standard solutions:

  Stock standards: fatty acid methyl esters are dissolved in methanol by volumetric dilutions (10 mg of each fatty acid methyl ester/10 ml methanol).

  Working standards are prepared by diluting the stock standards with methanol at the final concentrations of 25, 50, 100, 200 µg/ml.

(c) Apparatus

Usual basic laboratory equipment

Gas chromatography apparatus consisting of:

  Gas chromatograph, e.g. HR 6800 Dani with flame ionization detector 682 (FID), coupled with integrator, e.g. CDS 111 C Varian and equipped with capillary column SP 2340 (100% bis-cyanopropyl polysiloxane), 30 m × 0.25 mm ID, film thickness 0.20 µm,

  Recorder, e.g. Speedomax, Leeds and Northrup.

5.2.4 Sample collection

Venous blood samples (4–5 ml) in the post-absorbitive state are collected into sodium heparinate vacutainers and then centrifuged; 0.5 ml aliquots of plasma are used for analysis.

5.2.5 Procedure

(a) Lipid extraction

One millilitre of water is added to 0.5 ml of plasma and then 4 ml of methanol, 4 ml of chloroform and 4 ml of 0.1% BHT in chloroform are added in the above order. The solutions are mixed after each addition and equilibrated for two hours at 4°C. The lower phase is removed, evaporated under N_2 at 35°C in a rotavapor, and redissolved in chloroform-methanol (2:1 v/v) [8].

(b) Thin-layer chromatography of phospholipids

Samples (300 µl) are applied to the thin-layer chromatography plates previously washed by double runs with diethylether and then activated for two hours at 100°C. The solvent system used is petroleum ether, diethylether, acetic acid (70:30:1 v/v). The spots of phospholipids remaining at the origin are visible under ultraviolet light by spraying with 0.2% 2′, 7′-dichlorofluorescein. The spots are scraped into glass-stoppered flasks, where the products are subjected to the methanolysis procedure.

(c) Preparation of methyl esters

Fatty acids of phospholipids are transesterified with 10 ml of 4% H_2SO_4 in methanol at 75°C for 30 minutes. Fatty acid methyl esters are extracted using diethylether. The organic extract is neutralized with a saturated solution of sodium bicarbonate, washed twice with water, and dried over anhydrous sodium sulphate. The methyl esters are stored at −4°C under nitrogen.

(d) Technique

The methyl esters (1–3 µl) from samples and working standards are subjected to gas chromatography.

The chromatographic conditions are:

  Detector temperature FID: 280°C

Injector temperature: 280°C

Gas flow rates: air 300 ml/min; hydrogen 40 ml/min; nitrogen 35 ml/min; helium 1 ml/min

Injection system: 'splitting' – split ratio 40:1.

The analysis conditions are:

120°C isotherm for 5 min, then 4°C/min up to 170°C, isotherm for 25 min and then 4°C/min up to 210°C

Attenuation: 2 × 10 to the electrometer and × 4 to the integrator

Recording paper speed: 0.5 cm/min.

Under these conditions analyses of fatty acids from C 12:0 to C 22:6 n-3 are completed in 55 min. The fatty acids separated and identified are the following:

C 12:0, C 14:0, C 14:1 n-5, C 16:0, C 16:1 n-7, C 17:0, C 18:0, C 18:1 n-9, C 18:2 n-6, C 18:3 n-6, C 20:0, C 18:3 n-3, C 20:1 n-9, C 20:2 n-6, C 20:3 n-9, C 20:3 n-6, C 22:0, C 20:4 n-6, C 22:1 n-9, C 20:5 n-3, C 22:3 n-9, C 22:4 n-6, C 22:5 n-6, C 24:1 n-9, C 22:5 n-3, and C 22:6 n-3.

The identification of fatty acid methyl esters is performed by comparison with the retention times of standard fatty acid methyl esters.

The fatty acids C 20:3 n-9 and C 22:3 n-9 are identified by comparing the samples with the pattern of plasma phospholipid fatty acids of rats fed with an essential fatty-acid-free diet.

The working standards are used for the plotting of the calibration curve.

(e) Calculation

The quantitative analysis is carried out using 'normalization procedure' with response factors (RF) always equal to 1.

5.2.6 Performance characteristics

(a) Range of linearity

The linearity is assessed using the calibration curve within the concentration range examined. A correlation coefficient of 0.999 is obtained from linear regression analysis.

(b) Detection limit

Amounts of 5 ng of each fatty acid methyl ester injected can be quantitatively detected under these conditions.

(c) Recovery

Recovery of each fatty acid is determined by the internal standard method by adding known amounts of pentadecanoic acid methyl ester as internal standard to the similarly known amounts of each fatty acid methyl ester.

(d) Reproducibility

To evaluate precision the coefficient of variation (CV) within day and between days can be calculated from specimens of the standard mixtures (10 replicates at each level).

Table 5.1 Regression equations for indices (Y) of normal male human serum lipids [1]

$$Y = A \ (age) + B$$

N =	Total lipid 103			Phospholipids 102			Cholesteryl esters 101			Triglycerides 105			Free fatty acids 98		
	A	B	SD	A	B	SD	A	B	SD	A	B	SD	A	B	SD
Double-bond index	−0.0006	1.45	0.15	0.0003	1.66	0.13	0.0005	1.34	0.11	0.0007	0.93	0.12	−0.0009	1.06	0.09
C 18:2n-6 + C 20:4n-6 − C 20:3n-9	−0.0164	33.32	6.03	−0.0263	30.62	3.62	−0.0335	53.05	6.22	0.0492	15.28	6.10	0.0267	14.59	4.94
Total n-6 acids	−0.0221	38.33	6.55	−0.0303	37.85	3.94	−0.0332	55.79	5.83	0.0561	16.25	6.37	0.0256	15.40	4.93
n-6 metabolites	0.0066	11.67	3.35	0.0135	16.73	3.11	0.0348	9.92	3.38	0.0169	1.87	1.42	0.0011	1.77	2.08
Total n-3 acids	−0.0057	4.09	1.73	0.0088	4.67	1.80	0.0059	1.44	2.11	0.0015	1.35	1.20	0.0042	0.93	1.16
n-3 metabolites	−0.0055	3.60	1.71	0.0095	4.38	1.72	0.0056	1.02	2.08	−0.0002	0.56	0.93	−0.0003	0.41	0.68
Total n-9 acids	0.0326	23.92	4.79	0.0104	14.86	2.60	0.0173	24.23	3.39	−0.0199	44.23	6.12	0.0392	40.20	5.55
n-9 metabolites	0.0046	1.41	1.01	0.0068	1.42	1.04	0.0035	0.43	0.50	0.0059	0.52	0.59	0.0000	0.31	0.46
Total PUFA	−0.0232	43.83	7.42	−0.0147	43.94	4.36	−0.0238	57.66	5.85	0.0635	18.11	6.90	0.0298	16.64	5.27
Total monoenoic acids	0.0325	26.05	6.11	0.0028	15.20	2.93	0.0212	28.36	4.71	−0.0054	49.19	5.25	0.0484	44.75	5.48
Total saturated acids	−0.0059	30.11	3.52	0.0166	40.77	3.23	0.0095	13.98	2.15	−0.0582	33.04	4.55	−0.0805	39.28	5.39
C 18:2n-6 / C 20:4n-6	−0.0115	3.91	1.16	−0.0080	2.10	0.55	−0.0309	6.83	2.35	−0.1797	33.70	54.47		—	
C 20:3n-9 / C 20:4n-6	−0.0003	0.13	0.08	0.0003	0.10	0.07	0.0000	0.03	0.04	−0.0008	0.22	0.26	−0.0007	0.63	0.46

Table 5.2 Regression equations for indices (Y) of normal female human serum lipids [1]

$$Y = A \text{ (age)} + B$$

N =	Total lipid 101			Phospholipids 99			Cholesteryl esters 96			Triglycerides 98			Free fatty acids 95		
	A	B	SD	A	B	SD	A	B	SD	A	B	SD	A	B	SD
Double-bond index	−0.0001	1.18	0.15	0.0006	1.47	0.15	0.0005	1.09	0.08	0.0003	0.65	0.09	−0.0005	0.76	0.08
C 18:2n-6 + C 20:4n-6 − C 20:3n-9	−0.0304	34.66	4.53	−0.0285	31.33	3.69	−0.0756	55.71	5.67	−0.0027	18.45	4.80	0.0336	14.98	4.41
Total n-6 acids	−0.0341	39.47	4.91	−0.0283	38.82	3.62	−0.0639	57.93	5.28	−0.0028	19.55	4.93	0.0346	15.62	4.51
n-6 metabolites	0.0076	11.79	3.20	0.0103	17.90	3.36	0.0368	10.03	3.37	0.0055	2.30	1.33	0.0052	1.78	1.78
Total n-3 acids	−0.0006	3.94	1.73	0.0106	5.49	2.44	0.0059	1.37	1.25	0.0015	1.33	0.68	−0.0037	1.82	1.55
n-3 metabolites	0.0013	3.32	1.75	0.0086	5.26	2.37	0.0051	0.93	1.23	−0.0002	0.47	0.38	−0.0030	0.96	1.28
Total n-9 acids	0.0285	23.71	3.34	0.0075	14.47	2.55	0.0120	23.64	3.20	0.0055	43.31	4.49	0.0430	40.77	5.89
n-9 metabolites	0.0110	0.97	1.01	0.0016	1.53	0.84	0.0033	0.41	0.49	0.0039	0.47	0.47	0.0046	0.17	0.51
Total PUFA	−0.0237	44.38	5.53	−0.0161	45.84	4.22	−0.0547	59.72	4.97	0.0027	21.35	5.33	0.0355	17.60	4.86
Total monoenoic acids	0.0218	26.44	4.45	0.0091	14.42	2.69	0.0258	27.24	3.93	0.0262	47.97	3.89	0.0417	45.71	5.46
Total saturated acids	0.0050	29.10	3.08	0.0088	39.54	4.07	0.0267	13.48	2.41	−0.0295	30.99	3.95	−0.0744	37.08	5.30
C 18:2n-6 / C 20:4n-6	−0.0112	3.85	1.03	−0.0042	1.86	0.54	−0.0303	6.64	2.13	−0.2901	29.64	30.97		—	
C 20:3n-9 / C 20:4n-6	0.0003	0.08	0.08	−0.0003	0.12	0.07	0.0002	0.02	0.04	−0.0003	0.12	0.12	−0.0017	0.51	0.47

The mean of coefficients of variation calculated by us is 3.0 ± 1.9 for within day and 4.3 ± 2.7 for between days (Mean $\pm$ SD).

5.2.7 Reference values

According to Holman *et al.* [1] the distribution of percentage of fatty acids has a relative value, also some components demonstrate infrequent occurrence, non-relevance to EFA consideration and/or very low concentrations. Consequently, the authors propose the following indices for the fatty acid composition of phospholipids, cholesteryl esters, triglycerides, and free fatty acids: the double-bond index, the sum of C 18:2 n-6 and C 20:4 n-6 minus C 20:3 n-9, the total n-6 acids, the total n-6 metabolites, the total n-3 acids, the n-3 metabolites, the total n-9 acids, the n-9 metabolites, the total polyunsaturated fatty acids, the total monoenoic acids, the total saturated acids and the ratios C 18:2 n-6 / C 20:4 n-6 and C 20:3 n-9 / C 20:4 n-6.

In Tables 5.1 and 5.2 the regression equations for the above indices are reported in so-called normal male and female human serum lipids, where each

$$\text{index value} = \text{A (age)} + \text{B}$$

In infants Cooke *et al.* [9] proposed for the triene/tetraene ratio (=y) the equation

$$y = 0.14 + 0.07 \, x$$

where x is the postnatal age in days.

Because Holman *et al.* [1] studied hospital patients who may have suffered from diseases that had hitherto unnoticed effects on fatty acid metabolism, Manku *et al.* [6] examined a group of truly normal young adults (32 male and 18 female students recruited from Acadia University, Wolfville, Nova Scotia; mean age of each group, 20 years) and reported the fatty acid composition of red blood cells (total phospholipid, phosphatidylcholine, phosphatidylethanolamine) and total plasma phospholipids (Table 5.3). In the same Table they included the values of fatty acids in total plasma phospholipids from the study of Holman *et al.* calculated for the 20-year-old age group.

5.2.8 Interpretation

Holman *et al.* [1] in their study observed that the ratio C 20:3 n-9 / C 20:4 n-6 was 0.1 ± 0.08 in serum phospholipids for both sexes, and a value above 0.2 was considered the upper limit of 'normalcy'. At birth this ratio was equal to 0.16 and diminished significantly and progressively during the first eight months; this suggested a marginal reserve of EFA at birth and may have significance in the nutrition of premature or very young infants [10].

In this connection, in a study on development of essential fatty acid deficiency in premature infants given fat-free parenteral nutrition, Cooke *et al.* [9] have defined essential fatty acid deficiency as a ratio of C 20:3 n-9 / C 20:4 n-6 in plasma phospholipids greater than 0.4.

According to Cunnane *et al.* [11] the amount of arachidonic acid in maternal plasma phospholipids was lower than that of linoleic acid; but the reverse was true in fetal plasma. Compared with linoleic acid, arachidonic acid is preferentially transferred to the fetal circulation by the isolated perfused term placenta. In leukocytes from pregnant women at term, significantly more ^{14}C-linoleic acid and ^{3}H-arachidonic acid remained in the form of intracellular free fatty

Table 5.3 Percentage of the total amount of fatty acids present in blood

| Fatty acid | Red blood cells (Manku et al. study, [6]) (Mean ± SEM) | | | Plasma total phospholipids (Mean ± SD) | | |
	Total phospholipid	Phosphatidyl-choline	Phosphatidyl-ethanolamine	Manku et al. study [6]	Holman et al. study [1] female	male
C 18:2n-6	9.78 ± 0.24	16.01 ± 0.27	6.22 ± 0.27	21.45 ± 2.81	20.14 ± 3.72	20.24 ± 3.57
C 20:3n-6	1.37 ± 0.05	1.86 ± 0.06	0.84 ± 0.06	3.06 ± 0.60	3.38 ± 1.42	3.46 ± 1.02
C 20:4n-6	15.13 ± 0.29	12.49 ± 0.25	21.46 ± 0.35	11.36 ± 1.67	11.89 ± 2.45	11.08 ± 2.34
C 22: 4n-6	5.54 ± 0.20	1.87 ± 0.13	5.41 ± 0.15	0.73 ± 0.26	1.62 ± 0.78	1.47 ± 1.06
C 22:5n-6	3.99 ± 0.15	0.77 ± 0.09	—	1.12 ± 0.67	0.58 ± 0.72	0.46 ± 0.36
C 20:5n-3	0.65 ± 0.03	—	0.76 ± 0.07	1.01 ± 0.36	1.19 ± 0.62	1.06 ± 0.73
C 22:5n-3	2.53 ± 0.13	1.42 ± 0.08	3.52 ± 0.14	0.93 ± 0.27	0.71 ± 0.51	0.73 ± 0.59
C 22:6n-3	4.20 ± 0.15	3.85 ± 0.13	5.47 ± 0.22	3.54 ± 0.89	2.33 ± 1.27	1.80 ± 1.14
C 18:1n-9	14.83 ± 0.24	17.16 ± 0.24	19.39 ± 0.34	13.50 ± 2.20	13.06 ± 2.34	13.51 ± 2.60
C 16:0	20.68 ± 0.26	23.60 ± 0.32	15.42 ± 0.35	23.90 ± 7.02	26.81 ± 4.41	27.33 ± 3.55
C 18:0	14.71 ± 0.22	18.07 ± 0.31	9.87 ± 0.36	11.61 ± 1.32	12.59 ± 1.75	13.37 ± 2.18

acid, and less of both fatty acids was incorporated into the phospholipid fractions; this suggested that increased levels of free essential fatty acids in maternal leukocytes may facilitate EFA transfer to the fetus. But in some disorders of pregnancy such as pre-eclampsia, increased levels of arachidonic acid have been observed in phospholipid and cholesteryl ester (i.e. by Ogburn *et al.* [12]), while pre-eclamptic placentas had significantly lower proportions of arachidonic acid in the non-esterified fatty acid and triglyceride components.

Highly significant correlations (r=0.5) were found between the polyunsaturated:saturated fatty acid ratio of the adipose tissue and the corresponding variable in the diet in a study of Plakké *et al.* [4]; sex and age were not taken into consideration, since according to the authors their influence on adipose tissue fatty acid composition of adults was negligible. Calculating the effect of within-person variability in food intake on the correlation coefficient between diet and physiological variables, Beaton *et al.* [13] have estimated a coefficient between the long-term average dietary P/S ratio and the adipose tissue P/S ratio of the order of 0.85.

Jacobsen *et al.* [5] found significant correlations between percentage saturated, monounsaturated, and polyunsaturated fatty acids in adipose tissue and their corresponding values in plasma free fatty acids between polyunsaturated fatty acids in the diet, and in adipose tissue in a group of men participating in a primary coronary prevention programme (The Oslo study).

5.3 SEPARATION AND DETERMINATION OF PLASMA LIPIDS AND LIPOPROTEINS

5.3.1 Introduction

Plasma cholesterol and (in some countries) triglycerides are risk factors for the development of coronary heart disease (CHD) [14, 15]. More recently it has been shown that low-density lipoprotein (LDL) cholesterol also directly relates to the incidence of CHD, while high-density lipoprotein (HDL) cholesterol is inversely related to it [16]. The determination of the lipoprotein cholesterol levels in plasma is therefore of relevance to identify the 'risk' of a subject. Furthermore recent trials using the lipid-lowering drugs cholestyramine [17] and gemfibrozil [18] have shown that a reduction of cholesterol by 20% brings about a 40% reduction of the incidence of morbidity and mortality for CHD.

The plasma triglyceride levels are also believed to be a risk factor for CHD, although this relationship is not as clear as that found for cholesterol [14, 15]. In some epidemiological studies triglyceride levels are significantly associated with risk, whereas in other studies this is not the case. Certain genetic disorders may be expressed with triglyceride elevation and may confer increased risk. Therefore, measurement of plasma triglycerides is important in the routine clinical laboratory as well as in the research laboratory.

In this chapter the procedures most currently used in determining total plasma cholesterol and triglycerides will be outlined as well as the fractionation of plasma lipoproteins with special emphasis on determination of the LDL and HDL cholesterol.

SECTION I   PLASMA OR SERUM CHOLESTEROL DETERMINATION

Cholesterol, a constituent of cell membranes, is the most common sterol in human tissue and fluids. About 70% of cholesterol in plasma is esterified.

It would be almost pointless to review the historical development of cholesterol assay or to review all methodologies available. This subject has been covered in detail [19, 20].

Measurement of total cholesterol includes both free and esterified forms. In serum or plasma about two-thirds of total cholesterol is esterified. This observation has some analytical implications, the colour development is, in fact, greater for esterified cholesterol in some colorimetric reactions.

Several chemical methods exist for determining total cholesterol; they are briefly reviewed here.

1. *Single-step method.* No handling of the samples is required; this allows for a single reagent. However, these procedures may present both positive and negative errors caused by the interference of proteins, vitamins, turbidity, and differences in chromogenicity of free and esterified cholesterol.
2. *Two-step method.* These procedures require an organic phase extraction step that removes many of the substances that may interfere with the assay. Since no saponification occurs the differential response of free and esterified cholesterol remains, especially in the Liebermann–Burchard reaction [21].
3. *Three-step method.* These procedures involve, in addition to the extraction of cholesterol, a saponification step that hydrolyses esterified cholesterol. The method of Abell *et al.* (1952) belongs to this classification and is currently considered a reference method [22].
4. *Enzymatic procedures.* The majority of the tests performed today are concerned with measuring total cholesterol. For this reason and because of the urgent demand for speed and ease in processing a large number of samples, many simple and rapid determinations for cholesterol have been introduced.

Enzymatic methods for determining cholesterol have recently emerged to compete with the classic Liebermann–Burchard reaction. The original work involved preliminary chemical saponification of the sample to produce free cholesterol, which reacts with cholesterol oxidase. This causes the breakdown of cholesterol to cholest-4-en-3-one and hydrogen peroxide, after which several different reaction systems have been used to produce the final results.

The commercial kits currently available offer a total enzymatic procedure utilizing the enzyme cholesterol esterase. This enzyme is specific for cholesteryl esters, splitting the ester into free cholesterol and free fatty acids. The cholesterol oxidase reaction then follows. The amount of colour produced is directly proportional to the amount of cholesterol.

These enzymatic procedures are amenable to automation. The harsh reagents involved in chemical determinations are no longer used; moreover the interference of other constituents is greatly reduced because of the specificity of the enzymes. A few cholesterol analogues may interfere, but the magnitude of interferences present in the chemical determinants is low.

The first step in the enzymatic method for cholesterol determination uses the enzyme cholesterol esterase to hydrolyse the cholesterol ester present in the serum:

$$\text{Cholesteryl ester} + H_2O \xrightarrow{\text{cholesterol esterase}} \text{cholesterol} + \text{free fatty acids} \quad (1)$$

In the second step the enzyme cholesterol oxidase oxidizes the cholesterol generated in step 1 to cholest-4-en-3-one and hydrogen peroxide:

$$\text{Cholesterol} + O_2 \xrightarrow{\text{cholesterol oxidase}} \text{cholest-4-en-3-one} + H_2O_2 \quad (2)$$

The hydrogen peroxide produced is used to combine with compounds to form coloured products that can be measured spectrophotometrically.

$$2H_2O_2 + \text{phenol} + \text{4-aminophenazone} \xrightarrow{\text{peroxidase}} \text{quinonlimine dye} + 4H_2O \quad (3)$$

or

$$H_2O_2 + \text{methanol} \xrightarrow{\text{catalase}} \text{formaldehyde} + H_2O \quad (4)$$

$$\text{Formaldehyde} + \text{acetylacetone} \longrightarrow \text{3,5-diacetyl-1,4-dihydrolutidine}$$

Reaction (3) is the basis of the majority of the kits currently on the market [23]. Reaction (4) has the advantage of not being subject to bilirubin interference.

When enzymatic kits that assay with the quinonlimine dye as a chromogen are used, blanking can cause problems with turbid samples for manual procedures. For automated procedures, since tygon tubing will absorb the dye, glass tubing must be used after formation of the dye.

Standards may also be a problem with some automated procedures when pumping devices are used. All samples and standards must be of the same viscosity in order for the pump to deliver the same quantity for each. However, since primary cholesterol standards can only be dissolved in organic solutions, a reference serum should be selected. Care must be taken to find the right set point for a reference serum. Because of the presence of different interfering factors, as stabilizers, processing, and additives in the reference serums and the reagents, the same set points cannot always be used for kits obtained from the different manufacturers. Interfering substances also make it difficult to attain a set point for an enzymatic method by running the reference material on a reference method. Finally, some variations in results of different methods are probably due to measurements at different wavelengths. A range of 450–560 nm has been proposed, with 500 nm being the maximum absorbance of the dye. Commonly suggested wavelengths for taking measurements are 505–520 and 525 nm.

Note 1.

A number of substances may interfere with cholesterol analyses. These constituents may be present in the serum or in the reagents.

For methods using the Liebermann–Burchard reagents, interference is often caused by bilirubin, or haemoglobin in high concentrations, by the enhanced colour formed from cholesterol esters, and by glyoxylic acid impurity in the acetic acid used. Methods based on the iron salt reagents show the above interferences and some additional ones caused by sodium azide and bromide, although the colour difference from cholesteryl ester can be nearly eliminated at certain wavelengths.

Enzymatic procedures suffer interference from bilirubin, haemolysis, lipaemia, and ascorbic acid. Reports in the literature vary as to the amount of interference and whether the change is a positive or negative one.

Bilirubin is the most commonly found substance that interferes in cholesterol analysis. When it reacts with the Liebermann–Burchard or iron-type reagents, bilirubin is oxidized to form stable biliverdin. Since the absorbance of biliverdin is greater than that of the compound formed from cholesterol, a positive interference results, which increases as bilirubin increases. The interference is greater for the Liebermann–Burchard reaction than for the iron reaction, although sample purification steps and use of the proper wavelength can help to minimize interference. Bilirubin interferes with the enzymatic methods by acting as a competing substrate and destroying the peroxide generated by the cholesterol oxidase reaction, causing a lowering of the cholesterol value.

5.3.2 Procedure

Manual method. This method refers to the use of the enzymatic Boehringer kit.

(a) Technique

Turn on the spectrophotometer and adjust the wavelength to 500 nm.

Label tubes for water blank, calibrators, control materials, and specimens.

Dispense 2.0 ml of enzymatic cholesterol reagent into each of the tubes and place them in an ice bath.

Equilibrate specimens to room temperature. Add 20 µl of water, calibrator, control material, or supernatant to the appropriate tubes and mix thoroughly. (Add proportionately larger volumes for low-cholesterol specimens: 100 µl for HDL supernatants.) Mix specimens thoroughly before pipetting to assure homogeneity.

Transfer tubes to a water bath at 37°C for 10 min.

Cool tubes to room temperature and within 15 min read absorbance after adjusting spectrophotometer to zero with the water blank.

(b) Calculation

Cholesterol in specimens and control materials are calculated in relation to the calibrator.

$$\text{Cholesterol unknown} = \frac{\text{absorbance of unknown}}{\text{absorbance of calibrator}} \cdot \text{cholesterol calibrator}$$

SECTION II PLASMA OR SERUM TRIGLYCERIDE DETERMINATION

Until 1957 triglycerides were estimated by the substraction method, i.e. triglycerides = total lipids − (cholesterol+phospholipids). This indirect method was used until Van Handel and Zilversmit [24] published a direct method whereby the phospholipids are removed from the lipid extract by an adsorbant and the triglycerides are determined from the amount of glycerol released by saponification with KOH.

Triglyceride determination was also considerably simplified by using chemical or enzymatic methods of glyceride glycerol, which is then converted to the equivalent mass of an average triglyceride. Alternatively, concentration may be expressed on a molar basis.

Triglycerides analysis has recently been simplified by the introduction of enzymatic methods, which have been automated to provide the analyst with quick and direct procedures. They will be examined here in some details.

The enzymatic methods are based on the determination of the glycerol portion of the triglyceride molecules after hydrolysis (chemical or enzymatic) to remove the fatty acids. Methods employing the enzymatic determination of glycerol have been used for many years [25]. The recent development of a hydrolysis using enzymes (lipase) has made possible methods that are direct, rapid, and specific. Furthermore, the completely enzymatic systems eliminate the use of caustic reagents, extraction solvents, high-temperature baths and adsorption mixtures for phospholipid removal. Much recent work has been addressed to the development of lipase reagents that completely hydrolyse triglycerides. Whitlow and Gochman [26] have reported a microbiological source of lipase that is used without added protease. The role played by the protease enzyme is unknown, yet these enzymes are necessary to attain full hydrolysis of triglycerides [27].

A major problem in the completely enzymatic methods currently used is the inconsistent quality of the enzymes available. A check against a reference procedure is suggested to assure that reliable results are obtained. Good-quality control sera (at high, low, and normal values) and linearity checks will also help to determine lot-to-lot variance. Another important consideration is shelf-life and the stability of the reagents. These time periods vary considerably from manufacturer to manufacturer. Linearity checks are a convenient way to detect reagent deterioration.

The method described by Bucolo and David [27] in common use today is based on the following sequence of reactions:

$$\text{Triglycerides} \xrightarrow[\text{chymotrypsin}]{\text{lipase}} \text{glycerol and fatty acids} \tag{1}$$

$$\text{Glycerol} + \text{ATP} \xrightarrow{\text{glycerol kinase}} \text{glycerol-3-phosphate} + \text{ADP} \tag{2}$$

$$\text{ADP} + \text{phosphoenolpyruvate} \xrightarrow{\text{pyruvate kinase}} \text{ATP} + \text{pyruvate} \tag{3}$$

$$\text{Pyruvate} + \text{NADH} + \text{H} \xrightarrow{\text{lactic dehydrogenase}} \text{lactate} + \text{NAD} \tag{4}$$

$$\text{Glycerol phosphate} + \text{NAD} \xrightarrow{\text{glycerol phosphate dehydrogenase}} \tag{5}$$
dihydroxyacetone phosphate + NADH + H

NADH + H$^+$ + 2-(p-iodophenyl)-3-(p-nitrophenyl)-5-phenyltetrazolium

$$\text{(oxidized)} \quad \xrightarrow[\quad\quad\quad]{\text{diaphorase}} \quad \text{2-(p-iodophenyl)-3-(p-nitrophenyl)} \quad\quad\quad (6)$$

$$\text{-5-phenyltetrazolium (reduced) (formazan)} + \text{NAD}^+$$

The decrease in absorbance of NADH is measured at 340 nm. In order to blank this method the procedure is repeated using a buffer in place of the lipase reagent, the disappearance of NADH fluorescence can also be read at 460 nm after excitation at 355 nm.

A procedure introduced by Megraw *et al.* [28] uses reactions steps (1) and (2) then steps (5) and (6) to form formazan, which is measured in the 500–550 nm range.

Note 2.
For an accurate triglyceride determination, the free glycerol of the sample should be subtracted from the total glycerol (both free and that produced from saponification of the triglycerides) by a blanking procedure. In fact quantitative analysis for triglycerides in serum and plasma is commonly done by hydrolysing the triglycerides and then determining glycerol enzymatically or chemically. When this is done, not only glycerol derived from triglycerides but also the unesterified 'free' glycerol is measured. To account for this free glycerol analytically makes the methods cumbersome and inconvenient. Either two analyses must be performed, one before and one after the hydrolysis step, or the two serum constituents have to be separated by extraction or by solvent partition. However, free glycerol is 0.007–0.12 mmol/1. Individuals suffering from stress, patients with liver or kidney disease, and diabetic subjects are likely to be unpredictable in this blanking procedure.

5.3.3   Procedure

Manual method. This method refers to the use of the Boehringer kit.

(a) Technique

Pipette 1.0 ml of the enzymatic triglyceride reagent into appropriate test tubes.
Add 10 µl of specimen or glycerol standard.
Mix well and incubate at 37°C for at least 10 min.
Cool the samples at room temperature.
Measure the sample, also standard absorbance at 500 nm, vs a reagent blank in which deionized water is substituted for sample.

(b) Calculation

Triglycerides in specimens and control materials are calculated in relation to the calibrator.

SECTION III   SEPARATION OF PLASMA LIPOPROTEINS

For the isolation of lipoproteins several methods are currently available that permit the analysis of the individual components of the lipoproteins fractions.
The most representative methods are summarized in Table 5.4.

5.3.4   Ultracentrifugation

Since the efforts of Gofman *et al.* [29] ultracentrifugation has become a reference method in separating plasma lipoproteins.

Table 5.4 Lipoprotein separation from plasma

1. Ultracentrifugation
   a. preparative
   b. zonal
   c. analytical
2. Precipitation with polyanions or phosphotungstic acid
3. Column chromatography
4. Electrophoresis
5. Affinity chromatography

Preparative sequential centrifugation is the most frequent approach. It takes advantage of the flotation properties of the different lipoprotein classes. Therefore very-low-density lipoproteins (VLDL), low-density lipoproteins (LDL), and high-density lipoproteins (HDL) are separated by increasing sequentially the density of the sample from 1.006 to 1.21 g/ml [29] (Table 5.5). Several samples can be processed using adequate rotors, but the procedure is time-consuming and certainly not applicable to all patients. Furthermore, to obtain a reproducible analysis of lipoproteins several factors must be controlled, in particular rotor speed, temperature, recovery of lipoproteins, acceleration, and braking. The equipment is expensive and so is the disposable material. This method has been modified by the combination of precipitation of LDL with heparin-Mn^{2+} or phosphotungstic acid Mg^{2+} (Table 5.6).

Table 5.5 Separation of lipoproteins by ultracentrifugation

Plasma 1.006 g/ml | top layer
    105 000 *g* | VLDL
    20 h
    10°C

    bottom 1.063 g/ml | top layer
        105 000 *g* | LDL
        20 h
        10°C

        bottom 1.21 g/ml | top layer
            105 000 *g* | HDL
            22 h
            10°C

Separation of lipoproteins recommended by the Lipid Res. Clin.

plasma 1.006 g/ml top layer
    105 000 *g* | VLDL
    18 h
    0°C

    bottom   precipitation
    LDL + HDL ⟶ with   supernatant
                heparin/$MnCl_2$ HDL Chol*

VLDL Chol = total chol − (LDL + HDL Chol)
LDL Chol = (LDL + HDL Chol) − HDL Chol

* Chol = cholesterol

Table 5.6 Precipitation of VLDL + LDL

a. Heparin + MnCl$_2$
b. Phosphotungstic acid + MgCl$_2$
c. Dextran sulphate + MgCl$_2$

Besides preparative ultracentrifugation, zonal ultracentrifugation has recently gained importance [30]. This method allows separation of lipoproteins by a single spin; however, very few samples can be processed per day and diluted lipoprotein preparations are obtained. The advantage of the method is that the lipoproteins are eluted from the rotor according to their rate of flotation. It is therefore possible to identify the abnormal behaviour of some lipoprotein classes, a factor usually missed by preparative ultracentrifugation.

5.3.5 Precipitation with polyanions and phosphotungstic acid

The problems related to the determination of cholesterol and triglycerides in ultracentrifugally separated samples are twofold: firstly salts may interfere with some commercially available kits; these must be removed by dialysis or column chromatography. Secondly, evidence has shown that some breaking down of lipoprotein and loss of apoproteins may occur during centrifugation.

The precipitation of plasma lipoproteins by sulphated polysaccharides was first reported in the mid-1950s and precipitation methods were developed initially for the preparative isolation of serum lipoproteins. During the past 30 years these methods have been developed further and have been adapted for lipoprotein quantitation [31, 32]. They are rapid, and relatively inexpensive to perform. Lipoproteins can generally be separated from each other within 10 min to 2 h, depending on the precipitation conditions and lipoprotein class of interest; these methods can therefore be readily applied for screening, clinical analysis, and other purposes for which rapid analyses or screening of a large number of samples is required. It should be noted that certain non-lipid-containing plasma proteins can also be precipitated under conditions used for lipoprotein separation. This is not a problem when lipoprotein–cholesterol or other lipid component is measured, but must be considered if lipoprotein–protein is analysed.

Despite the speed and simplicity of the precipitation methods, they have not been widely used except for the measurement of HDL. This has apparently resulted from a combination of factors that are not particularly related to the adequacy of the precipitation methods for the analysis of other lipoprotein classes. Firstly, the lipoproteins have been classically defined in terms of their behaviour in the ultracentrifuge, and for the most part have been measured in research laboratories that have access to this equipment. One widely used procedure for the measurement of the major lipoprotein classes uses a combination of ultracentrifugation and polyanion precipitation to prepare lipoprotein-containing fractions [33].

Secondly, for many purposes adequate estimates of VLDL- and LDL-cholesterol concentrations can be obtained from measurements of total cholesterol, triglycerides, and HDL-cholesterol using this formula:

$$|\text{LDL-chol}| = |\text{total chol}| - |\text{HDL-chol}| - \frac{\text{TG}}{5}$$

where $|TG|/5$ corresponds to an estimation of $|$ VLDL-chol $|$ and all measurements are expressed in milligrams/decilitre [34, 35].

5.3.6   Sample collection

A number of factors related to blood drawing and storage of the samples before analysis can influence lipoprotein analyses [34, 36]. Such factors include changes in the subject's posture prior to venepuncture, prolonged venous occlusion during blood drawing, large osmotic shifts of water between red cells and plasma produced by certain anticoagulants, and various enzymatic and structural and compositional changes that occur during storage. For these reasons the condition of patients should be noted, posture should be standardized as much as possible for blood drawing, and lipoprotein fractions should be prepared as soon after venepuncture as possible. Cholesterol itself is stable during long periods of storage, and in general, if the lipoprotein–cholesterol analyses must be delayed, it is preferable to store the separated fractions rather than unfractionated plasma or serum.

The subject should have fasted for 12 h prior to venepuncture. Water can be taken.

The sitting position is most commonly used for drawing blood and should be used. The subject should sit quietly for 10 min before blood is drawn. Blood can be obtained from an antecubital vein or some other convenient arm vein. A tourniquet can be used, but should be released prior to drawing blood. Blood can be drawn with a syringe and then transferred to the appropriate tubes, which then also serve as centrifuge tubes when the cells are removed. If a syringe is used, the needle should be removed before transferring the blood, to prevent haemolysis.

5.3.7   Procedure

(a) Sample preparation

Lipoproteins can be analysed either in plasma or serum, but most workers prefer to use EDTA plasma (see below).

Plasma. Disodium EDTA should have a final concentration of 1–1.5 mg/ml. The blood must be mixed gently by inversion five or six times and immediately cooled to 2–4°C in an ice bath. As soon as possible, preferably within 3 h, centrifuge the sample at 4°C for 30 min at 1500 g. Transfer the plasma to a clean storage vial that can be closed to prevent evaporation, and store at 4°C. If several tubes of blood are drawn, the storage vial should be large enough to permit the plasma to be pooled and mixed.

Serum. Blood should be collected as described above but without the anticoagulant. Allow the sample to stand at room temperature for 45 min in a glass tube. Transfer the serum to a storage vial as above, cool to 2–4°C. If the analyses must be delayed, add EDTA (final concentration 1×10^{-3} M) to the serum to inhibit oxidative changes in the lipoproteins. This is not necessary if the analyses are to be performed promptly.

(b) Lipoprotein precipitation

Lipoproteins can be selectively precipitated with a variety of agents, including combinations of particular polyanions and divalent cations (e.g. heparin sulphate, dextran sulphate, or sodium phosphotungstate in combination with Mn^{2+}, Mg^{2+}, Ca^{2+}), anionic detergents such as sodium decylsulphate, polyethylene glycol, protamine, tetracyclines, and others. Of these, perhaps the most widely used to precipitate apo-B-containing lipoproteins have been sulphated polysaccharide–divalent cation combinations. The specific precipitants used, conditions of reagent concentration, temperature, and time vary depending on the lipoprotein class of interest. The lipoprotein specificity and completeness on precipitation are affected by a number of factors including pH, ionic strength, the presence of other serum proteins, the presence of polyions such as sucrose, and the lipid-to-protein ratio of the lipoprotein. In general, precipitation with sulphated polysaccharides occurs more readily (i.e., at lower precipitant concentrations) at low ionic strength and in the absence of other serum proteins.

SECTION IV   HDL CHOLESTEROL DETERMINATION

A wide variety of precipitating agents have been used to remove apo-B-containing lipoproteins from serum or plasma.

5.3.8 Heparin–MnCl₂ method

The heparin–$MnCl_2$ method of Burstein *et al.* [31, 37] has been perhaps the widest used and most intensively evaluated of the precipitation methods for HDL, and much of the epidemiological data that relates HDL cholesterol concentration to cardiovascular risk has been accumulated using this method [38].

5.3.9 Chemicals

(a) Chemicals

$MnCl_2$. $4H_2O$ p.a.

Heparin (porcine intestinal mucosa). Heparin is a polydisperse sulphated polysaccharide that is obtained from several sources, generally bovine lung or porcine intestinal mucosa. The preparations from lung and intestine differ somewhat in size, chemical structure, and lipoprotein-precipitating properties [39], although porcine intestinal heparin from various manufacturers has been reported to give equivalent HDL cholesterol measurements. Heparin sodium can be obtained as a powder or as an injectable solution in 0.15 M NaCl.

NaCl p.a.

(b) Solutions

$MnCl_2$. $4H_2O$, 1.0 M: The crystalline reagent is slightly deliquescent and should therefore be stored in a tightly closed container. Dissolve 19.791 g $MnCl_2$. $4H_2O$ in distilled H_2O, transfer quantitatively to a 100-ml volumetric flask, and dilute to volume with distilled H_2O. The solution should be stored in the refrigerator and prepared fresh every month.

Heparin (porcine intestinal mucosa). The dry powder is dissolved in 0.15 M NaCl to a concentration of 35 mg/ml. Injectable heparin sodium is generally provided with concentrations expressed in USP units of anticoagulability per millilitre. Dilute the solution to a final concentration of 5000 USP units/ml with 0.15 M NaCl. This provides a concentration of about 35 mg/ml. The solution stored in the refrigerator; in the author's experience, can be used for at least a month.

5.3.10   Procedure

The conditions for this method were originally developed for serum, but the method has been widely used in EDTA plasma.

Allow the samples to reach room temperature, then measure 2.0 ml of sample into a transparent 15 ml conical centrifuge tube. Add 80 μl of heparin (35 mg/ml) to each sample and mix thoroughly but smoothly to avoid foaming. If a vortex mixer is used, mix the sample intermittently several times to avoid layering of the reagent. Add 100 μl of 1.0 M $MnCl_2$ to each sample and mix as above. A heavy white precipitate will form immediately. Place the samples in an ice bath and allow them to stand for 30 min, then sediment the precipitate by centrifuging at 1500 g for 30 min at 4°C. The precipitate should be packed tightly at the bottom of the tube and the supernatant should be clear. Using a Pasteur pipette equipped with a rubber bulb, carefully remove an aliquot of the clear supernatant for cholesterol analysis. If the analysis will not be performed immediately, the supernatant should be stored in a container that can be sealed to prevent evaporation. The supernatants can be stored at 4°C for a few days before analysis, but should be frozen, preferably at −70°C or lower, if longer periods of storage are required.

Cholesterol in the heparin–Mn^{2+} supernatant can be analysed by either chemical or enzymatic methods (see below). The measured cholesterol concentration is multiplied by the factor 1.09 to correct for the sample dilution that results from the addition of the reagents.

More complete precipitation of apo-B-containing lipoproteins can be achieved using a higher concentration of $MnCl_2$. Based on extensive evaluations of the heparin–$MnCl_2$ method, the use of 0.092 M $MnCl_2$ was recommended for use in EDTA plasma [32]. Under these conditions, unprecipitated apo-B-associated cholesterol was reduced to 0.5 mg/dl or less, even in samples that were stored at 4°C for several days. Some HDL is also precipitated, but the loss is less than 1 mg/dl HDL cholesterol [32]. If this modification is used, the procedure is performed as described above, except that 2.0 M $MnCl_2$ is substituted for 1.0 M $MgCl_2$. Note that 0.046 M $MnCl_2$ should be used with serum, since larger amounts of HDL are precipitated at the higher $MnCl_2$ concentration and HDL cholesterol is therefore underestimated.

Samples with elevated triglycerides. Two kinds of difficulties can arise in samples with high triglyceride levels. One fairly common problem is that in which the heparin–Mn^{2+} lipoprotein complex does not sediment completely, and the supernatant remains turbid. This occurs most frequently in samples with triglyceride levels exceeding 300–400 mg/dl, but can occur in the presence of lower triglyceride levels also [32]. Since most plasma cholesterol is associated with apo-B-containing lipoproteins, even small amounts of turbidity can lead to grossly inaccurate HDL cholesterol measurements. Several approaches have been used with hypertriglyceridaemic samples. First, triglyceride-rich lipo-proteins are removed by ultracentrifugation and the precipitation then performed on the d 1.006 g/ml fraction. HDL-cholesterol values measured in this fraction are slightly lower than those in unfractionated plasma, due in part to losses incurred in preparing the ultracentrifugal fraction. In another approach, the turbid heparin–MnCl$_2$ supernatant is filtered through 0.22-μm filters to remove the unsedimented lipoprotein complexes, and HDL cholesterol is analysed in the filtrate [40]. In a third approach, turbid plasma is diluted with 0.15 M saline before being treated with heparin–MnCl$_2$. This reduces the triglyceride and plasma protein concentrations of the sample, and generally produces clear heparin–MnCl$_2$ supernatants. Dilutions greater than twofold are not recommended, however, because the HDL cholesterol concentrations become too low to measure accurately, and dilution errors become excessive. The fourth approach has been simply to centrifuge the turbid supernatant at higher speed, which usually clears the supernatant. In hypertriglyceridaemic samples, however, some of the precipitate may float to the top of the tube rather than sediment; this can make it difficult to recover the clear HDL-containing fraction. Finally, the incidence of turbid supernatants is about threefold lower when the precipitation is performed with 0.092 M MnCl$_2$ rather than 0.046 M reagent.

Incomplete sedimentation of the heparin–MnCl$_2$–lipoprotein complex is usually evident when it occurs. The more serious difficulties are encountered when the precipitated lipoproteins are sedimented satisfactorily but apo-B-containing lipoproteins are incompletely precipitated. Incomplete precipitation should be suspected in samples with HDL cholesterol concentrations that exceed about 80 mg/dl, and the analyses should be confirmed in these samples. In samples with apparent HDL cholesterol concentrations in the normal range, however, there may be no reason to suspect that a particular analysis was in error. For example, in incomplete precipitation of apo-B-containing lipo-proteins from a sample with an HDL cholesterol concentration of 55 mg/dl, the error would go undetected. It is therefore advisable to assess routinely the completeness of precipitation of apo-B-containing lipoproteins in a subset, perhaps 5% or 10%, of samples with HDL cholesterol concentrations in the normal range.

Analysis of stored samples. Lipoproteins are subject to a variety of alterations during storage, including auto-oxidation, changes in composition mediated by lipase or lecithin cholesterol acyltransferase, exchange of cholesteryl esters and triglycerides between HDL and other plasma lipoproteins, bacterial contamination, proteolytic cleavage, and others. These changes apparently influence the precipitability of the lipoproteins. For example, the apo-B-containing lipoproteins become increasingly more difficult to precipitate completely, and HDL becomes progressively easier to precipitate as the length of storage increases [41]. The net effect of these opposing trends depends on the cholesterol concentration. In samples with low HDL cholesterol levels the incomplete precipitation of apo-B-containing lipoproteins apparently predominates and there is a tendency for the apparent HDL cholesterol concentrations to increase with storage. In samples with high HDL cholesterol concentrations, the inappropriate prenipitation of HDL cholesterol concentrations tend to decrease somewhat in stored samples. These effects are most marked when samples are stored at refrigerator temperatures, but also observable in samples that are stored at $-20°C$ and to some extent at $-70°C$ as well. At refrigerator temperatures the effects were observable but small in samples stored up to 4 days, but became more pronounced after one and two weeks of storage. In our experience it is best to precipitate samples as soon as possible after they are drawn, preferably on the day of venepuncture. If necessary the heparin–$MnCl_2$ supernatants can be stored at $-70°C$ for at least one year prior to analysis of HDL cholesterol [42].

Enzymatic cholesterol analysis. The sources of inaccuracy and imprecision discussed above relate to the preparation of the HDL-containing fractions, and the information provided was based on the analysis of lipid extracts of samples using chemical cholesterol methods such as those based on the Liebermann–Burchard reaction. Under these conditions the precipitation reagents do not interfere with the cholesterol analyses. In recent years chemical methods have been largely replaced by enzymatic analysis of cholesterol, which can be performed directly in serum or plasma. $MnCl_2$, however, interferes with the enzymatic analysis of cholesterol and gives falsely high HDL cholesterol values in heparin–$MnCl_2$ supernatants [43, 44]. The mechanism of the interference is uncertain, but may be due in part to the precipitation of Mn^{2+} by phosphate-containing buffers that are commonly used in the enzyme reagents, and in part to the direct interference of Mn^{2+} with one or more of the enzymatic reactions themselves. Several approaches have been used to avoid this problem. In one, interference was eliminated by including EDTA ($4 \times 10^{-3}M$) in the enzymatic reaction system to chelate Mn^{2+} [43]. Workers using a 2.5-fold higher concentraon of the chelating agent, however, reported that EDTA itself interferes with enzymatic cholesterol analysis [45]. In another recently described modification, Mn^{2+} is first removed from the heparin–$MnCl_2$ supernatant by precipitation with $HCO\bar{3}$. This procedure is as follows.

Prepare the heparin-$MnCl_2$ supernatant as described above. Accurately measure a convenient aliquot (0.50 or 1.0 ml) of the heparin–Mn^{2+} supernatant into a 1–4 ml polypropylene microcentrifuge tube. Add 0.1 vol of 1 M $NaHCO_3$, mix well, and allow the sample to stand at room temperature for at least 30 min. A white precipitate of $Mn(HCO_3)_2$ forms immediately and precipitation is complete within this period. If the cholesterol analyses are not to be performed immediately the samples can be sealed to prevent evaporation and stored for two or three days in the refrigerator. The $Mn(HCO_3)_2$ precipitate is then sedimented by centrifuging for 10 min at 10 000 g in a benchtop microcentrifuge, and cholesterol is measured in the clear supernatant.

With this modification the measured HDL cholesterol values must be multiplied by 1.199 to correct for dilution by the heparin, $MnCl_2$, and $NaHCO_3$ reagents.

5.3.11 Dextran sulphate–$MgCl_2$ method

As mentioned earlier, a variety of precipitants have been used to remove apo-B-containing lipoproteins, the more common of which include dextran sulphate–Mg^{2+}, phosphotungstate–Mg^{2+}, polyethylene glycol, and heparin–Ca^{2+}. The completeness with which these agents remove apo-B-containing lipoproteins and leave HDL in solution differ somewhat, and can lead to results for HDL cholesterol that are as much as 5–10% higher or lower than those obtained with heparin and $MnCl_2$. With the advent of completely enzymatic cholesterol methods, there has been a growing interest in developing these procedures further, and recent modifications of methods that use the three non-heparin precipitants mentioned above give HDL cholesterol values that are quite similar to those obtained with the heparin–$MnCl_2$ method. The dextran sulphate–$MgCl_2$ method is described here because of its usefulness with enzymatic cholesterol methods and for the use by several lipid research clinics in Europe.

5.3.12 Chemicals

(a) Chemicals

NaN_3 p.a.
Gentamicin sulphate
Chloramphenicol
Dextran sulphate
$MgCl_2 . 6H_2O$ p.a.

(b) Solutions

Preservative solution: dissolve 5.0 g NaN_3, 50 mg gentamicin sulphate, and 100 mg chloramphenicol in distilled H_2O and adjust to 100 ml with H_2O.

Dextran sulphate (M_r 50 000 ± 5000), 20 g/litre: the dry reagent is stored at 4°C in a desiccator. Dissolve 2.0 g dextran sulphate in 80 ml distilled, deionized H_2O and adjust to pH 7.0 with HCl. Transfer the solution quantitatively to a 100-ml volumetric flask. Add 1.0 ml of the preservative solution and adjust to volume with H_2O. Store the solution at 4°C.

$MgCl_2 . 6H_2O$, 1.0 M: this reagent is hygroscopic and should be stored in a tightly closed container or a desiccator. Dissolve 20.3 g $MgCl_2 . 6H_2O$ in 80 ml and adjust to pH 7.0 with a solution of NaOH. Dilute to 100 ml with H_2O as described above and store the solution at 4°C.

Accurately measure equal volumes of the dextran sulphate and $MgCl_2$ solutions into a suitable container and mix. Store at 4°C. The working solution is stable for at least four months.

5.3.13 Procedure

The method can be used with either EDTA plasma or serum.

Allow the samples to reach room temperature. Using a volumetric pipette or device of similar accuracy, place a 1.0-ml sample in a transparent test tube or conical centrifuge tube. Add 100 μl working reagent and mix thoroughly. The final reagent concentrations are 0.91 mg/ml dextran sulphate and 0.045 M $MgCl_2$. Allow the mixture to stand at room temperature for 10 min, then sediment the precipitate by centrifuging at 1500 *g* for 30 min at 4°C. Using a Pasteur pipette, carefully remove an aliquot of the clear supernatant for cholesterol analysis. If necessary, the supernatant can be stored at 4°C in a sealed container for a few days before analysis.

The precipitants do not interfere either with chemical cholesterol methods such as the Liebermann–Burchard reaction, or any of the available enzymatic cholesterol methods, and any of these methods can be used to measure cholesterol in the dextran sulphate–$MgCl_2$ supernatants. The measured cholesterol values are multiplied by 1.10 to correct for dilution by the reagent.

Note 3.

This method was modified from earlier procedures that used dextran sulphate preparations of higher (M_r 500 000) or lower (M_r 15 000) molecular weight. The higher molecular weight material apparently precipitated a significant amount of HDL and the lower molecular weight preparations incompletely removed apo-B-containing lipoproteins. The use of dextran sulphate of M_r 50 000 gave HDL cholesterol values that averaged 1–2 mg/dl lower than those obtained with the heparin–$MnCl_2$ method, in part because of the presence of less residual apo-B-containing lipoproteins in the dextran sulphate–$MgCl_2$ supernatants. The method precipitated slightly more apo A-I than heparin–$MnCl_2$, but this accounted for only about 0.5 mg/dl HDL cholesterol.

Based on paired comparisons of the dextran sulphate–$MgCl_2$ and heparin–$MnCl_2$ methods in EDTA plasma, the two methods were highly correlated (r = 0.98) and gave similar results over the concentration range 25–75 mg/dl.

Samples with elevated triglycerides. As with the heparin–$MnCl_2$ method, turbid sulphate–$MgCl_2$ supernatants are occasionally encountered and can give grossly inaccurate HDL cholesterol values. This occurs most frequently in samples with high triglyceride levels, but occurs less than half as often with this method as with heparin–$MnCl_2$. When it does occur, clear supernatants can be prepared by ultrafiltration, sample dilution, or preliminary removal of triglyceride-rich lipoproteins by ultracentrifugation at d 1.006 g/ml.

5.4 THE ARACHIDONIC ACID CASCADE IN THE VASCULAR SYSTEM

5.4.1 Introduction

The formation of oxygenated metabolites of arachidonic acid (AA, 20:4 Δ 5, 8, 11, 14, n-6), through the two major enzymatic pathways cyclo and lipoxygenases, is a complex system involved in the modulation of a number of cell responses in biological compartments. These products are currently termed 'eicosanoids', and the overall process of activation of AA metabolism is named 'AA cascade'. Several types of cell elements within the vascular system (e.g. platelets, leukocytes, and cells of the vessel walls) produce eicosanoids under appropriate stimulation, thus contributing to the modulation of several functional parameters in the circulation.

AA and/or other 20-carbon polyunsaturated fatty acids (PUFA), such as eicosapentaenoic acid, EPA, 20:5 Δ 5, 8, 11, 14, 17 n-3, which play a key role as precursors of eicosanoids, are metabolically derived from the 18-carbon essential fatty acids (EFA), linoleic acid (18:2 Δ 9, 12) and α linolenic acid (18:3 Δ 9, 12, 15) respectively, provided by the diet, or are directly supplied with it. The conversion of the 18-carbon EFA, especially of α linolenic to the long-chain PUFA, however, is relatively inefficient and EPA accumulates in tissues only after dietary administration of the compound. The relationships between dietary fatty acids and the eicosanoid precursors provide the basis for the impact of dietary fatty acids on the eicosanoid cascade.

Eicosanoids produced in the circulation modulate parameters such as platelet aggregation, vascular resistance, leukocyte migration and others, which are relevant for the homeostasis of the vascular system in physiological conditions and may also play a role in the onset of pathological states such as arterial thrombosis and inflammation.

The above considerations provide the conceptual framework to the interest of nutritionists and epidemiologists in the impact of dietary lipids, especially fatty acids, not only on plasma lipid and lipoprotein levels and metabolism, but also on the production of eicosanoids in the vascular compartment, and hence on functions of cells in the circulation. In addition, recent data on imbalances of eicosanoid formation in vascular pathology, such as atherosclerosis induced by hyperlipidaemia, may indicate nutritional approaches to the control of altered eicosanoid production in these pathological conditions.

5.4.2. Sites and mechanisms of eicosanoid production

The pathways of the oxidative AA metabolism in specific cell types have been elucidated in the last decade and it is now well established that several cells in the circulation (with the exception of lymphocytes and red blood cells), or cells lined on vessel walls, such as endothelial elements, produce various types of eicosanoids, as summarized in Table 5.7. It is also clear that each type of cell has a certain degree of specialization in the production of AA metabolites, resulting in different patterns of eicosanoids, and that biochemical requirements differ among different cells. Platelets, for instance, convert very efficiently even very low concentrations of AA to cyclo and lipoxygenase products, whereas neutrophils require cell activation steps based on second mediators pathways such as G-proteins, inositol phosphate formation, and other signal-transduction events in order to initiate the formation of lipoxygenase products.

The biosynthesis of eicosanoids can be considered a two-step process, the first step producing a chemically reactive intermediate (e.g. the endoperoxides produced by the cyclo-oxygenase, and the leukotriene A_4 produced by the 5-lipoxygenase), and the second, mediated by specific enzymes such as the thromboxane and cyclo-oxygenase synthetases, the endoperoxide isomerases and the leukotriene A_4 hydrolase and C_4 synthase. It has become evident that the two steps of eicosanoid synthesis can take place in two separate cell types. The chemically reactive intermediate produced in the initial cell must have a sufficient stability in order to leave the cell, traverse the aqueous milieu between cells, and to enter in the second cell, where it is converted to the biologically active product. This type of interaction between cells, which can be considered a form of cell-to-cell communication, is a transcellular form of AA metabolism recently termed 'transcellular eicosanoid biosynthesis' [46]. This process can

Table 5.7 Eicosanoid metabolites produced by specific human blood or vascular cells

Cell types	Oxygenases	
	Cyclo (CO)	*Lipo (LO)*
Circulating elements		
Platelets	$PGH_2, TxA_2,$ $PGE_2, F_{2\alpha}, D_2$	12-LO (12-HETE)
Neutrophils		5-LO ($LTA_4, LTB_4,$ 5-HETE)
15-LO (15-HETE)		
Eosinophils		5-LO (LTA_4, LTC_4) 15-LO (15-HETE)
Monocytes*	$TxB_2, PGE_2,$ 6 keto-$PGF_{1\alpha}$	5-LO ($LTA_4, LTB_4,$ LTC_4)
Lymphocytes	No product	
Red blood cells	No product	
Vessel wall elements		
Endothelial cells:		
Umbilical vein	$PGI_2, F_{2\alpha},$ D_2, PGE_2	
Capillaries	PGE_2 or PGD_2 or $PGF_{2\alpha} > PGI_2$	
Smooth muscle cells	PGI_2	

* Monocyte/macrophage

extensively modify the eicosanoid profile presented in Table 5.7, since the eicosanoid product from one cell modulates the biosynthesis of eicosanoids by vicinal cells.

Most studies on eicosanoid synthesis are carried out on stimulated cell preparations *in vitro* and are based on direct quantitation of the primary prostaglandins or of specific metabolites. Production *in vivo* is assumed also to be the consequence of cellular stimulation and to reflect the activation of a given cell source. For the above considerations, however, the production of eicosanoids *in vivo* will reflect the multiple intercellular co-operation processes, where only the 'donor' cell undergoes activation and the 'recipient' cell carries out the final transformation to the end product. The contribution of each cell to the final product will thus be difficult to evaluate.

A key process responsible for triggering eicosanoid production is considered to be the stimulation of the release of precursor(s) fatty acid(s) from cell phospholipid pools, through activation of phospholipases. Phospholipase (PLase) activities may directly release the fatty acid from the 2-position of the glycerol backbone of phospholipids (PLase A_2), or sequential steps may take place involving the initial formation of diacylglycerol (DAG), e.g. from phosphoinositides through PLase C, followed by DAG hydrolysis through a DAG-lipase. The activation of these lipolytic pathways may be the result of receptor stimulation and requires the participation of G-proteins.

5.4.3 Approaches to the study of eicosanoid production in the vascular system

Formation of eicosanoids by cells present in blood is generally studied by measuring the products generated by homogeneous preparations of individual cell types, incubated in the presence of the fatty acid precursor(s) or challenged with adequate stimuli. The most simple biochemical approach is to incubate the cell preparations with labelled AA and to measure the labelled products thus formed, after separation by chromatographic techniques. It should be considered, however, that under these experimental conditions various factors may affect the amounts and profiles of eicosanoids produced. For example, the concentration of AA required by platelets for the synthesis of oxygenated metabolites is much lower than that required by leukocytes; the exogenous substrates do not equilibrate with the endogenous eicosanoid precursor and may have different access to the synthetic enzymes, since these have been shown in various cells to have different subcellular localizations (Table 5.8).

Table 5.8 Subcellular localization of major AA metabolizing enzymes

Enzymes	Product(s)	Site(s)	Cell
Prostaglandin Endoperoxide synthase	PGG_2 and PGH_2	ER, NM	Fibroblast
Thromboxane synthase	12-HHT TxA_2	DTM	Platelet
Prostacyclin synthase	PGI_2	PM NM	SMC
PGH to PGD Isomerase	PGD_2	C	rat brain, spleen
PGH to PGE Isomerase	PGE_2	ER	sheep vesicular glands
12-LO	12-S-HPETE	C, M	platelets
15-LO	15-S-HPETE	C	neutrophils
5-LO	5-HPETE	C	RBL-1
Dehydrase LTA hydrolase	LTA_4	"	"
Glutathion transferase	LTC_4	P	"

C, cytoplasm; DTM, dense tubular membranes; ER, endoplasmic reticulum; M, membrane fractions; NM, nuclear membrane; P, particulate; PM, plasma membrane; RBL, rat basophilic leukaemia cells; SMC, smooth muscle cells.

An alternative approach is to evaluate the formation of various products after challenge with appropriate stimuli, such as catecholamines, thrombin, collagen, etc. in the case of platelets. The concentration ranges and the additive or interacting activities of various agonists on the same type of cell make it difficult to relate, from the quantitative and the qualitative points of view, the effects observed *in vitro* with the situation in the intact animal. Measurements made in isolated cell preparations thus provide information on the 'capacity' of cells to activate the eicosanoid system upon appropriate stimulation, rather than indicate the actual involvement in pathophysiological processes. It should be considered, in addition, that there are sources of error in this type of measurements, since trauma during sampling can result in the *ex vivo* formation of prostaglandins [47].

More accurate information on the formation and release of eicosanoids into the vascular compartment in the intact animal can be obtained by evaluating the enzymatic metabolites of unstable products such as thromboxane A_2 (TxA_2) in plasma [48]. Additional analytical errors may confound measurements of eicosanoids in biological fluids, reflecting poor specificity of the assays. Measurements of plasma TxB_2 and 6-keto-$PGF_{1\alpha}$ by radioimmunoassay (RIA) are often an order of magnitude higher than those found by direct physico-chemical methods [49]. This may in part reflect cross-reactivity of the antibody at low levels of plasma metabolites in the presence of other eicosanoids in relatively high concentrations. Traumatic and analytical errors can be avoided by measurements of the urinary enzymatic metabolites of eicosanoids, and by assays based on the use of gas chromatography combined with mass spectrometry. Determinations of various enzymatic metabolites of TxA_2, i.e. 2, 3-dinor-thromboxane B_2 [50], and 11-dehydro-thromboxane B_2 [48], and of 2, 3-dinor-6-keto-prostaglandin $F_{1\alpha}$ [51] have been described. These method-ological approaches have shown that plasma levels of TxB_2 and 6-keto-$PGF_{1\alpha}$ are in the low pg/ml range rather than in the much higher (one hundredfold or more) ranges obtained by RIA determinations [51, 52].

Concerning the products of the lipoxygenase pathway, the leukotrienes (B_4 and C_4) are potent mediators of inflammation and many play a role in acute inflammatory processes occurring in the vascular compartment (e.g. shock, endotoxaemia). Formation of these products by isolated polymorphonuclear cells upon appropriate and adequate stimulation is currently studied. On the other hand evaluation of leukotriene formation *in vivo* is difficult since these compounds may be rapidly metabolized through cell-bound enzyme in various organs [53] (e.g. C_4 to D_4 and E_4) and rapidly excreted [54]. LTC_4 has a very short plasma half-life (30 s) [55] and LET_4 is considered the major urinary metabolite of LTC_4 [56].

5.4.4 Vascular eicosanoids, atherosclerosis, and dietary fatty acids

Eicosanoids have well-known vascular and haemostatic actions that may influence the onset and development of the atherosclerotic process and/or of its major complications, the thromboembolic events. Formations of the potent vasoconstricting and platelet-aggregating thromboxane A_2, the major cyclo-oxygenase product made by platelets, and of the vasodilating and antiaggregatory product prostacyclin, made by vessel walls, have been shown to be modified in hypercholesterolaemic subjects. Platelet responses to proaggregatory agents are often enhanced in type IIa hypercholesterolaemic subjects [57], and this is associated with greater formation of TxB_2, as assessed by a greater accumulation of the product in platelet suspensions from type IIa subjects, after stimulation with aggregating agents [58]. Also, the excretion of the urinary metabolites of thromboxane was enhanced in patients with unstable angina [59] and in patients with angiographic evidence of coronary thrombosis [60]. On the other hand, there is evidence of an imbalance in the prostacyclin/thromboxane system in several vascular diseases, and decreased production of prostacyclin by atherosclerotic vascular tissue has been demonstrated both in experimental animals and in man. Aortae from rabbits made atherosclerotic by cholesterol feeding, after a transient increase show a long-lasting reduction [61], and smooth muscle cells obtained from atherosclerotic lesions consistently produce less prostacyclin, possibly because of the high formation of lipoxygenase products, which inhibit prostacyclin generation [62]. In contrast, there have been also reports of increased release of prostacyclin by isolated perfused aortae of hypercholesterolaemic rabbits [63] and of enhanced urinary excretion of prostacyclin metabolites in patients with severe diffuse atherosclerosis [64]. Prostacyclin biosynthesis has also been reported to increase, in coincidence with an increase of thromboxane A_2, in patients with unstable angina [59].

Concomitantly with the evidence of an altered balance of vascular eicosanoids in hypercholesterolaemia and in various clinical forms of atherosclerotic disease, several studies have shown that dietary fatty acids also modulate the formation of the eicosanoids that play a role in thrombogenesis, i.e. thromboxane and prostacyclin. These effects may be considered in defining strategies for the dietary control of factors involved in vascular pathologies.

High levels of linoleic acid in the diet are known to exert a cholesterol-lowering effect [65] and the administration of linoleic-acid-rich diets has been reported to reduce platelet reactivity in animals [66], and in man [67]. A study in moderately hypercholesterolaemic population groups has shown that the administration of diets with high linoleic acid for a period of six weeks resulted in reduction of both plasma cholesterol (especially LDL cholesterol) levels and platelet thromboxane formation [68]. This effect may be related to reduction of platelet arachidonate as a consequence of partial replacement by linoleic acid. No effect on platelets was observed, however, in a study carried out in hypertriglyceridaemic subjects fed diets with high linoleic acid content for a period of only three weeks [69]. This may be related to the relatively short duration of the treatment, which, in effect, did not modify the AA content of platelets.

In summary, it appears that the administration of diets rich in linoleic acid, supplementing or replacing saturated fat, leads to some reduction of platelet reactivity. In fact, platelet aggregation to low doses of aggregating agents may be inhibited and these cells appear also to be less reactive, as evidenced by an increase in the clotting time and reduction in circulating aggregates. It is not clear, however, whether the effects of high dietary linoleic acid on platelet functions are dependent upon concomitant changes of plasma cholesterol or are directly centred on platelet biochemistry.

A greater interest in the effects of dietary fatty acids on platelet function derived from the observations of Dyerberg *et al.* [70] of a very low incidence of thrombotic episodes in populations, such as the Eskimos, consuming very high levels of marine products, rich in very-long-chain PUFA derived from α linolenic acids (n-3 fatty acids). More specifically the presence of the 20:5 member of this series, EPA, in marine fat and in plasma and in tissues of fish-consuming subjects has been considered the key factor responsible for the very low tendency of their platelets to aggregate. When n-3 fatty acids are included in the diet, EPA and the other long-chain PUFA present in high concentrations in marine fat, 22:6, DHA, compete with AA in several ways. EPA and DHA inhibit the formation of AA from linoleic acid; they compete with AA for the 2-position in membrane phospholipids, thus reducing the cellular levels of this fatty acid [71]; and EPA competes with AA as the substrate for the cyclo-oxygenase, inhibiting the production of TxA_2 by platelets and producing only small amounts of physiologically inactive thromboxane A_3 [72]. On the other hand the formation of prostaglandin I_2 is not markedly inhibited [73, 74] and the activity of a new prostaglandin, prostaglandin I_3 [73], synthesized from EPA, is added to that of prostaglandin I_2. The result of these changes in vascular eicosanoid formation is a new haemostatic balance toward reduced platelet aggregation.

EPA is also metabolized by a 5-lipoxygenase to the class of leukotrienes. Leukotrienes derived from AA (4-series leukotrienes) have a strong chemo-attraction to circulating polymorphonuclear leukocytes and monocytes, and are involved in inflammatory, allergic, and immune responses [75]. Leukotrienes participate also in the vascular response to ischaemia [76]. EPA, which accumulates in cell membrane phospholipids, thus replacing AA and inhibiting the production of LTB_4 from arachidonic acid, forms a leukotriene B_5, less active than the B_4 isomer [77]. These effects may explain the anti-inflammatory effects of n-3 enriched oils. In addition to the above actions, the administration of oils rich in n-3 fatty acids to experimental animals, resulted in reduced formation of lipid-derived second mediators, the inositol phosphates, by platelets after stimulation [78]. This indicates that dietary fatty acids may contribute to modulate also early biochemical events involved in the responses of cells to various types of stimulation.

In summary, the eicosanoid cascade appears to be altered in conditions of vascular pathology such as atherosclerosis, with a balance between the various products that may lead to thrombotic events. Dietary fatty acids contribute to modify favourably both plasma cholesterol levels and the generation of prothrombotic eicosanoids in the vascular compartment. In addition to increasing the amount of PUFA in the diet up to 7–8% of the energy (en%), in association with reducing saturated fat below 10 en% and elevating mono-unsaturated fatty acids up to 15 en%, as recommended by various health organizations, we should include n-3 fatty acids as important components of the diet and an adequate supply of natural antioxidants in order to prevent oxidation of these rather unstable products. The consequent rise of the n-3/n-6 fatty acid ratio would result in a more favourable balance among vasoactive eicosanoids and in a reduced tendency toward thrombosis.

REFERENCES

1. Holman, R.T., Smythe, L. and Johnson, S. (1979) Effect of sex and age on fatty acid composition of human serum lipids. *Am. J. Clin. Nutr.*, **32**, 2390–9.
2. Angelico, F., Amodeo, P., Borgogelli, C. *et al.* (1980) Red blood cell fatty acid composition in a sample of Italian middle-aged men on free diet. *Nutr. Metab.*, **24**, 148–53.
3. Reeves, V.B., Matusik, E.J. and Kelsay, J.L. (1984) Variations in plasma fatty acid concentrations during a one-year self-selected dietary intake study. *Am. J. Clin. Nutr.*, **40**, 1345–51.
4. Plakké, T., Berkel, J., Beynen, A.C. *et al.* (1983) Relationship between the fatty acid composition of the diet and that of the subcutaneous adipose tissue in individual human subjects. *Hum. Nutr. Appl. Nutr.*, **37A**, 365–72.
5. Jacobsen, B.K., Trygg, K., Hjermann, I. *et al.* (1983) Acyl pattern of adipose

tissue triglycerides, plasma free fatty acids and diet of a group of men participating in a primary coronary prevention program (The Oslo study). *Am. J. Clin. Nutr.*, **38**, 906–13.

6. Manku, M.S., Horrobin, D.F., Huang, Y.S. and Morse, N. (1983) Fatty acids in plasma and red cell membranes in normal humans. *Lipids*, **18**, 906–8.

7. McMurchie, E.J., Margetts, B.M., Beilin, L.J. *et al.* (1984) Dietary-induced changes in the fatty acid composition of human cheek cell phospholipids: correlation with changes in the dietary polyunsaturated/saturated fat ratio. *Am. J. Clin. Nutr.*, **39**, 975–80.

8. Galli, G., Edwards, K.D.G. and Paoletti, R. (1970) Serum phospholipid alterations and their control by chlorophenoxyisobutyrate and betabenzalbutyrate in puromycin aminonucleoside induced nephrotic syndrome in the rat. *Life Science*, **9**(II), 524–34.

9. Cooke, R.J., Zee, P. and Yeh, Y.Y. (1984) Essential fatty acid status of the premature infant during short-term fat-free parenteral nutrition. *J. Pediatr. Gastroenterol. Nutr.*, **3**, 446–9.

10. Hunt, C.E., Engel, R.R., Modler, S. *et al.* (1978) Essential fatty acid deficiency in neonates: Inability to reverse deficiency by topical applications of EFA-rich oil. *J. Pediatr.*, **92**, 603–7.

11. Cunnane, S.C., Meadows, N.J., Keeling, P.W.N. *et al.* (1985) Lipid incorporation of linoleic and arachidonic acids by peripheral blood leucocytes in human pregnancy at term. *Nutr. Res.*, **5**, 373–9.

12. Ogburn, P.L., Williams, P.P., Johnson, S.B. and Holman, R.T. (1984) Serum arachidonic acid levels in normal and pre-eclamptic pregnancies. *Am. J. Obstet. Gynecol.*, **148**, 5–9.

13. Beaton, G.H., Milner, J., Corey, P. *et al.* (1979) Sources of variance in 24-hour dietary recall data: implications for nutrition study design and interpretation. *Am. J. Clin. Nutr.*, **32**, 2546–59.

14. Carlson, L.A. (1963) Determination of serum triglycerides. *J. Ather. Res.*, **3**, 334–9.

15. Gotto, A.M. Jr. (1978) Status report: plasma lipids, lipoproteins, and coronary heart disease. *Ather. Rev.*, **4**, 17–28.

16. Castelli, W.P., Doyle, J.T., Gordon, T. *et al.* (1977) HDL cholesterol and other lipids in coronary heart disease. The cooperative lipoprotein phenotyping study. *Circulation*, **55**, 767–72.

17. Lipid Research Clinics coronary primary prevention trial results. (1984) *JAMA*, **251**, 351–74.

18. Frick, M.H., Elo, O., Haapa, K. *et al.* (1987) Helsinki heart study: Primary-prevention trial with gemfibrozil in middle-aged men with dyslipidemia. *N. Engl. J. Med.*, **317**, 1237–45.

19. Eberhagen, D. (1969) Betrachtungen zur Bestimmung des Cholesterins in Klinisch Chemichen Laboratorium. *Klin. Chem. Klin. Biochem.*, **7**, 167–76.

20. Zak, B. (1980) Cholesterol methodology of human studies. *Lipids*, **15**, 698–704.

21. Borke, R.W., Diamondstone, B.I., Velapoldi, R.A. and Menis, O. (1974) Mechanism of the Liebermann–Burchard and Zak color reactions for cholesterol. *Clin. Chem.*, **20**, 794–800.

22. Abell, L., Levy, B.B., Brodie, B.B. and Kendall, F.E. (1952) A simplified method for the estimation of total cholesterol in serum and demonstration of its specificity. *J. Biol. Chem.*, **195**, 357–66.

23. Trinder, P. (1969) Determination of glucose in blood using an alternative oxygen acceptor. *Ann. Clin. Biochem.*, **6**, 24–7.

24. Van Handel, E. and Zilversmit, D.B. (1957) Micromethod for the direct determination of plasma triglycerides. *J. Lab. Clin. Med.*, **50**, 152–7.

25. Garland, P.B. and Randle P.J. (1962) A rapid enzymatic assay for glycerol. *Nature*, **196**, 978–88.

26. Whitlow, K. and Gochman, H. (1978) Continuous flow enzymic method evaluated for measurement of serum triglycerides with use of an improved lipase reagent. *Clin. Chim. Acta*, **24**, 2018–22.

27. Bucolo, G. and David H. (1973) Quantitative determination of serum triglycerides by use of enzymes. *Clin. Chem.*, **19**, 476–82.

28. Megraw, R.E., Dunn, D.E. and Biggs, H.G. (1979) Manual and continuous flow colorimetry of triacyglycerols by a full enzymatic method. *Clin. Chem.*, **25**, 273–8.

29. Gofman, J.W., Lindgren, F.T. and Elliot, H. (1949) Ultracentrifugal studies of lipoproteins of human serum. *J. Biol. Chem.*, **179**, 793–7.

30. Patsch, J.R., Sailer, S., Kostner, G. *et al.* (1974) Separation of the main lipoprotein density classes from human plasma by rate-zonal ultracentrifugation. *J. Lipid Res.*, **15**, 356–66.

31. Burstein, M. and Scholnick, H.R. (1973) Lipoprotein–polyanion–metal interaction. *Advances in Lipid Research*, **11**, 68–108.

32. Warnick, G.R. and Albers J.J. (1978) A comprehensive evaluation of the heparin–manganese precipitation procedure for estimation of high density lipoprotein cholesterol. *J. Lipid Res.*, **19**, 65–73.

33. Fredrickson, D.S., Levy, R.I. and Lindgren, F.P. (1968) A comparison of irritable abnormal lipoprotein patterns as defined by two different techniques. *J. Clin. Invest.*, **47**, 2446–57.

34. Alper, C. (1974) in *Clinical Chemistry, Principles and Techniques*, 2nd edn (eds R.J. Henry, D.C. Cannon and J. Winkelman), Harper, New York.

35. Bachorik, P.S. (1979) in *Report of the High Density Lipoprotein Methodology Workshop* (ed. K. Lippel) NIH Publ. No. 79–1661, Bethesda (MD).

36. Bachorik, P.S. (1982) Collection of blood samples for lipoprotein analysis. *Clin. Chem.*, **28**, 1375–8.

37. Burstein, M. and Samaille, J. (1960) Sur un dosage rapide du cholesterol lié aux α-et aux β-lipoproteins du serum. *Clin. Chim. Acta*, **5**, 609–13.

38. Heiss, G., Johnson, N.J., Reiland, S. *et al.* (1980) The epidemiology of plasma high-density lipoprotein cholesterol levels. The Lipid Research Clinics Program Prevalence Study. *Circulation*, **62** [suppl 4], 116–36.

39. Mayfield, C., Warnick, G.R. and Albers, J.J. (1979) Evaluation of commercial heparin preparations for use in the heparin–Mn^{2+} method for measuring cholesterol in high-density lipoprotein. *Clin. Chem.*, **25**, 1309–13.

40. Warnick, G.R. and Albers, J.J. (1978) Heparin–Mn^{2+} quantitation of high density lipoprotein cholesterol. An ultrafiltration procedure for lipemic samples. *Clin. Chem.*, **24**, 900–4.

41. Gidez, L.I., Miller, G.J., Burstein, M. *et al.* (1982) Separation and quantitation of subclasses of human high density lipoproteins by a simple precipitation procedure. *J. Lipid Res.*, **23**, 1206–23.

42. Bachorik, P.S., Walker, R.E. and Kwiterovich, P.O. (1982) Determination of high density lipoprotein–cholesterol in human plasma stored at −70°C. *J. Lipid Res.*, **23**, 1236–42.

43. Steele, B.W., Koehler, D.F., Azar, M.M. *et al.* (1976) Enzymatic determinations of cholesterol of high-density lipoprotein fractions prepared by a precipitation technique. *Clin. Chem.*, **22**, 98–101.

44. Bachorik, P.S., Walker R.E. and Virgil, D.G. (1984) High-density lipoprotein cholesterol in heparin–$MnCl_2$ supernatants determined with the down enzymatic method after precipitation of Mn^{2+} with HCO_3^{-1}. *Clin. Chem.*, **30**, 839–42.

45. Demacker, P.N.M., Vos-Janssen, H.E., Hijmans, A.G.M. *et al.* (1980) Measurement of high density lipoprotein cholesterol in serum: comparison of six isolation methods combined with enzymic cholesterol analysis. *Clin. Chem..*, **26**, 1780–6.

46. Maclouf, J., Fitzpatrick, F.A. and Murphy, R. (1989) Transcellular biosynthesis of eicosanoids. *Pharmacol. Res.*, **21**, 1–7.

47. FitzGerald, G.A., Pedersen, A.K. and Patrono, C. (1983) Analysis of thromboxane and prostacyclin biosynthesis in cardiovascular disease. *Circulation*, **67**, 1174–5.

48. Catella, F., Healy, D., Lawson, J.A. and FitzGerald, G.A. (1986) 11-Dehydro-thromboxane B_2: a quantitative index of thromboxane A_2 formation in the human circulation. *Proc. Natl. Acad. Sci. (USA)*, **83**, 5861–5.

49. Schweer, H., Kammer, J. and Seyberth, H.W. (1985) Simultaneous determination of prostanoids in plasma by gas chromatography–negative ion chemical ionization–mass spectrometry. *J. Chromatogr.***338**, 273–80.

50. Lawson, J.A., Brash, A.R., Doran, J. and FitzGerald, G.A. (1985) Measurement of urinary 2, 3-dinor-thromboxane B_2 and thromboxane B_2 using bonded-phase phenylboronic acid columns and capillary gas chromatography–negative ion chemical ionization mass spectrometry. *Anal. Biochem.*, **150**, 463–76.

51. FitzGerald, G.A., Brash, A.R., Falardeau, P. and Oates, J.A. (1981) Estimated rate of prostacyclin secretion into the circulation in normal man. *J. Clin. Invest.*, **68**, 1272–6.

52. Patrono, C., Ciabattoni, C., Pugliese, F. *et al.* (1986) Estimated rate of thromboxane secretion into the circulation of normal man. *J. Clin. Invest.*, **77**, 590–3.

53. Keppler, D., Hagmann, W., Rapp, S. *et al.* (1985) The relation of leukotrienes to liver injury. *Hepatology*, **5**, 883–91.

54. Hammarstrom, S. (1983) Leukotrienes. *Ann. Rev. Biochem.*, **52**, 355–77.

55. Denzlinger, C., Rapp, S., Hagman, W. and Keppler, D. (1985) Leukotriene as mediators in tissue trauma. *Science*, **230**, 330–2.

56. Orning, L., Kaijser, L. and Hammarstrom, S. (1985) In vivo metabolism of leukotriene C_4 in man. *Biochem. Biophys. Res. Commun.*, **139**, 214–20.

57. Carvalho, A.C.A., Colman, R.W. and Lees, R.S. (1974) Platelet function in hyperlipoproteinemia. *N. Engl. J. Med.*, **290**, 434–8.

58. Tremoli, E., Maderna, P., Colli, S. *et al.* (1984) Increased platelet sensitivity and thromboxane B_2 formation in type II hyperlipoproteinaemic patients. *Eur. J. Clin. Invest.*, **14**, 329–33.

59. FitzGerald, D.J., Roy, L., Catella, F., and FitzGerald, G.A. (1986) Platelet activation in unstable coronary disease. *N. Engl. J. Med.*, **315**, 983–9.

60. Hamm, C.W., Lorenz, R.L., Weber, P.C. *et al.* (1986) Subgroups of patients with unstable angina identified by biochemical evidence of thrombous formation. [Abstract], *Circulation*, **74** [suppl II], 305.

61. Beetens, J.R., Coene, M.C., Verheyen, A. *et al.* (1986) Biphasic response of intimal prostacyclin production during the development of experimental atherosclerosis. *Prostaglandins*, **32**, 319–28.

62. Moncada, S., Gryglewski, R.J., Bunting, S. and Vane, J.R. (1976) A lipid peroxide inhibits the enzyme in blood vessels microsomes that generates from prostaglandin endoperoxides the substances (prostaglandin X) which prevents platelet aggregation. *Prostaglandins*, **12**, 715–26.

63. Tremoli, E., Socini, A., Petroni, A. and Galli, C. (1982) Increased platelet aggregability is associated with increased prostacyclin production by vessel walls in hypercholesterolemic rabbits. *Prostaglandins*, **24**, 397–404.

64. FitzGerald, G.A., Smith, B., Pedersen, A.K. and Brash, A.R. (1984) Prostacyclin biosynthesis is increased in patients with severe atherosclerosis and platelet activation. *N. Engl. J. Med.*, **310**, 1065–8.

65. AHA Special Report. (1984) Recommendations for the treatment of hyperlipidemia in adults. A joint statement of the Nutrition Committee and the Council on Arteriosclerosis of the American Heart Association. *Arteriosclerosis*, **4**, 445A–68A.
66. Hornstra, G. and Lussenburg, R.N. (1975) Relationship between the type of dietary fatty acid and arterial thrombosis tendency in rats. *Atherosclerosis*, **22**, 499–516.
67. Renaud, S., Dumond, E., Godsey, F. *et al.* (1978) Platelet functions in relation to dietary fats in farmers from two regions of France. *Thromb. Haemost.*, **40**, 518–31.
68. Tremoli, E., Petroni, A., Socini, A. *et al.* (1986) Dietary intervention in North Karelia, Finland and South Italy. Modifications of thromboxane B_2 formation in platelets of male subjects only. *Atherosclerosis*, **59**, 101–11.
69. Boberg, M., Gustafsson, I.B. and Vessby, B. (1986) High content of dietary linoleic acid does not reduce platelet reactivity in patients with hyperlipoprotein-aemia. *Eur. J. Clin. Invest.*, **16**, 28–34.
70. Dyerberg, J., Bang, H.O. and Hjorne N. (1975) Fatty acid composition of the plasma lipids in Greenland Eskimos. *Am. J. Clin., Nutr.*, **28**, 958–66.
71. Siess, W., Roth, P., Scherer, B. *et al.* (1980) Platelet-membrane fatty acids, platelet aggregation, and thromboxane formation during a mackerel diet. *Lancet*, **i**, 441–4.
72. Fischer, S. and Weber, P.C. (1983) Thromboxane A_3 (TxA$_3$) is formed in human platelets after dietary eicosapentaenoic acid (20:5 ω3). *Biochem. Biophys. Res. Commun.*, **116**, 1091–9.
73. Fischer, S. and Weber, P.C. (1984) Prostaglandin I_3 is formed in vivo in man after dietary eicosapentaenoic acid. *Nature*, **307**, 165–8.
74. Knapp, H.R., Reilly, I.A.G., Alessandrini, P. and Fitzgerald, G.A. (1986) In vivo indexes of platelet and vascular function during fish-oil administration in patients with atherosclerosis. *N. Engl. J. Med.*, **314**, 937–42.
75. Samuelsson, B. (1983) Leukotrienes: mediators of immediate hypersensitivity reactions and inflammation. *Science*, **220**, 568–75.
76. Mullane, K.M., Salmon, J.A. and Kraemer, R. (1987) Leukocyte-derived metabolites of arachidonic acid in ischemia-induced myocardial injury. *Fed. Proc.*, **46**, 2422–33.
77. Goldman, D.W., Pickett, W.C. and Goetzl, E.J. (1983) Human neutrophil chemotactic and degranulating activities of leukotriene B_5 (LTB$_5$) derived from eicosapentaenoic acid. *Biochem. Biophys. Res. Commun.*, **117**, 282–8.
78. Medini, L., Colli, S., Mosconi, C. *et al.* (1990) Diets rich in n-9, n-6 and n-3 fatty acids differentially affect the generation of inositol phosphates and of thromboxane by stimulated platelets, in the rabbit. *Biochem. Pharmacol.*, **39**, 129–33.

6 Protein nutriture methodology

6.1 Introduction   *D.J. Millward*   165
6.2 Indicators of nutritional status: general aspects *D.J. Millward*   167
6.3 Plasma proteins   *D.J. Millward*   169
6.4 Urinary creatinine   *D.J. Millward*   173
6.5 3-Methyl-histidine   *D.J. Millward*   175
6.6 IGF-1 (insulin-like growth factor-1, somatomedin C)
    D.J. Millward   178

6.1 INTRODUCTION

6.1.1 Protein nutrition, dietary protein deficiency, and body protein depletion

The state of protein nutrition can be defined in terms of protein deficiency and/or depletion. However, the difference between deficiency and depletion must be emphasized. To avoid ambiguity it is probably best if deficiency is strictly limited to situations of insufficient dietary protein, and depletion is limited to insufficient body protein. When used in these contexts they are independent terms and may be, in some circumstances, unrelated. Thus, protein depletion can result from factors other than protein deficiency, and protein deficiency, when defined in relation to requirements for safe levels of protein intakes or P:E ratios, will not induce depletion in all individuals. No attempt will be made here to list the various dietary factors which, if deficient, induce protein depletion, since failure of growth in children and a reduction of lean body mass in adults is a general response to inadequate food intake. In these cases measurements of lean body mass and of total body nitrogen provide the most basic assessment of the state of protein nutrition.

6.1.2 Groups at risk from protein deficiency

Notwithstanding the separate problem of defining protein requirements unequivocally, it is nevertheless useful to note the implications of the current FAO/UNU/WHO energy and protein requirement recommendations in terms of the relative risks of various groups from protein deficiency. With protein deficiency limited to situations when diets are inadequate in protein but adequate in energy (and all other nutrients), then the protein:energy ratio of the diet becomes the appropriate descriptor. Because energy requirements (defined as a multiple of BMR) decrease (per kg) with increasing body weight, whereas after early childhood protein requirements are relatively constant, the P:E ratio of the requirements (and the likelihood that a particular diet is protein deficient) increases, whilst with age (from 5 at the age of 1 year to 9.7 for an elderly woman).

6.1.3 Physiological consequences of protein deficiency

(a) Kwashiorkor

This is traditionally viewed as a consequence of protein deficiency, the link being hypoalbuminaemia, which is viewed as the main cause of the oedema of kwashiorkor. Indeed hypoalbuminaemia is often described clinically as kwashiorkor-like in patients without oedema [1]. However, this causal relationship is increasingly being challenged, notwithstanding the known role of albumin in regulating plasma oncotic pressure and fluid balance, and the fact that hypoalbuminaemia is a very frequent accompaniment to oedema. The fact that loss of oedema during treatment of malnourished children occurs in advance of any change in albumin concentrations [2] can only be interpreted as indicating that oedema and hypoalbuminaemia are independent characteristics of kwashiorkor. This means that it is difficult to sustain arguments that oedema, and therefore kwashiorkor, is a symptom of protein deficiency, or even that oedema is a diagnostic indicator of protein deficiency.

As to the aetiology of hypoalbuminaemia, there is no doubt that hypoalbuminaemia can be induced by a reduction in the P:E ratio of the diet, and the recent observations of Lunn and Austin [3] in animals confirm this. However, their arguments that a reduced P:E ratio should be viewed as a consequence of excessive energy intake (which induces metabolic disturbances associated with a hyperthyroid state), rather than inadequate protein intake, are highly contentious. They are, in any case, unrelated to most clinical situations of infant malnutrition where there is seldom evidence of excessive energy intakes and low levels of T_3 are found [4].

The fact that hypoalbuminaemia is a consequence of the acute-phase response, and the almost invariable association of kwashiorkor with infection and dietary toxins and pathogens which can provoke the acute-phase response, means that the hypoalbuminaemia of kwashiorkor can equally be considered to be, to a greater or lesser degree, a response to infection and environmental stress.

Although the relationship of oedema to the other symptoms of kwashiorkor including hypoalbuminaemia, remains obscure, what information that does exist indicates that the traditional link between kwashiorkor and protein deficiency, which in many parts of the world was never based on hard evidence, is not really justifiable [5].

(b) Stunting

Reduced growth in height has been identified as a consequence of protein deficiency, the evidence for this being the several supplementation studies that have been reviewed by Golden [5]. Thus height for age should certainly be identified as a potential indicator of protein deficiency.

One new development in this field relates to work on IGF-1 (somatomedin C) as a nutritionally sensitive regulator. As discussed below, this raises the possibility that IGF-1 levels can provide an index of nutritional status. Given the fact that bone growth is a target for IGF-1, reduced IGF-1 in response to dietary protein deficiency may be an important measurable component of the mechanism of stunting.

6.1.4   Determination of protein depletion

If it is accepted that protein depletion can result from a slowing of growth, i.e. stunting, as well as a loss of protein from individual compartments, then assessment of protein depletion should involve use of both internal and external standards. Internal standards relate to body compartments in terms of relative compartment size, N/body weight, muscle mass:body weight, etc., whilst external standards relate to absolute compartment protein content in terms of age-related standards.

6.2   INDICATORS OF NUTRITIONAL STATUS: GENERAL ASPECTS

6.2.1   Plasma proteins

The primary cause for concern with the use of plasma proteins as indicators of protein depletion and deficiency is the role of the acute-phase response in their regulation. Thus albumin, prealbumin, transferrin, and retinol-binding protein are all negative acute-phase reactants. Although the relative importance of the acute-phase response, as opposed to nutritional factors, in the regulation of plasma proteins has yet to be systematically evaluated in many clinical situations, those studies that have been reported do demonstrate the importance of non-nutritional factors.

6.2.2   Muscle mass from creatinine excretion

Regardless of whether protein depletion results from protein deficiency or some other cause, there is no doubt that reduced muscle mass is a major component of the depletion, and determination of muscle mass is of prime importance.

The 24-hour creatinine excretion has long been regarded as a measure of muscle mass. The rationale is that creatinine is derived non-enzymatically from creatine phosphate and quantitatively excreted, and since most (95%) of body creatine is in muscle, the excretion rate is proportional to the creatine pool size, in turn an index of muscle mass. From the available evidence, the creatinine concentration per gram of muscle is not affected by nutritional factors but is sensitive to temperature, so will rise in fever [6].

Many authors have measured LBM independently and have found a good correlation with muscle mass estimated from creatinine output [7]. However, it could not be assumed that muscle and non-muscle mass will always vary together [6]. Both in man and experimental animals, severe undernutrition causes a relatively greater loss of muscle than of visceral tissues.

6.2.3   Muscle protein turnover from urinary 3-methyl-histidine excretion

It is often assumed that the rate of whole body or organ protein turnover can be used as a nutritional indicator since there is ample evidence that it is nutritionally variable. The rate of excretion of urinary 3-methyl-histidine (3MH) is viewed as an easy non-invasive method of estimating the protein turnover rate in one key tissue-skeletal muscle [8]. However the usefulness of urinary 3-methyl-histidine excretion needs careful consideration since its significance is generally poorly understood. There are several circumstances where changes in the urinary 3MH:creatinine ratio are very misleading indicators of the changes in muscle protein turnover. The only reliable alternative involves measurement of muscle protein turnover rates directly during a constant infusion of [^{13}C] leucine from isotope incorporation into muscle protein sampled by biopsy. However, the requirement for both GCMS and isotope-ratio MS facilities rules out such studies from routine application.

Given these limitations on measurement of muscle protein turnover, a better alternative may be to focus on muscle function as an indicator of nutritional status since, although this has not been specifically related to dietary protein intake, there is increasing recognition that it is undoubtedly responsive to overall nutritional state.

6.2.4 IGF-1, (Insulin-like growth factor-1, somatomedin C) and nutritional status

There is a growing interest in IGF-1 as an indicator for nutritional status in general and protein deficiency in particular. Since IGF-1 responds more slowly to changes in food intake than insulin, corticosteroids, or growth hormone, it is more likely to yield useful information. The importance of these new observations about IGF-1 and nutritional status is that, as indicated above, they offer a potential mechanism to explain the relationship between dietary protein concentration and growth in height. For this link to exist it would need to be demonstrated that IGF-1 responded more to dietary protein intake than to energy or any other nutrient.

This has not yet been demonstrated since the RIA for IGF-1 has only recently become generally available. However, as will be discussed, difficulties can be anticipated with interpreting changes in marginally malnourished children, since concentrations are in any case much lower than in adults, reducing the potential sensitivity of the measurement in such age groups. In addition IGF-1 is a negative acute-phase reactant so that stress is likely to be a confounding factor, as with plasma proteins. At the moment it would be premature to suggest that IGF-1 could be a specific indicator of dietary protein intakes but there is no doubt that investigation of the relationship between nutritional status and IGF-1 is well worthwhile and potentially very exciting.

6.2.5 Plasma aminoacids

The significance of plasma free aminoacid levels has been extensively evaluated over the years in the context not only of the determination of protein nutritional status, but also of the determination of requirements for essential aminoacids and the evaluation of protein quality, (see [9–15]).

In the context of protein nutritional status, most work has related to examination of the changes in the free aminoacid patterns in the plasma of malnourished young children. Holt *et al.* [16] showed that plasma aminograms from children suffering from kwashiorkor showed a similar pattern: reduced levels of most essential aminoacids, with unaffected or even raised levels of several of the inessential group. A simplified field assessment to diagnose protein–calorie malnutrition involving plasma free aminoacid levels was then proposed by Whitehead and Dean [17]. These authors suggested that the ratio of plasma levels for glycine, serine, glutamine, and taurine (N) to plasma levels of leucine, isoleucine, valine and methionine (E) may be useful in diagnosing kwashiorkor. Normal values for the N:E ratio were found to be <2.0, with the ratio in children suffering from kwashiorkor exceeding this value (e.g. 5–10). Subsequently it was observed that the N:E ratio in marasmic children was in the normal range [18], suggesting the use of this ratio to diagnose differentially kwashiorkor and marasmus.

The reason for these changes in aminoacid patterns has never been entirely explained. Studies in experimentally protein-malnourished pigs have attempted to relate the increases in alanine and glycine to the reduced demands for gluconeogenesis, and the fall in the branched-chain aminoacids to their limitation on protein deposition resulting from a protein-deficient diet [19]. Thus, the abnormal ratio is less apparent in the final stages of protein deficiency when food intakes fall and the calorie deficiency increases demand for gluconeogenesis and induces tissue catabolism, with release of essential aminoacids.

In recent years there has been generally much less interest in these measurements, possibly because of the recognition that the original dietary hypothesis of kwashiorkor as protein deficiency and marasmus as energy deficiency could often not account for the symptoms observed. It is certainly the case that the very marked changes seen clinically have never been reproduced in experimental animals [19]. Some efforts have been made to relate the changes to the hormonal imbalances observed in children with kwashiorkor and the consequences of these changes to the maintenance of serum albumin [20]. Although Young and Scrimshaw [11] considered the N:E ratio to be generally useful for this purpose, they suggested caution in interpreting the results, primarily because of the influence of infections and recent protein intake on free aminoacid levels. The original paper chromatographic methods for measuring aminoacid ratios [17] have now been superseded by automated ion exchange or other high-performance chromatographic techniques, and no particular method will be described.

6.3 PLASMA PROTEINS

6.3.1 Purpose and scope   Of the various classes of plasma proteins (transport, immunological, and acute-phase) albumin and the transport proteins (thyroid-binding prealbumin (PA), retinol-binding protein (RBP), and transferrin (TF)) have been most widely studied as indicators of the nutritional state [21]. Fibronectin (FB), an opsonic glycoprotein, is a more recent addition to the catalogue. The shorter half-life and smaller pool size of PA, RBP, TF, and FB means that they can exhibit more rapid changes in concentrations and can thus be more sensitive indices of the immediate nutritional state than albumin. In children with kwashiorkor, one week of treatment induces a doubling of PA and RBP with no change in albumin or any measurable anthropometric indicator of nutritional status [22]. Therefore distinction needs to be made between indicators of immediate as opposed to long-term nutritional state. Obviously TF is sensitive to iron status (increasing in response to a deficiency [23]), and RBP will change in response to alterations in vitamin A status [24].

6.3.2 Principle of the methods

A commercially available method is described for albumin that can be used manually or automated. For other proteins, reference is made only to the types of methods in general use.

(a) Plasma transport proteins

In almost all cases the determination of plasma protein concentrations involves automated methods. Of these the most widely used methods are based on immunological techniques (see [25]). Mancini single radial immunodiffusion can be done with commercially available antibody-coated plates [26]. Electro-immunoassay by the Laurel 'rocket' method is faster and more accurate [27], although this requires monospecific antibodies. In the absence of this, crossed immunoelectrophoresis (two-dimensional immunoelectrophoresis) can be employed [28, 29] although this is more cumbersome and less accurate. Trace components can be measured by radioimmunoassay. It should be recognized that all immunological methods may overestimate the functional levels of some proteins, since degradation or dissociation products can give positive reactions.

(b) Fibronectin

This is determined by automated laser nephelometry [30], (Hyland Diagnostics, Deerfield, Ill.) with commercially available human fibronectin, and goat antiserum (CalBiochem-Behring, San Diego, Calif.).

(c) Albumin

This is usually measured with an automated dye-binding technique of which the most popular is based on bromocresol green (e.g. Technicon SMA-20, Sigma Diagnostics). However, a drawback of most dye-binding procedures is lack of specificity, which may lead to overestimation of albumin in samples with low albumin levels. This has been attributed to non-specific binding with various acute-phase proteins within the globulin fractions of serum. Improved specificity occurs with the dye bromocresol purple (BCP). BCP binds instantly with human serum albumin to produce a colour that remains unchanged on standing. The method described is that outlined in a commercially available kit based on BCP (Sigma 625), which derives from the method of Pinnel and Northam [31].

This can be cross-checked with any of the above mentioned methods or with cellulose acetate electrophoresis [32].

Human serum albumin reacts specifically with BCP to form a stable blue-purple colour complex with an absorption maximum at 600 nm. The intensity of the colour is proportional to the albumin concentration in the sample.

6.3.3 Chemicals and apparatus

(a) Plasma transport proteins

1. *Chemicals.* (See [25–29].)
2. *Solutions.* (See [25–29].)
3. *Apparatus.* (See [25–29].)

(b) Fibronectin

1. *Chemicals.* Commercially available human fibronectin and goat antiserum can be obtained from CalBiochem-Behring, San Diego, Calif.
2. *Solutions.* (See [30].)

3. *Apparatus*. Automated laser nephelometry [31] involves equipment from Hyland Diagnostics, Deerfield, Ill.

(c) Albumin

1. *Chemicals*. Bromocresol purple albumin reagent is available prepared from Sigma.
2. *Solutions*. Protein standard solutions are available prepared from Sigma; 0.85% saline is required.
3. *Apparatus*. Any spectrophotometer capable of accurately measuring absorbance at 600 nm.

6.3.4   Sample collection

Serum separated from cells by any conventional procedure is suitable. Albumin is stable in serum for at least one week at room temperature (18–26°C), 1 month at 2–6°C and indefinitely when frozen. Plasma containing heparin or EDTA is also suitable for analysis.

6.3.5   Procedure

(a) Plasma transport proteins

(See [25–29].)

(b) Fibronectin

(See [30].)

(c) Albumin

To tubes labelled Blank, Standard, and Test add 1.0 ml of albumin reagent (BCP).
To standard add 0.01 ml albumin standard.
To Test add 0.01 ml serum or plasma.
To Blank add 0.01 ml 0.85% saline.
Mix after each addition.
Read absorbance of Standard and Test vs Blank as reference at 600 nm.
Colour forms immediately and is stable for at least 30 min.

6.3.6.   Performance characteristics

(a) General considerations

1. *Plasma transport proteins*. (See [25–29].)
2. *Fibronectin*. (See [30].)
3. *Albumin*. The procedure is relatively free from interference by icterus, haemolysis, or lipaemia, or drugs known to bind to albumin.

(b) Range of linearity

1. *Plasma transport proteins*. (See [25–29].)
2. *Fibronectin*. (See [30].)
3. *Albumin*. Linear to 6 g/dl.

(c) Detection limit

1. *Plasma transport proteins*. (See [25–29].)
2. *Fibronectin*. (See [30].)
3. *Albumin*. An absorbance change of 0.13 corresponds to 1 g/dl albumin on typical spectrophotometers.

(d) Recovery

1. *Plasma transport proteins*. (See [25–29].)

2. *Fibronectin.* (See [30].)
3. *Albumin.* 94–99%.

(e) Reproducibility

1. *Plasma transport proteins.* (See [25–29].)
2. *Fibronectin.* (See [30].)
3. *Albumin.* CV reported as between 2.1% and 3.4%.

(f) Comparability

1. *Plasma transport proteins.* (See [25–29].)
2. *Fibronectin.* (See [30].)
3. *Albumin.* Good correlation (r=0.996) of values with this and other methods as long as human albumin is used as calibrator. Bovine albumin is not suitable.

6.3.7 Reference values

It is recommended that normal values are established for each laboratory, bearing in mind that variables include age, sex and, in the cases of proteins such as haptoglobin and a_1-PI phenotypic, differences exist.

6.3.8 Interpretation

Although the effort put in to the search for sensitive nutritional indicators continues unabated, there is increasing concern about the interpretation of changes in plasma protein concentrations.

Most plasma proteins are surprisingly resistant to severe energy deficiency or starvation. This is well established for albumin, which can be well maintained in response to prolonged dietary food restriction. Keys reported that six months of semi-starvation reduced total circulating albumin by only 2% [33]. In marasmic children, albumin levels are often well maintained. In healthy students a three-day fast resulted in significant changes in only two (out of twelve) proteins: albumin, which increased and RBP, which fell [34]. However, the undoubted and exhaustively documented sensitivity of albumin synthesis and of plasma concentrations to dietary protein and aminoacid supply in animals and in man [21], has naturally enough tended to confirm the assumption that hypoalbuminaemia is the primary diagnostic symptom of protein deficiency. This in turn has been the main evidence for the theory that kwashiorkor, almost invariably associated with hypoalbuminaemia, reflects protein deficiency. This is an attitude that has been maintained even though dietary surveys have often failed to substantiate such an aetiology. One possible explanation for this relates to the second major concern for the use of albumin and any other plasma protein as an indicator of protein depletion and deficiency. Albumin and the transport proteins are all negative acute-phase reactants so that their concentrations will be subject to non-nutritional factors associated with infection, trauma, and any acute illness that provokes an acute-phase response [35].

The increase in the acute-phase proteins is accompanied by reductions in the synthesis and plasma concentrations of albumin, prealbumin, retinol-binding protein, transferrin [25, 35] and fibronectin [30]. Although the relative importance of the acute-phase response, as opposed to nutritional factors, in the regulation of plasma proteins has yet to be systematically evaluated in many clinical situations, those studies which have been reported clearly demonstrate the importance of non-nutritional factors. Thus, in a recent study of paediatric oncology patients, plasma albumin was shown to be very poorly correlated with body weight and muscle and fat mass but was highly associated with fever [36]. In the case of prealbumin and transferrin, although there is no doubt that they are sensitive acute indicators of positive nitrogen balance in protein-energy supplemented hospital patients [37], it may be that the wide range of individual values (5-fold for PA and 2.5-fold for transferrin, which was independent of serum iron) is a reflection of the involvement of the acute-phase response in their regulation. In the same way, while fibronectin has been shown to exhibit an acute increase in response to nutritional support, individual values vary over a wide (5-fold) range and are not correlated with nitrogen balance [30]. The fact that fibronectin concentration was highly correlated with transferrin does suggest common regulatory factors of which the acute-phase response seems most likely.

Although the effect of infection and stress on plasma protein concentration has long been recognized, particularly in the specific case of protein-losing enteropathies [38], its general importance has almost certainly been underestimated in comparison to dietary causes.

Indeed, it is possible that in some circumstances the development of hypoproteinaemia through intestinal loss could be the cause, rather than a symptom, of overall protein depletion. In Crohn's disease, where gastrointestinal loss is known to be the main cause of hypoproteinaemia, there is a very good correlation with plasma albumin (and prealbumin to a lesser extent) and mid-arm circumference and other anthropometric indicators [39]. In this case the hypoproteinaemia is a direct consequence of a functional defect that impairs food utilization and induces protein depletion and, as such, is a much less equivocal indicator. In most other circumstances, however, the separate influence of nutrition and other stresses is much more difficult to evaluate. This means that the usefulness of plasma proteins as unequivocal indicators of previous nutritional state is considerably limited [40]. However, such measurements are useful as monitors of the efficacy of nutritional support.

6.4 URINARY CREATININE

6.4.1 Purpose and scope

Approximately 2% of the creatinine pool is converted to creatine per day. The arithmetic is therefore as follows:

Creatine = 2.5 g per kg muscle.
Conversion of 2% per day produces 50 mg creatinine excreted per day per kg muscle.

The validity of this factor depends on two assumptions: constancy of creatine concentration and constancy of its fractional rate of conversion to creatinine. Both assumptions need further investigation.

Caveats: (a) Meat and fish in the diet contain significant amount of creatine, which will enlarge the creatine pool and increase the excretion of creatinine; (b) an increase in body temperature will increase the rate of conversion of creatine to creatinine; (c) in some conditions (pregnancy, injury) creatine is excreted in addition to creatinine. Creatine is converted to creatinine by heating and some conversion will occur even at room temperature if urine is left standing; (d) renal diseases with impaired creatinine clearance.

6.4.2 Principle of the method

The traditional method, which is simple and highly reproducible, is by reaction with alkaline picrate and measurement at 520 nm, (the Jaffe reaction). The most recent method with HPLC gives results on urine that are only 60% of those by the Jaffe method [41]. The discrepancy requires further investigation.

6.4.3 Chemicals and apparatus

(a) Chemicals

Hydrochloric acid (HCl) 37% p.a.
Sodium chloride (NaCl) p.a.
Brij 35 (polyethylene glycol dodecylether) p.a.
Sodium hydroxide (NaOH) p.a.
Picric acid ($C_6H_3N_3O_7$) p.a.
Creatinine ($C_4H_7N_3O$) p.a.
Bidistilled water.

(b) Solutions

6 N Hydrochloric acid: 500 ml HCl 37% made up to 1000 ml with water.
30% Brij 35: 30 g Brij 35 dissolved in water to make 100 ml.
1.8% Sodium chloride: 1.8 g sodium chloride dissolved in water to make 100 ml with previous addition of 0.1 ml of 30% Brij 35.
0.5 N Sodium hydroxide: 20 g NaOH dissolved in water to make 1000 ml.
Picric acid saturated solution.
Creatinine standards: 0.018–1.326 mmol/l in water with 1 ml of 30% Brij 35.

(c) Apparatus

Usual basic laboratory equipment.
Technicon autoanalyser SMA 6/60.

6.4.4 Sample preparation

Twenty-four-hour urine is collected in vials containing 2 ml of 6 N HCl. An aliquot of the sample is filtered with vacuum through a No. 4 sintered glass funnel, and frozen at –20°C. The urine is diluted 1/10 with bidistilled water.

6.4.5 Procedure

The sample stream, segmented with air, is diluted with 1.8% sodium chloride. This diluted stream then enters the donor side of the dialyser. The analytical stream consists of water segmented with air. After emerging from the dialyser the analytical stream is joined with 0.5 N NaOH. These two components are mixed and then joined with saturated picric acid. The three components are mixed, and phased to the colorimeter. The absorbance of the analytical stream is measured at 505 nm in a 15-mm lg by 1.5 ID flowcell.

Calculation

A standard calibration curve is made plotting the absorbance value against the concentration of creatinine. Quantification of samples is done by comparing the absorbance value of the sample against that of the standard. Range of linearity: Beer law applies in the range of 0.018–1.326 mmol/l of creatinine.

6.4.6 Performance characteristics

(a) Detection limit

0.018 mmol/l of creatinine can be quantitatively detected.

(b) Recovery

The recovery is about 95%.

(c) Reproducibility

The day-to-day constancy of creatinine excretion has been much studied. On a meat-free diet with careful timing of collections the within-subject variability per day-to-day is ~ 7% [7]. On an uncontrolled diet it is somewhat greater – 10% [6]. It should be noted that in some specific groups the variation in daily excretion can be very marked. Thus in obese women on a meat-free diet the CV of the daily excretion was up to 34% [42], raising doubts about the value of 24-h creatinine excretion rates. However, after allowing for daily variability by calculating mean weekly excretion rates, that value was poorly correlated with lean body mass calculated from whole body potassium, body water, or body density. This means that either muscle is a variable component of the lean body mass in the obese or that creatinine excretion is not a good indicator of muscle mass in this case. However, in the non-obese it is generally considered that larger variations are suggestive of errors. Comparison with PABA excretion has shown that in free-living subjects a significant proportion of 24-h collections is likely to be incomplete. It is recommended that in order to estimate muscle mass from creatinine excretion, three 24-h collections should be made. The results should be rejected if the coefficient of variation of the three samples is greater than 10%.

6.4.7 Reference values

Reference values are population specific. As an example see Joossens *et al.* [43].

6.4.8 Interpretation

The data are expressed in mmols of creatinine in 24-h urine. One gram (8.84 mmol) of creatinine excreted is equivalent to 20 kg of muscle tissue [44, 45].

Uric acid, purines, and chromogen compounds can produce some interference with the method.

6.5 3-METHYL-HISTIDINE

6.5.1 Purpose and scope

3-Methyl-histidine (3MH) is formed as a post-translational modification of actin and some species of myosin heavy chain and, since it cannot be re-incorporated into protein or metabolized in the human, is excreted quantitatively. It must be emphasized that it is a dynamic indicator reflecting the overall rate of degradation of 3MH-containing proteins. The overall rate of 3MH excretion is a function not only of the amount of protein but also its fractional turnover rate. The suggestion is sometimes made that 3MH excretion can be used as an index of muscle mass. This implies that muscle protein turnover is constant (which is known to be untrue) and such use is unjustifiable.

In fact most studies express results as the 3MH:creatinine ratio. Although this results in problems in some circumstances (see below), it is nevertheless the more appropriate index, comparable to the fractional muscle turnover rate.

6.5.2 Principle of the method

3MH can be measured by routine ion-exchange chromatography, although modification is necessary to deal with the close proximity of the much larger histidine peak. One method involves separation on cation exchange resin with pyridine buffers, but in our experience this is not quantitative so that recovery must be estimated [46]. Ward [47] described the use of a ninhydrin-orthophthalaldehyde colorimetric reagent, which is reasonably specific for 3MH, reacting with 50% reactivity with arginine and ammonia, and to a much lower extent with any other aminoacids. With this reagent 3MH in urine can be resolved in a three-hour run although pretreatment with histidine decarboxylase is still recommended to remove most of the histidine. Fluorometric techniques allow increased sensitivities and the inclusion of formaldehyde prior to reaction with orthophthaldehyde decreases histidine fluorescence by 80% and increases that of 3MH [46]. When fluorescamine is used with a modification that renders it specific for imidazoles, the additional inclusion of formaldehyde can result in elimination of significant fluorescence from all other constituents in urine so that separation of 3MH from other aminoacids is not necessary [48]. With automation 6–7 samples can be measured per hour. This method is described below. Similar through-put can be obtained by HPLC on a reverse-phase column (Partisil 10 ODS 3) with methanol as solvent following precolumn derivitization with fluorescamine [46]. In this case both colorimetric or fluorometric monitoring can be used.

6.5.3 Chemicals and apparatus

(a) Chemicals

These are as described by Murray *et al.* [48].

(b) Solutions

5% glutaraldehyde/2.5% formaldehyde.
Buffer 1: 0.1% potassium tetraborate pH 9.0.(with 2.0 ml/l Brij 35).
Buffer 2: 0.05% potassium tetraborate pH 9.0 (with 2.0 ml/l Brij 35).
Fluorescamine: 0.02% in acetonitrile.
2M Hydrochloric acid (with 2.0 ml/l Brij 35).
Wash: 0.5 ml/l Brij 35.

(c) Apparatus

Autoanalysis manifold as described by Murray *et al.* [48]. Fluorometer fitted with Corning 7–60 (primary) and Wratten 2A (secondary) filters.

6.5.4 Sample collection

No pre-treatment of urine is required.

6.5.5 Procedure

As described by Murray *et al.* [48].

6.5.6 Performance characteristics

(a) General considerations

Interference. Urea fluorescence is accounted for by running pre-acidification blanks. Ammonia interference is removed by incorporation of dialyser in manifold. Allows for measurement on undiluted urine.

(b) Range of linearity, detection limit, and recovery

As described by Murray *et al.* [48].

(c) Reproducibility

CV reported as 1.8%, which is better than ion-exchange methods.

(d) Comparability

Good correlation ($r=0.994$) of measurements of undiluted and untreated urine with values obtained by ion-exchange chromatography.

6.5.7 Reference values

As described by Murray *et al.* [48].

6.5.8 Interpretation

The main difficulty in evaluating the 3MH:creatinine ratio as a dynamic indicator is the uncertainty associated with the origin of the 3MH. One obvious origin is diet (meat and meat products in food), which can increase the 3MH:creatinine ratio threefold [46]. However, this can be controlled for, at least in clinical contexts. The main uncertainty relates to its cellular origin in the body. Whilst the bulk of the body pool of actin is in skeletal muscle, it does occur in smooth muscle and most non-muscle cell types in the form of microfilaments. Platelets are an obvious example. Furthermore, turnover of non-skeletal muscle actin is much faster than the muscle pool [47]. The turnover rate in intestinal smooth muscle is 20 times that in skeletal muscle and studies of whole body 3MH kinetics in the rat indicate that actin pools with even faster turnover occur elsewhere [47]. As a result of this, in the rat more than half the excretion derives from non-skeletal muscle sources. This problem would not be insurmountable if all tissue pools of actin exhibited parallel changes in turnover rate or pool size, but unfortunately this does not occur.

These problems are best illustrated by specific clinical examples. Marked muscle wasting in dystrophic children is associated with reduced creatinine and 3MH excretion, but the 3MH:creatinine ratio is increased. This has in the past been widely interpreted as indicating increased muscle proteolysis [49]. However, direct measurements with stable isotopes indicate that muscle protein turnover is reduced so that the 3MH:creatinine ratio suggests the opposite change in muscle turnover to what has occurred [49]. The severe muscle wasting and consequent change in body composition has increased the relative size of the non-muscle 3MH pool, so that it is inappropriate to use creatinine as an index of the 3MH pool size. There is unfortunately no alternate reference point, so that no useful information can be obtained from the 3MH excretion rate.

Changes in the urinary 3MH:creatinine ratio can also occur in response to specific increases in turnover rates in non-muscle sources. This has been documented in surgical patients, where 3MH release from the leg has been shown to be depressed when the urinary 3MH:creatinine ratio is increased [49]. Whilst the source of the increased urinary 3MH has not been identified, it may well be related to platelet activity or the acute-phase response, since very high excretion rates are observed during infection [50]. Destruction of muscle tissue during injury or infection is often quoted as a likely reason for the increased excretion of 3MH in these circumstances but there are no specific reasons for dramatic increases in actin degradation during muscle destruction.

Another complicating factor not generally appreciated is the fact that although actin turnover is normally much slower than the average rate for muscle [51], its rate can change independently from the overall rate in muscle. This is indicated by quite marked differences in the relative net release of phenylalanine and 3MH from the perfused hind limb in the fed versus the fasted state [52]. This means that even if the urinary excretion was a function of muscle turnover, it would be a marker for an unrepresentative protein.

Clearly the use of 3MH is very problematical. The tantalizing aspect of its use is that in some circumstances it does appear to indicate the correct change. One such case is steroid-induced muscle wasting, where changes in the urinary 3MH excretion do occur in parallel to muscle proteolysis [53]. Furthermore, in uninfected undernourished children the reduced 3MH:creatinine ratio [50] is consistent with the reduced whole-body protein turnover. However, what is unknown in this case is the extent to which the changes in body composition (which are to some extent comparable to the changes in dystrophic children and which should increase the ratio), result in an underestimation of the actual changes in muscle protein turnover. It is often argued that even though 3MH excretion does include a substantial component derived from non-muscle sources, the turnover of the whole body actin and myosin pool is a useful indicator comparable to the whole-body protein turnover rate. Given the observation that increased turnover in some small non-muscle actin pool can mask a fall in turnover in the major pool in skeletal muscle, it is clear that the interpretation of the significance of the absolute rate of urinary 3MH excretion, or the 3MH:creatinine ratio, is very difficult, and investigators should be very clear in their objectives when making this measurement.

6.6 IGF-1 (INSULIN-LIKE GROWTH FACTOR-1, SOMATOMEDIN C)

6.6.1 Purpose and scope

As already indicated there is a growing interest in IGF-1 as an indicator for nutritional status, particularly with respect to protein. IGF-1 is identical to somatomedin C and A [54, 55] and is responsible for mediating the growth-promoting action of growth hormone, with connective tissue cells of the skeleton and several other cells as targets. It is therefore a primary regulator of bone and probably general somatic growth as well as exhibiting a broad range of anabolic properties. However, the relative importance of its action on different body tissues compared with other anabolic hormones such as insulin and thyroid hormones are not completely understood. It is produced in the liver, as well as in fibroblasts and possibly other sites, so that its action can be endocrine, autocrine, or paracrine [55]. The action of IGF-1 seems to involve more complex control than that of insulin, since IGF in the plasma is bound to a carrier protein, which no doubt explains its much greater half-life in comparison to insulin, and its activity can be modulated by peptide inhibitors as well as other circulating hormones and metabolites. Thus the relationship between the concentration of IGF-1 and the IGF-like action on a target is complex. Nevertheless, there are certainly broad correlations between height growth and

IGF-1 concentrations. The best known examples are the markedly reduced levels in human pygmies and Laron dwarfs. In addition IGF-1 concentrations are increased during the pubertal growth spurt. However, the relationship between IGF-1 and growth rates is by no means straightforward, since during development highest levels are seen in young adults, with quite low levels in infants and young children [56].

There is no doubt that IGF-1 levels are sensitive to nutritional state. In grossly malnourished children concentrations are very low indeed, i.e. opposite changes to the increased levels of growth hormone [57]. In adults changes accurately reflect changes in nitrogen balance, since concentrations fall during fasting, reduced levels being observable after 24 hours. During refeeding, concentrations rise in response to the provision of dietary energy and protein [58, 59]. Studies in rats have demonstrated similar relationships between dietary energy and protein intakes and IGF-1 concentrations, with a particularly good correlation between the dietary protein concentrations and IGF-1 levels in growing rats fed the diets *ad lib* [60]. This indicates that dietary protein concentration may be an important specific determinant of the IGF-1 level.

6.6.2 Principle of the method

IGF-1 can be measured by conventional equilibrium RIA (simultaneously adding tracer, antibody, and standards or unknown), although the presence of binding proteins in serum results in a displacement curve that is not always parallel to a standard curve. This problem can be circumvented by non-equilibrium conditions by incubating the antibody with the sample prior to the addition of tracer. The commercially available kit from Nichols Institute Diagnostics utilizes this approach and derives from the development work of Underwood and Van Wyk.

Alternatively, the problem of the presence of binding proteins in serum can be avoided by acid extraction of the serum prior to assay. This markedly increases the sensitivity (three-fold) and allows equilibrium conditions to be used.

Individual laboratories who prepare their own IGF-1 and antibody utilize this approach. The method described below is an outline of the procedure in the commercially available kit from Nichols.

6.6.3 Chemicals and apparatus

All chemicals, solutions, and apparatus are provided in SMC RIA kit, Nichols Institute Diagnostics, 26441 Via De Anza, San Juan Capistrano CA 9265 USA.

6.6.4 Sample collection

Blood is collected in EDTA and plasma rapidly separated or serum cooled immediately and frozen. Assay requires 50 µl of 1:20 dilution.

6.6.5 Procedure

As described with the kit.

Note 1.
In the absence of internationally recognized standards, pooled serum from young normal adults is used and assigned a value of 1 unit per ml.

Expected values (according to Underwood [56]) are:

Normal adults (i.e. arbitrarily defined as 1 U/ml)
    95% confidence limits: −0.4–2.0 U/ml
Cord blood 0.42 U/ml
Young children (3–6 years) 0.6 U/ml
Adolescents 2–3 U/ml

6.6.6 Performance characteristics

(a) General considerations

Specificity: no cross-reactivity with hGH, porcine glucagon, hTSH, hLH; <0.02% with prolactin, porcine insulin; >0.03% with porcine proinsulin.

(b) Range of linearity

Standard curve and serial dilutions of sample are parallel.

(c) Detection limit

As defined by that quantity of the standard which will reduce maximal binding of ^{125}ISM-C by 10%: i.e. between 2.3 and 4.2 mU/ml SM-C. Thus, 0.1 U/ml SM-C can be detected.

(d) Recovery

Recovery is 94–98%.

(e) Reproducibility

Intra-assay variance CV = 5.0%; Inter-assay variance CV = 9.4%.

(f) Comparability

(See General considerations.)

(g) Validity

(See General considerations.)

6.6.7 Reference values

Reference standards are in general population specific; as an example we quote the values reported by Underwood [56].

Normal adults (i.e. arbitrarily defined as 1 U/ml)
    95% confidence limits: −0.4–2.0 U/ml
Cord blood 0.42 U/ml
Young children (3–6 years) 0.6 U/ml
Adolescents 2–3 U/ml

6.6.8 Interpretation

Plasma IGF-1 concentrations exhibit little diurnal variability so should not be sensitive to immediate dietary state. The maximum values observed in young adults tend to decline with age and are slightly higher in females. Increases are observed in pregnancy (up to 2 SD above normal range). Values are low in hypopituitary patients and in some cases of hypothyroidism, and increased markedly in acromegalics.

In a range of malnourished adult hospital patients values were on average 38% of normal [61]. In children the fact that concentrations are lower means that the detection of nutritionally mediated changes is more difficult – the normal range for children under five years overlaps with hypopituitary patients. However, in severely malnourished children concentrations are invariably as low as in hypopituitary patients [57] and increase on refeeding. There is as yet little information on marginally malnourished children or adults.

Recently Phillips [61], an enthusiastic supporter of the use of IGF-1 as a nutritional indicator, has examined the relationship between IGF-1, albumin, transferrin, and lymphocyte count amongst hospitalized patients classified as malnourished, in an attempt to evaluate the usefulness of these four factors as nutritional indices. More patients had reduced IGF-1 levels than any of the other three indicators. Furthermore, when the response of these indicators to nutritional supplementation was examined, a greater increase in IGF-1 was observed than in any of the other indicators, with IGF-1 levels correlated with intakes of both calories and protein during the previous 24 hours.

One note of caution is the unreferenced comment in a recent review by Underwood [56] that IGF-1 levels do fall in inflammatory disease. This means that similar problems may exist in separating nutrition from illness as determinants of IGF-1, as previously discussed for the plasma proteins.

REFERENCES

1. Gassull, M., Cabre, E., Vilar, L. *et al.* (1984) Protein–energy malnutrition: an integral approach and a simple new classification. *Hum. Nutr. Clin. Nut.*, **38C**, 419–31.
2. Golden, M.H.N. (1982) Protein deficiency, energy deficiency and the oedema of malnutrition. *Lancet*, **i**, 1261–5.
3. Lunn, P.G. and Austin, S. (1983) Dietary manipulation of plasma and albumin concentration. *J. Nutr.*, **113**, 1791–802.
4. Payne-Robinson, H.M., Betton, H. and Jackson, A.A. (1984) Free and total T3 and T4 in malnourished Jamaican infants. *Biochem. Soc. Trans.*, **12**, 511–2.
5. Golden, M.H.N. (1985) The consequence of protein deficiency in man and its relationship to the features of kwashiorkor, in *Nutritional Adaptation in Man* (eds K. Blaxter and J.C. Waterlow), John Libbey, London, pp. 169–88.
6. Heymsfield, S.B., Arteaga, C. and McManus, C. (1983) Measurement of muscle mass in humans: validity of the 24-hour urinary creatinine method. *Am. J. Clin. Nutr.*, **37**, 478–94.
7. Forbes, G.B. and Bruining, G.J. (1976) Urinary creatinine excretion and lean body mass. *Am. J. Clin. Nutr.*, **29**, 1359–66.
8. Young, V. and Munro, H.N. (1978) 3-methyl histidine and muscle protein turnover: an overview. *Fed. Proc.*, **37**, 2291–300.
9. Leathem, J.H. (1968) *Protein Nutrition and Free Amino Acid Patterns*, Rutgers University Press, New Brunswick, New Jersey, pp. 56–65.
10. Berry, H.K. (1970) Plasma amino acids, in *Newer Methods of Nutritional Biochemistry* (ed A.A. Albanese) Vol. IV, Academic Press, New York, pp. 173–86.
11. Young, V. and Scrimshaw, N.S. (1972) The nutritional significance of plasma and urinary amino acids, in *Protein and Amino Acid Function* (ed. E.J. Bigwood), Pergamon Press, New York, pp. 69–81.
12. Eggum, B.O. (1973) The levels of blood amino acids and blood urea as indicators of protein quality, in *Proteins in Human Nutrition* (eds J.W.G. Porter and B.A. Rolls), Academic Press, New York, pp. 176–89.
13. McLaughlan, J.M. (1974) Nutritional significance of alterations in plasma amino acids and serum proteins, in *Improvements in Protein Nutriture*, National Academy of Sciences, Washington (DC), pp. 221–38.
14. Bodwell, C.E. (1975) Biochemical parameters as indexes of protein nutritional value, in *Protein Nutritional Quality of Foods and Feeds, Part 1. Assay Methods – Biological, Biochemical, and Chemical* (ed. M. Friedman), Marcel Dekker, New York, pp. 59–75.

15. Bodwell, C.E. (1977) Biochemical indices in humans, in *Evaluation of Proteins for Humans* (ed. C.E. Bodwell), Avi Publishing Co., Westport (Connecticut), pp. 279–81.

16. Holt, L.E., Snyderman, S.E., Norton, P.M. *et al.* (1963) The plasma aminogram in kwashiorkor. *Lancet*, ii, 1343–4.

17. Whitehead, R.G. and Dean R.F.A. Serum amino acids in kwashiorkor. II. An abbreviated method of estimation. *Am. J. Clin. Nutr.*, 14, 320–9.

18. McLaren, D.S., Kamel, W.W. and Ayyoub, N. (1965) Plasma amino acids and the detection of protein–calorie malnutrition. *Am. J. Clin. Nutr.*, 17, 152–61.

19. Whitehead, R.G. and Grimble, R.F. (1970) Changes in the concentration of specific amino acids in the serum of experimentally malnourished pigs. *Br. J. Nutr.*, 24, 557–64.

20. Lunn, P.G., Whitehead, R.G., Hay, R.W. and Baker, B.A. (1973) Progressive changes in serum cortisol, insulin and growth hormone concentrations and their relationship to the distorted amino acid pattern during the development of kwashiorkor. *Br. J. Nutr.*, 29, 399–421.

21. James, W.P.T. and Coward, W.A. (1981) Metabolism of plasma proteins in man, in *Nitrogen Metabolism in Man* (eds J.C. Waterlow and J.M.L. Stephen), Applied Science Publishers, London, pp. 457–73.

22. Ingenbleek, Y., Van Den Schreick, H.G., De Nayer, P. and De Visscher, M. (1975) Albumin, transferrin and the thyroxine-binding pre-albumin/retinol binding protein complex in assessment of malnutrition. *Clin. Chim. Acta*, 63, 61–7.

23. Delpeuch, F., Cornu, A. and Chevalier P. (1980) The effect of iron deficiency anaemia on two indices of nutritional status, prealbumin and transferrin. *Br. J. Nutr.*, 43, 375–9.

24. Large, S., Neal, G., Glover, J. *et al.* (1980) The early changes in retinol-binding protein and prealbumin concentrations in plasma of protein–energy malnourished children after treatment with retinol and an improved diet. *Br. J. Nutr.*, 43, 393–402.

25. Koj, A. (1984) Metabolic studies of acute phase proteins, in *Pathophysiology of Plasma Protein Metabolism* (ed. G. Mariani), Plenum Press, New York, pp. 86–99.

26. Smith, S.J., Bos, G., Esserveld, M.R. and van Eijk, H.G. (1977) Gebranding. *Clin. Chim. Acta*, 81, 75–81.

27. Weeke, B. (1973) Rocket immunoelectrophoresis. *Scand. J. Immunol.*, 2 [Suppl 1], 37–46.

28. Clarke, H.G., Minchen, Q., Freeman, T. and Pryse-Phillips, W. (1971) Serum protein changes after injury. *Clin. Sci.*, 40, 337–42.

29. Abd-el-Fattah, M. *et al.* (1981) Kinetics of the acute-phase reaction in rats after tumor transplantation. *Cancer Res.*, 41, 2548–52.

30. Kirby, D.F., Marder, R.J., Craig, R.M. *et al.* (1985) The clinical evaluation of plasma fibronectin as a marker for nutritional depletion and repletion and as a measure of nitrogen balance. *J. Parent. Enteral Nutr.*, 9, 705–8.

31. Pinnell, A.E. and Northam, B.E. (1978) New automated dye-binding method for serum albumin determination with bromocresol purple. *Clin. Chem.*, 24, 80–95.

32. Watson, D. and Nankiville, D.D. (1964) Determination of plasma albumin by dye-binding and other methods. *Clin. Chim. Acta*, 9, 359–65.

33. Keys, A., Brozek, J., Henschel, A. *et al.* (1950) *The Biology of Human Starvation* Vol 1, University of Minnesota Press, Minneapolis.

34. Broom, J., Fraser, M.H., McKenzie, K. *et al.* (1986) The protein metabolic response to short-term starvation in man. *Clin. Nutr.*, 5, 63–5.

35. Sganga, G., Siegel, J.H., Brown, G. *et al.* (1985) Reprioritization of hepatic plasma protein release in trauma and sepsis. *Arch. Surg.*, 120, 187–99.

36. Merritt, R.J., Kalsch, M., Roux, L.D. *et al.* (1985) Significance of hypoalbuminemia

in pediatric oncology patients – malnutrition or infection? *J. Parent. Enteral Nutr.*, **9**, 303–6.

37. Tuten, M.B., Wogt, S., Dasse, F. and Leider Z. (1985) Utilization of prealbumin as a nutritional parameter. *J. Parent. Enteral Nutr.*, **9**, 709–11.

38. Lunn, P.G., Whitehead, R.G. and Coward W.A. (1979) Two pathways to kwashiorkor? *Trans. R. Soc. Trop. Med. Hyg.*, **73**, 438–43.

39. Harries, A.D. and Rhodes, J. (1984) Efficiency of anthropometric indicators in the assessment of protein nutrition in Crohn's disease. *Hum. Nutr. Clin. Nutr.*, **39C**, 155–8.

40. Golden, M.H.N. (1982) Transport proteins as indices of protein status. *Am. J. Clin. Nutr.*, **35**, 1159–65.

41. Chasson, A.L., Grady, H.T. and Stanley, M.A. (1961) Determination of creatinine by means of automatic chemical analysis. *Am. J. Clin. Pathol.*, **35**, 83–8.

42. Webster, J.D., Hesp, R. and Garrow, J.S. (1984) The composition of excess weight in obese women estimated by body density, total body water and total body potassium. *Hum. Nutr. Clin. Nutr.*, **38C**, 299–306.

43. Joossens, J.V., Claessens, J., Geboers, J. and Claes, J.H. (1980) Electrolytes and creatinine in multiple 24-hours urine collections (1970–1974), in *Epidemiology of Arterial Pressure* (eds H. Kesteloot and J.V. Joossens), Martinus Nijhoff, The Hague, pp. 45–63.

44. Ryan, R.J., Williams, J.D. and Ansell, B.M. (1957) The relationship of body composition to oxygen and creatinine excretion in healthy and wasted men. *Metabolism*, **6**, 365–9.

45. Graystone, J.E. (1986) Creatinine excretion during growth, in *Human Growth* (ed. D.B. Cheek), Lea and Febiger, Philadelphia, pp. 192–8.

46. Huszar, G., Golenwsky, G., Maiocco, J. and Davis, E. (1983) Urinary 3-methyl histidine excretion in man: the role of protein bound and soluble 3-methyl histidine. *Br. J. Nutr.*, **49**, 287–94.

47. Ward, L.C. (1978) A ninhydrin-orthophalaldehyde reagent for the determination of 3-methyl histidine. *Anal. Biochem.*, **88**, 598–604.

48. Murray, A.J., Baccaro, F.J. and Thomas, F. (1982) A rapid method for the analysis of 3-methyl histidine in human urine. *Anal. Biochem.*, **116**, 537–44.

49. Rennie, M.J. and Millward, D.J. (1983) 3-methylhistidine excretion and the urinary 3-methylhistidine/creatinine ratio are poor indicators of skeletal muscle protein breakdown. *Clin. Sci.*, **65**, 217–25.

50. Tomkins, A.M., Garlick, P.J., Schofield, W.N. and Waterlow, J.C. (1983) The combined effects of infection and malnutrition on protein metabolism in children. *Clin. Sci.*, **65**, 313–24.

51. Millward, D.J. and Bates, P.C. (1983) 3-methylhistidine turnover in the whole body, and the contribution of skeletal muscle and intestine to urinary 3-methylhistidine excretion in the adult rat. *Biochem. J.*, **214**, 607–15.

52. Li, J.B. and Wassner, S.J. (1984) Effects of food deprivation and refeeding on total protein and actomyosin degradation. *Am. J. Physiol.*, **246**, E32–E37.

53. Odedra, B.R., Bates, P.C. and Millward, D.J. (1983) Time course of the effect of catabolic doses of corticosterone on protein turnover in rat skeletal muscle and liver. *Biochem. J.*, **214**, 617–27.

54. Froesch, E.R. and Zapf, J. (1985) Insulin-like growth factors and insulin: comparative aspects. *Diabetologia*, **28**, 485–93.

55. Van Wyk, J.J. (1984) The somatomedins: biological actions and physiological control mechanism, in *Hormonal Proteins and Peptides*, Vol XII (ed. C. Li), Academic Press, New York, p. 81.

56. Underwood, L. (1985) Somatomedin-C in clinical diagnosis. *ICPR* (Sep/Oct), 13–17.

57. Smith, I.F., Latham, M.C. and Azubuike, J.A. (1981) Blood plasma levels of cortisol, insulin, growth hormone and somatomedin in children with marasmus, kwashiorkor, and intermediate forms of protein energy malnutrition. *Proc. Soc. Exp. Biol. Med.*, **167**, 607–11.

58. Isley, W.L., Underwood, L.E. and Clemmons, D.R. (1983) Dietary components that regulate serum SM-C levels in humans. *J. Clin. Invest.*, **71**, 175–82.

59. Clemmons, D.R., Klibanski, A., Underwood, L.E. *et al.* (1981) Reduction of plasma immunoreactive somatomedin C during fasting in humans. *J. Clin. Endocrinol. Metab.*, **51**, 1247–50.

60. Prewett, T.E.A., D'Ercole, A.J., Switzer, B.R. and van Wyk, J.J. (1982) Relationship of serum immunoreactive somatomedin-C to dietary protein and to dietary protein and energy intake. *J. Nutr.*, **112**, 144–50.

61. Unterman, T.G., Vazquez, R.M., Slas, A.J. *et al.* (1985) Nutrition and somatomedin. XIII. Usefulness of somatomedin-C in nutritional assessment. *Am. J. Med.*, **78**, 228–35.

7 Vitamin nutriture methodology

7.1   Introduction   *F. Fidanza and G.B. Brubacher*   186

7.2   Vitamin A   191

     Section I   Vitamin A (retinol) in plasma by HPLC
J.P. Vuilleumier, H.E. Keller and F. Fidanza   191

     Section II   Vitamin A (retinol) in plasma and serum by
HPLC-micromethod   *J. Schrijver, A.J. Speek
and H. van den Berg*   195

     Section III   β-Carotene in plasma by HPLC
J.P. Vuilleumier, H.E. Keller and F. Fidanza   200

7.3   Vitamin D (25-OHD) in serum by competitive protein-
binding assay   *H. van den Berg, J. Schrijver and P.G. Boshuis*   203

7.4   Vitamin E (α-tocopherol)   *J.P. Vuilleumier, H.E. Keller
and F. Fidanza*   209

7.5   Vitamin K_1 214

     Section I   Phylloquinone (vitamin K_1) in serum or
plasma by HPLC   *M.J. Shearer*   214

     Section II   Trans-vitamin K_1 (phylloquinone) in serum
by HPLC-micromethod   *P.M.M. van
Haard, A.J.M. Peitersma and T. Postma*   220

7.6   Thiamin   228

     Section I   Erythrocyte transketolase activity
J.P. Vuilleumier, H.E. Keller and F. Fidanza   228

     Section II   Erythrocyte transketolase activity –
micromethod   *R. Bitsch*   233

     Section III   Total thiamin in whole blood by HPLC
J. Schrijver, A.J. Speek and H. van den Berg   235

     Section IV   Thiamin in urine   *H. Heseker and A. Speitling*   241

7.7   Riboflavin   244

     Section I   Erythrocyte glutathione reductase activity
J.P. Vuilleumier, H.E. Keller and F. Fidanza   244

     Section II   Erythrocyte glutathione reductase activity –
micromethod   *R. Bitsch*   248

     Section III   Flavin adenine dinucleotide (FAD) in whole
blood by HPLC   *J. Schrijver, A.J. Speek and
H. van den Berg*   251

     Section IV   Riboflavin in urine by HPLC   *H. Heseker and
A. Speitling*   256

7.8   Niacin   258
        Section I   Niacin in whole blood by microbiological assay
                     *J. Schrijver, N. van Breederode and H. van den
                     Berg*   258
        Section II   Niacin metabolites in urine by HPLC
                     J. Sandhu and D. Fraser   263
7.9   Vitamin B$_6$ 266
        Section I   Erythrocyte aspartate transaminase
                     *J.P. Vuilleumier, H.E. Keller and
                     F. Fidanza*   266
        Section II   Pyridoxal 5'-phosphate (PLP) in whole blood
                     by HPLC   *J. Schrijver, A.J. Speek and H. van
                     den Berg*   271
        Section III Pyridoxal 5'-phosphate in plasma by
                     radioenzymatic assay using tyrosine
                     decarboxylase apoenzyme   *H. van den
                     Berg, H.A.J. Mocking and J. Schrijver*   276
        Section IV   4-Pyridoxic acid in urine by HPLC
                     H. Heseker and A. Speitling   280
7.10 Folic acid (5-Me-THF) in serum and erythrocytes by
        radioassay   *K. Pietrzik and M. Hages*   283
7.11 Vitamin B$_{12}$ (total cobalamins) in serum by competitive
        protein-binding assay   *H. van den Berg and J. Schrijver*   290
7.12 Biotin   296
        Section I   Biotin in whole blood by microbiological assay
                     *J. Schrijver, N. van Breederode and H. van den
                     Berg*   296
        Section II   Biotin in plasma or urine by RIA   *R. Bitsch*   300
7.13 Pantothenic acid in whole blood by microbiological assay
        J. Schrijver, N. van Breederode and H. van den Berg   304
7.14 Vitamin C   309
        Section I   Vitamin C in plasma and buffy coat layer of
                     blood by dinitrophenyl hydrazine assay
                     C. Bates   309
        Section II   Total vitamin C in whole blood and plasma
                     by HPLC-micromethod   *J. Schrijver, A.J.
                     Speek and H. van den Berg*   315

7.1   INTRODUCTION   The *Manual for Nutrition Surveys* of the Interdepartmental Committee on Nutrition for National Defense [1, 2] can be considered to be the first attempt to provide a description and standardization of methods for vitamin nutriture assessment.

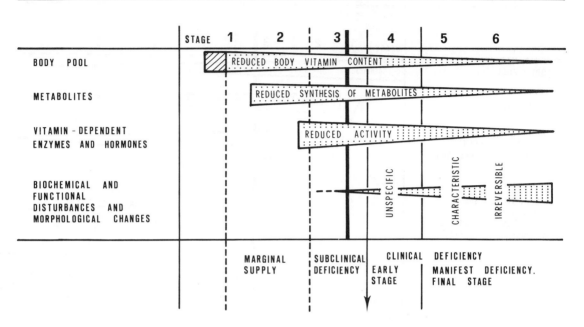

Fig. 7.1 Stages of vitamin deficiency steady-state conditions (a stationary phase) [5].

In the volume on *The vitamins: Chemistry, Physiology, Pathology, Methods* edited by Sebrell and Harris [3] some methods for the biochemical detection of deficiency are given, and methods for vitamin nutriture evaluation are reported also in the book by Sauberlich *et al* [4] on *Laboratory Tests for the Assessment of Nutritional Status*.

The biochemical methods described also in other recent manuals are the most appropriate ones for vitamin nutriture assessment. They do not provide, in general, accurate estimates of individual vitamin intake, but may give good estimates of mean vitamin intake in a specific group of the population.

As Brubacher [5] pointed out, we can have stationary and dynamic cases. In the stationary case (Fig. 7.1), there is a long-term constancy of vitamin intake and requirement. In the case of excessive intake, various mechanisms guarantee homeostasis within the cell. But confounding variables are present that can impair the results. In the dynamic case the situation is much more complex and at the very least there is a time-lag phenomenon. The first event that is observed when the intake is decreased (Fig. 7.2) is a lowering of body stores, followed in time by lower concentration of metabolites, a reduction in the activity of vitamin-dependent enzymes, and hormonal disturbance of the metabolism. During a repletion period (Fig. 7.3) the same sequence will have an opposite direction.

In cases of variable vitamin intake during a given period, the biochemical variables with a large time-lag reflect the mean vitamin intake per unit time and

DEPLETION   PERIOD

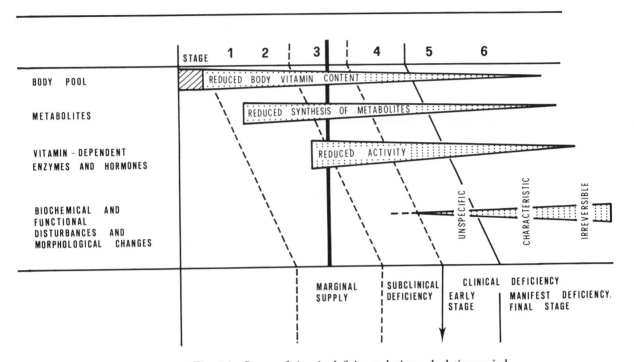

Fig. 7.2   Stages of vitamin deficiency during a depletion period.

are more useful than variables with a small time-lag. Thus in general it can be stated that measurement of the active vitamin form in blood cells usually better reflects body status than serum or plasma levels or urinary vitamin excretion.

If we correlate the actual vitamin intake with biochemical variables either no or rather low correlations are observed. To explain this various hypotheses have been made. The methods for dietary surveys are in general not as accurate as biochemical methods. In addition dietary surveys providing data on nutrient intake have to rely on food composition tables and sometimes the nutrient content in the tables does not correspond to the actual amount consumed. In food tables the nutrient values are in general for raw and individual foods and they do not take into consideration nutrient/nutrient interactions, heating losses, and bioavailability in general. Also important confounding factors (excluding those concerning the biochemical methods for nutriture assessment) are the individual metabolic conditions, drug/nutrient interactions, smoking habits, and other environmental and social factors.

Some of the above-mentioned factors will be examined for specific vitamins, in order to have a better interpretation of the results. On this last point it is reported here what was suggested at our Workshop in Colombella (Perugia) in 1986 (see Introductory Note [3]).

In principle there are two possibilities for describing the outcome of an investigation.

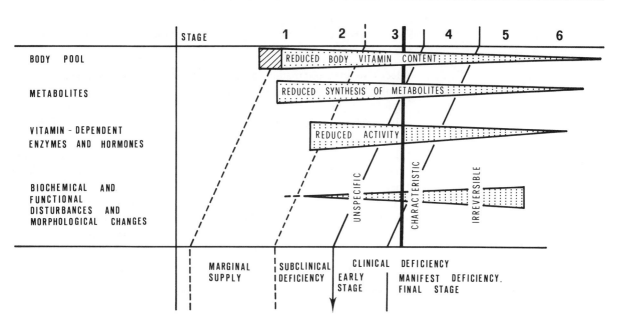

Fig. 7.3 Stages of vitamin deficiency during a repletion period.

1. The descriptive method.

   By using this method the results of an investigation are compared with the results found in a healthy reference population. It is therefore necessary that the description of the full method contains information with regard to a defined reference population.

   This information should be given preferably in percentiles, or in cases where a normal distribution can be assumed, with the characteristics of a normal distribution.

2. Subdivision into subgroups that require a judgement by the investigator.

   Since nutritionists are asked by health authorities to give a judgement on the outcome of an investigation, it is compulsory to establish interpretative guidelines.

   A reasonable basis for establishing such guidelines consists of classification of the results into risk groups and of construction of cut-off points. It seems reasonable to distinguish between three risk groups:

   High risk. If the result of an investigation shows that an appreciable percentage (10% or more; to be defined) falls into this risk group the population may be at risk and health authorities may take action.

   Low risk. If more than 70% (or another criterion) of the results found in a certain population falls into this category, there is practically no risk for the population, and the authorities have no need to take action at the community level.

Moderate risk. This category lies between the high- and the low-risk groups. If an appreciable proportion of the results falls into this category it is advisable to analyse the situation in more detail.

3. Construction of cut-off points.

For construction of cut-off points the following procedure should be adhered to.

Select a defined population group according to sex and age, etc.

Supplement this group during a sufficiently long period of time with at least 1 RDA of the vitamin in question, or make sure by some other method that each member of this population group receives at least 1 RDA.

Assess the vitamin status by the method chosen.

Take the 2.5 percentile as the cut-off point between the high-risk and the moderate-risk category and the 30th percentile as the cut-off point between moderate-risk and low-risk category. (This procedure can only be used for variables that show an upper limit.) A better way for constructing cut-off points between the high-risk and the moderate-risk category consists in determining the biochemical value which corresponds to the earliest determinable biochemical, physiological, or behavioural functional changes and morphological alterations. Examples are:

First sign of impaired dark adaptation and plasma retinol (physiological change).

Elevated alkaline phosphatase and plasma 25-hydroxycholecalciferol (biochemical change).

H_2O_2–induced haemolysis and plasma tocopherol (physiological biochemical function).

Hypersegmentation of granulocytes and plasma folic acid (morphological alteration).

The Group recommended further research for construction of cut-off points using functional parameters like physical working capacity, cognitive functions, psychological indices, immunological response, etc. Because particular physiological conditions can influence the assessment and evaluation of vitamin nutriture, one must take them into consideration.

In pregnancy the most important factors are the increase of vitamin requirements, the increase of plasma volume and the change in hormonal status. Most of the indices of vitamin intake drop to a lower level in particular at the end of pregnancy if no supplementation is provided. This is attributable not only to a higher vitamin requirement, but also to an increased plasma volume that reaches a peak during the second trimester of pregnancy.

Finally hormonal changes may lead to either an increase or a decrease in the synthesis of certain proteins. Increase of transport proteins could cause a higher plasma level, suggesting a better vitamin status than is actually present.

On the other hand the increase of erythrocyte apoenzymes would lead to an increase of the activation coefficient, suggesting a lower vitamin status than that which really exists [6].

In elderly people nutritional surveys have revealed that the most borderline vitamin deficiency concerns vitamin C, followed by vitamin B_6, thiamin, vitamin E, and with lesser frequency vitamin D and folic acid. This has been ascribed to problems of vitamin supply in groups of elderly at risk [7].

Even though the vitamin requirements of the elderly do not seem to be very different from the requirements of younger people, allowance should be made for the higher individual variability in old age.

In conclusion, in spite of the numerous above-mentioned factors affecting the vitamin nutritional status, including many individual confounding variables, biochemical tests are the best indicators of the vitamin nutriture, rather than the assessment of the daily intake by dietary surveys.

At the moment more recent and accurate methods are available that can be considered promising for the assessment of vitamin status, but many of them need still further investigation for a better standardization.

7.2 VITAMIN A

Three methods for Vitamin A nutriture assessment are described: the HPLC method for plasma retinol determination, the micromethod for plasma vitamin A, and the HPLC method for plasma β-carotene.

Recently a very promising method based on conjunctival cytology has been proposed [8]. This can identify individuals with physiologically significant preclinical vitamin A deficiency. Specimens can be obtained quite easily, stored for a very long time under field conditions, and only an ordinary microscope is needed for interpretation.

SECTION I VITAMIN A (RETINOL) IN PLASMA BY HPLC

7.2.1 Purpose and scope

The best method for vitamin A nutritional status assessment is determination of retinol concentration in the liver, where it is stored mostly as retinyl palmitate. However the plasma determination is usually carried out because of the difficulty of obtaining liver biopsy material. Vitamin A is present in plasma as retinol bound to the retinol-binding protein (RBP) and forming a water-soluble complex. Accordingly to determine total plasma retinol it is necessary to free it from this carrier protein using an appropriate ethanol concentration for this purpose.

Vitamin A is present only in limited quantities in plasma except in certain circumstances, such as after elevated vitamin A dosages or in certain disease states (severe liver disease, severe protein–energy malnutrition) [9, 10].

The vitamin A plasma level is regulated by a homeostatic mechanism, which means that it can be considered an indicator of vitamin A intake only if the intake is less than adequate [5].

The plasma level of this vitamin also reflects the mean vitamin intake over a given period rather than its daily fluctuation, since there is a big time-lag between the actual intake and the plasma level change, which depends principally on the liver stores. If the protein intake is very low, RBP synthesis is reduced, which induces a lowering of the vitamin A plasma level even with a satisfactory intake. On the other hand, in the case of A hypervitaminosis the retinol plasma level is only slightly enhanced whereas the retinyl palmitate level is increased much more. Assessment of the latter is considered indicative of vitamin A hypervitaminosis together with the molar ratio of retinol to retinol-binding protein, which in this situation is greater than 1. According to Smith and Goodman [11] vitamin A toxicity occurs when very high amounts of vitamin A are present in cell membranes in association with lipoproteins, rather than being bound to the retinol-binding protein, which also protects tissues from the surface-active properties of the vitamin.

Because vitamin A deficiency is a major public health problem in many parts of the world the International Vitamin A Consultative Group (IVACG) has also recently published a manual of *Biochemical Methodology for the Assessment of Vitamin A Status* [12] and a collection of *Reprints of Selected Methods for the Analysis of Vitamin A and Carotenoids in Nutrition Surveys* [13].

7.2.2 Principle of the method

Retinol is freed from retinol-binding protein by adding ethanol to diluted plasma and extracting it with n-hexane. The extract is separated by straight-phase HPLC on a silica gel column. Detection is carried out at an adequate wavelength [14].

7.2.3 Chemicals and Apparatus

(a) Chemicals

Ethanol (C_2H_5OH) p.a.
n-Hexane (C_6H_{14}) p.a.
2-Propanol (C_3H_8O) p.a.
(all-E)-Retinol of crystalline purity, e.g. Fluka, purity: 95% (all-E) and 5% 13 Z isomer, cat. No. 95144
Butylhydroxytoluene (BHT) p.a.

(b) Solutions

HPLC mobile phase: n-hexane/2-propanol (97:3 v/v).
Retinol standard solutions for HPLC:
  Stock standard: 60 mg (all-E)-retinol and 1 g BHT (butylhydroxytoluene) are dissolved in n-hexane to make 100 ml. The stock solution can be stored for one month in the dark.
  Standard dilution: 10 ml of stock solution are made up to 100 ml with n-hexane.
  Working standard: 1 ml of standard dilution is made up to 100 ml with n-hexane.

Standard dilution and working standard are prepared fresh every day. The working standard is checked photometrically in a quartz 10 mm cuvette at 325 nm (maximum absorbance). The absorbance should be 0.104.

(c) Apparatus

Glass tubes (4 ml capacity, 7 × 100 mm) for shaking and centrifugation; adjustable pipettes; Vortex; microlab dispenser; mechanical shaker.
HPLC apparatus consisting of:
  Merck Hibar prepared column, 250–4 mm, filled with LiChrosorb Si 60, 5 μm
  Altex model 110 A pump with pulse suppressor and manometer WIKA 0–250 bar

Automatic injector, e.g. Waters WISP 710 A with BCD board for signal receptor from the integrator

Waters Fixed Wavelength Detector Model 440 with filter 313 nm

W+W recorder Model 314 (single-channel)

Integrator, e.g. Spectra-physics, Model 4270.

7.2.4   Sample collection

Blood is collected by vein puncture into herapin-lined vacutainer tubes.

7.2.5   Procedure

(a) Sample preparation and extraction

The heparinated whole blood is centrifuged at a low speed for plasma separation. Plasma can be stored frozen (–20°C) for several months. (Retinol content in frozen plasma at –20°C was practically unchanged after five years).

The deep-frozen plasma is thawed and mixed to disperse possible precipitates. 200 µl of plasma is pipetted in a 4 ml centrifuge tube and diluted with 200 µl of water. While shaking on a Vortex-shaker, 400 µl of ethanol are added and the tube shaken for ten seconds. 800 µl of n-hexane are added from a microlab dispenser. The tube is sealed with a polyethylene stopper, shaken for five minutes on a mechanical shaker, and centrifuged at 2000 g for five minutes.

From the hexane phase appropriate volumes are transferred into sample conical vials (5 × 40 mm) and protected from light (brown glass or wrapped with dark material).

(b) Calibration

Freshly prepared reference solution of (all-E)-retinol, suitably diluted in n-hexane and partitioned between aqueous ethanol and hexane, as for plasma samples, are used as external standards. It is assumed that the distribution between the two phases is the same irrespective of the presence of plasma or water.

Calibration is repeated when one-sided drifts of the values for the control plasma exceeding 3% of the mean are found.

Human and bovine plasma are pooled to give a retinol level between 1.40 and 2.79 µmol/l. Aliquot volumes in excess of 750 µl are transferred to plastic vials and frozen at –80°C until required for analysis.

An extract of control plasma, usually 3 ml hexane corresponding to 750 µl plasma, is distributed into micro-injection vials, which are kept at –20°C. These controls are inserted in the 1st, 24th and 48th position of the sampler rings. They are prepared fresh daily.

(c) HPLC

The entire chromatographic procedure is carried out at room temperature.

One hundred microlitres of sample extract is subjected to isocratic straight-phase HPLC. The flow rate of the mobile phase is about 1.9 ml/min (working pressure 8.5 MPa).

Retention time is about five minutes. Should this time change, the flow rate is modified accordingly.

The effluent of HPLC column is passed through the photometer set at 313 nm (the actual maximum absorbance is at 325 nm if a monochromator is available).

In this set-up the recorder tracing is used as control. The peak integration is done by an integrator that prints the results according to the calibration parameters programmed.

(d) Calculation

The resulting peak area calculated by the integrator is compared to the corresponding peak area of the standard solution, which has been treated exactly as the plasma sample (external calibration).

7.2.6 Performance characteristics

(a) Detection limit

The practical detection limit without changing the operating conditions is 0.07 µmol/l plasma.

(b) Reproducibility

The coefficient of variation of duplicate assays is 3.3% (N = 189; range 0.63 − 3.07 µmol/l) for plasma, 2.2% (N = 6; x̄ = 1.85 µmol/l) for whole blood. When blood was collected from the same individual at six days time-lag between collections, the coefficient of variation was 15% (N = 6; x̄ = 1.85 µmol/l) [15].

Actual true recovery is not possible at the moment because retinol bound to RBP is not available. However, repeated extractions have shown that practically all retinol is contained in the first extract and none in the subsequent extract.

(c) Validity

Comparison of the retinol assay by HPLC (assay x) and the former manual method (assay y) gave a correlation coefficient of 0.980 and a linear regression equation y = −0.0182 + 1.02x (N=189), in µmol/l [15].

7.2.7 Reference values

The reference values are in general population specific. For example, the average retinol level of 150 adult blood donors of both sexes from Basel (Red Cross Centre) is 2.09 µmol/l (men = 2.31 µmol; women = 1.86 µmol/l) [16]. The cumulative frequency distribution is given in Table 7.1.

Table 7.1 Cumulative frequency distribution of plasma retinol (N = 150 blood donors)

Percentile	Retinol µmol/l
Min	1.12
5	1.26
25	1.72
50	2.09
75	2.43
95	2.94
Max	3.11
Mean	2.09
SD	0.49

7.2.8 Interpretation

Confounding variables, which limit the use of the vitamin A plasma level determination, should also be considered: zinc and copper nutriture, alcohol intake, lipid status, age, and sex, besides the already mentioned protein nutriture. Several diseases (chronic infections, cystic fibrosis, sprue, liver diseases) and drugs (neomycin, cortisone, phenobarbitone, oral contraceptives) also affect the vitamin A status [10]. Finally, the effects of other vitamins on vitamin A nutritional status, in particular that of viatmin E, which protects retinol against its oxidative destruction and of vitamin C on the effects of vitamin A toxicity, should be taken into account [16].

SECTION II   VITAMIN A (RETINOL) IN PLASMA AND SERUM BY HPLC-MICROMETHOD

7.2.9 Purpose and scope

Vitamin A generally comprises retinol, retinal, and retinoic acid and is found in various tissues and plasma [17–20]. High levels are especially found in the liver, where it is stored mainly as retinyl fatty acid esters (the storage pool increasing with age). Provitamin A carotenoids (e.g. β-carotene) serve as precursors of vitamin A (conversion mainly in the small intestine). Together with other carotenoids they contribute to the colour of tissues (e.g. skin). In addition to its function in vision vitamin A plays an important yet incompletely understood role in the differentiation and maintenance of epithelial membranes and in spermatogenesis, bone growth, and mucopolysaccharide synthesis.

The clinical manifestations of vitamin A deficiency in vision are well recognized [21]. The most reliable index of the vitamin A status would be the amount of vitamin A in the liver. As this is unpractical, vitamin A is routinely investigated by its analysis in plasma or serum [17], although this level is kept quite constant by the liver as long as the liver store is not depleted ($> 20 \, \mu g/g$ of liver). At concentrations below $0.70 \, \mu mol/l$ serum ($< 20 \, \mu g/100 \, ml$), the vitamin A status is probably decreased; below $0.35 \, \mu mol/l$ serum ($< 10 \, \mu g/100 \, ml$) deficiency is most probable. However, low levels can be found not reflecting retinol deficiency (see below).

Plasma/serum carotenoids are poor indicators of the vitamin A status. They merely reflect recent dietary intake (from green leafy vegetables and fruit and absorption in the gut). Levels below $0.7 \, \mu mol/l$ indicate low (recent) intake of carotenoids. Retinol in plasma is transported to the target tissues as its retinol-binding protein-prealbumin (RBP-PA) complex.

The levels of RBP and PA in plasma are of limited value (normal levels: RBP 30–60 mg/l and PA 100–400 mg/100 ml serum) as they are influenced by a number of factors not related to vitamin A status such as infection [22]. Recently the analysis of vitamin A in tear fluid has been described [23]. Whether this level has prognostic value is not yet known. The dark adaptation test can be used to detect a developing vitamin A deficiency. Night-blindness appears to be the first clinical sign of vitamin A deficiency. However, routine use is not simple; neither is conjunctival impression cytology [24]. The relative dose response test seems a promising method, although it is not practical on a large scale. If a single dose of vitamin A results in an increase of serum retinol of less than 10%, the status is normal, at 10–20% inconclusive, and at >20% a deficiency is most likely. The method is based on the observation that in vitamin-A-deprived states, RBP synthesis continues in hepatocytes in excess to holo-RBP that is released. When vitamin A becomes available, it binds to RBP and is promptly released into the blood [25].

Primary deficiency has repeatedly been described in fast-growing children, especially in relation to infections (measles), as a result of protein–energy malnutrition, and on a low-fat diet, resulting in the various stages of xerophthalmia and finally blindness [21]. Secondary deficiency may result from malabsorption, lipoproteinaemia, zinc deficiency, liver disorders, long-term drug use (cholestyramine, neomycin, mineral oil, antacid, cortisone, phenobarbitone, caffeine), and alcohol abuse [26, 27]. Clinical signs include degenerative changes in the eyes and skin.

Several methods have been described for the analysis of retinol [12]. Direct colorimetric, spectrophotometric, and fluorometric methods are, however, not very specific. In recent years, this drawback has resulted in the use of high-performance liquid chromatography (HPLC) with UV or fluorometric detection. In general the HPLC methods require at least 100 μl of plasma. In addition, many methods incorporate evaporation of the extracting solvent and redissolving of the residue, since the extraction and HPLC solvents are not compatible. This step, even if performed under nitrogen, may cause loss of vitamin A and, moreover, it makes large-scale routine analysis more time-consuming. To reduce handling of samples and account for limited amounts of biological material, a micromethod should be used. A specific example for the analysis of vitamin A in only 5 μl samples using HPLC is described below [28].

7.2.10 Principle of the method

After precipitation of the plasma or serum proteins with ethanol, vitamin A is extracted by n-hexane. Following separation on a straight-phase HPLC column, all-*trans* retinol is detected fluorometrically and is quantitated from peak area by integration using an external standard.

7.2.11 Chemicals and apparatus

(a) Chemicals

Ethanol (100%) p.a.
Butylated hydroxytoluene (BHT), e.g. Baker, cat. No. 8098
n-Hexane p.a.
Methylene chloride p.a.
2-propanol p.a.
Dimethyl acetamide p.a.
Sodium chloride (NaCl) p.a.
Polygosil 60–5, Marcherey-Nagel, cat. No. 71101
All-*trans* retinol, e.g. Fluka, cat. No. 95144
Water: quartz-bidistilled every 2–3 days.

(b) Solutions

0.9% (w/v) NaCl: 9 g NaCl dissolved in water to make 1000 ml.
n-Hexane + 0.25% (w/v) BHT (2.5 g/l).
HPLC mobile-phase consisting of n-hexane : methylene chloride : 2-propanol
   = 900 : 90 : 12, to which 0.25% (w/v) BHT is added.
Vitamin A stock standard solution for HPLC : about 50 mg of the vitamin A

standard is dissolved in a calibrated receiver made of brownish glass in 100 ml 100% ethanol. The concentration of all-*trans* retinol in this solution is calculated from the absorption of a 100-fold dilution in ethanol at 325 nm measured in a suitable spectrophotometer and using the molar absorption coefficient of 52 480 (molecular weight of all-*trans* retinol = 286.5, [29]). A working standard solution is prepared by a dilution of the stock standard solution with n-hexane to a concentration of about 50 nmol/l. This solution and the stock standard solution are stored in the dark at −20°C and are stable for at least one month.

(c) Apparatus

Tubes made of brownish glass (e.g. 17 × 110 mm) suited for centrifugation; adjustable (micro-) pipettes; dispensers; Vortex.

Refrigerated laboratory centrifuge; spectrophotometer; 1 cm quartz cuvettes.

HPLC apparatus consisting of:

Knauer stainless steel column, 125 × 4.6 mm diameter, filled with Polygosil 60–5

Constant-flow pump

Automatic injector (or injection valve)

Fluorescence detector, e.g. Kratos Fluoromat filter fluorometer, model FS 950, provided with light source FSA 111 (330–375 nm), excitation band filter FSA 403 (365 nm), emission cut-off filter FSA 428 (470 nm) and a flow cell of 28 µl; in general, several other fluorometers might be used if the instrument provides the correct excitation light and photomultiplier sensitivity; in case a fluorometer is not available, a sensitive UV detector can be used set at a wavelength of 325 nm.

Recorder

Integrator.

7.2.12   Sample collection

All procedures during sample treatment are carried out under subdued light conditions. The anticoagulant (citrate, EDTA, or heparin) used in the collection of whole blood does not influence the analytical procedures. Whole blood samples collected in vacuum tubes can be stored in the refrigerator (4°C) for a couple of days without appreciable loss of vitamin A, provided the tube is kept closed during storage. Plasma and serum are separated by centrifugation for 10 min at 1500 *g* and 4°C. Plasma and serum samples can be stored in the refrigerator for several months (preferably at temperatures <−20°C) without appreciable loss of vitamin A, except when EDTA is used as anticoagulant.

7.2.13   Procedure

(a) Sample extraction

An amount of 5 µl of well-mixed plasma or serum is put into a 50 × 6 mm glass tube containing 95 µl 0.9% (w/v) NaCl.

The contents are mixed with 100 µl of absolute ethanol containing 1.5 g/l BHT and thereafter thoroughly vortex-mixed for 1 min with 200 µl of n-hexane containing 0.25 g/l BHT.

The tube is centrifuged for 5 min at 1000 *g* and 4°C, and stored in the dark at −20°C for HPLC analysis within 24 h.

(b) Calibration

Before analysis, a few aliquots of the working standard solution are injected to equilibrate the chromatographic system (constant peak height). In routine analysis each series of five sample extracts is preceded by this external standard. The linearity of the chromatographic system is controlled every month by a range of different standard concentrations, corresponding to original levels of 0–5 µmol all-*trans* retinol per litre serum or plasma.

(c) HPLC

The entire chromatographic procedure is carried out at ambient temperature. Extracts in the HPLC injector are protected from UV light. Aliquots of 100 µl of the n-hexane extract are subjected to straight-phase HPLC. The flow rate of the mobile phase is about 1.2 ml/min. In general, the retention time of all-*trans* retinol is about 5 min, the total run time about 6–7 min. Fluorescence is detected using the wavelength couple 325/470 nm (or suitable filters as indicated in HPLC apparatus). The elution profiles are displayed on the recorder set at 10 mV full-scale and a recording speed of 2 mm/min. The recorder as well as the integrator are connected directly to the fluorometer.

(d) Calculation

The concentration of all-*trans* retinol in the original sample is calculated from integration based on the peak area ratio sample/standard. In cases of failure of the integrator, peak heights are used. By the extraction method described, all-*trans* retinol is released quantitatively. The equation for calculation of all-*trans* retinol concentration in plasma or serum will be:

$$\text{all-}trans \text{ retinol (µmol/l)} = \frac{A_s \cdot C_{st} \cdot D}{A_{st}}$$

where A_s = peak area of the sample, A_{st} = peak area of standard, C_{st} = concentration of working standard solution in µmol/l, and D = correction factor for dilution. For 5 µl plasma/serum, $D = \dfrac{200}{100} \cdot \dfrac{100}{5} = 40$.

7.2.14 Performance characteristics

(a) Range of linearity

Using dilutions of plasma or serum samples (aliquots of 5–100 µl of sample made up to 100 µl with 0.9% (w/v) NaCl) results in comparable retinol levels in the range up to about 5 µmol/l.

(b) Detection limit

Assuming the signal-to-noise ratio should be at least 3, the HPLC method described here shows a detection limit as low as 0.05 µmol/l (injected amount about 1.25 nmol or 3.6 µg all-*trans* retinol).

(c) Recovery

Recovery can be determined in each series by analysis of aliquots of pooled plasma or serum and aliquots of the same pooled plasma or serum to which all-*trans* retinol has been added. For that purpose, all-*trans* retinol is dissolved in a minimum amount of dimethyl acetamide. To correct for volume changes, the same amount of dimethyl acetamide is added to pooled plasma or serum. Pooled and recovery samples are stored at –20°C in the dark for a period generally not exceeding three months. For an addition of 0.7 µmol/l all-*trans* retinol, the recovery is complete with a CV for a singular analysis as low as 7%.

(d) Reproducibility

In our laboratory the precision of the method is determined in each series by analysis of three aliquots of pooled plasma or serum (see also 7.2.14(c)). For a pool with an average level of about 0.7 µmol/l plasma the overall CV of a single sample run in an arbitrary series can be as low as 5.0%.

(e) Validity

In general, vitamin A levels obtained by colorimetric (Carr and Price) and UV methods are comparable to those obtained by HPLC with fluorometric detection. However, the former methods may be interfered with by known and unknown sample components (e.g. carotenoids interfere with the colorimetric method). Up till now no interference has been observed with the HPLC method. Possible isomers of all-*trans* retinol (e.g. 9-*cis* and 13-*cis* retinol) are clearly separated from the all-*trans* isomer.

7.2.15 Reference values

Reference values are, in general, population-specific. For example, the average (± SD) vitamin A level for 207 apparently healthy volunteers (blood donors from the centre of the Netherlands) with an average age (± SD) of 37 ± 11.2 years (range 18–64 yrs), was 2.00 ± 0.46 µmol/l serum [30]. The cumulative frequency distribution is given in Table 7.2. An influence of age on the level of all-*trans* retinol in serum was not observed. However, the vitamin A level of women was significantly ($P < 0.001$) lower than that of men (averages 1.9 and 2.2 µmol/l serum for women and men respectively). Furthermore, the vitamin A concentration in serum of women using oral contraceptives (average 2.2 µmol/l) was significantly higher than that of women not using this drug (average 1.7 µmol/l).

For 122 apparently healthy Dutch free-living elderly people with an average age of 72 ± 3.8 years (range 65–89 years) [31], the average all-*trans* retinol level (1.55 ± 0.44 µmol/l plasma) was significantly lower than that of the group of blood donors.

Table 7.2 Cumulative frequency distribution of plasma all-*trans* retinol (N = 207 volunteers)

Percentile	Vitamin A µmol/l
Min	0.70
5	1.30
25	1.70
50	2.00
75	2.20
95	2.80
Max	3.30
Mean	2.00
SD	0.46

7.2.16 Interpretation

Levels of all-*trans* retinol in plasma or serum in the range of 0.35–0.70 µmol/l are considered as indicative of vitamin A depletion of the liver; below 0.35 µmol/l deficiency is very likely.

SECTION III β-CAROTENE IN PLASMA BY HPLC

7.2.17 Purpose and scope

The principal carotenoids found in human plasma or serum are β-carotene, α-carotene, lycopene and small quantities of an oxycarotenoid, the xanthophyll named cryptoxanthin.

At the intestinal mucosa level, carotenes are mostly transformed into retinaldehyde by a 15,15′-carotene dioxygenase. β-Carotene yields two molecules of retinaldehyde, other carotenes only one. Retinaldehyde is also reduced to retinol. An appreciable quantity of retinol derived from carotenes is incorporated in esterified chylomicra with long-chain fatty acids. A certain amount of carotenoids pass through the intestinal mucosa cell membrane without change [9]. Carotenes are stored in different body tissues, in particular adipose tissue and in small amounts in the liver, where most of them are transformed into retinaldehyde [10].

In the past determination of serum β-carotene was used to assess its nutritional status particularly in people with high vegetable intake and low intake of preformed vitamin A [9]. More recently it has become evident that carotene can play an important role in the prevention of some types of cancers, particularly lung cancer [32]. Some studies have also shown regression in development of premalignant lesions, (actinic keratosis, leukoplakia) [33] and of different epithelial cancers in relation to consumption of high doses of β-carotene or retinol [34].

This beneficial activity seems to be ascribed to synergistic links between various essential antioxidants involved in a multilevel defence system against oxygen radicals [35].

Determination of β-carotene concentration and the study of its pharmaco-kinetic activity and metabolism will be useful in monitoring cancer patients or healthy individuals taking part in chemoprevention trials. These clinical studies on the cancer–β-carotene hypothesis should nevertheless incorporate a more discriminatory analysis of carotenoids in food, biological fluids, and tissues.

7.2.18 Principle of the method

β-Carotene is liberated from protein by the addition of ethanol to diluted plasma and extracted with n-hexane. The extract is separated by straight-phase HPLC on a silica gel column. Detection is carried out at an appropriate wavelength [36].

7.2.19 Chemicals and apparatus

(a) Chemicals

Ethanol (C_2H_5OH) p.a.
n-Hexane (C_6H_{14}) p.a.
Dioxane ($C_4H_8O_2$) p.a.
β-Carotene, e.g. Fluka, 97% (UV), cat. No. 22040

Dichloromethane (CH_2Cl_2) p.a.
Butylhydroxytoluene (BHT) p.a.

(b) Solutions

HPLC mobile phase: n-hexane/dioxane (1000 : 10 v/v).
Carotene standard solutions for HPLC:
Stock standard: 25 mg β-carotene are dissolved in approximately 5 ml dichloromethane and made up to 100 ml with n-hexane.
Standard dilution (containing 2.5 mg/dl): 10 ml stock standard are made up to 100 ml with n-hexane.
Working standard (containing 100 µg/dl): 4 ml of standard dilution are made up to 100 ml with n-hexane.

All the solutions are unstable and should be prepared fresh every day. The stock standard is stable up to one week if 35 mg per cent of butylhydroxytoluene (BHT) is added.

The working standard is checked photometrically in a 10 mm cuvette at 453 nm (maximum absorbance), the absorbance should be 0.235.

(c) Apparatus

Glass tubes (4 ml capacity, 7×100 mm) for shaking and centrifugation; adjustable pipettes; Vortex; microlab dispenser; mechanical shaker.
HPLC apparatus consisting of:
Merck Hibar prepared column 250–4 mm filled with LiChrosorb Si 60, 5 µm
Altex Model 110 A pump with pulse suppressor and manometer WIKA 0–250 bar
Automatic injector, e.g. Waters WISP 710 A with BCD board for signal receptor from the integrator
Waters Fixed Wavelength Detector Model 440 with filter 436 nm
W + W recorder Model 314 (single-channel)
Integrator, e.g. Spectra-physics, Model 4270.

7.2.20 Sample collection

Blood is collected by vein puncture into heparin-lined vacutainer tubes.

7.2.21 Procedure

(a) Sample preparation and extraction

The heparinated whole blood is centrifuged at low speed for plasma separation. Plasma can be stored frozen ($-20°C$) for a maximum of six months.

The deep-frozen plasma is thawed and mixed to disperse possible precipitates. Two hundred microlitres plasma is pipetted into a 4 ml centrifuge tube and diluted with 200 µl water. While shaking on a Vortex shaker, 400 µl ethanol are added and the tube shaken for ten seconds. Eight hundred microlitres n-hexane are added by a microlab dispenser. The tube is sealed with a polyethylene stopper, shaken for five minutes on a mechanical shaker and centrifuged at 2000 *g* for five minutes.

From the hexane phase an appropriate aliquot is transferred into sample vials protected from light (brown glass or wrapped with black material).

(b) Calibration

Freshly prepared reference solutions of β-carotene suitably diluted in n-hexane and partitioned between aqueous ethanol and hexane, as for plasma samples, are used as external standards. It is assumed that the distribution between the two phases is the same irrespective of the presence of plasma or water.

Calibration is repeated when one-sided drifts of the values for the control plasma exceeding 3% of the mean are found.

Human and bovine plasma are pooled to give a β-carotene level between 500 and 1000 μg/l. Aliquot volumes in excess of 750 μl are transferred to plastic vials and frozen at –80°C until required for analysis.

An extract of control plasma, usually 3 ml hexane corresponding to 750 μl plasma, is distributed into micro-injection vials, which are kept at –20°C. These controls are inserted in the 1st, 24th and 48th positions of the sampler rings. They are prepared fresh daily.

(c) HPLC

The entire chromatographic procedure is carried out at room temperature.

One hundred microlitres of sample extract is subjected to isocratic straight-phase HPLC. The flow rate of the mobile phase is about 0.9 ml/min. Retention time is about 3.7 min. Should this retention time change the flow rate is modified accordingly.

The effluent of HPLC column is passed through the photometer set at 436 nm (the actual maximum absorbance is at 452 nm, if a monochromator is available).

In this set-up the recorder tracing is used as control. The peak integration is done by an integrator which prints the results according to the calibration parameters programmed.

(d) Calculation

The resulting peak area of β-carotene calculated by the integrator is compared to the corresponding peak area of the standard solution, which has been treated exactly as the plasma sample (external calibration).

7.2.22 Performance characteristics

(a) General considerations

The carotene assay, which is used in human as well as in animal studies, separates the oxygen-containing carotenoids such as xanthophylls, which do not appear on the recorder diagram, from the hydrocarbon pigments, the carotenes. Within the carotene group, however, selectivity is limited. If present, α-carotene would not be separated from β-carotene, but lycopene, the main carotene in tomatoes, would. The great majority of human plasma specimens collected in our laboratory show additional peaks following the carotene peak, the principal one probably being lycopene. Methods are available for separation and determination of various carotenes if needed [37, 38].

(b) Range of linearity

This is 0.09 – 35 μmol/l.

(c) Detection limit

The practical detection limit without changing the operating conditions is 0.05 μmol/l of plasma.

(d) Reproducibility

The variation coefficient of duplicate assay for plasma samples is 3.0% (N=188; range 0.07–6.6 μmol/l), and for whole blood is 2.4% (N=6; $\bar{x}$ = 1.4 μmol/l).

When blood was collected from the same individual at six days time-lag between collections, the variation coefficient was 6.8% (N=6; $\bar{x}$ = 1.4 µmol/l) [36].

Actual true recovery is not possible at the moment because carotene cannot be introduced into plasma. However, repeated extractions have shown that practically all the β-carotene was present in the first extract and none in the subsequent extracts.

(e) Validity

Comparison of the β-carotene assay by HPLC (assay x) and the former manual method [15] (assay y) gave a correlation coefficient of 0.994 and a linear regression equation y = 0.011 + 1.03x (N=188) in µmol/l [36].

7.2.23 Reference values

The reference values are, in general, population specific. For example the average β-carotene level of 150 adult blood donors of both sexes from Basel (Red Cross Centre) was 0.70 µmol/l (men = 0.60 µmol/l, women = 0.83 µmol/l) [36]. The cumulative frequency distribution is given in Table 7.3.

Table 7.3 Cumulative frequency distribution of plasma β-carotene (N = 150 blood donors)

Percentile	β-carotene µmol/l
Min	0.13
5	0.21
25	0.42
50	0.58
75	0.86
95	1.43
Max	3.26
Mean	0.70
SD	0.47

7.3 VITAMIN D (25-OHD) IN SERUM BY COMPETITIVE PROTEIN-BINDING ASSAY

7.3.1 Purpose and scope

25-Hydroxyvitamin D (25-OHD) is the most abundant circulating metabolite of vitamin D, with a relatively long half-life (about 20 days). Its content in serum or plasma is generally considered a reliable indicator of the vitamin D nutritional status [9, 39, 40]. Under conditions of normal solar exposure, 25-hydroxycholecalciferol (25-OHD$_3$) is the only, or by far the most predominant, form in the circulation. In healthy adults its concentration in serum (plasma) varies from 20 to 130 nmol/l and shows a strong seasonal variation. Vitamin D$_2$ metabolites are present only after vitamin D$_2$ supplementation or therapy. In general, non-hydroxylated vitamin D is present in only relatively low concentrations (< 20 nmol/l) [40, 41]. Next to 25-OHD, 24,25-(OH)$_2$D and 1,25-(OH)$_2$D metabolites are also present in serum (plasma) in relatively low concentrations (1–10 nmol/l and 40–140 pmol/l, respectively). The dihydroxy metabolites are not considered as reliable indices of the vitamin D nutritional status.

Competitive protein binding (CPB) assay and high-performance liquid chromatography (HPLC) with UV detection can be used for quantification of the serum or plasma 25-OHD content [40, 41].

7.3.2 Principle of the method

The vitamin D metabolites 25-OHD$_2$ and 25-OHD$_3$ in plasma are bound to a specific binding protein (DBP). After extraction of serum (plasma) with a mixture of dichloromethane, methanol and water, 25-OHD is isolated by chromatography on a small silica column. The 25-OHD content is quantified by a CPB assay using diluted rat serum as a source of the binder [42]. After incubation of the extract in the presence of tritium (^{3}H)-labelled 25-OHD$_3$, the free and bound molecules are separated by a dextran-coated charcoal precipitation step. The amount of bound ^{3}H-labelled 25-OHD is estimated by counting the radioactivity of the supernatant fraction obtained after charcoal precipitation. The radioactivity counted is a measure of the 25-OHD content in the original serum (plasma) sample. The binding protein present in rat serum has nearly equal affinity for 25-OHD$_2$ and 25-OHD$_3$.

7.3.3 Chemicals and apparatus

(a) Chemicals

Dichloromethane p.a.
Methanol p.a.
n-Hexane p.a.
Diethylether, peroxide-free (freshly distilled)
Ethanol, absolute
Nitrogen gas, oxygen-free
Scintillation fluid, e.g. Opti-Fluor (Packard Instruments)
Bovine serum albumin (BSA); each batch should be checked before use as being free from DBP activity (i.e. non-specific binding in the CPB assay should be $< 5\%$)
Disposable prepacked extraction columns Silica gel, e.g. Baker Chemicals, 3-ml cartridges
Barbitone sodium p.a.
25-hydroxy[26,27-methyl-^{3}H]vitamin D$_3$ (specific radioactivity approximately 160 Ci/mmol), e.g. Amersham, cat. No. TRK 655
25-hydroxyvitamin D standard, e.g. Duphar (Weesp, The Netherlands)
Norit A
Dextran T70, e.g. Pharmacia
Water: Quartz-bidistilled every 2–3 days
Sodium chloride p.a.
Sodium azide p.a.

(b) Solutions

Buffer solutions of sodium barbitone:

Stock solution: 20.6 g sodium barbitone dissolved in 1000 ml water, add sodium azide (0.01 M) or thimerosal (0.02%; w/v) as a preservative.

Working buffer I: Dilute stock solution 1:10 with water, add 9.0 g NaCl per litre. Adjust to pH 8.6.

Working buffer II: Add 0.2 g BSA per 100 ml working buffer I.

Binder solutions of normal rat serum:

Stock solution: Pooled normal rat serum (e.g. from Wistar rats) is diluted 1:300 with working buffer I and stored in small (e.g. 1 ml) aliquots at –80°C. Under these conditions the stock solution can be stored for at least one year.

Working solution: Before each assay an aliquot of the binder stock solution is diluted with working buffer II. The degree of dilution depends on the affinity of the batch of rat serum used and should be such that in the assay approximately 50% of the added undiluted radioactive $[^3H]25\text{-}OHD_3$ is bound to the binding protein (i.e. B_0/T = about 50%). In general the final dilution will vary between 20 000 and 40 000. The dilution factor remains constant for one specific batch of rat serum.

Tracer solutions:

Assay tracer solution: After evaporation of the benzene/alcohol solvent 25-hydroxy[26,27-methyl-^3H]vitamin D_3 is dissolved in ethanol to obtain a concentration of 60 pg (approx. 13 000 c.p.m.) per 10 µl. The radio-purity is checked at regular intervals (every two months) by HPLC (HPLC column: Polygosil Si 60, 5 µm (Macherey–Nagel); 4.6 × 250 mm i.d. Eluent: Hexane/iso-propanol 97:3 (v/v)).

Recovery tracer solution: Dilute the assay tracer solution with ethanol to a concentration of about 12 pg/10 µl. Tracer solutions are stored at –20°C.

25-Hydroxyvitamin D_3 standard solutions:

Stock standard: Every 6 months the content of a new ampoule containing 25 mg of 25-OHD is dissolved in 40.0 ml ethanol and the concentration checked spectrophotometrically (molar absorption coefficient is 18 200 at 264 nm; $E_{1\%,1\ cm}^{264\ nm} = 454.2$).

For each assay standard dilutions are prepared from the stock standard containing 300, 200, 150, 100, 50, 25, and 0 pg 25-OHD_3/50 µl ethanol respectively.

Dextran-coated charcoal (DCC) solution:

An amount of 6 g of Norit (e.g. Norit A) is suspended in 150 ml working buffer (I). Dissolve 0.6 g Dextran T70 in 50 ml working buffer. The dextran solution is slowly added, with stirring, to the charcoal suspension. This solution is stored at 4°C for not more than four weeks.

Before and during the addition of the DCC-solution to the assay tubes, the suspension should be thoroughly mixed using a magnetic stirrer.

(c) Apparatus

Microlitre pipettes, 0–50 µl, 50–200 µl, 200–1000 µl, e.g. Eppendorff, Finn repeating pipette

Repeating dispenser with 500 µl syringe; e.g. Hamilton

Liquid transfer system, e.g. Seripettor (Boehringer), 1–5 ml

Disposable borosilicate culture tubes, 12 × 75 and 13 × 100 mm

Pyrex culture tubes, 16 × 150 mm

Magnetic stirrer
(Multi-)Vortex-type mixer
'Baker' 10 Extraction System (Baker Chemicals)
Refrigerated centrifuge
Counting vials, e.g. 6 ml polypropylene minivials (Baker)
Liquid scintillation counter.

7.3.4   Sample Collection

Serum or plasma should be prepared by centrifugation of the blood samples. No significant difference between the 25-OHD concentrations in heparinized plasma, EDTA-containing plasma, or serum has been observed. Uncentrifuged blood can be kept at room temperature for as long as three days without a significant change in the 25-OHD content.

At −20°C, plasma or serum samples are stable for at least six months [43].

7.3.5   Procedure

(a) Sample extraction

An aliquot of 10 µl of the recovery tracer is added (using a repeating dispenser) to 50 µl serum or plasma in a Pyrex culture tube, followed by 0.5 ml distilled water, 1.25 ml dichloromethane, and 2.5 ml methanol respectively.

After mixing using a multivortex for two minutes, 1 ml water and 1.25 ml dichloromethane are added. After vortexing again for one minute the mixture is centrifuged for 15 min at 1 500 *g* and 4°C.

The bottom layer is transferred to a disposable glass tube (13 × 100 mm) and evaporated to dryness at 37°C under a stream of nitrogen gas. The residue is dissolved in 100 µl hexane/ether, 2:1 (v/v).

(b) Chromatography

The silica extraction columns are pretreated with 3 ml hexane/ether (2:1, v/v). The sample extract is quantitatively applied to the column by washing the tube twice with 100 µl hexane/ether (2:1).

The column is flushed with 3 ml hexane/ether (2:1) and subsequently with 5 ml diethylether to elute 25-OHD from the column.

The ether eluate is evaporated to dryness using nitrogen gas and the residue is dissolved in 500 µl ethanol.

(c) Recovery counting

To estimate the recovery of the added radioactive 25-OHD, a 100 µl aliquot of the extract is counted in 4 ml scintillation fluid. To measure the radioactivity of the recovery tracer added, 10 µl of the recovery tracer and 90 µl ethanol are transferred in duplicate into counting vials and subsequently counted.

(d) Competitive protein-binding assay

Aliquots of 50 µl standard (0–300 pg), control, and unknown samples are transferred in duplicate to appropriate test tubes. For estimation of the non-specific binding (NSB) the highest and lowest standard concentration, as well as two random sample extracts are transferred in duplicate into (extra) test tubes.

To all tubes 10 µl assay-tracer (60 pg) is added using the repeating dispenser.

For determination of the total radioactivity (total count) transfer in duplicate 10 µl assay-tracer solution and 50 µl ethanol to a counting vial.

With the exception of the NSB tubes, to all tubes 500 µl binder solution is

added. To the NSB tubes 500 µl working buffer II (buffer + 0.2% BSA) is
added.

After mixing vigorously using a multivortex all tubes are incubated overnight at
4°C.

Note 1.

An incubation period of at least one hour is sufficient, but overnight
incubation offers the possibility to split up the assay over two consecutive
days.

After incubation 200 µl of the dextran-coated charcoal suspension is added to
all tubes. After vigorously mixing on a multivortex all tubes are incubated for
30 min at 4°C.

Centrifuge all tubes at 1 500 g for 15 min at 4°C. Transfer 500 µl of the
supernatant to a counting vial; after addition of 4 ml scintillation liquid the
radioactivity is determined.

(e) Calculations

The radioactivity of the standard and sample tubes is corrected for the non-
specific binding by subtracting the NSB counts. The corrected counts are
then expressed in percentage binding relative to the maximal bound counts
($B/B_0 \times 100$; B_0 is the corrected counts for the '0'-standard). The percentages
of bound radioactivity ($B/B_0 \times 100$) calculated for the standards are plotted
against the 25-OHD concentration (or pg/tube). By reference to the standard
curve the concentration of 25-OHD in the serum and control samples can then
be calculated, allowing for the serum volume assayed and correcting for the
losses in the extraction and chromatography procedure. Transformation of the
standard data to fit straight standard curves, i.e. by plotting the logit of B/B_0
($=\log [B/B_0]/[1-B/B_0]$) against the log 25-OHD_3 concentration, is useful and
offers increased speed. Automated data calculation programs for simple hand-
held calculators up to sophisticated data processing packages to run on on-line
(personal) computer systems are now easily available at relatively low cost [44].

Calculation % recovery: Counts (c.p.m.) in aliquot $\times$ 5 $\times$ 100/total counts
(c.p.m.) recovery tracer added.

*(f) Variations and
modifications*

For chromatographic purification a variety of solvent systems are appropriate,
such as chloroform/methanol, hexane/isopropanol/ether and ethylacetate/
cyclohexane. Some authors have proposed the omission of the chromatographic
step. Although good correlation between chromatographic (direct) and non-
chromatographic assays has been reported, direct assays overestimate the
serum 25-OHD content by about 20%; this is due to the contribution of 24,25-
and 25,26-$(OH)_2D$ [45]. It seems that chromatography is essential to obtain
accurate results [46, 47]. Interlaboratory comparisons indicate lower specificity
and precision using direct assays [48, 49]. The non-specific interference in the
direct assay can be eliminated by using specific antibodies against 25-OHD and
preparing the standard curve in 25-OHD-free serum [45]. However, this
antibody is not routinely available.

Various chromatographic supports have been applied like Sephadex
LH-20 and silica gel. More recently the use of 'single-step solid phase'

systems has been described with Extrelut columns [50] or Sep-Pak C18 cartridges [51].

In principle, a variety of vitamin-D-binding protein (DBP) sources can be used (human (pregnancy) serum, rat kidney cytosol, rat serum, etc.). This protein from various species shows similar characteristics [40, 41]. The relative displacement potency of 25-OHD$_2$ and 25-OHD$_3$ is identical for mammalian DBP, while that for avian DBP is about 15-fold less for 25-OHD$_2$ [40, 48].

More recent commercial reagent kits for 25-OHD are available, e.g. from IRE-Medgenix (Belgium) and INC (Immuno Nuclear Corporation, Stillwater, Minnesota). Performance of these kits seems adequate, although a slight overestimation of serum 25-OHD content may occur due to omission of a chromatographic separation step from the kit protocol. Kits using only ethanol extraction without purification of the extract will give unreliable results.

In principle HPLC–UV can be used as an alternative for the CPB assay. As indicated sensitivity is limited, requiring sample volumes over 1 ml. Although valid results can be obtained, HPLC–UV methods are relatively laborious and expensive compared to the CPB assay [48].

7.3.6 Performance characteristics

(a) Range of linearity

Within the range of the standard curve good parallelism was established after serial sample dilution. Extracts of samples with concentrations outside the standard range should be appropriately diluted with ethanol.

(b) Detection limit

The detection limit (defined as the amount 25-OHD$_3$ giving 10% displacement of the tracer, i.e. a B/B$_0$ of 90%) amounts to 12 pg/tube, corresponding with a serum (plasma) concentration of about 2.4 ng/ml (6 nmol/l).

(c) Recovery

Mean tracer recovery: 89 ± 5% ($\bar{x}$ ± SE; N = 150). After addition of increasing amounts of 25-OHD$_3$ to serum (15–100 nmol/l were added) recovery rates between 93 and 103% ($\bar{x}$ ± SE: 95 ± 5%) were obtained.

(d) Reproducibility

In our laboratory the precision of the method is determined in each series by analysis of three aliquots of pooled human serum. The within-assay coefficient of variation (CV) is about 4–7%; between-assay CV 7–10% (average pool level: 24, 58, and 103 nmol/l serum respectively).

(e) Validity

The accuracy of both competitive protein binding assays and HPLC has been established (see also Variations and modifications, p. 207).

7.3.7 Reference values

Reference values are, in general, population specific. For example, the average 25-hydroxyvitamin D level for 207 healthy volunteers (blood donors from the centre of the Netherlands) with an average age of 37 ± 11.2 years (range 18–64 years) was 61 ± 27 nmol/l serum. The cumulative frequency distribution is given in Table 7.4.

An effect of age, gender, or oral contraceptive use was not observed [30]. In

Table 7.4 Cumulative frequency distribution of serum 25-hydroxyvitamin D (N = 207 volunteers)

Percentile	*25-OHD nmol/l*
Min	10.0
5	23.3
25	41.1
50	58.0
75	76.0
95	115.2
Max	180.0
Mean	61.1
SD	27.4

newborns and children during the first year of life, serum 25-OHD levels may vary considerably, but are generally lower compared with adults [52]. Serum or plasma 25-OHD concentrations during summer may be two or three times higher than those during winter [42]. For 115 apparently healthy Dutch free-living elderly people with an average age of 72 ± 3.8 years (range 65–89 years), the 25-OHD level (39 ± 16 nmol/l plasma) was significantly ($P < 0.001$) lower than that of the group of blood donors [31].

7.3.8 Interpretation

Serum or plasma 25-OHD levels below 12.5 nmol/l (5 ng/ml) are indicative for vitamin D deficiency and often associated with signs or symptoms of osteomalacia or rickets.

7.4 VITAMIN E (α-TOCOPHEROL)

7.4.1 Purpose and scope

In lymph and blood, α-tocopherol is bound to all lipoproteins, in particular the β-lipoprotein fraction. Its plasma levels are highly correlated with total lipids, β-lipoproteins, and cholesterol. Accordingly the ratio of plasma tocopherol to lipids can be considered a better index of vitamin E nutriture and a more reliable expression of adequacy than the value of tocopherol alone. Vitamin E is also transported into erythrocytes: their vitamin E concentration seems to reflect rapid changes in plasma levels of the vitamin. Tocopherol uptake and concentration in tissues vary proportionally to the logarithm of intake. Adrenal and pituitary glands, testes, platelets, and adipose tissue have the highest vitamin E concentration [53].

Vitamin E, as an essential antioxidant, can play an important role in the body's multilevel defence system against oxygen radicals. Epidemiological prospective studies show an inverse correlation between the α-tocopherol of plasma levels and lung, breast, and gastrointestinal cancer prevalences. Of course the other essential antioxidants like vitamin A, carotene, vitamin C, and selenium, are also involved in this preventive effect [54] and their antioxidant properties are synergistic with vitamin E.

Vitamin E may also reduce the activation of various carcinogens to epoxides, inhibit the formation of nitrosamines, and enhance both the humoral and cellular (lymphocytic and leukocytic) immune response [53].

It has also been shown that vitamin E is potentially beneficial for coronary heart disease. The vitamin E concentration within lipoproteins (α-tocopherol: cholesterol ratio) shows the most prominent inverse correlation with CHD mortality. The possible antiaggregant effect of vitamin E has been attributed to an influence of arachidonic acid on the metabolic pathway [55].

There is no homeostatic mechanism for vitamin E and in the low intake range a correlation between intake and plasma level has been observed. But this is not the case with a very high intake. Unfortunately neither can a plasma level corresponding to adequate vitamin E intake be defined [5].

Among the methods of nutriture assessment of this vitamin the most commonly used are plasma or serum tocopherol level determination. An analysis of red blood cells content in vitamin E and a hydrogen peroxide haemolysis test have no advantage over the plasma or serum tocopherol level assays and are more difficult to execute. Platelet tocopherol determination has also been suggested, but its usefulness in man has not been satisfactorily verified. The recent analysis of adipose tissue biopsy may offer a good index of long-term vitamin E intake assessment because of the very slow turnover of α-tocopherol in adipose tissue [53].

The method described here is only for plasma α-tocopherol, which is the most representative carotene in plasma; α-tocotrienol, if present, can be separated from α-tocopherol [36].

7.4.2 Principle of the method

α-Tocopherol is first freed from lipoproteins by addition of ethanol to diluted plasma and then extracted with n-hexane. The extract is separated by straight-phase HPLC on a silica gel column. The detection is carried out at an adequate wavelength.

7.4.3 Chemicals and apparatus

(a) Chemicals

Ethanol (C_2H_5OH) p.a.
n-Hexane (C_6H_{14}) p.a.
Ethylacetate ($C_4H_8O_2$) p.a.
α-Tocopherol, e.g. Fluka 99% (UV), cat. No. 89550.

(b) Solutions

HPLC mobile phase: n-hexane/ethyl acetate (1000:75).
α-Tocopherol standard solutions for HPLC:
  Stock standard: 50 mg α-tocopherol are dissolved in n-hexane to make 100 ml.
  Standard dilution (5 mg/dl): 10 ml stock standard made up to 100 ml with n-hexane.
  Working standard (1 mg/dl): 10 ml of standard made up to 50 ml with n-hexane.

The solutions are not stable and should be prepared immediately before use.

The working standard is checked photometrically at 292–294 nm (maximum absorbance) in a 10 mm quartz cuvette. The absorbance should be 0.085.

(c) Apparatus

Glass tubes (4 ml capacity, 7 × 100 mm) for shaking and centrifugation; adjustable pipettes; Vortex; microlab dispenser; mechanical shaker.

HPLC apparatus consisting of:

Merck Hibar prepared column 250–4 mm filled with LiChrosorb Si 60, 5 μm

Altex Model 110 A pump with pulse suppressor and manometer WIKA 0–250 bar

Automatic injector, e.g. Waters WISP 710 A with BCD board for signal receptor from the integrator

Perkin Elmer Fluorescence Spectrophotometer Type 650–10 LC (290/330 nm)

W + W Recorder Model 314 (single-channel)

Integrator, e.g. Spectra-physics, Model 4270.

7.4.4 Sample collection

Blood is collected by vein puncture into heparin-lined vacutainer tubes.

7.4.5 Procedure

(a) Sample preparation and extraction

The heparinated whole blood is centrifuged at low speed for plasma separation. Plasma can be stored frozen (–20°C) for several months (α-tocopherol content in frozen plasma was practically the same after two years).

The deep-frozen plasma is thawed and mixed to disperse possible precipitates; 200 μl of plasma is pipetted in a 4 ml centrifuge tube and diluted with 200 μl of water.

While shaking on a Vortex-shaker, 400 μl of ethanol are added and the tube shaken for 10 seconds; 800 μl of n-hexane are added from a microlab dispenser.

The tube is sealed with a polyethylene stopper, shaken for five minutes on a mechanical shaker and centrifuged at 2000 *g* for five minutes.

From the hexane phase an appropriate aliquot is transferred into sample conical vials (5 × 40 mm) protected from light (e.g. brown glass or wrapped with black paper).

(b) Calibration

Freshly prepared reference solutions of α-tocopherol suitably diluted in n-hexane and partitioned between aqueous ethanol and hexane as for plasma samples, are used as external standards. It is assumed that the distribution between the two phases is the same irrespective of the presence of plasma or water.

Calibration is repeated when one-sided drifts of the values for the control plasma exceeding 3% of the mean are found.

Human and bovine control plasma are pooled to give an α-tocopherol level between 12.8 and 23.2 μmol/l.

Aliquot volumes in excess of 750 μl are transferred to plastic vials and frozen at –80°C until required for analysis.

An extract of control plasma, usually 3 ml hexane corresponding to 750 μl plasma, is distributed into micro-injection vials which are kept at −20°C. These controls are inserted in the 1st, 24th and 48th positions of the sampler rings. They are prepared fresh daily.

(c) HPLC

The entire chromatographic procedure is carried out at room temperature. One hundred microlitres of sample extract is subjected to isocratic straight-phase HPLC. The flow rate of the mobile phase is about 1.7 ml/min (working pressure 8.0 MPa). Retention time is about 3.5 min. Should this retention time change, the flow rate is modified accordingly.

The effluent of HPLC column is passed through the fluorimeter set at excitation 298 nm, emission 328 nm. With other fluorimeters the optimal excitation and emission wavelength have yet to be found. In this set-up the recorder tracing is often used for control purposes. The peak integration is done by an integrator that prints the results according to the calibration parameters programmed.

Note 2.
The other tocopherols are outside the recorder diagram of α-tocopherol. Interfering carotenoids can be eliminated by chromatography through a column of floridin earth as with the former photometric assay [56], which would not separate the tocopherols.

(d) Calculation

The resulting peak area calculated by the integrator is compared to the corresponding peak area of the standard solution which has been treated exactly as the plasma sample (external calibration).

7.4.6 Performance characteristics

(a) Range of linearity

This is 0.25 − 140 μmol/l.

(b) Detection limit

The practical detection limit without changing the operating conditions is 0.2 μmol/l.

(c) Reproducibility

The coefficient of variation of duplicate assays for plasma is 1.8% (N=109; range 4.6–41.8 μmol/l), for whole blood 3.1 (N=6, $\bar{x}$=28.1 μmol/l). When blood is collected from the same individual at six days time-lag between collections, the coefficient of variation was 10.5% (N=6, $\bar{x}$=28.1 μmol/l).

(d) Validity

Comparison of the α-tocopherol assay by HPLC (assay x) with the former manual method (assay y) [56] gave a correlation coefficient of 0.997 and a linear regression equation y = 0.07 + 0.98x (N=109), in μmol/l.

7.4.7 Reference values

The reference values are, in general, population specific. For example the average α-tocopherol level of 150 adult blood donors of both sexes from Basel (Red Cross Centre) was 29.3 μmol/l (men = 30.4 μmol/l, women = 28.1 μmol/l) [36]. The cumulative frequency distribution is given in Table 7.5.

Table 7.5 Cumulative frequency distribution of plasma α-tocopherol (N = 150 blood donors)

Percentile	α-tocopherol μmol/l
Min	17.6
5	20.0
25	24.4
50	28.1
75	33.2
95	43.1
Max	52.2
Mean	29.3
SD	6.7

7.4.8 Interpretation

Without additional information no interpretation of the plasma levels of α-tocopherol seems possible. Several authors, for instance Horwitt *et al.* [57], Brubacher *et al.* [58], or Lehmann [59] have questioned the usefulness of these figures as an indicator of vitamin E status, because strong correlations exist between plasma lipid variables like cholesterol, triglycerides, β-lipoproteins, etc., and plasma tocopherol. Brubacher *et al.* [58] have found a relatively high correlation between plasma-β-lipoproteins and α-tocopherol level. This correlation can be confirmed by comparison of a set of assays with the corresponding β-lipoprotein values (Table 7.6).

Table 7.6 Correlation between α-tocopherol and β-lipoproteins

Subjects	N	Correlation coefficient r	Linear regression
Male donors	75	0.790	y = 2.935 + 0.525 x
Female donors	75	0.752	y = 1.203 + 0.523 x
Total	150	0.777	y = 1.442 + 0.545 x

y = g β-LP/l plasma
x = μmol α-tocopherol/l plasma

These correlations and the fact that in a-β-lipoproteinaemia the plasma level of vitamin E is decreased to below the sensitivity limit of the assay, allows the interpretation that the β-lipoproteins behave like α-tocopherol carriers. The load of α-tocopherol on the carrier protein may be expressed by the ratio of milligrams α-tocopherol per litre to grams β-lipoproteins per litre plasma.

It is obvious that an insufficient intake of vitamin E will be reflected in a lower than average ratio of α-tocopherol to β-lipoproteins.

In epidemiological studies on coronary heart disease (CHD) the α-tocopherol: cholesterol ratio [55] expressed in μmol/mmol is now preferred. In a 12-population study [55] this ratio showed the highest correlation with CHD. This highly significant correlation seems to be independent of the risk of CHD mortality attributable to hypercholesterolaemia.

Some pathologies such as chronic enteropathies conditioning malabsorption, haemolytic anaemia, protein–energy malnutrition, prematurity, spontaneous myopathies, or cholestatic liver disease with neurological complications can influence the vitamin E nutritional status.

The toxic or negative effect of different drugs (oral contraceptives, anthracyclines, aspirin, acetaminophen), and heavy metals can also be considered confounding variables [53].

7.5   VITAMIN K$_1$

SECTION I   PHYLLOQUINONE (VITAMIN K$_1$) IN SERUM OR PLASMA BY HPLC

7.5.1   Purpose and scope

Until recently vitamin K status could only be defined in terms of the specific lowering in plasma of the four vitamin K-dependent clotting factors (II, VII, IX and X) and detected by coagulation assays which measure their procoagulant activity in plasma. Some coagulation assays (e.g. prothrombin time) reflect the combined deficiency of the vitamin K-dependent factors whereas others measure the functional activity of individual factors. Such assays of procoagulant activity have two disadvantages. First they lack sensitivity so that only an overt deficiency state is detected. Secondly they lack selectivity and cannot by themselves distinguish between a nutritional deficiency and certain acquired deficiency states such as those produced by various antagonists (e.g. coumarin drugs) of vitamin K. In the newborn the problem of interpretation of coagulation assays is compounded by the 'physiological hypoprothrombinaemia' which is a feature of normal neonatal haemostasis.

The introduction of immunoassays for the abnormal des γ-carboxy forms of prothrombin, secreted into the plasma when the supply or metabolism of vitamin K is impaired, offer a more sensitive method of detecting vitamin K deficiency but their specificity is again uncertain even in the absence of known antagonists. Also because des γ-carboxy prothrombin may circulate in plasma for some time after correcting vitamin K deficiency, its detection may reflect a past rather than an existing deficiency. As with other fat-soluble vitamins the measurement of plasma levels of vitamin K offers a potentially more direct method of assessing vitamin K status but this has been hampered by analytical problems associated with the measurement of low plasma concentrations of a wide range of molecular forms.

Despite these problems, assays based on high-performance liquid chromatography are now becoming routine though as yet only for phylloquinone (vitamin K$_1$), the predominant dietary source of the vitamin. Several problems remain: there is as yet only limited information on plasma levels, particularly for large population groups, and the normal ranges obtained by different laboratories are still quite variable (probably due to methodological differences).

Nevertheless there is encouraging evidence that plasma levels of phylloquinone do reflect the status of vitamin K and that the finding of subnormal plasma levels is a useful diagnostic indicator for subclinical vitamin K deficiency that may not be apparent from clotting indices [60, 61].

A variety of HPLC methods for phylloquinone now exist. Original methods based on UV detection have been largely abandoned and most laboratories employ either electrochemical or fluorometric detection which can detect as little as 25 pg of phylloquinone. The method described here is based on dual-electrode electrochemical detection in the redox mode using a 'coulometric' detector.

7.5.2 Principle of the method

Phylloquinone in plasma is associated with lipoproteins. The vitamer is extracted with hexane after flocculation of proteins with ethanol. This hexane extract is subjected to an intensive multi-stage purification procedure to remove interfering lipids before final analysis by reversed-phase HPLC and electrochemical detection (HPLC–EC). The electrochemical detector has a 'coulometric' design using a cell with two porous graphite electrodes arranged in series. The principle of the detection method is to reduce the quinone moiety of phylloquinone at the upstream (generator) electrode and to detect the electrolysis current generated by the oxidation of the hydroquinone product at the downstream (detector) electrode. Quantitation is based on the method of peak height ratios after the addition to the sample of another K vitamin (menaquinone-6) as an internal standard.

7.5.3 Chemicals and apparatus

(a) Chemicals

Phylloquinone (2-methyl-3-phytyl-1,4-naphthoquinone), e.g. Sigma, cat. No. V3501

Menaquinone-6 (2-methyl-3-farnesyl-farnesyl-1,4-naphthoquinone), e.g. Hoffmann–La Roche

Hexane (C_6H_{14}) HPLC grade

Dichloromethane (CH_2Cl_2) HPLC grade

Methanol (CH_3OH) HPLC grade

Diethylether ($C_4H_{10}O$) (peroxide free), p.a.

Ethanol (C_2H_5OH) AR grade

Glacial acetic acid ($C_2H_4O_2$) AR grade

Sodium acetate, anhydrous ($C_2H_3NaO_2$) AR grade

Ethylenediaminetetra-acetic acid (EDTA) AR grade

Nitric acid (HNO_3) AR grade

Nitrogen gas (oxygen free) for evaporating solvents from samples

Helium gas for degassing the mobile phase for reversed-phase HPLC–EC (not always necessary)

HPLC grade water.

(b) Solutions

Semi-preparative HPLC mobile phase: 3–6% (v/v) of 50% water-saturated dichloromethane in hexane.

Analytical HPLC mobile phase: 3–5% (v/v) of 0.05 M acetate buffer (pH 3.0) in methanol and containing EDTA at a final concentration of 0.1 mmol/l.

Standard solutions of phylloquinone and menaquinone-6 for chromatographic calibration:

Stock standards: prepared in ethanol at concentrations of about 5×10^{-2} mmol/l and stored at –20°C. The concentrations are determined accurately by UV absorption spectroscopy (EmM at 248 nm = 18.9 for both phylloquinone and menaquinone-6).

Working standards: accurately prepared 100-fold dilutions of each calibration stock standard in ethanol (5×10^{-4} mmol/l) of phylloquinone and menaquinone-6 respectively. These are stable indefinitely at $-20°C$.

From these individual working standards a series of analyte/internal standard mixtures are prepared in ethanol for chromatographic injection and calibration of the final analytical HPLC stage: these contain a known weight ratio of phylloquinone to the internal standard of menaquinone-6, (range 0.1–4.0) and a final concentration of menaquinone-6 of about 10^{-4} mmol/l. 10–20 µl of these solutions are directly injected into the chromatograph.

The working internal standard solution of menaquinone-6 in ethanol (for addition to the plasma sample) is prepared by accurate dilution of the working calibration solution of menaquinone-6 (5×10^{-4} mmol/l) and has a typical concentration of 5×10^{-6} mmol/l.

Solutions for the mobile phase for HPLC–EC:

5 M Acetate buffer (pH 3.0): 5 M glacial acetic acid (30.03 g $C_2H_4O_2$ dissolved in water to make 100 ml) is adjusted to pH 3.0 with 5 M sodium acetate (41.02 g $C_2H_3NaO_2$ dissolved in warm water to make 100 ml). 5 M stock solutions are stored at 4°C.

0.1 M Ethylenediaminetetra-acetic acid: 37.2 g EDTA made up to 100 ml with water and stored at 4°C.

6 M nitric acid: 417 ml made up to 1000 ml with water.

(c) Apparatus

Usual basic laboratory equipment.

Water bath and gas-manifold arrangement in fume cupboard to hold tubes for evaporation of solvents under a stream of nitrogen at 50°C.

Equipment for HPLC. Two dedicated systems are recommended for the semi-preparative and analytical stages respectively.

The semi-preparative stage requires a standard reciprocating pump and a UV photometer.

The analytical stage requires a high-quality pump (to minimize the noise associated with electrochemical detection and pulsations in solvent delivery) and is designed for a specific detector (model 5100 A Coulochem from Environmental Sciences Associates) equipped with a model 5011 dual electrode analytical cell. The mobile phase for electrochemical detection is recycled and if necessary degassed with helium.

Each system requires a syringe-loading injection valve, e.g. Rheodyne model 7125 and a chart recorder or integrator.

Sep-Pak silica cartridges (Waters Associates).

Semi-preparative HPLC column: Spherisorb-5-nitrile, particle size 5 µm (Phase Separations), dimensions 250 × 5 mm (i.d.).

Analytical HPLC column: Spherisorb octyl, particle size 5 µm (Phase Separations), dimensions 250 × 5 mm (i.d.).

7.5.4 Sample collection

Venous blood samples (preferably taken after an overnight fast to avoid influence of recent dietary intake) are collected into plain tubes (serum) or tubes containing EDTA or heparin (plasma). The sample should be shielded from strong light. At $-20°C$ serum or plasma samples are stable for at least one year.

7.5.5   Procedure

(a) Hexane extraction

One to two millilitres of serum or plasma is pipetted into a glass, stoppered centrifuge tube and 2 volumes of ethanol including an appropriate volume (typically 0.5 ml) of the menaquinone-6 internal standard solution added. After brief vortex mixing to flocculate proteins, 4 volumes of hexane are added and the contents mixed vigorously by alternate handshaking and vortex mixing for five minutes. The mixture is then centrifuged at $1500\,g$ for 10 minutes to separate an upper hexane layer (containing vitamin K and other lipids) from a lower aqueous–ethanolic layer and precipitated proteins. Finally the upper hexane layer is transferred with a Pasteur pipette to a glass-stoppered tube and the hexane extract evaporated to dryness under a stream of nitrogen at 50°C.

(b) Sorbent extraction

The lipid extract is dissolved in 2 ml of hexane and introduced into a 10 ml glass syringe that has a Luer end fitting. A Sep-Pak silica cartridge is then attached to the Luer nozzle and the hexane solution pushed through to load the extract at the head of the cartridge. The tube originally containing the lipid extract is rinsed with a further 2 ml of hexane and this pushed through the cartridge in the same way. After loading the lipid extract, the cartridge is eluted with successive volumes of 10 ml of hexane (eluate discarded) and 10 ml of 3% (v/v) diethylether in hexane. The latter eluate (containing phylloquinone and the internal standard) is collected into a glass-stoppered tube and evaporated to dryness under nitrogen.

(c) Semi-preparative HPLC

The mobile-phase composition is adjusted until the retention of a standard solution containing phylloquinone and menaquinone-6 is constant with the retention of phylloquinone in the range of 8–10 minutes. The internal standard, menaquinone-6 elutes after phylloquinone in this normal phase system [62]. After equilibration and before injecting the samples the valve injector is washed thoroughly with mobile phase and a solvent blank injected to ensure that no standard is carried over with succeeding sample injections. To inject the sample, the vitamin K fraction isolated by sorbent extraction is dissolved in 70 µl of mobile phase and the total volume injected into the column. The eluate fraction that encloses phylloquinone and the internal standard is collected into a glass-stoppered, tapered tube and evaporated to dryness under nitrogen.

Flow rate: 1 ml/min.

Detection: UV absorbance detector, wavelength 254 or 270 nm.

As precautions for this technique, great care needs to be taken to avoid cross-contamination of samples (from syringes or injection valve) with the standard solution used to determine the retention time of phylloquinone and menaquinone-6.

Since the collection of the eluate from sample injections is carried out 'blind' (the amounts of phylloquinone and internal standard are too low for detection at this stage) care should also be taken to ensure complete collection of both components. Sufficient allowance is normally obtained by starting the eluate collection one minute (i.e. 1 ml) before the leading edge of the phylloquinone peak and one minute after the trailing edge of the menaquinone-6 peak.

(d) Analytical HPLC

The mobile-phase composition is adjusted until the retention of phylloquinone and menaquinone-6 are about 8 and 10 minutes respectively. On each day of analysis the chromatograph needs to be run under operating conditions until the initial baseline drift has stabilized and the sensitivity is maximal. This normally takes 0.5–1 hour. During this time the sensitivity is checked periodically by injecting a phylloquinone standard. After equilibration the column is calibrated by injecting 10–20 μl of the working calibration standards and recording the chromatograms. The samples (i.e. the fractions from the semi-preparative HPLC stage) are then dissolved in ethanol (50–70 μl) with brief warming (50°C) and vortex mixing to ensure complete solution of the lipids. A suitable volume (typically 20 μl) is then injected onto the column and the chromatogram recorded.

Flow rate: 1 ml/min.

Detection: Series dual-electrode electrochemical detection with the upstream electrode set at –1.3 V and the downstream electrode set at 0 V or +0.05 V.

As precautions for this technique, the applied potentials should be designed to give maximum selectivity rather than maximum sensitivity. If changes in the electrode response cause a shift in the hydrodynamic voltammogram, some adjustments to the potentials may be necessary [63, 64]. To minimize the background current several precautions are necessary. Firstly only reagents (including water) of the highest chemical purity should be used for the mobile phase. Secondly the HPLC pump and stainless steel fittings in contact with the mobile phase should be passivated with 6 M nitric acid before use. The addition of 0.1 mM EDTA to the mobile phase further improves the stability and delays electrode passivation, presumably by preventing the reaction and deposition of metal ions at the electrode surface. The column packing material should preferably be packed into a pre-passivated empty column and new columns washed thoroughly with the mobile phase before attaching to the system. In the long term, high stability and low background currents are best achieved by recycling the mobile phase. Helium degassing of the mobile phase has been found to greatly improve the sensitivity of some ageing cells but not of others. Extreme loss of sensitivity due to electrode passivation may be restored by a cell washing procedure [63, 64].

(e) Calculation

To quantify the plasma concentration of phylloquinone, the peak heights of phylloquinone and menaquinone-6 given by standards and samples are first measured and the peak height ratios (PHR) of phylloquinone to menaquinone-6 calculated. A linear calibration graph may then be obtained (using regression analysis) which relates the PHRs of the standards against their known weight ratios. From this data the PHR given by the sample may be converted to an equivalent weight ratio. Multiplication of this weight ratio by the amount of internal standard originally added gives the amount of phylloquinone in the volume of plasma extracted.

7.5.6 Performance characteristics

(a) Range of linearity

To detect endogenous plasma concentrations of phylloquinone the detector is set to maximum sensitivity (gain setting 9900) giving a full-scale recorder deflection of 10 nA. The calibration graphs are entirely linear over this range. Keeping the injection volume constant (20 µl or less) the linearity range for peak height measurements extends at least fivefold beyond this normal working range.

(b) Detection limit

Although the detection sensitivity and baseline noise was subject to day-to-day variation, the minimum limit of detection generally ranged from 10 to 20 pg (20–40 fmol) based on a signal-to-noise ratio of 3. When extracting 2 ml of plasma and injecting 20 µl from 50 µl at the final analytical HPLC stage, the detection limit was within the range 20–40 pg/ml (44–89 pmol/l).

(c) Recovery

The relative recovery may be assessed by adding known amounts of phylloquinone (in ethanolic solution) to plasma; amounts ranging from 0.1 to 5.0 ng (0.2–11.1 pmol) are added to 1–2 ml of plasma and the samples analysed according to the described procedure. After allowing for the endogenous amount of phylloquinone in the plasma sample (measured separately) the added amounts were found to be accurately measured by the procedure.

Owing to the multi-stage design of the assay the absolute recovery of the phylloquinone (determined by external standardization) was found to vary considerably, but averaged about 70%.

(d) Reproducibility

The precision of the method was evaluated by determining both within-run and between-run coefficients of variation. The within-run precision estimated [65] by running 37 routine unknowns (mean concentration 0.7 ng/ml or 1.3 nmol/l) in duplicate was 12.4%. The between-run coefficients of variation for replicate analyses of two plasma pools over a six-month period were 11.5% (N = 37) and 17.9% (N = 30) at concentrations of 1.1 ng/ml (2.4 nmol/l) and 0.3 ng/ml (0.7 nmol/l) respectively.

(e) Validity

The validity of the assay should be first assessed from recovery experiments as described in section 7.5.6(c). The peak purity of phylloquinone may be assessed by comparing the hydrodynamic voltammograms of sample and standard chromatographic peaks [63]; it would be necessary to extract a larger volume of plasma to do such experiments. In our laboratory further evidence of validity is the comparability of plasma values by this method with a previously developed UV detection method [64].

7.5.7   Reference values

Plasma assays of phylloquinone have only recently become available and there are as yet relatively few controlled studies of healthy population groups. For this reason each laboratory needs to establish its own reference range. In our laboratory values obtained to date [61] yielded a range in 45 fasting adult individuals subjects of 0.17–0.68 ng/ml (0.38–1.51 nmol/l) with a median of 0.37 ng/ml (0.82 nmol/l). In 22 non-fasting individuals the values tended to be slightly higher, ranging from 0.15 to 1.55 ng/ml (0.33–3.44 nmol/l) with a median of 0.53 ng/ml (1.18 nmol/l). By the same method but extracting larger volumes, values in cord plasma from healthy newborns were very low, ranging from 4 to 45 pg/ml (9–100 pmol/l) with a median of 16 pg/ml (36 pmol/l).

7.5.8 Interpretation

Although the internal standard menaquinone-6 is a naturally occurring K vitamin of the K_2 series, analyses without its addition showed that menaquinone-6 was undetectable in normal subjects when 1–2 ml of plasma was extracted. Although a small peak of menaquinone-6 has been occasionally detected in patients with hyperlipidaemia, such patients also have grossly raised levels of phylloquinone [61] and the height of the menaquinone-6 peak was less than one-tenth that of phylloquinone. Therefore, provided sufficient internal standard is initially added to maintain an ideal PHR of around unity, any error in the measurement of phylloquinone introduced by the presence of such small amounts of endogenous menaquinone-6 is in practice negligible.

Although the relationship of plasma concentrations of vitamin K_1 to total tissue stores (i.e. including menaquinones) has not yet been established, evidence to date does suggest that low plasma levels reflect a reduced vitamin K status. Substantially reduced plasma levels have been detected in patients with a reduced vitamin K_1 intake (malnourishment or parenteral feeding), and impaired absorption (chronic gastrointestinal disease) or impaired plasma transport (abetalipoproteinaemia). An association has been shown between low plasma levels and susceptibility to antibiotic-induced hypoprothrombinaemia. Low values have also been found in osteoporotic patients. An extremely low normal range (4–45 pg/ml) is a physiological feature in newborn babies and may account for their increased susceptibility to vitamin K deficiency.

Apart from the diagnosis of hypovitaminosis K from low plasma levels, the finding of normal values may usefully differentiate a nutritional deficiency from a mild congenital deficiency of the vitamin-K-dependent factors or an acquired deficiency produced by antagonists to vitamin K. Elevated plasma levels of vitamin K_1 may be seen in hyperlipoproteinaemia, particularly in hypertriglyceridaemia.

SECTION II TRANS-VITAMIN K_1 (PHYLLOQUINONE) IN SERUM BY HPLC-MICROMETHOD

7.5.9 Purpose and scope

The recognized primary function of trans-vitamin K_1 and presumably of menaquinones in man is the mediation of gamma-carboxylation of glutamic acid residues from calcium- and phospholipid-binding proteins, which are the precursors of coagulation factors II, VII, IX, X, anti-coagulation and fibrinolysis-promoting factors C and S, osteocalcin of bone and dentine, and atherocalcin among others [66–70]. Carboxylation of glutamic acid residues is coupled to the proposed cycling of vitamin K_1 through the 2,3-epoxide and hydroquinone forms of the vitamin. The total body pool of vitamin K_1 in the human adult is about 100 µg and comprises almost completely the hepatic pool [67]. However, depletion of vitamin K_1 occurs within 72 h after termination of oral intake and after beginning broad-spectrum antibiotic therapy. The assumption of there being no appreciable storage pool means therefore that man is dependent on a continuous dietary supply of vitamin K_1. Although menaquinones synthesized in the gut are hardly found in adult serum or cord blood plasma [71, 72], but constitute a major part of the hepatic storage pool [73], they may still add nothing to the total vitamin K activity. Menaquinones are apparently not sufficiently utilized to prevent various signs of vitamin K deficiency in subjects with insufficient dietary intake of vitamin K_1 [60]. In contrast, the maternal plasma as well as the placenta contain considerable amounts of menaquinone-4 [72]. Since the placenta also contains very high concentrations of calcium, it was suggested [72] that vitamin K is involved within the placenta in regulating bone formation in the fetus. If too much calcium accumulates in fetal bones, head-moulding and overlapping of cranial bones may occur, making delivery more difficult.

With the exception of the neonate the diet content of vitamin K_1 barely influences its level in the serum [71], contrary to vitamin K_1 epoxide levels.

Effects of high vitamin K_1 intake on haematological parameters do show a lag-time which becomes maximal after three consecutive days ingestion of vitamin-K_1-enriched foods.

As regards newborns, the levels of vitamin-K-dependent clotting factors are low compared to those of their mothers and adults in general, so placing the newborn at haemorrhagic risk. When bleeding occurs the newborn responds to supplementation of vitamin K, but coagulation factors do not change significantly [74]. However, when bleeding occurs it is usually common practice to give a supplement of both vitamin K_1 and fresh-frozen plasma, the latter containing the necessary clotting factors.

It seems an anachronism that newborns are either vitamin-K-deficient or in precarious vitamin K balance at birth.

There are several methods of determining vitamin K in serum or plasma (for reviews, see [62, 75, 76]). Comparison of physiological levels [75] reveals that the methods for vitamin K_1 quantification currently available give results in the same range. The most often used is an HPLC method applying electrochemical reduction in combination with fluorometry. Problems of matrix incompatibility with chromatographic systems have been solved [75, 77, 78], and in several clinical diagnostic centres the reduction-fluorometry approach has been followed with success. Because of limited amounts of biological material available a micromethod should be used. A specific example for the analysis of vitamin K_1 in 1000 µl serum samples, using HPLC, is described below [77].

7.5.10 Principle of the method

After wetting and precipitating serum (lipo-)proteins by methanol, vitamin K_1 is extracted by methylene chloride in a monophasic design. Following clean-up on a C 18 cartridge, fractionation occurs on a straight-phase HPLC column with UV monitoring. The selected fraction, containing trans-vitamin K_1 is separated on a reversed-phase column and trans-vitamin K_1 detected fluorometrically after post-column electrochemical reduction. Quantification occurs from peak height by integration using standard addition and internal standard correction for losses.

7.5.11 Chemicals and apparatus

(a) Chemicals

Acetonitrile (C_2H_3N) p. Chr., e.g. Merck, cat. No. 30
n-Hexane (C_6H_{14}) p.a., e.g. Merck, cat. No. 4367
Methylene chloride (CH_2Cl_2) p. Chr., e.g. Merck, cat. No. 6044
Methanol (100%) (CH_3OH) p. His., e.g. Baker, cat. No. 8047

Ethanol (100%) (C_2H_5OH) p.a., e.g. Merck, cat. No. 983

1,4-Dioxane ($C_4H_8O_2$) p. Chr., e.g. BDH, cat. No. 15224

Sodium chloride (NaCl) p.a., e.g. Baker, cat. No. 0278

Sodium perchlorate ($NaClO_4 . H_2O$) p.a., e.g. Merck, cat. No. 6564

Vitamin K_2, menaquinone-30, kindly donated by Hoffmann–La Roche

Trans-vitamin K_1 (impure, 2-methyl-3-phytyl-1,4-naphthoquinone), e.g. Sigma, cat. No. V3501

Water: deionized and quartz-bidistilled every 2–3 days

Cartridges: Sep-Pack C 18, e.g. Millipore–Waters, cat. No. 51910

LiChrosorb Si 60, 5 μm, e.g. Merck, cat. No. 9388

Hypersil C 8, 5 μm (spherical), e.g. Shandon, cat. No. 58005020.

(b) Solutions

0.9% (w/v) NaCl: 9 g NaCl are dissolved in water to make 1000 ml.

HPLC straight-phase eluent consisting of n-hexane:1,4-dioxane = 99.75:0.25.

HPLC reversed-phase eluent consisting of methanol:water = 100:0.5, to which 0.42% (w/v) sodium perchlorate is added.

Standard solutions of vitamin K_1:

Vitamin K_1 stock standard: about 45 mg of the vitamin K_1 standard are dissolved in 100 ml 100% methanol in a calibrated brownish glass receiver. The concentration of vitamin K_1 (cis and trans isomers) in this solution is calculated from the absorption of a 100-fold dilution in methanol at 248 nm in a suitable spectrophotometer using the molar absorption coefficient 19 900 (molecular weight of trans-phylloquinone = 450.7).

The presence of cis-vitamin K_1 was corrected by equiretention chromatography of both geometric isomers.

Working standard is prepared by diluting the stock standard with methanol to a concentration of 100 nmol/l. This solution and the stock standard solution are stored in the dark at −20°C and are stable for at least twelve months.

Standard solutions of menaquinone-30:

Stock internal standard: about 45 mg of the menaquinone are dissolved in 10 ml 100% methanol and handled as the vitamin K_1 standard.

Working standard is prepared by diluting the stock standard with methanol to a concentration of 100 μmol/l. This solution and the stock standard are stored in the dark at −20°C and are stable for at least twelve months.

(c) Apparatus

Dark room under dim red light maintained at 20°C.

Vacuum tubes, e.g. Vacutainer, Becton–Dickinson, red top 6490, for blood collection; blackened or non-transparent disposable overtubes for light-protected sample transportation.

Glass tubes, e.g. 100 × 16 mm o.d., suitable for centrifugation; polyethylene stoppers with double rims; calibrated glass and adjustable (micro-)pipettes; dispenser, e.g. Seripettors from Boehringer (adapted with Luer unions for cartridge elution); Vortex; calibrated glass receivers.

Heating block maintained at 40°C; nitrogen-evaporation assembly.

Refrigerated laboratory centrifuge; spectrophotometer, 1-cm quartz cuvettes.

Calibrated syringes for HPLC injection and sample handling, e.g. Kloehn, with Teflon Luer hub and suited for Valco-type injection needle, e.g. Kloehn.

HPLC apparatus consisting of:

Home-made stainless steel column, nitric acid washed, 250×4.6 mm i.d., packed upwards with LiChrosorb Si 60, 5 μm. Retention volume of an unretained solute was determined using benzene, eluting with methanol, which is also the packing solvent

Home-made stainless steel column, nitric acid washed, 200×4.6 mm i.d., packed upwards with Hypersil C 8, 5 μm, using acetone as a packing solvent

Two constant-flow pumps (or one with eluent switchover, using isopropanol as the intermediate eluent)

Injection valve(s) with fixed 250 μl loop, e.g. Valco, type C6W, or automatic injector

Variable-wavelength UV detector, e.g. Applied Biosystems, model Spectroflow 773 or 757, provided with prefixed light source and operating-hours indicator (wavelength 248 nm, sensitivity range 0.005, filter rise time 2 seconds)

Spectrofluorometer, e.g. Perkin–Elmer, model LS-4, with a xenon-arc source (excitation wavelength 330 nm, emission wavelength 435 nm, slit widths 15 and 20 nm respectively, attenuation 5)

Any other device should show a signal-to-noise ratio for the Raman band of pure water of at least 50 (excitation 350 nm, emission 395 nm, both slits 5 nm)

Electrochemical detector, e.g. ESA–Coulochem, model 5100, provided with dual-cell reaction model 5010 (–0.9 V, gain 1×1, both), preceded by both a 0.5 μm filter and the common graphite filter unit

Inert gas blanketing device for degassing the reversed-phase eluent

Recorder

Integrator.

Glassware, thoroughly cleaned and used solely for vitamin K₁ analysis.

7.5.12 Sample collection

All procedures during sample treatment are carried out under dim red light conditions in a dark room maintained at 20°C. Whole blood samples, collected in vacuum tubes can be stored in the refrigerator at 4°C for a couple of days without appreciable loss of vitamin K₁, provided the tube is placed in a non-transparent overtube and kept closed during storage. Serum is separated by centrifugation for 10 min at 2000 g and 4°C. Serum samples can be stored at room temperature up to six days or in a refrigerator (preferably at –20°C) up to eight months, without appreciable loss of vitamin K₁, if protected from sunlight and fluorescent light.

7.5.13 Procedure

(a) Sample extraction

1000 μl of well-mixed serum is transferred into a 100×16 mm o.d. glass tube, containing 100 μl 100 μmol/l working internal standard menaquinone-30.

Tubes receiving samples to be spiked contain in addition 25 μl 100 nmol/l working standard vitamin K₁.

The contents are gently vortex-mixed with 1000 µl 0.9% (w/v) NaCl.

The contents are next gently mixed (stoppered) with 3 ml 100% methanol and left for 10 min to enhance protein wetting and denaturation.

Thereafter, 3 ml methylene chloride is added and the contents of the stoppered tube gently mixed for 1 min.

1000 µl water is added and the contents again gently mixed. The final diluted volume ratios sample:methanol:methylene chloride are now 1:1:1.

Centrifuge for 10 min at 2000 g and 4°C.

The upper phase is slowly aspirated. After puncturing the protein layer with an air bubble released from the tip of a long needle, 2 ml of the lower phase is sucked into a syringe. The syringe is quickly tilted and the contents transferred to the bottom of a clean glass tube.

After evaporation under a stream of dry nitrogen, the residue is dissolved, gently mixing in 100 µl methylene chloride and 900 µl acetonitrile.

(b) Clean-up

The extract solution is sucked into a syringe and loaded into the Sep-Pak C 18 cartridge via the short end at a rate of 1 drop per second.

From another syringe 1.5 ml acetonitrile is added and the eluate discarded.

Next, the cartridge is eluted with 8 ml acetonitrile and the eluates collected in a glass tube.

The contents of the tube are evaporated for 30 min until critically dry. The residue is dissolved in 300 µl of straight-phase eluent.

(c) Fractionation

The cleaned-up extract solution is subjected to straight-phase HPLC. The chromatographic procedures are carried out at 20°C and samples protected from light. The HPLC is open-ended and parts are cleaned thoroughly to prevent any interference. Before fractionation, a few 250 µl aliquots of working standard, reconstituted and diluted with eluent are injected to equilibrate the chromatographic system (constant peak height) and to establish the time-range of eluting trans-vitamin K_1. In routine analysis, each series of ten cleaned-up sample extracts is preceded by this calibration procedure. The flow rate of the eluent is 2 ml/min. The linearity of the chromatographic system is checked every month using five different standard concentrations, corresponding to the original levels of 0–20 nmol trans-vitamin K_1/l serum.

Aliquots of 250 µl of cleaned-up extract solution are injected into the straight-phase column. At this stage vitamin K_1 levels can be monitored while fractionating.

Within the relative established time-range, the fraction containing trans-vitamin K_1 is taken and blown critically dry under nitrogen. If necessary, the fraction can be stored overnight under hexane at −20°C.

(d) Quantification of trans-vitamin K_1

The entire chromatographic procedure is carried out at 20°C. The eluent is freshly prepared, sonicated in vacuo for 10 min, flushed with nitrogen on-line with HPLC for 2 h before measurements are started and continuously degassed further. The flow rate of the eluent is 1 ml/min. Before analysis, a few 250 µl aliquots of the working standard, diluted with 100% methanol to make a solution with a trans-vitamin K_1 concentration of 10 nmol/l, are injected to equilibrate the chromatographic system (constant peak height). In routine analysis, each series of five samples is preceded by a native sample and the same sample spiked with 2.5 nmol/l trans-vitamin K₁. Linearity of the chromatographic system is checked for every series by three different spiked standard concentrations, corresponding to the original levels of 0–5 nmol vitamin K₁/l serum.

The residue obtained from the fractionated straight-phase eluate is reconstituted with 300 μl 100% methanol. Aliquots of 250 μl are subjected to reversed-phase HPLC. In general, the retention time of trans-vitamin K₁ is about 5 min, the total run time 10 min. The post-column coulometric reduction reactor (both cells) is operated at –0.9 V and preceded by a 0.5 μm high-pressure filter and standard carbon filter. Fluorescence is detected on-line with the reactor using the wavelength couple 330/435 nm (as indicated in HPLC apparatus). The elution profiles are displayed on the dual-pen recorder set at 5 and 10 mV full scale and a recording speed of 5 mm/min. The recorder signal entrances and integrator are connected directly to the spectrofluorometer.

(e) Calculation

The concentration of trans-vitamin K₁ in the original sample is calculated from integration based on the peak heights in the native and spiked samples, normalized to peak height of the internal standard in the native sample. The whole method described releases trans-vitamin K₁ almost quantitatively. The equation for calculating trans-vitamin K₁ concentration in serum is:

$$\text{trans-vitamin K}_1 \text{ (nmol/l)} = \frac{H_s}{H_{ss} \cdot (H_{iss}/H_{is}) - H_s} \cdot C_{sst} \cdot PPP \cdot RCP$$

where: H_s = peak height of the sample on the reversed-phase system; C_{sst} = increase in concentration by spiking with working standard solution (= 2.5 nmol/l); PPP = peak purity percentile, a factor correcting for the true amount of trans-vitamin K₁ in the commercial standard (e.g. = 1.18); RCP = recovery correction percentile, a factor correcting for recovery (e.g. = 1.08); H_{ss} = peak height of the spiked sample; H_{iss} = peak height of the internal standard in the spiked sample on the straight-phase system; H_{is} = peak height of the internal standard in the native sample on the straight-phase system.

7.5.14 Performance characteristics

(a) Range of linearity

Analysing 0.2–2.0 ml serum of specimens containing 1–20 nmol/l trans-vitamin K₁, the results revealed no serum volume dependency.

(b) Detection limit

Assuming a signal-to-noise ratio of at least 3, the HPLC method described here shows a detection limit as low as 20 pg (on column) trans-vitamin K₁ or 0.05 nmol/l (1 ml serum analysed).

(c) Recovery

Recovery can be determined in each series by analysing aliquots of samples spiked with trans-vitamin K₁ in the range 0–10 nmol/l and standard trans-vitamin K₁ solutions added with water.

The general equation of the graphs of peak heights (y = mm) versus concentrations (x = nmol/l) is y = a + bx, where a and b represent the intercept and slope, respectively. Recovery is achieved by dividing the b-values for the standard-addition graphs by the corresponding graphs for the vitamin spiked with water. The analytic recovery of trans-vitamin K_1 from serum is 92%.

(d) Reproducibility

In our laboratory, precision of the method is verified by analysing aliquots of pooled serum preceding each series of five patient samples, with a minimal number of three aliquots each day.

For a serum pool with an average level of about 1.2 nmol/l trans-vitamin K_1 the overall CV of a single run in an arbitrary series can be as low as 5.0%. We have three persons qualified for the vitamin K_1 assay who work a three-week schedule.

(e) Validity

We have been using this HPLC method routinely now for four years and no interferences have been observed.

Turning the reactor off results in a zero signal at the relevant retention time (or better, at the chromatographic address k). Chromatograms obtained from various sources, e.g. breast milk, formula milk, and vegetables show various other peaks besides that of trans-vitamin K_1. For these samples, in case of doubt, duplicate specimens are analysed with the reactor turned off.

Menaquinones, if present, are removed in the clean-up and fractionation steps or clearly separated from their trans-vitamin K_1 congener. The electrochemical reactor is routinely cleaned off-line once every four months by eluting in consecutive order 10 ml water, and 6 mol/l sodium hydroxide, water, isopropanol, methylene chloride, hexane, isopropanol, water, and methanol.

7.5.15   Reference values

Reference values are, in general, population-specific. For example, the non-parametrically calculated reference values, expressed as 0.025 and 0.975 population percentiles for 163 apparently healthy volunteers (90 men and 73 women blood donors from the local Red Cross Centre), age range 18–65 years, are 0.7–4.9 nmol/l serum.

For 107 off-line outpatients the reference values are 0.8–5.3 nmol/l serum. The cumulative frequency distribution for the donor population is given in Table 7.7. No influence from age on the level of trans-vitamin K_1 in serum was observed, either by ourselves or others [75, 77, 78]. However, the vitamin K_1 levels of 42 women immediately after delivery (reference values 0.1–2.0 nmol/l) were significantly lower (P < 0.001) than those of non-pregnant women or men of comparable age. Their coagulation parameters were normal [74]. Newborns, both term and preterm, have undetectably low levels of vitamin K_1 in cord blood, (levels < 0.0005 nmol/l serum) even when the routine sample amounts are worked up 100 times. On the third postnatal day all newborns have detectable serum levels of vitamin K_1, depending on the type of feeding. Breast-fed newborns have serum levels of vitamin K_1 in the range 0.03–6.0 nmol/l. Serum vitamin K_1 levels of formula-fed newborns on the third postnatal day are 0.4–6.0 nmol/l, which is statistically significant (P < 0.05) with respect to those of breast-fed infants. The vitamin K_1 content of breast milk samples at seven postnatal days are 1.3–8.9 nmol/l, whereas formula milk (Almiron M2(r), Nutricia, Zoetermeer, The Netherlands) contains 150–160 nmol vitamin K_1/l solution.

Table 7.7 Cumulative frequency distribution of serum trans-vitamin K_1 (N = 163 volunteers)

Percentile	Trans-vitamin K_1 nmol/l
Min	0.3
1	0.4
5	0.7
10	0.8
25	1.0
50	1.5
75	2.1
90	3.4
95	4.9
99	7.2
Max	9.3
Mean	1.87
SE	0.11

7.5.16 Interpretation

In adult humans the most frequent causes of vitamin K deficiency diseases are malfunction of the gastrointestinal tract, reduced bile excretion, liver diseases, antibiotics, and other medications. Dietary deficiency of vitamin K is rare among humans. Levels of trans-vitamin K_1 in serum in the range 0.35–0.70 nmol/l are considered indicative of vitamin K_1 depletion in the body; below 0.35 nmol/l deficiency is very likely.

In non-supplemented newborns even levels of 0.2 nmol/l are found along with normal coagulation parameters.

Extremely high serum levels of vitamin K_1 are found after vitamin K_1 treatment (e.g. 1 mg Konakion parenterally), but coagulation factors II and X remain almost constant.

At birth measurement of vitamin K_1 reveals undetectable levels in cord blood serum even when 100 times the routine sample amounts are worked up (levels 0.0005 nmol/l serum). These findings accentuate the very large concentration gradient differences between the mother and fetus. This suggests a protecting role by the placenta during fetal life, which would inhibit mutagenic events during a period of rapid fetal cell proliferation due to high levels of vitamin K_1 [79]. Other hypotheses are the above-mentioned self-contained placental role in fetal bone metabolism, or at least a storage role for postnatal life. In species other than man, mothers eat the placenta before giving breast milk.

Thus, supplementing the newborn with vitamin K, which is standard practice in various parts of the world, means intervention by man in a natural phenomenon.

The question remains about the placenta's role in setting priorities in the gamma-carboxylation of the proteins involved in haemostasis (clotting factor synthesis) and bone metabolism (mineralization of the skeleton in the growing fetus).

7.6 THIAMIN

Four methods will be described for thiamin nutriture assessment: erythrocyte transketolase activity, the very common macro- and micro-methods; HPLC for total thiamin in whole blood; and urine thiamin to provide information on the recent thiamin intake.

SECTION I ERYTHROCYTE TRANSKETOLASE ACTIVITY

7.6.1 Purpose and scope

In 1958 Brin showed that transketolase activity is a useful test for thiamin nutriture assessment, giving information on adequate, less-than-adequate or deficient intake [80]. Transketolase is a thiamin-dependent enzyme that plays an essential role in the glucose oxidative pathway [81]. The transketolase activity in haemolysed erythrocytes (ETK) is measured either by disappearance of pentose or appearance of hexose (ThDP effect) [82]. In the case of thiamin deficiency the quantity of hexose appears to be reduced. When thiamin diphosphate (ThDP) is added to the reaction mixture the enzyme activity is markedly enhanced in thiamin-deficient haemolysates but not in thiamin adequate samples [83].

This procedure makes it possible to measure total apoenzyme (which can be considered as an estimate of coenzyme content in conditions of excess apoenzyme), according to the following equation:

$$\text{Total apo-ETK} + \text{ThDP}_o + \text{ThDP suppl} = (\text{ETK} + \text{ThDP}) + \text{excess ThDP}.$$

In conditions where the total apoenzyme content is constant and independent of the thiamin nutritional status, the quotient

$$\frac{\text{ETK}\,(+\text{ThDP})}{\text{ETK}_o} = \alpha\,\text{ETK or ETK-AC}$$

can be considered a measure of the coenzyme content of the erythrocytes [6].

According to Brin *et al.* [82] one limitation of the ThDP effect is that it is related not only to the amount of holoenzyme present, but rather to the proportion of the total apoenzyme.

The original method has been modified by measuring the sedoheptulose generated in the enzyme reaction [84–86]. Subsequently the colour reaction with cysteine and sulphuric acid was replaced by a sulphuric acid only treatment as proposed by Kunovits [87]. This test is carried out on washed erythrocytes to reduce the interference of colour reaction from plasma components and because practically all the enzyme is located in the erythrocyte.

For an indication of the thiamin nutriture, activation with thiamin diphosphate alone is not sufficient because in some conditions such as low thiamin intake the amount of apoenzyme as well as the amount of holoenzyme decreases. The result is a normal activation at a low basal activity. Accordingly, basal activity should be carried out together with the activation test. But standardization of apoenzyme activation is at present not possible [88, 89].

For both the activation test and basal activity a time-lag between actual intake and full response has been observed [90].

7.6.2 Principle of the method

Washed erythrocytes are haemolysed with saponin, buffered, and split into two subsamples. To one sample, substrate alone is added, and to the other substrate plus thiamin diphosphate. After adequate incubation time, samples are deproteinized and the sedoheptulose formed is measured colorimetrically by sulphuric acid reaction [91].

7.6.3 Chemicals and apparatus

(a) Chemicals

Citric acid, anhydrous ($C_6H_8O_7$) p.a.
Sodium citrate dihydrate ($C_6H_5Na_3O_7$. $2H_2O$) p.a.
Glucose ($C_6H_{12}O_6$) p.a.
Sodium chloride (NaCl) p.a.
Saponin p.a.
Potassium phosphate, dibasic trihydrate (K_2HPO_4 . $3H_2O$) p.a.
Potassium chloride (KCl) p.a.
Magnesium sulphate, heptahydrate ($MgSO_4$. $7H_2O$) p.a.
Cocarboxylase (ThDP chloride), crystallized, e.g. Boehringer Mannheim, 99%, cat. No. 5891
Ribose-5-phosphate disodium salt, e.g. Sigma, 99–100%, cat. No. R7750
Potassium hydroxide (KOH) p.a.
Trichloroacetic acid ($C_2HCl_3O_2$) p.a.
Sulphuric acid (H_2SO_4) p.a.
Sedoheptulose anhydride, e.g. Sigma, cat. No. 3375
Distilled water.

(b) Solutions

ACD stabilizer: citric acid 38 mmol (7.3 g), sodium citrate 74.8 mmol (22.0 g), D glucose . H_2O 123.6 mmol (24.5 g) in water to make 1000 ml.
0.9% NaCl.
Saponin solution, 0.025%: 25 mg saponin dissolved in water to make 100 ml (prepared shortly before use).
Buffer pH 7.4:
  K_2HPO_4 . $3H_2O$, 15.7 mmol (3.58 g)
  KCl, 124.2 mmol (9.26 g)
  NaCl, 4.8 mmol (0.28 g)
  $MgSO_4$. $7H_2O$, 1.2 mmol (0.296 g)
  in water to make 1000 ml and pH adjusted to 7.4.
Activation buffer, thiamin diphosphate, 4 mmol/l: 19.15 mg thiamin diphosphate are dissolved in 10 ml of buffer pH 7.4; fresh daily.
KOH, 1 mol/l: 56.11 g dissolved in water to make 1000 ml.
Substrate solution, ribose-5-phosphate (R-5-P), 24.3 mmol/l: 100 mg ribose-5-phosphate disodium salt are dissolved in 15 ml buffer pH 7.4. The pH is readjusted to 7.4 with KOH 1 mol/l. Storage in aliquots at –20°C.
Trichloroacetic acid: 918 mmol/l (15% w/v).

Sulphuric acid, 14.2 mol/l: 790 ml of concentrated H_2SO_4 are slowly poured into 210 ml of H_2O.

Sedoheptulose anhydride: 0.3 μmol and 0.6 μmol in 0.5 ml buffer.

(c) Apparatus

Automatic pipetting device; centrifuge; glass test tubes of various dimensions; boiling water bath; incubation water bath at 37°C; Fibreglass filters (G4).

Photometer or colorimeter switching at two wavelengths.

7.6.4   Sample collection

Evacuated blood collection tubes lined with sodium heparin are used and specimens of approximately 4 ml blood are immediately transferred into sterile brown glass septum ampoules of 5 ml capacity containing 0.75 ml ACD stabilizer.

The vials are shipped at ambient temperature and then stored at 4–6°C until analysed.

The assays should be made within 10 days of blood collection.

7.6.5   Procedure

(a) Preparation of erythrocytes

The blood is washed three times with isotonic saline. The supernatant wash solution is drawn off together with the buffy layer.

A volume of saline slightly smaller than the volume of erythrocytes is added to the sediment, so that the measured haematocrit (Hct) of the suspension reaches a value of approximately 0.40.

(b) Technique

One millilitre of the suspension of washed erythrocytes is mixed with 3 ml of saponin solution. After 15 min standing, 0.4 ml aliquots of haemolysate are pipetted into 6 centrifuge tubes of 10 ml capacity.

To tubes 1–3 0.1 ml of buffer pH 7.4 is added. To tubes 4–6 0.1 ml of activation buffer is added. The tubes are incubated for 15 min in a reciprocating water bath at 37°C.

Thereafter 0.5 ml substrate solution is added to each tube in sequence and incubation is continued for exactly 20 min. The proteins are precipitated by adding 0.5 ml trichloroacetic acid in the same sequence as the substrate additions.

The precipitates are filtered off or centrifuged and 1.0 ml aliquots of the clear solutions are mixed with 5 ml sulphuric acid, which has been precooled in an ice bath.

The tubes are heated in a boiling water bath for exactly 2.5 min and returned to the ice bath.

The optical density A of the solutions is measured at 350 nm (absorbance minimum) and 405 nm (peak absorbance) in cells of 10 mm path length. The absorbance differences are calculated, corrected for the blank, and averaged.

A figure for the blank is obtained by subjecting to the above procedure graded amounts of haemolysates prepared by dilution of the regular preparation with water. The absorbances are plotted in ordinate versus haemolysate volumes in abscissa. A straight line through the points will intercept the y axis at an average absorbance value of 0.035.

This figure is used as mean blank correction for all determinations. Values for basal (ETK$_o$) and stimulated enzyme activity (ETK$_+$) may be obtained by calibration with sedoheptulose anhydride. The optimal heating time of the anhydride in sulphuric acid is 4 min instead of 2.5 min of sedoheptulose phosphate.

(c) Calculation

The enzyme activity is expressed as μmol sedoheptulose formed per second at 37°C by 1 litre of erythrocyte suspension of haematocrit 1.0. The values calculated without addition of coenzyme should be taken as arbitrary units (μkat/l), since assay conditions started with ribose-5-phosphate alone have not achieved enzyme saturation with xylulose-5-phosphate at the start of the run.

(d) Automation

This method has been automated with minor changes. With the most recent one, the COBAS-BIO, realized at Hoffman–La Roche, some of the drawbacks reported below under Reproducibility were eliminated, and in addition it was less time consuming and required fewer personnel.

7.6.6 Performance characteristics

(a) Range of linearity

This is −0.8 to 5.5 μkat/l (Hct 1.0).

(b) Reproducibility

As the stimulation tests are not amenable to standardization or to recovery experiments, the only way to check the process of *in vitro* coenzyme stimulation for consistency and reproducibility is by using reference samples. These are prepared from pools of washed erythrocytes that are divided into small aliquots and stored frozen at −80°C. Haemolysates are not stable under these conditions. Erythrocyte pools showing too low stimulation values may be adjusted by admixture of erythrocytes from dog or bovine blood, which usually show high stimulation.

The coefficient of variation for the enzyme activity without the addition of ThDP (ETK$_o$) is ± 5.3% for within-day analysis (mean value 2.75 μkat/l on six blood collections determined in duplicate) and ± 4.6% for day-to-day analysis on 45 blood collections determined in duplicate (mean value 2.63 μkat/l). The corresponding values for α-ETK are ± 2.2% (mean value 1.01) and ± 3.8% (mean value 1.12) [88].

The precision of the parameter, the ratio coefficient, compares favourably with the corresponding figures for basal and stimulated activity. As the value of α is affected by the variance of two reaction rate assays, one might expect it to be less precise than the values for basal or stimulated activity. In fact, the scatter of the latter figures reflects the reproducibility of the haemolysis step which, together with the haematocrit determination, introduces a great part of the overall variance. The coefficient on the other hand is calculated on the basis of two reaction rates measured in the same haemolysate. Their ratio is unaltered irrespective of a variable recovery of enzyme activity in different haemolysates of the same blood specimen, since both rates are affected in the same proportion. This feature probably constitutes the main advantage of the stimulation parameter over the basal activity, which is also dependent on the vitamin status [83, 88].

Alongside this advantage there is also a serious drawback. Reference standards for checking the process of stimulation, e.g. stable apoenzymes of known content are not available, so standardization of the stimulation effect is therefore difficult. The reference samples prepared from erythrocyte pools allow detection of gross variations but do not protect from slow drifts over longer time periods.

In addition the method is highly dependent on technical details. The enzyme starts working at non-saturated concentration in xylulose phosphate, and must be synthesized from ribose phosphate, which is added as only one part of the substrate, and during the running part of the sedoheptulose formation it is further transformed by the enzyme of the pentose phosphate shunt present in the haemolysate.

(c) Validity

No true validity test is available at the present time.

7.6.7 Reference values

The reference values are, in general, population specific. For example, the average ETK_o level of 150 adult blood donors of both sexes from Basel (Red Cross Centre) was 2.82 μkat/l [91]. The cumulative frequency distribution is given in Table 7.8. The average α-ETK level of the same group of individuals was 1.074 [88]. The cumulative frequency distribution is given in Table 7.9.

Table 7.8 Cumulative frequency distribution of ETK_o (N = 150 blood donors)

Percentile	*μkat/l (Hct 1.0)*
Min	1.34
5	1.99
25	2.45
50	2.73
75	3.12
95	3.69
Max	4.19
Mean	2.82
SD	0.51

7.6.8 Interpretation

Erroneous interpretation of the transketolase activity can be made when a reduced level of apoenzyme occurs during long-term thiamin deficiency or malnutrition as in chronic alcoholism in which the activity is low and only partially saturated by the addition of the coenzyme, indicating in this case a deficiency of coenzyme along with a lower level of apoenzyme. The same situation can be found in cases of genetic defects [81].

Conditions that reduce thiamin intake or absorption can also affect the thiamin status (in particular gastrointestinal acute or chronic diseases, other pathologies, or drugs inducing loss of appetite, increase of intestinal motility, vomiting or diarrhoea). In addition, high alcohol intake not only influences thiamin absorption but also its metabolism [92].

Table 7.9 Cumulative frequency distribution of α-ETK (N = 150 blood donors)

Percentile	α-ETK
Min	1.00
5	1.00
25	1.04
50	1.07
75	1.11
95	1.16
Max	1.24
Mean	1.074
SD	0.502

Increased losses of urinary thiamin (uncontrolled diabetes mellitus or diabetes insipidus and diuretics) can impair thiamin nutriture; in diabetes mellitus a deficiency of the apoenzyme has also been observed [81].

Age, stress, fevers, infections, and hyperthyroidism, which increase thiamin requirement, should be considered confounding variables.

SECTION II ERYTHROCYTE TRANSKETOLASE ACTIVITY – MICROMETHOD [93–95]

7.6.9 Chemicals and apparatus

(a) Chemicals

Sodium chloride (NaCl) p.a.
Saponin p.a.
Potassium phosphate, dibasic trihydrate ($K_2HPO_4 . 3H_2O$) p.a.
Potassium chloride (KCl) p.a.
Magnesium sulphate, heptahydrate ($MgSO_4 . 7H_2O$) p.a.
Cocarboxylase (ThDP chloride), e.g. Merck, cat. No. 2334
Ribose-5-phosphate, disodium salt, e.g. Sigma, 99–100%, cat. No. R7750
Trichloroacetic acid (TCA) p.a.
Sulphuric acid (H_2SO_4), 95–97% p.a.
Distilled water.

(b) Solutions

0.9% NaCl.
Saponin solution, 0.025%: 25 mg saponin dissolved in water to make 100 ml (prepared shortly before use).
Buffer pH 7.4:
   $K_2HPO_4 . 3H_2O$, 15.7 mmol (3.58 g)
   KCl, 124.2 mmol (9.26 g)
   NaCl, 4.8mmol (0.28 g)
   $MgSO_4 . 7H_2O$, 1.2 mmol (0.296 g)
   in water to make 1000 ml and pH adjusted to 7.4.

Activation buffer, thiamin diphosphate, 4 mmol/l: 19.15 mg thiamin diphosphate are dissolved in 10 ml of buffer pH 7.4; store at –20°C.

Substrate solution, ribose-5-phosphate (R-5-P), 24.3 mmol: 100 mg ribose-5-phosphate disodium salt are dissolved in 15 ml buffer pH 7.4 (corresponding to 3.6 mg ribose/ml); stored closed at –20°C.

Trichloroacetic acid: 918 mmol/l (15% w/v).

Sulphuric acid, 14.2 mol/l: 21 ml H_2O are mixed carefully with 79 ml sulphuric acid, 95–97%.

(c) Apparatus

Automatic pipetting device; centrifuge; glass test tubes of various dimensions including Eppendorf centrifuge vials; boiling water-bath; incubation water bath at 37°C.

Photometer or colorimeter, switching at two wavelengths (366 and 405 nm).

7.6.10   Sample collection

Blood may be obtained by puncturing a fingertip using sterilized disposable blood lancets. Heparinized blood (0.3 ml) (0.1 mg heparin per 10 ml total blood) is transferred into an Eppendorf centrifuge vial.

7.6.11   Procedure

(a) Sample preparation

The blood is carefully mixed with 0.8 ml 0.9% NaCl. After 5 min centrifugation (900 *g*) the supernatant together with the buffy layer is drawn off by sucking off with a Pasteur pipette connected to vacuum line and discarded.

The sediment (packed erythrocytes) is washed with 0.8 ml 0.9% NaCl twice more and resuspended in 0.9% NaCl (0.08 ml saline per 0.1 ml packed sediment).

For hemolysis, 0.1 ml of the suspension is mixed with 0.3 ml 0.025% saponin solution and left in the dark for about 15 min.

(b) Technique

Measurement of enzyme activity and ThDP effect in the haemolysate is performed in Eppendorf vials according to the following scheme:

Vial No.	Haemolysate (ml)	Buffer pH 7.4 (ml)	ThDP solution (ml)	Incubation 37°C (min)	R-5-P (ml)	Incubation 37°C (min)	Trichloro-acetic acid (ml)
1	0.2	0.05	—	15	0.25	20	0.25
2	0.2	0.05	—	15	0.25	20	0.25
3	0.2	—	0.05	15	0.25	20	0.25
4	0.2	—	0.05	15	0.25	20	0.25

Note that the enzyme reaction in each vial is stopped by adding trichloroacetic acid after exactly 20 min (stop-watch).

Each vial is centrifuged for 3 min and 0.2 ml of the supernatant added to 1.0 ml ice-cold 14.2 mol/l sulphuric acid.

Each sample is heated in a boiling water bath for exactly 2.5 min followed by refrigeration in iced water for 2 min.

The absorbance of the clear solution is measured in a photometer at 405 and 366 nm using water as reference.

(c) Calculation

The difference value $E_{405} - E_{366}$ (ΔE_{ETK}) of each sample is employed to calculate the enzyme activity. The transketolase activity is calculated as follows (mean ΔE of a duplicate):

$$\frac{\Delta E \cdot 1000}{0.05 \cdot 20} = \mu mol \text{ sedoheptulose-7-phosphate/l cell suspension} \cdot min.$$

The reactivation (ThDP effect) is calculated:

$$\frac{\Delta E_{ETK_+}}{\Delta E_{ETK_o}} - 1 \cdot 100 = \% \text{ reactivation}$$

$$\frac{\Delta E_{ETK_+}}{\Delta E_{ETK_o}} = \alpha \text{ ETK (activation coefficient)}$$

If the enzyme activity is expressed in katal according to SI the calculation of enzyme activity has to be changed as follows (divide by $10^6 \cdot 60$),

$$\frac{\Delta E}{60 \cdot 10^3} = \text{mole sedoheptulose-7-phosphate/litre cell suspension} \cdot sec$$
$$\text{(kat/litre cell suspension).}$$

7.6.12 Performance characteristics

Reproducibility

Coefficient of variation (CV), calculated from ETK–AC values of a heparinized whole blood pool: CV within day $= 3.7\%$; CV between days $= 10.4\%$.

7.6.13 Reference values

As in the macromethod, see p. 232.

7.6.14 Interpretation

As in the macromethod, see p. 232.

SECTION III   TOTAL THIAMIN IN WHOLE BLOOD BY HPLC

7.6.15 Purpose and scope

Virtually all thiamin present in blood is located within the erythrocytes and nearly all is in the form of its coenzyme thiamin diphosphate (ThDP) [96]. Therefore, the analysis of thiamin in whole blood (or erythrocytes) can represent a great advantage (next to the erythrocyte transketolase activation test: ETK–AC) in the evaluation of the vitamin B_1 status of individuals [31, 97].

In fact in some situations, thiamin analysis may be superior to ETK–AC. For instance, during long-term vitamin B_1 deficiency or malnutrition (as in alcoholism) the activation coefficient may become normal as a result of decreased synthesis of the apotransketolase [98, 99]. Also in cases of genetic defects or certain diseases (diabetes, polyneuritis, pernicious anaemia, or disorders of the gastrointestinal tract) the synthesis and/or the kinetic functions of the apoenzyme might be altered [100, 101]. Furthermore, heterogeneity has been described for the enzyme [102].

Although it seems warranted to determine ThDP, in general the amounts of ThDP and total thiamin will hardly differ in fresh whole blood samples.

Furthermore, the analysis of ThDP is hampered by the fact that even short-term storage of blood samples at room temperature, in the refrigerator, or even in the freezer may result in hydrolysis of ThDP. Therefore, if analysis of ThDP is requested it should be carried out immediately after sample collection.

In general, for different population groups a significant correlation has been found between the total thiamin content of whole blood and the ETK activity [31].

7.6.16　Principle of the method

Thiamin and its phosphate esters are extracted from whole blood (erythrocytes or any other biological fluid) using trichloroacetic acid. After adjusting the pH, the phosphate esters are hydrolysed to free thiamin by incubation with Taka-Diastase. Thereafter, thiamin is separated by straight-phase HPLC, oxidized on-line to thiochrome, and detected by its thiochrome fluorescence. Total thiamin is quantitated from peak area by integration using an external standard.

7.6.17　Chemicals and apparatus

(a) Chemicals

Trichloroacetic acid (TCA) p.a.
Acetic acid (HAc), glacial 100% p.a.
Sodium hydroxide (NaOH) p.a.
Ferric chloride ($FeCl_3$) p.a.
Potassium ferricyanide ($K_3Fe(CN)_6$) p.a.
Sodium chloride (NaCl) p.a.
100% ethyl alcohol, technical quality
Sodium phosphate, dibasic dihydrate ($Na_2HPO_4.2H_2O$) p.a.
Sulphuric acid (H_2SO_4) 95–97% p.a.
Hydrochloric acid (HCl) 37% p.a.
Taka-Diastase, Pfaltz and Bauer (Stamford, USA), cat. No. T 0040

Note 3.
Taka-Diastase from Pfaltz and Bauer (Stamford, USA) is a crude α-amylase preparation (registered trade mark for Aspergillus oryzae diastase) containing an aspecific but high phosphatase activity. Most types of Diastase or Clarase offered by several other suppliers are not suitable for hydrolysis of phosphate esters of vitamins due to a lack of (sufficient) phosphatase activity. Some phosphatase preparations (e.g. acid phosphatase) might be able to hydrolyse ThDP, but long incubation periods (overnight) are needed.

Thiamin hydrochloride, e.g. Sigma, cat. No. T 4625
Cocarboxylase (ThDP chloride), e.g. Sigma, cat. No. C 8754
Water: quartz-bidistilled every 2–3 days
Dialysis tube: weldless, 1.6 cm diameter, e.g. Visking, cat. No. 20.

(b) Solutions

TCA/$FeCl_3$ solution: 65 g TCA dissolved in water to make 1000 ml, followed by the addition of 1440 mg $FeCl_3$.
Sodium acetate buffer solution, pH 6.2: 160 g NaOH dissolved in 500 ml of

water. Thereafter, 272 g HAc is added under careful mixing and cooling. After cooling the volume is made up with water to 1000 ml.

Taka-Diastase solution (about 200 mg/ml): 6.0 g of Taka-Diastase is dissolved in 30.0 ml water and transferred into a 40 × 1.6 cm diameter dialysis tube equilibrated in water for about 10 min. After closing the tube with knots, dialysis is performed against water for about 24 h in a cool and dark place (4–8°C). During dialysis, water is renewed twice. The enzyme solution is collected and stored for not more than two weeks in the refrigerator (about 4°C).

NaOH 1.8 M: 72 g NaOH dissolved in water to make 1000 ml.

Thiochrome reagent 1.5 mM $K_3Fe(CN)_6$: 500 mg dissolved in 1.8 M NaOH to make 1000 ml.

Na_2HPO_4 0.13 M: 23.1 g $Na_2HPO_4.2H_2O$ dissolved in water to make 1000 ml.

KH_2PO_4 0.13 M: 17.7 g KH_2PO_4 dissolved in water to make 1000 ml.

H_2SO_4 0.15 M: 8.3 ml sulphuric acid dissolved in water to make 1000 ml.

TCA 0.4 M: 65 g TCA dissolved in water to make 1000 ml.

HPLC mobile phase, pH 7.4: this solution is prepared by mixing 750 ml of KH_2PO_4 0.13 M with 750 ml H_2SO_4 0.15 M, 1500 ml water, and 1100 ml ethyl alcohol.

Thiamin standard solution for HPLC: 100 mg thiamin hydrochloride/200 ml 0.15 M H_2SO_4. The concentration of the vitamin is determined using dilutions in 0.1 M HCl in the range 0–10 µg/ml. From the absorption at 248 nm in 1 cm quartz cuvettes, the standard concentration is calculated using the molar absorption coefficient of 13 400 (molecular weight of thiamin hydrochloride = 337.3) (ref. [29]). The original standard solution in H_2SO_4 is diluted with water to a concentration of 500 ng/ml. Thereafter, 15.0 ml of this solution is mixed with 375 ml 0.4 M TCA and 500 ml sodium acetate buffer. This solution is used as the external standard for HPLC analysis and is stored in aliquots for not more than four weeks at −20°C.

(c) Apparatus

Plastic tubes (e.g. 16 × 110 mm) suited for centrifugation; adjustable pipettes; dispensers; Vortex.

Waterbath; refrigerated laboratory centrifuge.

Spectrophotometer; 1 cm quartz cuvettes.

HPLC apparatus consisting of:

Radial-Pak Cartridges Si 10, 8 µm (silica straight-phase)

Waters 8 × 10 Module for Radial-Pak Cartridges

Constant-flow HPLC pump

Automatic injector (or injection valve)

Fluorescence detector, e.g. Kratos Fluoromat filter fluorometer, model FS 950, provided with light source FSA 110 (365 nm, blue filtered), excitation band filter FS 403 (365 nm), emission cut-off filter FS 428 (470 nm) and a flow cell of 28 µl. The optimal excitation wavelength for thiochrome is 367 nm, resulting in an optimal emission at 418 nm. In general, several other fluorometers might be used if the instrument provides the correct excitation light and photomultiplier sensitivity.

Reagent pump

Reaction coil: 1.2 × 1 mm diameter
Recorder
Integrator.

7.6.18   Sample collection

All procedures during sample treatment are carried out under subdued light conditions. The anticoagulant (citrate, EDTA, or heparin) used for collection of whole blood does not influence the procedures. Samples can be stored in the freezer for several months.

7.6.19   Procedure

(a) Sample extraction

Before extraction, whole blood or erythrocyte samples should be frozen (–20°C) and thawed three times for quantitative release of the contents of the blood cells. Freezing is performed during the night, while thawing is done slowly in running tap-water. The third thawing step is carried out on the day of analysis.

While vortexing, 1.0 ml of a well-mixed sample is carefully and slowly brought into a plastic tube containing 1.5 ml 0.4 M TCA. If less than 1.0 ml sample is available, the volume is adjusted to 1.0 ml using 0.9% (w/v) NaCl.
The tube is left for 30–60 min, with vigorously mixing half-way.
0.4 ml sodium acetate buffer is added and mixed thoroughly, followed by 0.1 ml of the Taka-Diastase solution.
The tube is incubated for 2 h at 45 ± 2°C in a water-bath. Half-way through this incubation the tube is vortexed thoroughly.
The tube is centrifuged for 15 min at 2 000 *g* and 4°C.
The supernatant is used for HPLC analysis (if necessary, sample extracts may be stored in the refrigerator or freezer for at least one week).

(b) Calibration

Before analysis, a few aliquots of the external standard solution are injected to equilibrate the chromatographic system (constant peak height). In routine analysis, each series of five sample extracts is preceded by the external standard.
    The linearity of the chromatographic system is controlled every month by a range of standard concentrations corresponding to original levels of 0–250 nmol thiamin/l whole blood.

(c) HPLC

The entire chromatographic procedure is carried out at room temperature. 120 µl sample extract is subjected to isocratic straight-phase HPLC. The flow rate of the mobile phase is about 3.2 ml/min (working pressure < 20 MPa). In general, the retention time of thiamin varies between 14 and 18 min, depending on the quality and history of the HPLC column. The retention time may be changed easily by varying the amount of ethyl alcohol in the mobile phase. The effluent of the HPLC column is mixed on-line with the thiochrome reagent delivered by the reagent pump (flow rate 0.3 ml/min). This results in the oxidation of thiamin to its thiochrome complex. The complex is detected fluorometrically. The elution profiles are displayed on the recorder set at 10 mV full-scale and a recording speed of 2 mm/min. The recorder as well as the integrator are connected directly to the fluorometer.

(d) Calculation

The concentration of thiamin in the sample is calculated by integration based on the peak area ratio sample/standard. In cases of failure of the integrator, peak heights are used.

By the extraction method described, thiamin and its phosphate esters are released quantitatively (according to results obtained with repeated extraction and, determination of the water content of the precipitate using ^3H_2O, see ref. [96]). Assuming the water content of whole blood being 85%, the equation for calculation of the total thiamin concentration in whole blood will be:

$$\text{total thiamin (nmol/l)} = \frac{A_s \cdot C_{st} \cdot D}{A_{st}}$$

where A_s = peak area of the sample, A_{st} = peak area of standard, C_{st} = concentration of standard in nmol/l, and D = dilution factor; for 1 ml of whole blood D is calculated according to: $D = [0.85 + 2.00] = 2.85$.

7.6.20 Performance characteristics

(a) Range of linearity

Using dilutions of whole blood samples (aliquots of 0.2–1.0 ml of sample made up to 1.0 ml with 0.9% (w/v) NaCl) results in comparable total thiamin levels in the range up to 200 nmol/l whole blood.

(b) Detection limit

Assuming the signal-to-noise ratio should be at least 3, the HPLC method described here shows a detection limit as low as 5 nmol total thiamin/l whole blood (injected amount about 0.2 pmol or 70 pg respectively).

(c) Recovery

Recovery is determined in each series by analysis of three aliquots of pooled whole blood and 2×3 aliquots of the same pooled whole blood to which ThDP has been added (two different levels of addition). For that purpose, ThDP is dissolved in 0.9% (w/v) NaCl. To correct for volume changes, the same volume of 0.9% (w/v) NaCl is added to pooled whole blood. The concentration of ThDP used is determined from the absorption of a solution in 0.1 M HCl in a 1 cm quartz cuvette at 248 nm, using the molar absorption coefficient of 13 400 (molecular weight of ThDP chloride = 460.8) (ref. [29]).

Pooled whole blood and recovery samples are stored at –20°C in the dark for a period generally not exceeding three months.

For a total of 63 series using additions of 54 and 108 nmol ThDP/l whole blood, the average recoveries for singular analysis were 99 ± 13% and 109 ± 7% respectively.

(d) Reproducibility

In our laboratory the precision of the method is determined in each series by analysis of three aliquots of pooled whole blood (see also Recovery, above). For a total of 63 series using the same pool (pool mean: 108 nmol total thiamin/l whole blood) the overall CV of a single sample run in an arbitrary series amounted to about 5%.

(e) Validity

Total thiamin levels obtained by the classical microbiological method seem not to deviate significantly from those obtained by HPLC methods. However, it is well known that performance characteristics of the microbiological methods are less optimal.

7.6.21　Reference values　Reference values are, in general, population specific. For example, the average total thiamin level for 207 healthy volunteers (blood donors from the centre of the Netherlands) with an average age of 37 ± 11.2 years (range 18–64 years) was 127 ± 22 nmol/l whole blood [30]. The cumulative frequency distribution is given in Table 7.10.

Table 7.10 Cumulative frequency distribution of total thiamin in whole blood (N = 207 volunteers)

Percentile	Thiamin nmol/l
Min	67.0
5	94.0
25	112.0
50	124.5
75	141.0
95	159.0
Max	197.0
Mean	126.7
SD	21.5

An influence of age, gender, or oral contraceptives on the level of total thiamin in whole blood was not observed.

For 124 apparently healthy Dutch free-living elderly people with an average age of 72 ± 3.8 years (range 65–89 years) [31], the total thiamin level (105 ± 23 nmol/l) was not significantly different from that of the group of blood donors.

On the same population (Dutch blood donors) various indices of thiamin status have been assessed. The correlation coefficients are reported in Table 7.11. Significant correlations were found between basal ETK and total ETK activities and the concentration of total thiamin in whole blood. This is not the case for ETK–AC.

Table 7.11 Correlation matrix of indices of the thiamin status (Pearson correlation coefficients)

Index	Thiamin	Basal ETK	Total ETK
Total thiamin	1.0000	–	–
Basal ETK	0.4201*	1.0000	–
Total ETK	0.3814*	0.9721*	1.0000
ETK–AC	–0.2898	–0.3997*	–0.1806

*Significant at $P < 0.001$ (df = 205); blood samples of Dutch blood donors (men and women, 18–65 years) were used for the investigation of the indices of the thiamin status.

7.6.22 Interpretation

Whole blood levels of total thiamin below 80 nmol/l most probably indicate a vitamin B$_1$ deficiency.

SECTION IV THIAMIN IN URINE

7.6.23 Purpose and scope

In subjects with an adequate thiamin status thiamin excretion in urine is in close correlation with its recent intake [4]. Therefore determination of thiamin content in urine is often used to assess short-term thiamin status. Under survey conditions a 24-h urine sample might not be feasible. In this case the thiamin concentration of fasting morning urine should be determined and related to its creatinine concentration. The sensitive reaction to recent vitamin intake results in a large day-to-day variability in the vitamin excretion. However thiamin-deficient subjects excrete only small amounts of this vitamin regardless of recent intake [103]. An established but modified method of determination is described here [104].

7.6.24 Principle of the method

Thiamin is mainly excreted in the urine as free thiamin. This is converted to thiochrome by reaction with potassium ferricyanide in an alkaline solution. Before the thiochrome fluorescence is measured, thiochrome is extracted with isobutanol.

The non-thiochrome fluorescence is measured after the destruction of thiochrome with a mixture of hydrochloric acid (HCl) and methanol.

7.6.25 Chemicals and apparatus

(a) Chemicals

Thiamin hydrochloride, purum
Sodium hydroxide (NaOH) p.a.
Potassium ferricyanide (K$_3$Fe(CN)$_6$) p.a.
Sodium acetate (CH$_3$COONa), anhydrous p.a.
Sulphuric acid (H$_2$SO$_4$), 96% p.a.
Isobutanol, 99% p.a.
Sodium chloride (NaCl), 99.8% p.a.
Methanol, 99.7% p.a.
Hydrochloric acid (HCl), 37% (fuming) p.a.
Distilled water.

(b) Solutions

1% K$_3$Fe(CN)$_6$: 1 g K$_3$Fe(CN)$_6$ dissolved in water to make 100 ml.
10 N NaOH: 40 g NaOH dissolved in water to make 100 ml.
2.5 N CH$_3$COONa: 20.5 g CH$_3$COONa dissolved in water to make 100 ml.
0.2 N H$_2$SO$_4$: 5.5 ml 96% H$_2$SO$_4$ made up to 1000 ml with water.
0.5 N H$_2$SO$_4$: 13.75 ml 96% H$_2$SO$_4$ made up to 1000 ml with water.
1 N HCl: 82.58 ml 37% HCl made up to 1000 ml with water.
Thiochrome reagent: 70 ml 10 N NaOH + 20 ml 1% K$_3$Fe(CN)$_6$ (prepare every day).
Thiochrome-destroying reagent: 4 ml 1 N HCl + 3 ml methanol.
Thiamin stock standard: before preparing a standard solution, the thiamin hydrochloride is dried. 56 mg thiamin hydrochloride is dissolved in 0.2 N

H_2SO_4 to make 100 ml (=50 mg thiamin/100 ml 0.2 N H_2SO_4). The stock standard can be stored in 1-ml aliquots for about four weeks at –20°C. This stock standard is diluted with 0.2 N H_2SO_4 to a concentration of 50 µg/dl (working standard).

(c) Apparatus

Adjustable pipettes; test tubes; refrigerated laboratory centrifuge; cuvettes. Fluorescence detector, e.g. Perkin Elmer, LS-3B.

The excitation wavelength for thiochrome is 375 nm, the emission wavelength 418 nm.

7.6.26 Sample collection

After collecting 24 h urine in clean 2.5 l containers and measuring the volume (or drawing a fasting sample) an aliquot of 2 ml is diluted with 2 ml 0.5 N H_2SO_4 and frozen at –20°C. The sample may be stored for at least three months.

7.6.27 Procedure

(a) Technique

0.5 ml of a thawed thiamin standard is diluted with 0.5 ml 0.2 N H_2SO_4. Diluted standard sample and urine sample are both treated in the same way as follows:

2 ml of distilled water and 0.2 ml sodium acetate are added to 1 ml diluted standard or 1 ml diluted urine sample, mixing thoroughly.

3 ml of thiochrome reagent are added to the tube, mixing for 30 s.

Thereafter 1.5 g sodium chloride and 4 ml isobutanol are added, mixing for 90 s.

After a short centrifugation, about 3.5 ml of the supernatant is transferred to a cuvette.

The thiochrome complex is detected fluorometrically. A blank with isobutanol is run with every measurement. After detecting with 375 nm/425 nm, 0.1 ml of the HCl/methanol mixture is added and the non-specific non-thiochrome fluorescence is measured. The thiochrome fluorescence can be calculated as follows:

$$Fl_{thio} = Fl_{total} - Fl_{non-thio}$$

where Fl_{thio} = thiochrome fluorescence; Fl_{total} = total fluorescence; $Fl_{non-thio}$ = non-specific non-thiochrome fluorescence.

(b) Calculation

The concentration of thiamin in the urine sample is calculated according to the equation:

$$\text{Total thiamin (µg/dl)} = \frac{ES - EB}{ESt - EB} \cdot 50$$

where ES = emission of the sample; EB = emission of the blank; ESt = emission of the standard.

The conversion factors for SI units are:
µg/dl · 29.65 = nmol/l

$\mu g/g$ creatinine $\cdot$ 0.3354 $=$ nmol/mmol creatinine
$\mu g/24$ hr $\cdot$ 2.965 $=$ nmol/day.

7.6.28 Performance characteristics

(a) Range of linearity

Linearity of the described method was observed from 5 to 150 $\mu g/dl$.

(b) Detection limit

The detection limit of the method described here is as low as 5 $\mu g/dl$ (150 nmol/l).

(c) Recovery

Recovery is performed by adding known amounts of thiamin to urinary samples. The actual recovery was estimated to be 97.5 $\pm$ 4%.

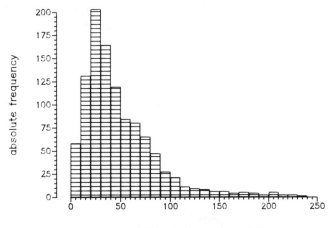

Fig. 7.4 Urinary thiamin concentration (frequency distribution) in a sample of 1081 healthy young men.

(d) Reproducibility

The precision of the method is determined in a ten-fold determination of aliquots of a pooled urine sample. The CV amounted to 3.1% in a continued series and to 3.9% in the day-to-day determination.

(e) Validity

No true validity test is available at the moment.

7.6.29 Reference values

The reference values are, in general, population specific. As an example, in 1081 healthy young men with an average age of 22.6 years (range 17–29 years) we found a mean fasting thiamin excretion of 48.8 $\pm$ 37.2 nmol thiamin/ mmol creatinine. The frequency distribution is shown in Fig. 7.4. Ninety-five per cent of the values are within the range of 5.0–157.0 nmol thiamin/mmol creatinine. The oral administration of 3 mg thiamin plus the usual dietary thiamin of about 1.54 mg results in a 2.6-fold increase of the average thiamin excretion.

7.7 RIBOFLAVIN

Four methods will be described for riboflavin nutriture assessment: Erythrocyte glutathione reductase activity, the very common up to now macro- and micro-methods; HPLC for flavin adenine dinucleotide in whole blood; urine riboflavin to provide information on the recent intake of riboflavin.

SECTION I ERYTHROCYTE GLUTATHIONE REDUCTASE ACTIVITY

7.7.1 Purpose and scope

Glatzle [105] proposed the stimulation of the erythrocyte glutathione reductase (EGR) by flavin adenin dinucleotide (FAD) as a test for riboflavin nutriture assessment.

NADPH$_2$-dependent glutathione reductase is a flavoenzyme with FAD as a prosthetic group. In cases of suboptimal concentration of FAD in haemolysed red blood cells its addition to the haemolysate stimulates the enzyme activity. This phenomenon is called FAD effect: it measures the extent to which the enzyme protein is undersaturated with coenzyme FAD. This procedure permits measurement of the total apoenzyme content according to the following equation:

$$\text{Total apo-EGR} + \text{FAD}_o + \text{FAD suppl} = (\text{EGR} + \text{FAD}) + \text{excess FAD}.$$

In conditions where the total apoenzyme content is constant and independent of the riboflavin nutritional status, the quotient

$$\frac{\text{EGR (+FAD)}}{\text{EGR}_o} = \alpha\text{-EGR or EGR-AC}$$

can be considered a measure of the coenzyme content in the erythrocyte: the higher the coefficient the lower the coenzyme content [6].

According to Glatzle if 'riboflavin deficiency symptoms occur only after long-term deficiency ... the disturbances of riboflavin-dependent enzyme systems ... would appear earlier. ... Consequently the detection of biochemical lesions seems to be appropriate for an early recognition of a riboflavin deficiency' [106].

In cases of people with intakes covering the requirements, the samples stimulated with FAD sometimes show lower activity than non-stimulated samples, which results in an α-EGR smaller than 1. This is probably due to some inhibitors present in the FAD solution.

To avoid EGR-AC values below 1.0, the technical suggestions of Garry and Owen [107] and of Thurnham and Rathakette [108] can be followed.

The classical stimulation test does not provide information on the basal EGR activity. Accordingly, together with the activation test, the basal activity should also be carried out.

Tillotson and Baker [109] have observed a lag in depletion effects, due to the finite rates of turnover of riboflavin in the body, and loss of riboflavin from the EGR enzyme *in vivo*, (where the rate presumably reflects the dilution of existing saturated RBCs with newly synthesized cells containing unsaturated EGR, due to deficiency in the bone marrow). Also Bates *et al.* [110] have shown that virtually complete repletion of deficient Gambian subjects can take place within three weeks from beginning supplementation (2 mg/day), whereas subsequent depletion on their home-food diet occurs much more gradually. Thus, only a partial return to pre-intervention levels was seen nine weeks after the withdrawal of the (2 mg daily) supplement. According to them it seems clear, both from theory and experience, that the rate of change depends on the magnitude of the intake, especially during the repletion phase. Thus a daily B_2 intake many times greater than the RDA will replete the tissues and unsaturated apo-EGR, much faster than a small daily increment in the intake.

7.7.2 Principle of the method	Washed erythrocytes are haemolysed with distilled water and the sample is split into two subsamples and mixed with substrate. FAD solution is added only to one sample. After a short pre-incubation period the decrease of NADPH is monitored in a kinetic assay [91].
7.7.3 Chemicals and apparatus	
(a) Chemicals	Citric acid anhydrous ($C_6H_8O_7$) p.a.
	Sodium citrate, dihydrate ($C_6H_5Na_3O_7 . 2H_2O$) p.a.
	D-Glucose, monohydrate ($C_6H_{12}O_6 . H_2O$) p.a.
	Sodium chloride (NaCl) p.a.
	Dipotassium phosphate, trihydrate ($K_2HPO_4 . 3H_2O$) p.a.
	Monopotassium phosphate (KH_2PO_4) p.a.
	Flavine adenine dinucleotide, disodium salt (FAD-Na_2), e.g. Boehringer Mannheim, cat. No. 104736
	Sodium hydrogen carbonate ($NaHCO_3$) p.a.
	Nicotinamide adenine dinucleotide phosphate, reduced (NADPH), tetra-sodium salt, e.g. Boehringer Mannheim 98%, cat. No. 107824
	Ethylenediamine tetra-acetate, dipotassium salt, dihydrate (EDTA-$K_2 . 2H_2O$) p.a.
	Sodium hydroxide (NaOH) p.a.
	Glutathione oxidized (GSSG), e.g. Boehringer Mannheim, cat. No. 105627
	Distilled water.
(b) Solutions	ACD-stabilizer: citric acid 38 mmol (7.3 g), sodium citrate 74.8 mmol (22.0 g), D-glucose . H_2O 123.6 mmol (24.5 g) in water to make 1000 ml.
	0.9% NaCl.
	Buffer pH 7.4: a solution of $K_2HPO_4 . 3H_2O$ 0.1 mol/l (22.82 g/l) is titrated with a solution of KH_2PO_4 0.1 mol/l (13.61 g/l) to pH 7.4.
	FAD-Na_2 (fresh daily), 0.29 mmol/l: 1.2 mg dissolved in water to make 5 ml.
	NADPH (fresh daily), 2.60 mmol/l: 2.17 g NADPH dissolved in 0.12 mol/l (10.08 g/l) $NaHCO_3$.
	EDTA-K_2 (storage in the refrigerator), 75 mmol/l: 30.34 g dissolved in water to make 1000 ml.
	GSSG (fresh daily), 7.13 mmol/l: 4.37 g GSSG dissolved in 8 mmol/l (0.32 g/l) NaOH.
(c) Apparatus	Automatic pipette device; centrifuge; glass test tubes of various dimensions.
	Photometer with thermostated cuvette holder at 35°C with Hg-lined filter at 334 nm or monochromator set at about 340 nm.

7.7.4   Sample collection

Evacuated blood collection tubes lined with sodium heparin are used and specimens of approximately 4 ml blood are immediately transferred into sterile brown glass septum ampoules of 5 ml capacity containing 0.75 ml ACD stabilizer.

The vials are shipped at ambient temperature and then stored at 4–6°C until analysed. The assays should be made within 10 days from blood collection.

7.7.5   Procedure

(a) Sample preparation

The blood is washed three times with isotonic saline. The supernatant wash solution is drawn off together with the buffy layer.

A volume of saline slightly smaller than the volume of erythrocytes is added to the sediment so that the measured haematocrit of the suspension reaches a value of approximately 0.4.

(b) Technique

The washed erythrocytes are centrifuged and 0.2 ml of the sedimented cells are pipetted into 3.8 ml of water in an ice bath.

After 30 min standing at 0°C the haemolysate is centrifuged, the clear supernatant separated from the cell debris and kept for 1 hour at 0°C in the dark.

The systems with and without FAD activation are made up in 2 cuvettes of 1 cm path length. The first cuvette contains 1.35 ml buffer pH 7.4 to which are added 50 µl of 0.29 mmol/l FAD, 200 µl of haemolysate, 100 µl of 2.60 mmol/l NADPH, and 50 µl of 75 mmol/l EDTA. In the second cuvette the 0.29 mmol/l FAD is replaced by 50 µl buffer pH 7.4.

The cuvettes are pre-incubated for 5 min at 35°C in the thermostated holder and the optical density monitored so that no drift is noted.

The reaction is then started by addition of 50 µl of 7.13 mmol/l GSSG and the decrease of absorbance monitored over 10 min. The final concentrations of reactants are: glutathione 0.2 mmol/l, NADPH 0.14 mmol/l, FAD 8 µmol/l.

Note 4.
To avoid α values below 1.0 and to ensure maximal reactivation of apoenzyme, Bates *et al.* [111] recommend the use of about 3 µM FAD, with about 30 min pre-incubation [108].

(c) Calculation

Straight lines are fitted to the points of the recorder diagram and their slope used for the calculation of the activation coefficient α-EGR. No figure for enzyme activity is calculated for this test, since the pipetting of erythrocyte sediment introduces too much variance.

(d) Automation

This method has now been automated in a few laboratories, using a Shimadzu or Eppendorf apparatus. At Hoffmann-La Roche the COBAS-BIO arrangement allows more analyses per day and requires fewer personnel.

7.7.6 Performance characteristics

(a) General considerations

In cases of individuals with an intake covering the requirement, the samples stimulated with FAD sometimes show lower activity than non-stimulated samples, which results in an α-EGR smaller than 1. This is probably due to some inhibitors in the FAD solution.

(b) Range of linearity

The range of linearity for EGR_o cannot be estimated.

(c) Reproducibility

As the stimulation tests are not amenable to standardization or to recovery experiments, the only way to check the process of *in vitro* coenzyme stimulation for consistency and reproducibility is by using reference samples. These are prepared from pools of washed erythrocytes that are divided into small aliquots and stored frozen at −80°C. Haemolysates are not stable under these conditions. Erythrocyte pools showing too low stimulation values may be adjusted by admixture of erythrocytes from dog or bovine blood, which usually show high stimulation.

The coefficient of variation of α-EGR is + 3.3% for within-day analysis (mean 1.07 on six blood collections determined in duplicate) and + 4.5% for day-to-day analysis (mean 1.14 on 45 blood collections determined in duplicate) [91].

(d) Validity

No true validity tests are available at the moment.

7.7.7 Reference values

The reference values are, in general, population specific. For example, the average α-EGR of 150 adult blood donors of both sexes from Basel (Red Cross Centre) was 1.06 [91]. The cumulative frequency distribution is given in Table 7.12.

Table 7.12 Cumulative frequency distribution of α-EGR (N = 150 blood donors)

Percentile	α-EGR
Min	0.91
5	0.95
25	0.99
50	1.03
75	1.09
95	1.24
Max	2.22
Mean	1.06
SD	0.13

7.7.8 Interpretation

In steady-state conditions, the EGR-AC can be considered a good index of riboflavin status, but in acute deficiency the rate of the response is not related to its final extent, and correlation with other riboflavin-sensitive variables is less satisfactory [112].

Prentice and Bates [113] have studied changes in liver enzymes in riboflavin-deficient animals and have shown a wide spectrum of changes ranging from rapid and major losses of activity in some enzyme activities to slower changes in others, and to complete 'depletion-resistance' of some flavoenzymes.

Among the confounding variables that can affect the sensitivity of the EGR-AC, individual and analytical variations have also to be considered. Glatzle *et al.* [106] in geriatric patients have found that the distribution of the activation coefficient appears decidedly skewed.

Increased EGR activity with a high degree of saturation with FAD has been reported in patients with severe uraemia, cirrhosis of the liver, biliary disorders, diabetes, thyroid diseases, and congenital heart disease [114]. In glucose-6-phosphate dehydrogenase deficiency the EGR-AC and basal EGR values are actually misleading because the biochemical lesion interferes specifically with EGR and/or red cell metabolism [115]. In iron deficiency anaemia it seems likely that EGR-AC (being independent of the Hb denominator) would be more informative than basal EGR activity (with Hb as an 'unreliable' denominator) [111].

Chronic alcoholism can be accompanied by riboflavin deficiency. In these cases a depressed gluthatione reductase activity can be found, resulting in an increase of EGR-AC [114].

Moreover, stress and various drugs (in particular contraceptives and chlorpromazine) can also induce a rise of EGR activation coefficients [114, 116].

Pyridoxine deficiency produces an increase in the riboflavin concentration but depresses the enzyme activity. Administration of pyridoxine to human individuals with clinical and enzymatic evidence of riboflavin deficiency provoked a marked fall in erythrocyte riboflavin concentration, and a slight improvement in glutathione reductase activity. This suggests that erythrocyte riboflavin concentration is a poor index of riboflavin status when there is associated pyridoxine deficiency [117].

In individuals with a defect of vitamin B_6 conversion to the corresponding coenzymatic form, high FAD activation coefficients have been observed. The riboflavin supplementation seems to reverse the inefficient conversion of both vitamins [118].

SECTION II   ERYTHROCYTE GLUTATHIONE REDUCTASE ACTIVITY – MICROMETHOD [119–121]

7.7.9 Chemicals and apparatus

(a) Chemicals

Citric acid anhydrous ($C_6H_8O_7$) p.a.
Sodium citrate ($C_6H_5Na_3O_7 . 2H_2O$) p.a.
D-Glucose, monohydrate ($C_6H_{12}O_6 . H_2O$) p.a.

Sodium chloride (NaCl) p.a.

Dipotassium phosphate, trihydrate ($K_2HPO_4 . 3H_2O$) p.a.

Monopotassium phosphate (KH_2PO_4) p.a.

Flavine adenine dinucleotide (FAD), disodium salt, e.g. Boehringer Mannheim, cat. No. 104736

Sodium hydrogen carbonate ($NaHCO_3$) p.a.

Nicotinamide adenine dinucleotide phosphate reduced (NADPH), tetrasodium salt, e.g. Boehringer Mannheim 98%, cat. No. 107824

Ethylendiamine tetra-acetate, disodium salt, dihydrate (EDTA-$Na_2 . 2H_2O$) p.a.

Sodium hydroxide (NaOH) p.a.

Glutathion oxidized (GSSG), e.g. Boehringer Mannheim, cat. No. 105627

Distilled water.

(b) Solutions

ACD stabilizer: citric acid 38 mmol (7.3 g), sodium citrate 74.8 mmol (22.0 g), D-glucose . H_2O 123.6 mmol (24.5 g) in water to make 1000 ml.

0.9% NaCl.

Buffer pH 7.4: a solution of $K_2HPO_4 . 3H_2O$ 67 mmol/l (15.22 g/l) is titrated with a solution of KH_2PO_4 67 mmol/l (9.07 g/l) to pH 7.4.

FAD-Na_2, 0.29 mmol/l: 1.2 mg dissolved in water to make 5 ml (fresh daily); store in the dark.

NADPH, 1.99 mmol/l: 1.66 g NADPH, tetrasodium salt, dissolved in 0.12 mol/l (10.08 g/l) $NaHCO_3$.

EDTA-Na_2, 80.6 mmol/l: 30 g dissolved in water to make 1000 ml. The solution can be stored in the refrigerator for 1 week.

GSSG, 7.5 mmol/l: 4.6 g GSSG dissolved in 8 mmol/l (0.32 g/l) NaOH (fresh daily).

(c) Apparatus

Automatic pipette device; centrifuge; glass test tubes of various dimensions.

Photometer with thermostated cuvette holder at 37°C with Hg-lined filter at 334 nm.

7.7.10 Sample collection

Heparinized blood (3 ml) are mixed with 0.75 ml ACD stabilizer by gentle shaking; it can be stored in a refrigerator at 4–6°C up to 1 week.

Haemoglobin has to be determined before ACD addition.

7.7.11 Procedure

(a) Sample preparation

Three millilitres of blood are gently mixed with 8 ml 0.9% NaCl in a graduated centrifuge tube and centrifuged for 5 min (900 *g*).

The supernatant is discarded by sucking off with a Pasteur pipette connected to a vacuum line.

The washing procedure is repeated twice more, discarding the supernatant each time.

The remaining sediment is suspended with 40 volumes of iced water in a centrifuge tube and kept in an ice bath for 30 min. After removing cell debris by centrifugation (15 min) the clear supernatant (haemolysate) is kept in a refrigerator for 1 hour.

(b) Technique

For the microassay the following solutions (and quantities) are pipetted into four Eppendorf vials as follows:

	No. 1 ml	No. 2 ml	No. 3 ml	No. 4 ml
Buffer pH 7.4	1.12	1.12	1.08	1.08
Haemolysate	0.16	0.16	0.16	0.16
NADPH	0.08	0.08	0.08	0.08
EDTA-Na$_2$	0.04	0.04	0.04	0.04
FAD	–	–	0.04	0.04

The reaction mixture is incubated at 37°C for 5 min. Thereafter at 5 min intervals (stop-watch), 0.04 ml of GSSG solution are added to each vial.

Each vial is well mixed and the absorption of each reaction mixture is measured at 334 nm in 1 cm cuvettes, using water as reference (E_1). Incubation of the samples at 37°C is continued.

Exactly 10 min after reading E_1, the absorption E_2 at the same wavelength is measured (stop-watch).

(c) Calculation

The calculation is performed as follows:

$$\Delta E = E_1 - E_2$$

The mean value of the duplicate measurements is applied to the equation:

$$\frac{\Delta E_{FAD_+}}{\Delta E_{FAD_o}} = \alpha EGR \text{ (activation coefficient)}$$

where ΔE_{FAD_+} = absorption difference of samples with FAD addition; ΔE_{FAD_o} = absorption difference of samples without FAD addition.

The EGR activity is expressed in μmoles substrate being changed per min per litre of erythrocyte suspension (packed sediment) at 37°C. The EGR activity is related to Hb content (g/1000 ml).

$$\frac{\Delta E \cdot 10^6 \cdot 1440 \cdot 150}{10 \cdot 6.0 \cdot 10^3 \cdot 3.9 \text{ Hb(g/l)}} = \text{μmole substrate/g Hb·min (U/g Hb)}$$

where $\Delta E/10$ = absorption decrease per min; 1440 = volume of the whole reaction mixture in μl; 3.9 = μl erythrocyte suspension in the reaction mixture; $6.0 \cdot 10^3$ = molar absorption coefficient of NADPH at 334 nm; 150 = mean haemoglobin content (g/l).

If the enzyme activity is expressed in katal according to SI the above equation is changed as follows (divide by $10^6 \cdot 60$):

$$\frac{\Delta E \cdot 24 \cdot 150}{10 \cdot 6.0 \cdot 10^3 \cdot 3.9 \text{ Hb(g/l)}} = \text{mole substrate/g Hb·sec (kat/g Hb)}$$

αEGR-values below 1.00 can result from an inhibition of the erythrocyte glutathion reductase (EGR) caused by excess FAD in the test assay.

7.7.12 Performance characteristics

Reproducibility

The within-day and day-to-day coefficient of variation of EGR activity in pooled blood samples ranged from 6% to 9%.

7.7.13 Reference values

These are as in the macromethod (p. 247).

7.7.14 Interpretation

This is as in the macromethod (p. 247).

SECTION III FLAVIN ADENINE DINUCLEOTIDE (FAD) IN WHOLE BLOOD BY HPLC

7.7.15 Purpose and scope

Vitamin B_2 may be present in tissues and biological fluids as its cofactors flavin adenine dinucleotide (FAD) and flavin mononucleotide (FMN) and as free riboflavin (Rb). In whole blood, these B_2 vitamers can be detected in plasma as well as in all blood cells. However, in normal situations FAD will be the predominant form in blood and is mainly present in the blood cells [31, 122, 123].

The analysis of FAD in whole blood (or erythrocytes) can represent a great advantage (next to the erythrocyte glutathione reductase activation test: EGR-AC) in the evaluation of the vitamin B_2 status. Especially in long-term evaluations, the level of FAD in blood may serve as a reliable indicator of the vitamin B_2 status of individuals [31, 123]. EGR is the major flavo-protein in erythrocytes using FAD as cofactor. Although the EGR-AC test is regarded as the best laboratory test for assessing vitamin B_2 nutritional status, in certain situations FAD analysis may be superior to EGR-AC. In patients with glucose-6-phosphate dehydrogenase deficiency, severe uraemia, or cirrhosis of the liver, increased EGR activity with a high degree of saturation with FAD has been reported [124]. Clinical signs of riboflavin deficiency have been seen in some cases with a deficiency of vitamin B_6, vitamin C, niacin, or iron, probably resulting from a decreased synthesis of the apoenzyme [117]. Higher activity has also been reported in iron deficiency anaemia [125].

In general, for different population groups a significant correlation has been found between FAD in blood and the basal and total EGR activities [31].

7.7.16 Principle of the method

The various forms of vitamin B_2 are extracted from whole blood (erythrocytes or any other biological fluid) using trichloroacetic acid. After adjusting the pH, the B_2 vitamers are separated by reversed-phase HPLC and detected by their native fluorescence. The individual forms are quantitated from peak area by integration using external standards.

7.7.17 Chemicals and apparatus

(a) Chemicals

Trichloroacetic acid (TCA) p.a.
Acetic acid (HAc), glacial 100% p.a.

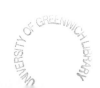

Sodium hydroxide (NaOH) p.a.

Methyl alcohol p.a.

Potassium phosphate, monobasic (KH_2PO_4) p.a.

Sodium chloride (NaCl) p.a.

Orthophosphoric acid (H_3PO_4, 85%, w/v) p.a.

Flavine adenine dinucleotide, disodium salt (FAD), e.g. Boehringer, cat. No. 104728

Riboflavin 5′-monophosphate, monosodium salt (flavin mononucleotide, FMN), e.g. Fluka, cat. No. 83810

Riboflavin (Rb), e.g. Hoffmann–La Roche

Water: quartz-bidistilled every 2–3 days.

(b) Solutions

TCA 10% (w/v): 100 g TCA dissolved in water to make up 1000 ml.

Sodium acetate buffer, pH 6.2: 160 g NaOH dissolved in 500 ml of water; thereafter, 272 g HAc is added under careful mixing and cooling. After cooling the volume is made up with water to 1000 ml.

0.9% (w/v) NaCl: 9.0 g NaCl dissolved in water to make 1000 ml.

HPLC mobile phase, pH 2.9: 0.3 M KH_2PO_4 and 20% (v/v) methyl alcohol; 40.82 g KH_2PO_4 dissolved in water to make 1000 ml and mixed with 250 ml methyl alcohol; the pH is adjusted to 2.9 using H_3PO_4.

Vitamin B_2 standard solutions for HPLC: as B_2 vitamers are light (UV) sensitive, all operations with standards, samples and extracts should be carried out under subdued light conditions.

Of each B_2 vitamer (FAD, FMN, Rb) an amount of 10 mg is dissolved in 200 ml water (stock standard). For riboflavin a temperature of about 50°C will increase its solubility. The concentrations in these solutions are determined using dilutions in 0.1 M phosphate buffer (pH 7.0) in the range 0–50 µg/ml.

From the absorption at 450 (FAD) and 445 (FMN and Rb) nm in 1 cm quartz cuvettes, the standard concentrations are calculated using the molar absorption coefficients of 11 300 (FAD) and 12 500 (FMN and Rb) (molecular weight of riboflavin = 376.4, of FMN-Na = 478.4, and of FAD-Na_2 = 829.6). However, this procedure may not be reliable for FMN, as available standards of FMN are not pure [29].

The three original solutions (10 mg/200 ml for each B_2 vitamer) are used to prepare an aqueous solution containing about 0.15 µg/ml Rb, 0.40 µg/ml FMN and 1.00 µg/ml FAD. An amount of 30 ml of this solution is diluted with 20 ml water and 90 ml 10% (w/v) TCA and the volume is adjusted with the sodium acetate buffer to 200 ml (working standard). This working standard is used as the external standard for HPLC analysis and is stored in aliquots for not more than four weeks at –20°C. After thawing an aliquot, refreezing should not be done as the vitamers will be destroyed.

(c) Apparatus

Plastic tubes (e.g. 16 × 110 mm) suitable for centrifugation; adjustable pipettes; dispensers; Vortex.

Refrigerated laboratory centrifuge.

Spectrophotometer; 1 cm quartz cuvettes.

HPLC apparatus consisting of:
  Column 125 × 4.6 mm diameter, filled with C 18 stationary phase (e.g. ODS
    Hypersil 5 μm)
  Constant-flow HPLC pump
  Automatic injector (or injection valve)
  Fluorescence detector, e.g. Shimadzu Fluorescence HPLC Monitor, model
    RF-530, provided with a xenon lamp, two monochromators, and a flow
    cell of 12 μl, the excitation wavelength is set at 462 nm, the emission
    wavelength at 520 nm
  Recorder
  Integrator.

7.7.18   Sample collection

All procedures during blood collection and sample treatment should be carried
out under subdued light conditions. The anticoagulant (citrate, EDTA or
heparin) used for collection of whole blood does not influence the procedures.

It is best, in the analysis of FAD in whole blood (or other biological material),
to use fresh samples. If storage is required, samples can be stored in the freezer
for several months. However, after thawing, a second freezing-thawing will
destroy the vitamers.

7.7.19   Procedure

(a) Sample extraction

Samples are thawed under subdued light conditions in running tap water on the
day of analysis.

While vortexing, 1.0 ml of a well-mixed sample is carefully and slowly brought
  into a plastic tube containing 3.0 ml 10% (w/v) TCA. If less than 1.0 ml
  sample is available, the volume is adjusted to 1.0 ml using 0.9% (w/v) NaCl.
The tube is left for 30–60 min in the dark at 4°C (refrigerator), with vigorously
  mixing half-way.
2.0 ml sodium acetate buffer is added and mixed thoroughly.
The tube is centrifuged for 15 min at 2000 *g* and 4°C.
The supernatant is used for HPLC analysis; if necessary, sample extracts may
  be stored in the refrigerator (not in the freezer!) for one week.

(b) Calibration

Before analysis, a few aliquots of the external standard solution are injected to
equilibrate the chromatographic system (constant peak height). In routine
analysis, each series of five sample extracts is preceded by the external standard.

The linearity of the chromatographic system is controlled every month
by a range of standard concentrations, corresponding to original levels of
0–900 nmol FAD/l whole blood.

(c) HPLC

The entire chromatographic procedure is carried out at room temperature
under subdued light conditions. 150 μl sample extract is subjected to isocratic
reversed-phase HPLC. The flow rate of the mobile phase is about 1.2 ml/min.
In general, the retention time of FAD is about 8 min, of FMN 15 min and of
Rb 20 min. In normal blood samples, the levels of FMN and Rb are quite low.
The retention times may be changed by varying the amount of methyl alcohol in

the mobile phase. The effluent of the HPLC column is passed through the fluorometer set at the wavelength couple 462/520 nm. The elution profiles are displayed on the recorder set at 10 mV full-scale and a recording speed of 2 mm/min. The recorder as well as the integrator are connected directly to the fluorometer.

(d) Calculation

The concentrations of the B_2 vitamers in the original blood sample are calculated by integration based on the peak area ratio sample/standard. In cases of failure of the integrator, peak heights are used.

By the extraction procedure described, an amount of about 6% of each B_2 vitamer is retained in the precipitate (according to results obtained with repeated extraction and determination of the water content of the precipitate using ^3H_2O, see Ref. [31]). Assuming the water content of whole blood being 85%, the equation for calculation of the FAD concentration in whole blood will be:

$$FAD \text{ (nmol/l)} = \frac{A_s \cdot C_{st} \cdot D}{A_{st}}$$

in which A_s = peak area of the sample, A_{st} = peak area of standard, C_{st} = concentration of standard in nmol/l, and D = dilution factor; for 1 ml of whole blood D is calculated according to the equation:

$$D = \frac{[0.85 + 5.00]}{[1.00 - 0.06]} = 6.22$$

7.7.20 Performance characteristics

(a) Range of linearity

Dilutions of whole blood samples (aliquots of 0.2–1.0 ml of sample made up to 1.0 ml with 0.9% (w/v) NaCl) result in comparable levels in the range up to about 500 nmol FAD/l whole blood.

(b) Detection limit

Assuming the signal-to-noise ratio to be at least 3, the HPLC method described here shows a detection limit as low as 20 nmol FAD/l, 15 nmol FMN/l, and 10 nmol Rb/l whole blood (injected amounts FAD: about 0.5 pmol = 400 pg, FMN: about 0.4 pmol = 180 pg, Rb: 0.2 pmol = 75 pg).

(c) Recovery

Recovery is determined in each series by analysis of three aliquots of pooled whole blood and 2 × 3 aliquots of the same pooled whole blood to which FAD has been added (two different levels of addition). For that purpose, FAD is dissolved in 0.9% (w/v) NaCl. To correct for volume changes, the same volume of 0.9% (w/v) NaCl is added to pooled whole blood. The concentration of FAD used is determined from the absorption of a solution in 0.1 M phosphate buffer (pH 7.0) in a 1 cm quartz cuvette at 450 nm, using the molar absorption coefficient of 11 300 [29].

Pooled whole blood and recovery samples are stored as aliquots in the dark at −20°C for a period generally not exceeding three months.

For a total of 18 series using addition of 35 and 63 nmol FAD/l pooled whole blood the average recoveries for singular analysis were $100 \pm 25\%$ and $100 \pm 14\%$ respectively.

(d) Reproducibility

In our laboratory the precision of the method is determined in each series by analysis of three aliquots of pooled whole blood. For a total of 18 series using the same pool (pool mean: 215 nmol FAD/l whole blood) the overall CV of a single sample run in an arbitrary series amounted to about 5%.

(e) Validity

The results obtained for total vitamin B_2 in whole blood by the direct fluorometric analysis of the extract or by the classical microbiological method show relatively good qualitative correlation with the FAD results obtained by the HPLC method. In principle, direct and microbiological methods result in higher levels, as the total level includes free riboflavin and its 5'-phosphate ester.

7.7.21   Reference values

Reference values are, in general, population specific. For example, the average FAD level in whole blood obtained from 206 healthy individuals (blood donors from the centre of the Netherlands) with an average age of 37 ± 11.2 years (range 18–64 years) was 280 ± 42 nmol/l [30]. The cumulative frequency distribution is given in Table 7.13. An influence of age or oral contraceptive use on the FAD level in whole blood was not observed. However, average FAD in whole blood of women was significantly ($P < 0.001$) lower than that of men by about 8%.

Table 7.13 Cumulative frequency distribution of FAD in whole blood (N = 206 volunteers)

Percentile	FAD nmol/l
Min	160
5	210
25	250
50	270
75	300
95	350
Max	450
Mean	280
SD	42

For 123 apparently healthy Dutch free-living elderly people with an average age of 72 ± 3.8 years (range 65–89 years), the average FAD level (294 ± 50 nmol/l) was not significantly different from that of the group of blood donors [31].

On the same population sample (Dutch blood donors) various indices of the riboflavin status have been assessed. The correlation coefficients are reported in Table 7.14. Significant correlations were found between basal EGR and total EGR activities and the concentration of FAD in whole blood. This is not the case for EGR-AC.

Table 7.14 Correlation matrix of indices of the riboflavin status (Pearson correlation coefficients)

Index	FAD	Basal EGR	Total EGR
FAD	1.0000		
Basal EGR	0.5065*	1.0000	
Total EGR	0.4725*	0.9076*	1.0000
EGR-AC	−0.2690	−0.5800*	−0.2012

* Significant at $P < 0.001$ (df = 204); blood samples of Dutch blood donors (men and women, 18–65 years) were used for the investigation of the indices of the riboflavin status.

7.7.22   Interpretation

Whole blood levels of FAD below 200 nmol/l most probably indicate a vitamin B_2 deficiency.

SECTION IV   RIBOFLAVIN IN URINE BY HPLC

7.7.23   Purpose and scope

The amount of riboflavin excreted in urine depends both on the amount ingested and the reserves already present in the body [4]. Correlations between riboflavin intake and urinary excretions of the vitamin have been established through carefully controlled human studies [103]. Therefore the determination of riboflavin concentration in urine is suitable for estimating recent riboflavin intake. In the case of riboflavin deficiency no substantial amounts of the vitamin are excreted. Riboflavin concentration is usually expressed as nmol riboflavin/24 h or as nmol riboflavin/mmol creatinine.

7.7.24   Principle of the method

Riboflavin is the most important flavin excreted by the body in significant amounts [126]. Without pre-processing an aliquot of the urine sample is injected into an HPLC apparatus, chromatographed, and fluorometrically detected with 445/530 nm. The method described here is based on the method of Gatautis and Naito [127] with some modifications.

7.7.25   Chemicals and apparatus

(a) Chemicals

Methanol, 99.7%, for HPLC
Acetonitrile, 99.7%, for HPLC
Riboflavin, purum
Distilled water
Water for HPLC.

(b) Solutions

Mobile phase: water/methanol (50/50 by volume), filtered and degassed with an ultrasonic apparatus.
Riboflavin stock standard (100 mg/l): add 10 mg riboflavin to 20 ml acetonitrile and dilute to 100 ml with water. Under dark conditions this standard solution is stable at 2–8°C for about four weeks.

Working standards prepared as follows:
   400 µl stock standard diluted with water to 100 ml = 40 µg/dl
   600 µl stock standard diluted with water to 100 ml = 60 µg/dl
   1000 µl stock standard diluted with water to 100 ml = 100 µg/dl
   To 500 µl of each calibration standard 500 µl methanol are added (analogous to the urine sample treatment).

(c) Apparatus

Adjustable pipettes; tubes; 2 ml autosample glass bottles; laboratory centrifuge. HPLC apparatus including:
   HPLC pump (Model 300B, Gynkotek)
   RP18 column (Hypersil, Shandon; 5 µm, 4.6 × 250 mm)
   RP18 pre-column (Bischoff, 2 cm)
   Fluorescence HPLC monitor (Model RF 530, Shimadzu)
   Integrator/Plotter (Model CR-2AX Shimadzu)
   Automatic sample injector (ASI-3 Talbot).

7.7.26 Sample collection

An aliquot of a collected 24 h urine is frozen at –20°C if analysis cannot be done within 24 h of collection of the specimen. The sample may be stored for at least three months. During urine preparation and subsequent procedures, specimen exposure to light must be kept to a minimum.

7.7.27 Procedure

(a) Sample preparation

Five hundred microlitres of a urine sample are diluted with 500 µl methanol, mixed thoroughly and centrifuged for 4 min to remove any sediment.

(b) Chromatography

A volume of 50 µl urine or working standard is injected into the chromatograph. The flow rate of the mobile phase is 1 ml/min. The plotter chart speed is set at 0.5 cm/min. Analysis can be done at room temperature. The pre-column packing should be replaced after about 100 injections.

(c) Detection

Riboflavin is then detected fluorometrically: fluorescence excitation, 445 nm; fluorescence emission, 530 nm.
   Analysis time averages about 5 min per sample.

(d) Calculation

The concentrations of riboflavin in urine samples are measured by integration of the peak area using the absolute calibration curve method with automatic baseline correction. The standard curves are used for the calculation of riboflavin concentrations. The conversion factors for SI units are:

   µg riboflavin/dl · 26.57 = nmol/l.
   µg riboflavin/24 h · 2.657 = nmol riboflavin/day.
   µg riboflavin/g creatinine · 0.3005 = nmol/mmol creatinine.

7.7.28 Performance characteristics

(a) Range of linearity

Linearity of this HPLC method was observed from 1 to 300 µg/dl.

(b) Detection limit

The detection limit of this simple, rapid, and precise quantitative procedure for measuring urinary riboflavin by HPLC is as low as 1 µg/dl (25 nmol/l).

(c) Recovery

The recovery rate is calculated by adding known amounts of riboflavin to urinary samples. The actual recovery rate was estimated to be 102 ± 3%.

(d) Reproducibility

The precision of the method is verified in a tenfold determination of a pooled urine sample. The within-day reproducibility (CV) amounted to 1.9% and day-to-day reproducibility to 2.5%.

(e) Validity

No true validity test is available at the moment.

7.7.29   Reference values

The reference values are, in general, population specific. In a random sample of healthy young men, average age 22.6 years (range 17–29 years), a mean fasting riboflavin excretion of 137 ± 108 nmol riboflavin/mmol creatinine was found. The frequency distribution is shown in Fig. 7.5. Ninety-five per cent of the values are within the range of 11–450 nmol riboflavin/mmol creatinine. Oral administration of 3.5 mg riboflavin plus the usual dietary riboflavin of about 2.3 mg results in a threefold increase in the average riboflavin excretion.

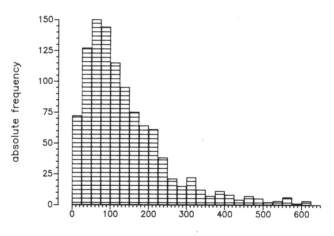

Fig. 7.5   Urinary riboflavin concentration (frequency distribution) in a sample of 1081 healthy young men.

7.8   NIACIN

SECTION I   NIACIN IN WHOLE BLOOD BY MICROBIOLOGICAL ASSAY

7.8.1   Purpose and scope

Niacin (vitamin PP or B-3, nicotinic acid and nicotinamide) is part of NAD(P), coenzymes of a number of enzymes catalysing redox reactions in which hydrogen is transferred. Niacin deficiency, which results in pellagra, still occurs in certain maize-eating populations like Yugoslavia and Egypt (bound niacin, e.g. niacytin, is biologically not available) and in those parts of India where jowar is a dietary staple [128, 129]. Furthermore, niacin deficiency would occur in association with alcoholism [130].

Niacin nutritional status may be evaluated by analysis of the vitamin and its metabolites N'-methyl-2-pyridone-5-carboxylamine and N'-methylnicotinamide (the excretion ratio being the most reliable indicator) in blood, plasma, and/or urine samples (in normal healthy individuals the ratio is within the range 1.3–4). Recently, several HPLC methods have been described. However, routine measurements of these metabolites are not yet fully evaluated [129].

At present, the microbiological assay is still a classical method to measure niacin in biological samples, although analysis of niacin or its components in blood has not proved reliable or practical [129].

The method described here uses *Lactobacillus plantarum* (ATCC 8014, formerly known as *L. arabinosus*) as the test organism and it shows comparable growth response for nicotinic acid, nicotinamide, and its coenzyme forms [131–133].

7.8.2 Principle of the method

Niacin is extracted from whole blood (plasma or any other biological fluid) by sterilization in hydrochloric acid. After pH adjustment and filtration, niacin in the extract is measured by its growth response towards *L. plantarum*.

7.8.3 Chemicals and apparatus

(a) Chemicals

Hydrochloric acid (HCl), 37% (v/v) p.a.
Sodium hydroxide (NaOH) p.a.
Sodium chloride (NaCl) p.a.
Ethyl alcohol, 96% (v/v) p.a.
Glycerol, specific weight 1.26 p.a.
Liquid nitrogen (N_2)
Antifoam emulsion, e.g. Sigma, cat. No. A-5757
Lactobacillus plantarum (ATCC 8014) from Difco, cat. No. 3211–30–3
Stock culture medium for *L. plantarum*: Bacto Lactobacilli Agar AOAC, dehydrated, Difco, cat. No. 0900–15–4
Inocula medium for *L. plantarum*: Bacto Lactobacilli Broth AOAC, dehydrated, Difco, cat. No. 0901-15-3
Assay medium for *L. plantarum*: Bacto Niacin Assay Medium, dehydrated Difco, cat. No. 0322-15-4
Niacinamide, e.g. Sigma, cat. No. N-3376; molecular weight: 122.1
Water: quartz-bidistilled every 2–3 days.

(b) Solutions

1 M HCl: 83 ml 37% (v/v) HCl made up to 1000 ml with water.
10 M NaOH: 40 g NaOH dissolved in water to make 100 ml.
2% (v/v) antifoam emulsion: 2 ml antifoam made up to 100 ml with water.
Sterile 0.85% (w/v) NaCl: 8.5 g NaCl dissolved in water to make 1000 ml and divided in glass bottles and sterilized (15 min, 121°C). The sterilized solution is stored in the refrigerator for not more than one week.
Sterile 20% (v/v) glycerol: 30 ml glycerol is mixed with 120 ml 0.85% (w/v) NaCl and sterilized (15 min, 121°C). This solution is stored in the refrigerator for not more than one week.

General information/procedures in microbiology: see Ref. [133].

Bacto Lactobacilli Agar AOAC: used for carrying stock cultures.

An amount of 48 g is suspended in 1 litre water and heated to boiling (2–3 min) to dissolve completely. The agar is divided in glass culture tubes (diameter 16–20 mm; 10 ml each), sterilized (15 min, 121°C) and stored in the refrigerator for not more than one month.

Stock cultures are prepared by stab inoculation of one or more tubes of sterile medium. Cultures are incubated for 18–24 h at 37°C, held constant at ± 0.5°C. The cultures are stored at 2–8°C. Transplants are made at monthly intervals in triplicate.

(This procedure is not necessary if *L. plantarum* is stored as described under Preparation of the inocolum, below.)

Bacto Lactobacilli Broth AOAC: used to prepare inocula.

An amount of 38 g is suspended in 1 litre water and heated to boiling (2–3 min). After preparation, the pH of the medium is adjusted to 6.75 using diluted HCl or NaOH solutions. Divided in 10 ml aliquots in glass culture tubes (diameter 16–20 mm), the culture medium is sterilized (15 min, 121°C) before use and stored in the refrigerator for not more than one week.

Bacto Niacin Assay Medium: used in the assay of niacin.

An amount of 7.5 g is suspended in 100 ml water and heated to boiling (2–3 min). A slight precipitate is dispersed by agitation. The suspension is quickly cooled in running tap water and the pH is adjusted to 6.75 using diluted HCl or NaOH solutions. The suspension is distributed in 2.5 ml amounts into test tubes. After addition of standard and test solutions, the volume is adjusted to 5 ml with water and the tubes are sterilized for 12 min at 121°C.

Preparation of the inoculum

Inocula are prepared by subculturing from the stock culture of *L. plantarum* (see above) to 10 ml of Bacto Lactobacilli Broth AOAC. After 18–20 h incubation at 37°C, 1 ml is diluted with 150 ml of the culture medium (see above). This suspension is incubated at 37°C for a period (in general at least 20 h) till the increase of the absorption measured at 660 nm in a 1 cm cuvette is not more than 0.1 absorption unit per hour. Thereafter the suspension is divided in tubes and centrifuged under aseptic conditions for 5 min at 2600 g and room temperature. The supernatant liquid is decanted and the cells are resuspended in 150 ml sterile NaCl solution and again centrifuged under aseptic conditions. The final inoculum suspension is prepared by suspending these cells in 150 ml sterile glycerol solution, followed by division in 1 ml aliquots into cryotubes and frozen in liquid nitrogen (–196°C). These samples can be stored in liquid nitrogen for years.

Standard solutions

Niacinamide (molecular weight = 122.1) is dissolved in water to obtain solutions containing 20 ng/ml and 50 ng/ml. These solutions are used to construct the standard calibration curve (see Calibration, below).

(c) Apparatus

Glass culture tubes of 50 ml (18 × 150 mm), suited for centrifugation, e.g. Gibco Europe, cat. No. 3–42110; glass bottles of 30 ml (for sample extraction); glass assay tubes (18 × 120 mm); cryotubes of 3.8 ml, e.g. Nunc, cat. No. 3–66524.

Adjustable pipettes; dispensers; Vortex; filtration paper.

Sterilization equipment (autoclave); stove (incubation cabinet); inoculum cabinet provided with UV tubelight.

Photometer provided with a 1 cm flow-through cuvette.

Hardware (e.g. glass tubes, pipettes etc) are sterilized after sealing in plastic bags by gamma-irradiation at 2.5 Mrad. After irradiation, sterility is guaranteed for about two years.

Dewar container, e.g. L'Air Liquide, cat. No. BT 40; containing about 40 litres liquid nitrogen for long-term storage of the inoculum samples of *L. plantarum* (see above). The temperature of the liquid phase is −196°C and of the gas phase −140°C.

7.8.4 Sample preparation

If storage is required, samples can be stored in the refrigerator for several months or in the freezer for much longer periods. Samples can also be stored as extracts in 1 M HCl in the freezer (see Sample extraction below).

7.8.5 Procedure

(a) Sample extraction

On the day of analysis, samples are thawed in running tap water.

An amount of 1 ml of whole blood (or 2 ml of plasma or serum or 1 ml of urine) is extracted in 15 ml 1M HCl in a 30 ml glass bottle during 20 min at 121°C.

After cooling in running tap water, the pH is adjusted to 4.5 using 10 M NaOH and the volume is made up with water to 50 ml.

The solution is filtered and adjusted to pH 6.75 using diluted HCl or NaOH solutions.

An amount of 5 ml of this filtrate is diluted with water to 25 ml (this step is not carried out for plasma, serum or urine samples).

This final extract is used in the microbiological assay (see below).

(b) Calibration

A calibration curve is prepared from the 20- and 50-ng/ml standard solutions directly into incubation tubes containing 2.5 ml of the niacin assay medium. The total volume is made up with water to 5.0 ml. The niacinamide concentrations in these tubes range from 0 to 200 ng/5 ml (8 different levels). All standard incubations are carried out in triplicate. An S-shaped curve is generally obtained when the observed absorptions are plotted against the concentrations.

Linearity hardly exists in microbiological assays. Therefore, sample extracts are assayed in duplicate and for three different volumes of the extracts (see Microbiological assay) and read from the S-shaped calibration curve.

(c) Microbiological assay

Duplicate samples of 1.0, 1.5 and 2.5 ml of the final extract are brought into tubes containing 2.5 ml of the assay medium. The volume is adjusted to 5.0 ml using water.

Glass tubes containing the standard curve and those containing the samples are sterilized (12 min at 121°C).

After cooling, each tube (with the exception of a blank) is inoculated with 100 μl diluted inoculum (about 120 µl of inoculum is diluted with 25 ml sterile 0.85% (w/v) NaCl solution).

The tubes are incubated in the stove at 37°C for a period resulting in an absorption at 660 nm (1 cm cuvette) of the tube containing the highest standard concentration (200 ng/5 ml) of about 0.6 (i.e. normally after about 18–20 h).

The content of each tube is mixed with 100 µl 2% antifoam and the absorption at 660 nm is read against the blank tube.

(d) Calculation

The concentrations of the original samples are calculated on the basis of the absorption at 660 nm using the calibration curve (see Calibration) and taking care of the proper dilution factors. (Readings from the calibration curve can be done by hand or by using a 6th degree orthogonal polynome for automatic calculations.)

7.8.6 Performance characteristics

(a) Range of linearity

A dilution of blood or urine in the range of 0.5 to 2.0 ml (made up with 0.9% (w/v) NaCl to 2.0 ml) has no effect on the observed concentration of niacin.

(b) Detection limit

Based on the calibration curve, the detection limit of the microbiological assay for a reliable analysis of niacin in whole blood is about 10 µmol/l (about 1.22 mg/l).

(c) Recovery

Recovery is determined in each series by analysis of an aliquot of pooled whole blood and an aliquot of the same pooled whole blood to which niacinamide has been added. For that purpose, niacinamide is dissolved in the NaCl solution. To correct for volume changes, the same volume of the NaCl solution is added to pooled whole blood. For 100 series the analytical recovery of 42 µmol niacin added per litre whole blood was 92 ± 5%.

Pooled whole blood and recovery samples are stored as aliquots in the dark at −20°C for a period generally not exceeding six months. Similar procedures apply to other biological samples.

(d) Reproducibility

In our laboratory the precision of the method is determined in each series by analysis of pooled whole blood (see also Detection limit above). For a total of 100 series using the same pool (pool mean: 36.3 µmol niacin per litre whole blood) the overall CV of a single sample, run in an arbitrary series amounted to 8%.

(e) Validity

The classical microbiological method for the analysis of niacin in biological fluids has not yet been validated using other methods of analysis (e.g. HPLC) [129].

7.8.7 Reference values

Reference values are, in general, population specific. For example, the average niacin level in whole blood obtained from 206 healthy volunteers (blood donors from the centre of the Netherlands) with an average age of 37 ± 11.2 years

Table 7.15 Cumulative frequency distribution of niacin in whole blood (N = 206 volunteers)

Percentile	Niacin μmol/l
Min	27.0
5	37.0
25	43.0
50	48.0
75	52.5
95	61.0
Max	80.0
Mean	48.4
SD	7.22

(range 18–64 years) was 48.4 ± 7.2 μmol/l [30]. The cumulative frequency distribution is given in Table 7.15.

For this group of volunteers the niacin level in whole blood of men was significantly (P < 0.001) higher than that of women (means 50.2 and 46.8 μmol/l respectively; SED = 0.91 μmol/l). Within the group of women a slightly lower (difference by about 6%, P < 0.05) level was found for those using oral contraceptives. No influence of age on the level of niacin in whole blood was observed.

7.8.8 Interpretation

Whole blood levels of niacin below 30 μmol/l might indicate a vitamin deficiency. This possibility is strengthened if the urinary level falls below 8 μmol/l. However, it is not known whether whole blood and urinary levels of niacin are reliable indicators of the niacin status in various conditions [129].

SECTION II   NIACIN METABOLITES IN URINE BY HPLC

7.8.9 Purpose and scope

The determination of N′-methyl nicotinamide (N′MN) and N′-methyl-2-pyridone-5-carboxamide (2-pyridone) in urine is the basis of the most widely-used of biochemical assays of niacin status. The ratio of these two substances is considered to provide an early indication of impending niacin deficiency [134] and is independent of the absolute recovery of either metabolite, so that a spot sample can be used. The assay is best achieved by high-pressure liquid chromatography, which is capable of permitting the quantitation of both substances from a single chromatographic run, using a single (standard type) UV detector and a peak integrator to measure peak ratios. The same separation is capable of yielding values for nicotinic acid and trigonelline (N′methyl nicotinic acid), if these also are required, and the procedure is far less laborious and more sensitive than older assay techniques for urinary niacin derivatives [135–141].

Trigonelline was detected in urine from rats fed a maize diet, but was totally absent from that of rats fed a casein diet. Consequently this metabolite can be considered a potentially useful indicator of the type of diet (cereal-rich vs cereal-poor), that is being ingested.

7.8.10 Principle of the method

Urine samples are mixed with isonicotinic acid internal standard (0.2 μmol/ml), extracted with chloroform, evaporated to dryness; the residue is then extracted with methanol, and aliquots are chromatographed on a 50-cm Partisil 10SCX column that is recommended for optimum separation characteristics, with a C18 reverse-phase precolumn, eluted isocratically with 15 mM potassium citrate pH 2.0 containing 5% v/v methanol. The effluent is monitored by absorption at 254 nm, the peaks being quantified by peak area using external calibration standards and corrections for inter-run recovery variations with an internal isonicotinic acid standard in each run.

7.8.11 Chemicals and apparatus

(a) Chemicals

Thymol crystals
Nicotinic acid ($C_6H_5NO_2$), e.g. Sigma, cat. No. 4126
Isonicotinic acid ($C_6H_5NO_2$), e.g. Sigma, cat. No. I1137
N′-methyl nicotinamide ($C_7H_8N_2O$), e.g. Sigma, cat. No. M4502
2-pyridone ($C_7H_8N_2O_2$): synthesized by the method of Pullman and Colowick [136] from N′-methyl nicotinamide
Chloroform ($CHCl_3$), e.g. BDH AnalaR reagents, cat. No. 10077
Methanol (CH_3OH), e.g. BDH AnalaR reagents, cat. No. 10158
Potassium citrate ($K_3C_6H_5O_7.H_2O$), e.g. BDH AnalaR reagents, cat. No. 10200
Hydrochloric acid (HCl), 37% (fuming) p.a.

(b) Solutions

Stock standard: 1 g N′-methyl nicotinamide and 1 g 2-pyridone are dissolved in water to make 1000 ml.
Working solutions: 5, 10, 25, 50, 100 μg/ml of N′-methyl nicotinamide and 2-pyridone are prepared diluting 200, 100, 40, 20, and 10 times the stock solutions (plus internal standard 0.2 μmol/ml).
Isonicotinic acid 10 mM solution (internal standard): 1.23 g isonicotinic acid are dissolved in water to make 1000 ml.
0.05 N HCl: 4.13 ml 37% HCl made up to 1000 ml with water.
Citrate buffer pH 2.0: a solution of $K_3C_6H_5O_7.H_2O$ 15 mM (4.78 g/l) is titrated with HCl 0.05 N to pH 2.0.
Citrate-methanol solution: 15 mM citrate buffer pH 2.0 containing 5% v/v methanol.

(c) Apparatus

Automatic pipette device; centrifuge; glass test tubes of various dimensions; vortex mixer; shaker for urine extraction.
HPLC apparatus comprising, e.g.:
Waters model 6000 A pump
U6K LOOP injector
Model 440 UV absorbance detector monitoring at 254 nm and 0.005 *A* full-scale deflection, with peak integrator
A Vydac-201, 33–44 μm C18 precolumn (Waters) is attached to a Partisil 10SCX main column (50 × 4.5 mm), from HPLC Technology,

Macclesfield, Cheshire, UK. Degassing can be achieved by water pump suction or sonication or helium purging; particle removal is performed by Millipore 0.45 μm filtration.

Desiccator containing silica gel and a molecular sieve, for evaporation of urine samples.

7.8.12 Procedure

(a) Sample preparation

One millilitre urine (samples preserved with thymol crystals) plus 20 μl 10 mM isonicotinic acid is extracted with 6 ml chloroform for 2 h at room temperature and is centrifuged for 30 min at 1300 *g*.

Five hundred microlitres of the upper phase is removed and is evaporated under reduced pressure in a desiccator at room temperature. The residue is extracted with 500 μl methanol for 30 s by vortex mixing.

(b) Technique

After centrifugation, 5 μl is injected directly into the HPLC system, eluted with citrate-methanol solution flowing at 2.5 ml/min.

Standard curves obtained with standard solutions provide the external calibration. The precolumn helps to remove impurities, which can become tightly bound to Partisil.

An additional aid to the maintenance of resolving power is to flush water through the column for 30 min, followed by methanol for 30 min, after 12 urine samples.

The detection is performed at the optical density of 254 nm, and 0.005 absorbance units of the full-scale deflection; then the peak areas are estimated by integration.

The throughput of the method is 10–12 samples per day (each chromatographic run takes 30 min).

(c) Calculation

$$C_u - C_{es} \cdot \frac{PA_u}{PA_{es}} \cdot \frac{PA_{is(u)}}{AA_{is(es)}}$$

where C_u = unknown concentration of the urine metabolite in the sample; C_{es} = known concentration of the urine metabolite in the calibration run; PA_u = peak area of the urine metabolite in the sample; PA_{es} = peak area of the same metabolite in the calibration run; $PA_{is(u)}$ = peak area of the internal standard in the sample; $PA_{is(es)}$ = peak area of the internal standard in the calibration run.

7.8.13 Performance characteristics

(a) Detection limit

The detection limit of the test is less than 10 ng of any of the substances studied.

(b) Recovery

The recovery of the metabolites added to urine sample is possible in the range of 81–89%.

(c) Validity

Niacin-deficient rats were shown to excrete about 15% the amount of N'-methyl nicotinamide and about 52% the amount of 2-pyridone of control animals, and the ratio of N'-methyl nicotinamide: 2-pyridone was reduced from 2.65 to 0.73. All these changes were significant at $P < 0.001$ by Student's t-test.

7.8.14 Interpretation

Proposed limits of acceptability [134, 137] are urinary 2-pyridone : N'-methyl nicotinamide ratio below 1.0, 'high risk'; above 1.0, 'medium to low risk'. Excretion of N'-methyl nicotinamide below 0.6 mg/6 h, 'medium risk'; below 0.2 mg/6 h, 'high risk'. Less than 20% of a test dose (50–200 mg nicotinamide) excreted in 24 h, 'high risk'. The first of these three indices is the least variable with age and other confounding factors.

7.8.15 Comments from the editor

More recently Shibata *et al.* [142] presented an HPLC method for simultaneous micro-determination of nicotinamide and its major metabolites, N'-methyl-2-pyridone-5-carboxamide and N'-methyl-4-pyridone-3-carboxamide. They claim that determination of the pyridones 2-py and 4-py urinary excretion can be considered the best method for assessing the niacin status of the Japanese students who were examined in this study. A wider application of the method is necessary.

7.9 VITAMIN B$_6$

Many methods have been proposed for the assessment of vitamin B$_6$ nutritional status in animals and humans.

The first method proposed for this purpose in population surveys was measurement of the xanthurenic acid excretion because vitamin B$_6$ is necessary for the conversion of tryptophan to nicotinic acid. A standardization of this method is not yet available [143].

A tryptophan load test was also performed, but, according to Coursin [144] this method does not permit diagnosis of early and severe stages of vitamin B$_6$ deficiency. It should also be interpreted with caution considering the numerous metabolic and hormonal factors involved in tryptophan metabolism.

Consequently the most appropriate methods for vitamin B$_6$ nutriture will be described here: erythrocyte aspartate transaminase activity, pyridoxal 5'-phosphate determination in plasma by radioenzymatic assay, pyridoxal 5'-phosphate determination in whole blood by HPLC, and urinary 4-pyridoxic acid determination.

SECTION I ERYTHROCYTE ASPARTATE TRANSAMINASE

7.9.1 Purpose and scope

Vitamin B$_6$ is metabolically active in humans as a coenzyme mainly in the form of pyridoxal 5'-phosphate (PLP) which is involved in most of the aminoacid metabolism reactions [145].

PLP in plasma and erythrocytes is transported by proteins, particularly albumin and haemoglobin, and its distribution between plasma and erythrocytes is controlled by competing protein binders. Very small reserves of this vitamin are present in the body. PLP bound to muscular glycogen phosphorylase represents the major vitamin body pool.

It has been reported that in B$_6$-deficient persons the activity of two particular enzymes – aspartate transaminase (EAST) and alanine transaminase (EALT) – which have PLP as the prosthetic group decreases in erythrocytes, leukocytes and serum.

The measurement of erythrocyte aspartate transaminase activity appears more sensitive than the other enzyme activity and more indicative of long-term vitamin B$_6$ nutritional status [146].

Weber *et al.* [147] were the first to propose the stimulation of erythrocyte aspartate transaminase by PLP as a test for vitamin B$_6$ nutriture. Stanulovic *et al.* [148] further improved the method.

This is a stimulation test that uses a classical kinetic pathway and measures basal enzyme activity and stimulated activity by addition of PLP. The total apoenzyme activity can be considered an estimate of coenzyme content in conditions of excess of apoenzyme, according to the following equation:

Total apo-EAST + PLP + PLP suppl = (EAST + PLP) + excess PLP.

In conditions where the total apoenzyme content is constant and independent of the vitamin B$_6$ nutritional status, the quotient

$$\frac{\text{EAST}\,(+\text{PLP})}{\text{EAST}_\text{o}} = \alpha\ \text{EAST or EAST-AC}$$

can be considered a measure of the coenzyme content of the erythrocytes [6], EAST$_\text{o}$ being the actual measured activity of the enzyme (basal activity).

7.9.2 Principle of the method

Washed erythrocytes are haemolysed with saponin, buffered, and split into two subsamples. To one sample substrate alone is added, to the other substrate and PLP. After a pre-incubation period, the enzyme reaction is started by addition of 2-oxoglutarate. The decrease of absorption is monitored for 10 min [91].

7.9.3 Chemicals and apparatus

(a) Chemicals

Citric acid p.a.
Sodium citrate, dihydrate ($C_6H_5Na_3O_7 . 2H_2O$) p.a.
D-Glucose monohydrate ($C_6H_8O_7 . H_2O$) p.a.
Sodium chloride (NaCl) p.a.
Saponin p.a.
L-Aspartic acid ($C_4H_7NO_4$), e.g. Fluka, cat. No. 11190
Triethanolamine hydrochloride ($C_6H_{15}NO_3 . HCl$), crystallized, e.g. Boehringer Mannheim, cat. No. 127426
Ethylenediamine tetra-acetic acid, disodium salt, dihydrate (EDTA-Na$_2$) p.a.
Sodium hydroxide (NaOH) concentrate p.a.
Malate dehydrogenase (MDH) suspension, e.g. Boehringer Mannheim, 1200 U/mg, cat. No. 127914
Nicotinamide adenine dinucleotide, disodium salt, (NaDH-Na$_2$) grade I 100%, e.g. Boehringer Mannheim, cat. No. 107735
Pyridoxal 5′-phosphate (PLP), e.g. Fluka, cat. No. 82870

2-Oxoglutarate crystallized, disodium salt, dihydrate ($C_5H_4O_5$-Na_2 . $2H_2O$) p.a.

(b) Solutions

ACD stabilizer: citric acid 38 mmol (7.3 g), sodium citrate 74.8 mmol (22.0 g), D glucose . H_2O 123.6 mmol (24.5 g) in water to make 1000 ml.

NaCl 0.9%.

Saponin 0.025%: 25 mg dissolved in isotonic solution to make 100 ml.

Buffer pH 7.5:

  L-Aspartic acid 250 mmol/l (33.28 g)

  Triethanolamine HCl 50 mmol/l (9.28 g)

  EDTA-Na_2 . $2H_2O$ 2.5 mmol/l (0.84 g)

    in water to make 1000 ml, the pH is adjusted to 7.5 by addition of NaOH. Store in the refrigerator.

Malate dehydrogenase, 50 µg/ml approx.: 60 U/ml prepared from MDH suspension diluted with buffer pH 7.5 (fresh daily).

NADH-Na_2, 11.2 mmol/l: 79.4 mg dissolved in buffer pH 7.5 to make 10 ml (fresh daily).

Pyridoxal 5′-phosphate, 7.5 mmol/l: 19.9 mg dissolved in buffer pH 7.5 to make 10 ml (fresh daily).

2-Oxoglutarate disodium salt, 0.2 mol/l: 0.452 g dissolved in water to make 10 ml. Store in the refrigerator.

(c) Apparatus

Automatic pipette device; centrifuge; glass test tubes of various dimensions.

Photometer with thermostated cell holder at 25°C and filter of 334 nm or monochromator set at 340 nm.

7.9.4   Sample collection

Evacuated blood collection tubes lined with sodium heparin are used and specimens of approximately 4 ml blood are immediately transferred into sterile brown glass septum ampoules of 5 ml capacity containing 0.75 ml of ACD stabilizer.

The vials can be shipped at room temperature and then stored at 4–6°C until analysed. The assays should be done within ten days of blood collection.

7.9.5   Procedure

(a) Preparation of erythrocytes

The blood is washed three times with isotonic saline. The supernatant wash solution is drawn off together with the buffy layer.

A volume of saline slightly smaller than the volume of erythrocytes is added to the sediment so that the measured haematocrit (Hct) of suspension reaches a value of approximately 0.4%.

(b) Technique

Mix 0.5 ml of the suspension of washed erythrocytes with 9.5 ml of saponin solution.

After 15 min standing at room temperature aliquots of 200 µl haemolysate are transferred into two cuvettes of 1 cm path length.

To one cuvette are added 2.0 ml of buffer pH 7.5, 50 µl of MDH solution and 50 µl of NADH solution. To the other cuvette, which measures the P5′-P stimulation, the same reagents are added, plus 20 µl of pyridoxal 5′-phosphate solution.

After incubation at 25°C for 30 min the reaction is started by the addition of 200 μl of 2-oxoglutarate solution.

The decrease of absorbance (ΔA) at 334 nm is monitored over 10 min. The final concentration of reactants are: aspartate 200 mmol/l, 2-oxoglutarate 16 mmol/l, MDH 1.0 mg/l approximately 1200 U/l, NADH 0.22 mmol/l, pyridoxal 5′-phosphate 60 μmol/l.

(c) Calculation

Straight lines are fitted to the points of the recorder diagram and their slope is used to calculate the activation coefficient

$$\alpha-\text{EAST}$$

A figure for the enzyme activity is calculated by the formula:

$$\frac{\Delta A}{\min} \cdot \frac{10^6}{6.15 \cdot 10^3} \cdot \frac{0.4}{\text{Hct}} \cdot \frac{2500}{10} = x \text{ arbitrary units}$$

where ΔA = decrease of absorbance; min = time of measuring; $6.15 \cdot 10^3$ = molar extinction of NADH at 334 nm; Hct = haematocrit of erythrocyte suspension; 2500 = final volume in μl; 10 = volume of erythrocyte suspension in μl.

The figure represents the enzyme activity contained in 1 litre of erythrocyte suspension of haematocrit 0.4 transforming x μmol of substrate per min at 25°C.

(d) Automation

This method has now been automated in a few laboratories. The most recent one, the COBAS-BIO, realized at Hoffmann–La Roche, is less time-consuming and requires fewer personnel.

7.9.6 Performance characteristics

(a) Range of linearity

This is 4–40 μkat/l (Hct 1.0).

(b) Reproducibility

As the stimulation tests are not amenable to standardization or to recovery experiments, the only way to check the process of *in vitro* coenzyme stimulation for consistency and reproducibility is by using reference samples. These are prepared from pools of washed erythrocytes which are divided into small aliquots and stored frozen at −80°C. Haemolysates are not stable under these conditions. Erythrocyte pools showing too low stimulation values may be adjusted by admixture of erythrocytes from dog or bovine blood, which usually show high stimulation. The coefficient of variation for enzyme activity without the addition of PLP (EAST_o) is ± 5.2% for within-day analysis (mean value 13.1 μkat/l on six blood collections determined in duplicate) and ± 2.7% for day-to-day analysis (mean value 12.6 μkat/l).

The corresponding values for α-EAST are ± 3.0% (mean value 1.78) and ± 2.1% (mean value 1.78).

The precision of the characteristic, the ratio coefficient, compares favourably with the corresponding figures for basal and stimulated activity. As the value of α is affected by the variance of two assays of reaction rate, one might expect it to be less precise than the values for basal or stimulated activity. In fact the scatter of the latter figures reflects the reproducibility of the haemolysis step which, together with the haematocrit determination, introduces a great part of the overall variance. The coefficient, on the other hand, is calculated on the basis of two reaction rates measured in the same haemolysate. Their ratio is unaltered irrespective of a variable recovery of enzyme activity in different haemolysates of the same blood specimen, since both rates are affected in the same proportion. This feature probably constitutes the main advantage of the stimulation parameter over the basal activity, which also depends on the vitamin status.

Despite this advantage, there is also a serious drawback: reference standards for checking the process of stimulation, e.g. stable apoenzymes of known content, are not available. Standardization of the stimulation effect is therefore difficult. The reference samples prepared from erythrocyte pools allow detection of gross variations but do not protect against slow drifts over longer time periods.

(c) Validity

No true validity test is available at the moment.

7.9.7   Reference values

The reference values are, in general, population specific. The average $EAST_o$ level of 150 adult blood donors of both sexes from Basel (Red Cross Centre) was 12.62 μkat/l [91]. The cumulative frequency distribution is given in Table 7.16. The average α-EAST level of the same group of individuals was 1.77. The cumulative frequency distribution is given in Table 7.17.

Table 7.16 Cumulative frequency distribution of $EAST_o$ (N = 150 blood donors)

Percentile	μkat/l(Hct 1.0)
Min	6.42
5	8.42
25	10.79
50	11.85
75	13.98
95	18.92
Max	25.46
Mean	12.62
SD	3.08

7.9.8   Interpretation

Many conditions can influence the vitamin B_6 status and subsequently the coenzyme stimulation of erythrocyte aspartate transaminase activity. Among these some diseases should be considered: renal and liver diseases, cancers, coeliac disease; stress, a diet with high levels of proteins, thiamin status, and finally drugs (isoniazide, penicillamine, semicarbazide, amphetamine, chlorpromazine, various anticonvulsants, oral contraceptive agents, etc.).

Table 7.17 Cumulative frequency distribution of α-EAST (N = 150 blood donors)

Percentile	α-EAST
Min	1.23
5	1.42
25	1.65
50	1.76
75	1.91
95	2.05
Max	2.21
Mean	1.77
SD	0.195

In supplementation studies it has been observed that large doses of vitamin B$_6$ lead to an increased enzyme protein synthesis; however, we have no explanation for this phenomenon at the moment.

In addition, in people who usually drink alcoholic beverages, the α values are low notwithstanding the vitamin B$_6$ deficiency.

Biochemical evidence of vitamin B$_6$ malnutrition has also been reported in the elderly and during pregnancy.

SECTION II PYRIDOXAL 5′-PHOSPHATE (PLP) IN WHOLE BLOOD BY HPLC

7.9.9 Purpose and scope

Vitamin B$_6$ may be present in tissues and biological fluids as its cofactors pyridoxal 5′-phosphate (PLP) and pyridoxamine 5′-phosphate (PMP), as pyridoxine 5′-phosphate (PNP), and as free pyridoxal, pyridoxamine, and pyridoxine [149]. In whole blood, these B$_6$ vitamers may be detected in plasma as well as in all blood cells. However, in normal situations PLP will be the predominant form in blood and about 60% is present within the blood cells [31, 149, 150].

A high number of enzymes (especially those in the metabolism of proteins) use PLP as cofactor. However, several PLP-enzymes show a high sensitivity to hormones and drugs. This may result in alterations in the distribution of the vitamin between tissues and between its numerous biochemical functions within a tissue. This partly explains the relative ease with which the results of the tryptophan load test (excretion of xanthurenic acid) are changed (e.g. in women using oral contraceptives) [151, 152].

The transaminase *in-vitro* activation tests (EAST-AC and EALT-AC) are often used in the assessment of the vitamin B$_6$ status [149, 151, 152]. However, cut-off levels for vitamin B$_6$ adequacy are still a matter of controversy. Plasma and whole blood PLP levels may indicate a depletion of vitamin B$_6$ reserves, as a good correlation has been observed between plasma PLP and tissue PLP levels in rats [153]. Therefore, PLP in plasma may serve as a good indicator of the circulating vitamin B$_6$ available to the tissues, and PLP analysis seems to be more reliable than both enzyme activation tests [154].

For determination of PLP both HPLC and (radio-)enzymatic (REA) methods are available. For determination in whole blood samples HPLC is the method of choice; for plasma the REA method is more suitable due to its higher sensitivity.

7.9.10 Principle of the method

PLP and PL are extracted from whole blood (plasma or any other biological fluid) using trichloroacetic acid. After conversion to their semicarbazones, these derivatives are separated by reversed-phase HPLC and detected by fluorescence. The individual forms are quantitated from peak area by integration using external standards.

7.9.11 Chemicals and apparatus

(a) Chemicals

Trichloroacetic acid (TCA) p.a.
Semicarbazide p.a.
Sodium hydroxide (NaOH) p.a.
Methyl alcohol p.a.
Potassium phosphate, monobasic (KH_2PO_4) p.a.
Sodium chloride (NaCl) p.a.
Ortho phosphoric acid (H_3PO_4, 85%, w/v) p.a.
Pyridoxal 5'-phosphoric acid, monohydrate ($PLP.H_2O$), e.g. Merck, cat. No. 7526
Pyridoxal hydrochloride (PL.HCl), e.g. Sigma, cat. No. P 9310
Water: quartz-bidistilled every 2–3 days.

(b) Solutions

TCA 5% (w/v): 50 g TCA dissolved in water to make 1000 ml.
Semicarbazide 0.5 M: 2.79 g dissolved in water to make 50 ml, prepared weekly.
NaOH 6% (w/v): 6 g NaOH dissolved in water to make 100 ml.
NaOH 0.1 M: 4 g NaOH dissolved in water to make 1000 ml.
0.9% (w/v) NaCl: 9.0 g NaCl dissolved in water to make 1000 ml.
HPLC mobile phase, pH 2.90: 0.05 M KH_2PO_4 and 2.5% (v/v) methyl alcohol. 6.8 g KH_2PO_4 dissolved in water to make 1000 ml and mixed with 25 ml methyl alcohol; the pH is adjusted to 2.90 using H_3PO_4.
Vitamin B_6 standard solution for HPLC: as B_6 vitamers are sensitive to intensive (UV) light, all operations with standards are carried out under subdued light conditions. PLP (and, if necessary, PL) is dissolved in 0.1 M NaOH. The concentration of PLP (and PL) is determined using dilutions in 0.1 M NaOH in the range 0–5 µg/ml. From the absorption at 388 nm (PLP) and 393 nm (PL) in 1-cm quartz cuvettes, the standard concentrations are calculated using the molar absorption coefficients of 6 550 (PLP) and 1700 (PL) (molecular weight of $PLP.H_2O$ is 265.2 and of PL.HCl is 203.6) (Ref. [29]).
   Equal volumes of the PLP and PL solutions are mixed and diluted with 5% (w/v) TCA to about 10 nmol/l. This solution is used as the external standard and stored in aliquots for not more than four weeks at –20°C. Before analysis, PLP and PL in this solution are converted to their semicarbazones as described under sample extraction below.

(c) Apparatus

Plastic tubes (e.g. 16 × 110 mm), suitable for centrifugation; adjustable pipettes; dispensers; Vortex.

Refrigerated laboratory centrifuge; water-bath.

Spectrophotometer; 1-cm quartz cuvettes.

HPLC apparatus consisting of:

Column 125 × 4.6 mm diameter, filled with C 18 stationary phase (e.g. ODS Hypersil 5 µm)

Constant-flow HPLC pump

Automatic injector (or injection valve)

Fluorescence detector, e.g. Kratos Fluoromat filter fluorometer, model FS 950, provided with light source FSA 110 (365 nm, blue filtered), excitation band filter FSA 403 (365 nm), emission cut-off filter FSA 428 (470 nm), and a flow cell of 28 µl.

Reagent pump

Reaction coil 1 m × 1 mm diameter

Recorder

Integrator.

7.9.12 Sample collection

It is best, in the analysis of PLP in whole blood (or other biological material), to use fresh samples. If storage is required, samples can be stored in the freezer for several months.

The anticoagulant (citrate, EDTA, or heparin) used for collection of whole blood does not influence the procedures.

7.9.13 Procedure

(a) Sample extraction

Frozen samples are thawed under subdued light conditions in running tap water at the day of analysis.

While vortexing, 1.0 ml of a well-mixed sample is carefully and slowly brought into a plastic tube containing 5.0 ml 6% (w/v) TCA. If less than 1.0 ml sample is available, the volume is adjusted to 1.0 ml using 0.9% (w/v) NaCl.

The tube is left for 30–60 min in the dark at 4°C (refrigerator), with vigorously mixing half-way.

The tube is centrifuged for 15 min at 2000 *g* and 4°C.

2.0 ml of the supernatant is brought into a plastic tube containing 0.1 ml 0.5 M semicarbazide. The tube is incubated for 15 min in a water-bath at 45°C (the external standard solution is treated likewise).

This solution is used for HPLC analysis. (If necessary, sample extracts may be stored in the refrigerator for at least one week.)

(b) Calibration

Before analysis, a few aliquots of the derivatized external standard solution are injected to equilibrate the chromatographic system (constant peak height). In routine analysis, each series of five sample extracts is preceded by the external standard.

The linearity of the chromatographic system is controlled every month by a range of standard concentrations, corresponding to original levels of 0–250 nmol PL(P) per litre whole blood.

(c) HPLC

The entire chromatographic procedure is carried out at room temperature. 100 µl sample extract is subjected to isocratic reversed-phase HPLC. The flow rate of the mobile phase is about 1.1 ml/min. In general, the retention time of PLP is about 8 min and of PL 11 min. In normal blood and plasma samples, the level of PL is quite low. The retention times may be changed by varying pH and/or the amount of methyl alcohol in the mobile phase. The effluent of the HPLC column is passed through the fluorometer and the elution profiles are displayed on the recorder set at 10 mV full-scale and a recording speed of 2 mm/min. The recorder as well as the integrator are connected directly to the fluorometer.

(d) Calculation

The concentration of PL(P) in the original sample is calculated by integration based on the peak area ratio sample/standard. In cases of failure of the integrator, peak heights are used.

By the extraction procedure described, an amount of about 12% of PL(P) is retained in the precipitate (results obtained with repeated extraction and determination of the water content of the precipitate using ^3H_2O, see Ref. [149]). Assuming the water content of whole blood being 85%, for plasma 95% and erythrocytes 71%, the dilution factor D of the original sample is:

$$D = \frac{[0.85 + 5.00]}{[1.00 - 0.12]} = 6.65 \text{ for whole blood;}$$

while for plasma and erythrocytes, these factors are 6.76 and 6.49, respectively and the equation for the calculation of the PL(P) concentration in whole blood is:

$$PL(P) \text{ (nmol/l)} = \frac{A_s \cdot C_{st} \cdot D}{A_{st}}$$

in which A_s = peak area of the sample, A_{st} = peak area of standard, C_{st} = concentration of standard in nmol/l, and D = dilution factor.

7.9.14 Performance characteristics

(a) Range of linearity

The HPLC method can be applied with reliable results to the analysis of sample aliquots of less than 1.0 ml and made up to 1.0 ml using 0.9% (w/v) NaCl. In that case the equations used in the calculation (see above) should be corrected on the basis of the sample volume used for analysis.

(b) Detection limit

Assuming the signal-to-noise ratio should be at least 3, the HPLC method described here shows a detection limit as low as 2 nmol PL(P) per litre whole blood or plasma (injected amounts PL(P): about 0.2 pmol = 40–55 pg).

(c) Recovery

Recovery is determined in each series by analysis of three aliquots of pooled whole blood and 2 × 3 aliquots of the same pooled whole blood to which PLP has been added (two different levels of addition). For that purpose PLP is dissolved in 0.9% (w/v) NaCl. To correct for volume changes, the same volume of 0.9% (w/v) NaCl is added to pooled whole blood. The concentration of PLP used is determined from the absorption of a solution in 0.1 M NaOH in a 1-cm quartz cuvette at 388 nm, using the molar absorption coefficient of 6 550 [29]. Pooled whole blood and recovery samples are stored as aliquots in the dark at −20°C for a period generally not exceeding three months.

For a total of 68 series using additions of 36 and 65 nmol PLP per litre whole blood, the average recoveries for singular analysis were $99 \pm 15\%$ and $98 \pm 9\%$ respectively.

(d) Reproducibility

In our laboratory the precision of the method is determined in each series by analysis of three aliquots of pooled whole blood. For a total of 68 series using the same pool (pool mean: 49 nmol PLP per litre whole blood) the overall CV of a single sample, run in an arbitrary series amounted to about 8%.

(e) Validity

A good correlation has been obtained between the PLP levels in plasma analysed by the HPLC method and those analysed by the radioenzymatic method using tyrosine decarboxylase apoenzyme (see next section).

7.9.15   Reference values

Reference values are, in general, population specific. For example, the average PLP level for 207 healthy volunteers (blood donors from the centre of the Netherlands) with an average age of 37 ± 11.2 years (range 18–64 years), was 65 ± 19 nmol/l whole blood [30]. The cumulative frequency distribution is given in Table 7.18.

Table 7.18 Cumulative frequency distribution of PLP in whole blood (N = 207 volunteers)

Percentile	PLP nmol/l
Min	15.0
5	39.4
25	52.8
50	62.0
75	74.0
95	98.0
Max	165.0
Mean	65.1
SD	19.2

For this group of volunteers, whole blood PLP decreased significantly ($P < 0.005$) with age, and levels in women were significantly lower (by about 10%, $P < 0.005$) than those in men. Oral contraceptive use did not influence the whole blood PLP level.

For 123 apparently Dutch free-living elderly people with an average age of 72 ± 3.8 years (range 65–89 years) [31], the average whole blood PLP level (53 ± 18 nmol/l) was significantly lower (by 15%, $P < 0.01$) than that of the group of blood donors.

On the same population sample (Dutch blood donors) various indices of vitamin B_6 status have been assessed. The correlation coefficients are reported in Table 7.19. Significant correlations were found between basal EAST and total EAST activities and the concentration of PLP in whole blood. This is not the case for EAST-AC.

Table 7.19 Correlation matrix of indices of the vitamin B_6 status (Pearson correlation coefficients)

Index	PLP			EAST	
	Blood	Plasma	RBC	Basal	Total
PLP					
blood	1.0000				
plasma	0.6889*	1.0000			
RBC	0.7561*	0.0621	1.0000		
Basal EAST	0.4120*	0.1823	0.3912*	1.0000	
Total EAST	0.2993	0.0387	0.3581*	0.7981*	1.0000
EAST-AC	−0.2222	−0.2571	−0.0837	−0.3800*	−0.2382

* Significant at P <0.001 (df=205); blood donors (men and women, 18–65 years) were used for the investigation of the indices of the vitamin B_6 status. (RBC = red blood cells).

7.9.16 Interpretation

Levels of PLP in whole blood below 20 nmol/l are generally considered as deficient. Hormonal effects may strongly affect the PLP level especially in plasma, but do not indicate a deficiency.

SECTION III PYRIDOXAL 5′-PHOSPHATE IN PLASMA BY RADIOENZYMATIC ASSAY USING TYROSINE DECARBOXYLASE APOENZYME

7.9.17 Purpose and scope

Vitamin B_6 may be present in tissues and biological fluids as its cofactors pyridoxal 5′-phosphate (PLP), and pyridoxamine 5′-phosphate (PMP). Furthermore, the vitamin can be present as pyridoxine 5′-phosphate (PNP), and as free pyridoxal, pyridoxamine, and pyridoxine [149]. In whole blood, these B_6 vitamers may be detected in plasma as well as in blood cells. However, in normal situations PLP will be the predominant form in blood and about 60% is present within the blood cells [31, 149, 150].

A high number of enzymes (especially those in the metabolism of proteins) use PLP as cofactor. However, several PLP enzymes show a high sensitivity to hormones and drugs. This may result in alterations in the distribution of the vitamin between tissues and between its numerous biochemical functions within a tissue. This partly explains the relative ease with which the results of the tryptophan load test (excretion of xanthurenic acid) are changed (e.g. in women using oral contraceptives) [151, 152].

The transaminase *in-vitro* activation tests (EAST-AC and EALT-AC) are often used in the assessment of the vitamin B_6 status [149, 151, 152]. However, cut-off levels for vitamin B_6 adequacy are still a matter of controversy. Plasma PLP levels may indicate a depletion of vitamin B_6 reserves, as a good correlation has been observed between plasma PLP and tissue PLP levels in rats [153]. Therefore, PLP in plasma may serve as a good indicator of the circulating vitamin B$_6$ available to the tissues, and PLP analysis seems to be more reliable than both enzyme activation tests [154].

Enzymatic assays for plasma PLP yield more uniform results or are more sensitive than other methods of analysis, including microbiological assays and HPLC techniques [155].

7.9.18 Principle of the method

The assay for plasma PLP is based on the coenzyme-dependent decarboxylation of tyrosine catalysed by L-tyrosine decarboxylase (LTD) [156, 157]. After deproteinization of the plasma sample, PLP is pre-incubated with the LTD apoenzyme. The amount of holoenzyme formed depends on the amount of PLP present in the plasma sample. The enzyme reaction is monitored by the use of L-[1-^{14}C]-tyrosine as the substrate, and measuring the amount of residual L-[1-^{14}C]-tyrosine after incubation, or trapping of $^{14}CO_2$ generated during the reaction.

7.9.19 Chemicals and apparatus

(a) Chemicals

L-tyrosine, e.g. Merck, cat. No. 8371
Pyridoxal 5′-phosphate.H$_2$O (PLP), e.g. Merck, cat. No. 7526
Sodium EDTA.2H$_2$O p.a.
Trichloroacetic acid (TCA) p.a.
Diethylether p.a.
Citric acid.H$_2$O p.a.
Sodium citrate.2H$_2$O p.a.
Tyrosine decarboxylase apoenzyme (TYDAPO), Sigma, cat. No. T 4629
L-[1-^{14}C]-tyrosine, S.A. 40–60 mCi/mmol, e.g. NEN, cat. No. NEC-170
Scintillation fluid, e.g. Atomlight, NEN, cat. No. NEF-968
Water, quartz-bidistilled every 2–3 days
Hydrochloric acid (HCl) p.a.

(b) Solutions

0.1 M Citrate buffer pH 6.0: 5.25 g citric acid.H$_2$O dissolved in water to make 250 ml. Dissolve 29.41 g sodium citrate.2H$_2$O and 2.5 g EDTA in 1000 ml water. Mix both solutions until pH is 6.0.
6 M HCl: Mix one volume water with one of volume of concentrated HCl (37%) (Be careful, add concentrated HCL to water; wear safety glasses).
5% (w/v) TCA: 5 g TCA dissolved in water to make 100 ml (be careful; wear gloves).
Enzyme solution:
L-tyrosine decarboxylase (LTD) suspension: Suspend about 50 U LTD in about 50 ml citrate buffer. Mix this suspension for about 1 h on a magnetic stirrer (prepare fresh).

Note 5.
One unit is the amount of enzyme that catalyses the decarboxylation of 1 μmol tyrosine per min in the presence of excess PLP. In our experience it is not necessary to purify the apoenzyme. However, every new batch of

apoenzyme is checked for the presence of contaminating endogenous PLP and pyridoxal kinase activity by evaluating the slope of the standard curve, blank value, and incubation studies with excess pyridoxal, respectively.

PLP standard solution:
Stock standard (10μg/ml): 100 mg PLP.H_2O is dissolved in water to make 100 ml. 1 ml of the stock solution is made up to 100 ml. This stock solution is calibrated by measuring the absorbance of the stock in 0.1 M NaOH at 388 nm ($\varepsilon = 6600$ cm^{-1}M^{-1}; $E_{1\%, 1 \text{ cm}}^{388 \text{ nm}} = 249$).
Working standard (5 ng/ml): 25 μl of the stock standard is made up to 50 ml with 0.1 M citrate buffer pH 6.0 (prepare fresh).

Tracer solution:
L-[1-^{14}C]-tyrosine solution: 130 mg L-tyrosine is dissolved in 250 ml citrate buffer by slightly heating to about 60°C. After cooling to room temperature, add 50 μl L-[1-^{14}C]-tyrosine. This solution, with radioactivity of ± 15 000 c.p.m./250 μl, is stored at 4°C. In case some precipitation occurs during storage, the solution is slightly heated until a clear solution is obtained (before using, the solution is cooled to room temperature).

(c) Apparatus

Microlitre pipettes, 0–50 μl; 200–1000 μl (e.g. Eppendorf, Finn repetitive pipettes).
(Refrigerated) centrifuge.
Spectrophotometer.
Borosilicate tubes, 13 × 100 mm.
Counting vials, e.g. 6-ml polypropylene minivials (Baker).
Multi-vortex type mixer.
Thermostated shaking water bath (37°C).
Liquid scintillation counter.

7.9.20 Sample collection

EDTA plasma samples should be prepared by centrifuging the blood samples. Plasma samples should be protected from light and stored in the freezer (–20°C) as soon as possible. Under these conditions samples can be stored for at least six months. Serum or heparinized plasma is not suitable due to inhibition of the tyrosine decarboxylase enzyme.

7.9.21 Procedure

(a) Sample extraction

Frozen samples are thawed under subdued light conditions in running tap water on the day of analysis.

Aliquots of 200 μl unknown and control plasma are transferred in duplicate to borosilicate test tubes.
While vortexing, add 800 μl 5% TCA and centrifuge the tubes for 20 min at 2000 *g* and 4°C.
Transfer the supernatant to another tube and extract three times with 2 ml diethylether (pre-saturated with water). The ether is aspirated using a suction device and after the final (third) extraction the sample is placed in a

water-bath (37°C) to evaporate residual ether traces (this step is performed in a fume hood).

(b) Enzymatic assay

The enzymatic assay is performed in a fume hood in plastic counting vials, placed in a shaking water-bath (37°C).

Add 0, 50, 100, 150, 200, 250, and 300 μl respectively of the PLP working solution in duplicate to 6-ml counting vials.
Add 200 μl of the TCA extract in duplicate to 6 ml counting vials.
Adjust the volume to 500 μl in all tubes using citrate buffer.
Add 200 μl LTD apoenzyme suspension and incubate for 45 min at 37°C.
Add 250 μl L-[1-^{14}C]-tyrosine to all tubes and incubate again for exactly 30 min at 37°C.
The reaction is stopped after exactly 30 min by the addition of 50 μl 6 M HCl. During addition of the HCl the air above the water-bath is sucked off using a hood connected with a peristaltic pump. The air is led through a solution containing 3 M KOH to trap the generated $^{14}CO_2$. After 30 min scintillator fluid is added to all vials and the radioactivity is counted in a liquid scintillation counter.

Note 6.
Alternatively, capped reaction tubes can be used with a suspended plastic centre well containing a small paper strip wetted with hyamine hydroxide to trap the generated radioactive CO_2 after injection of HCl through the stopper to terminate the reaction.

(c) Calculation

The absolute PLP content in the tube can be read from the standard curve. The plasma PLP concentration is calculated using the following formula:

$$\text{Plasma PLP (nmol/l)} = A \cdot \frac{1000}{B} \cdot \frac{1000}{C \cdot 1.05} \cdot \frac{1000}{265.2}$$

where A = ng PLP.H$_2$O read from the standard curve, B = amount (in μl) TCA extract used in the enzymatic assay, and C = amount (in μl) plasma used for TCA extraction (usually 200 μl).
N.B.: 1.05 is a correction factor to adjust for the volume effect due to deproteinization with TCA.

7.9.22 Performance characteristics

(a) Range of linearity

Within the range of the standard curve good parallelism was established after serial sample dilution. TCA extracts of samples with concentrations outside the standard range should be appropriately diluted with buffer.

(b) Detection limit

The detection limit, defined as the amount of PLP giving a significant difference in c.p.m. from the '0' standard amounts to 0.1 ng PLP.H$_2$O, corresponding to a plasma concentration of 10 nmol/l, when 200 μl plasma is used in the assay.

(c) Recovery

In standard addition experiments, recoveries > 90% were obtained.

(d) Reproducibility

In our laboratory the precision of the method is determined in each series by analysis of three aliquots of pooled human serum. The within-assay coefficient of variation (CV) is about 1–3%, between-assay CV 5–8% (average pool level: 32, 53, and 106 nmol/l serum, respectively).

(e) Validity

A good correlation has been obtained between the PLP levels in plasma obtained by the HPLC method (see previous section) and the radioenzymatic method (see also Ref. [155]).

7.9.23 Reference values

Reference values are, in general, population specific. For example the average plasma PLP level for 207 healthy volunteers (blood donors from the centre of the Netherlands) with an average age of 37 ± 11.2 years (range 18–64 years) was 48 ± 22.5 nmol/l plasma. The cumulative frequency distribution is given in Table 7.20.

Table 7.20 Cumulative frequency distribution of plasma PLP (N = 207 volunteers)

Percentile	Plasma PLP (nmol/l)
Min	15
5	21
30	32
50	43
75	59
95	86
Max	165
Mean	48
SD	22.5

Significant effects of gender $P < 0.005$) and age ($P < 0.005$) were observed for plasma PLP. Males have slightly higher values, while PLP decreases with age for men as well as for women [30]. During pregnancy plasma PLP levels are usually lower as compared to non-pregnant controls [158].

7.9.24 Interpretation

Levels below 15 nmol/l are generally considered as deficient.

SECTION IV   4-PYRIDOXIC ACID IN URINE BY HPLC

7.9.25 Purpose and scope

The main urinary metabolite of vitamin B_6 is 4-pyridoxic acid (4-PA). The 4-PA excretion decreases markedly during periods of vitamin B_6 deficiency. Therefore 4-PA excretion in urine is used to assess vitamin B_6 status. This section describes a simple and rapid method for a quantitative determination of urinary 4-PA using reversed-phase chromatographic separation and fluorescence detection.

7.9.26 Principle of the method

This HPLC method, developed by Gregory and Kirk [159], is based on the reversible association of 4-PA with a reversed-phase octadecylsilica column and subsequent fluorimetric detection at 320/415 nm.

7.9.27 Chemicals and apparatus

(a) Chemicals

Phosphoric acid (H_3PO_4), 85% p.a.
Methanol, 99.7% for HPLC
Potassium hydroxide (KOH) p.a.
Sulphuric acid (H_2SO_4), 96% p.a.
Trichloroacetic acid p.a.
4-Pyridoxic acid, purum.
Distilled and bidistilled water.

(b) Solutions

H_3PO_4 0.033 mol/l: 2.2 ml 85% H_3PO_4 made up to 1000 ml with water.
6 N KOH: 336.6 g KOH dissolved in water to make 1000 ml.
0.5 N H_2SO_4: 13.75 ml 96% H_2SO_4 made up to 1000 ml with water.
Trichloroacetic acid, 1.22 mol/l (20% w/v).
Mobile-phase buffer 0.033 mol/l H_3PO_4 + 5% methanol: a mixture of 100 ml methanol and 4.6 ml 85% phosphoric acid is diluted with 1700 ml water and adjusted with 6 N KOH to a pH of 2.2. This solution is diluted with distilled water to a final volume of 2000 ml with subsequent filtration and degassing with an ultrasonic apparatus.
4-Pyridoxic acid stock standard: prepared by dissolving 0.02 g 4-PA in 1000 ml bidistilled water.
Working standards prepared as follows:
5 ml stock standard are diluted with bidistilled water to 100 ml = 100 µg/100 ml.
10 ml stock standard are diluted with bidistilled water to 100 ml = 200 µg/100 ml.
25 ml stock standard are diluted with bidistilled water to 100 ml = 500 µg/100 ml.
To 90 ml of each working standard 10 ml 0.5 N H_2SO_4 are added (as for sample preparation).

(c) Apparatus

Adjustable pipettes; Eppendorf centrifuge; test tubes of various dimensions, including centrifuge Eppendorf vials.
HPLC apparatus including:
HPLC pump (Model 300B, Gynkotek)
Reversed-phase octadecylsilica column (5 µm, 4.6 × 250 mm)
Fluorescence HPLC monitor (Model RF 530, Shimadzu)
Integrator Plotter CR-2 AX (Shimadzu).

7.9.28 Sample collection

After collecting a 24-h urine sample and measuring the volume or drawing a fasting sample, an aliquot of 1.8 ml is diluted with 0.2 ml 0.5 N H_2SO_4 and frozen at −20°C. The sample may be stored for at least three months.

7.9.29 Procedure

(a) Sample preparation

Two hundred microlitres 20% TCA are added to 400 µl frozen urine sample and mixed thoroughly. After centrifuging for 5 min the supernatant is removed for analysis and kept in an ice bath until detection.

(b) Chromatography

The flow rate of the mobile phase was 2 ml/min. The plotter chart speed was set at 2 cm/min. Analysis is at room temperature. A volume of 50 µl was injected and chromatographed.

(c) Detection

4-PA is detected fluorometrically:
Fluorescence excitation: 320 nm;
Fluorescence emission: 415 nm;
Analysis time averages about 6 min per sample.

(d) Calculation

The concentrations of 4-PA in urine samples are calculated by integration of the peak area with an absolute calibration curve method and automatic baseline correction. The conversion factors for SI units are:

$$\mu g \ 4\text{-PA/dl} \cdot 54.6 = \text{nmol/l}$$
$$\mu g \ 4\text{-PA/24 h} \cdot 5.46 = \text{nmol/day}$$
$$\mu g \ 4\text{-PA/g creatinine} \cdot 0.6175 = \text{nmol 4-PA/mmol creatinine.}$$

7.9.30 Performance characteristics

(a) Range of linearity

Linearity of the described method was observed from 20 to 6000 µg/dl.

(b) Detection limit

The detection limit of the method described here is as low as 20 µg/dl (1 µmol/l).

(c) Recovery

The recovery rate is performed by adding known amounts of 4-pyridoxic acid to urinary samples. The actual recovery was estimated to be 103.1 ± 1.3%.

(d) Reproducibility

The precision of the method is verified by a tenfold determination of a pooled urine sample. The CV amounted to 1.9% in a continued series and to 2.5% in the day-to-day determination.

(e) Validity

No true validity test is available at the moment.

7.9.31 Reference values

The reference values are population specific. For example, in a random sample of healthy young men, average age of 22.6 years (range 17–29 years) a mean fasting 4-PA excretion of 340 ± 135 nmol 4-PA/mmol creatinine was found. The frequency distribution is shown in Fig. 7.6; 95% of the values are within the range 128–680 nmol 4-PA/mmol creatinine. Oral administration of 4.5 mg pyridoxine plus the usual dietary vitamin B_6 of about 2.1 mg results in a three-fold increase of the average 4-PA excretion.

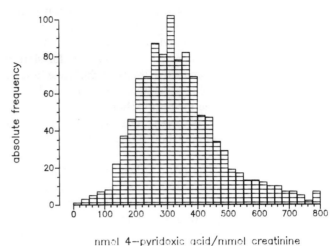

nmol 4−pyridoxic acid/mmol creatinine

Fig. 7.6   Urinary 4-pyridoxic acid concentration (frequency distribution) in a sample of 1081 healthy young men.

7.10   FOLIC ACID (5-Me-THF) IN SERUM AND ERYTHROCYTES BY RADIOASSAY

7.10.1   Purpose and scope

The measurement of folate concentrations in blood is of importance in establishing the aetiology of megaloblastic anaemias and assessing nutritional status. Deficiency of circulating folic acid levels is often observed during pregnancy, in alcoholics and in people eating diets without fresh fruits and vegetables.

To verify folic acid deficiency, it is also advisable to assay for RBC folic acid since RBC folate represents the real body stores and is less indicative of recent food intake than serum folate [160].

Until fifteen years ago serum and red cell folate levels were assayed by microbiological methods, which have several disadvantages. The techniques are tedious and require a degree of skill that limits their use in most laboratories. In addition antibiotics and antimetabolites interfere with the growth of the assay organism, and therefore the microbiological assay gives false results if the serum contains a high level of certain antibiotics or antifolates.

In 1971 Waxman *et al.* [161] reported a radioisotopic method for measuring serum folate. Since then many reports modifying this technique have appeared [162–164]. The radioassay is rapid, sensitive, and reproducible. Several authors have reported good statistical correlations between the microbiological and radioisotopic method for estimating serum folates [161, 163, 164], but when the red cell folate results were compared with the clinical and other laboratory findings the radioassay was more closely related to the folate status of the patients [165].

A higher response of folate polyglutamates than folate monoglutamates in the radioassay procedure makes this technique unsuitable for determination of the mixture derivates that are normally encountered in biological materials except serum and erythrocytes.

Improved radioassay kits for simultaneous determination of folic acid and vitamin B_{12} levels in the same assay tube have been developed. They allow either separate or joint folic acid and/or vitamin B_{12} assays. (For vitamin B_{12} see the next section, p. 290.)

We report here the procedure for folic acid only – the Diagnostic Products Corporation (DPC) Radioassay.

7.10.2 Principle of the method

The folate radioassay allows quantitative determination of all monoglutamate derivatives in serum and erythrocytes and is based on the principle of competitive protein binding.

An exact amount of different folate standards and serum or diluted whole blood is mixed with a buffer and a radioactively labelled folate derivative. Folate content is protected against oxidative destruction by adding a reducing agent such as dithiothreitol. Under the influence of heat or a denaturating reagent endogenous folate binding proteins are inactivated and bound folate is released.

Note 7.

Comparing assay values obtained with PGA (pteroylglutamic acid) calibrators and N-methyltetrahydrofolate calibrators in folic acid acid-free serum gives no clinically significant difference in the values at a buffer pH 9.3 [166]. This indicates that at pH 9.3 the more stable folic acid may be used as the standard in radioassays of endogenous folates.

The liberated serum folate and the radioactive folate then compete for the limited binding sites of a specific folate-binding protein, normally β-lactoglobulin, the folic-acid-binding protein in cows' milk. Following incubation the fraction of radioactive and non-radioactive material not bound by the binding proteins is adsorbed on processed charcoal or other special adsorbent substances and separated from the protein-bound fraction by centrifugation. The radioactivity in the bound fraction is determined by counting the supernatant. The data of the folate standards are plotted on a semilogarithmic graph to construct a standard dose response curve. The quantity of folate in the unknown sample is interpolated from the standard curve.

7.10.3 Chemicals and apparatus

(a) Chemicals

Beta-lactoglobulin binder, DPC No. DCT1
^{125}I Folic acid, DPC No. FOD2
Pteroylglutamic acid (PGA) p.a.
Dextran-coated charcoal, DPC No. CDS1.

(b) Solutions

Seven calibrators, containing different levels of folic acid (PGA) in a protein matrix (0, 0.5, 1, 3, 6, 12, and 24 ng/ml), DPC No. DCT3–9.

Borate-KCN Buffer pH 9.3, DPC No. BCN.
5% Dithiothreitol solution, DPC No. DTT1.

(c) Apparatus   Micropipettes calibrated between 100 and 500 µl; polyethylene or polypropylene disposable tubes with caps; vortex mixer; a covered boiling water-bath (100°C); centrifuge.
Gamma counter.

7.10.4 Sample collection

Blood is collected by vein puncture into heparin- or EDTA-lined vacutainers.

7.10.5 Procedure

(a) Sample preparation   For folic acid determination either serum, heparinized plasma or EDTA plasma may be used. Haemolysis must be avoided because folic acid is present in erythrocytes at concentrations many times higher than in serum. If the serum is to be analysed within 3–4 hours after collection it may be refrigerated (4°C), otherwise it must be kept frozen until just prior to analysis.

For red cell folic acid determinations the patient's haematocrit must be known in order to translate whole blood into red cell folic acid results, expressed as nanograms per millilitre of packed red cells.

To prepare the haemolysates, freshly obtained heparinized or EDTA whole blood is diluted by preparing a 1-in-21 dilution of the sample with a freshly prepared 1% ascorbic acid solution. It is important to prepare the 1% solution fresh daily. The haemolysate may be stored in the dark for exactly 90 minutes at room temperature.

After incubation the haemolysate must be frozen immediately (−20°C).

Frozen samples should be thawed at room temperature rather than with the help of a heat block or a water-bath. Repeated freezing and thawing of the samples should be avoided. As folic acid is light sensitive, avoid excessive exposure of samples to direct light.

(b) Technique   First a working solution must be prepared. For each assay tube 950 µl Borate-KCN Buffer, 50 µl of the ^{125}I folic acid solution and 20 µl of the dithiothreitol solution are mixed. It is advisable to multiply the volumes by a number greater than the number of tubes to be run.

Label two tubes for the total count, two for each standard including MB (maximum binding) and NSB (non-specific binding) and two for each patient sample and control.

Add 200 µl of the 0-calibration to NSB and MB tubes, and 200 µl of the calibrators 0.5 to 24 ng/ml, to the samples and controls in the corresponding tubes.

Add 1000 µl of the radioactive working solution to all tubes.

Cap the tubes, vortex, and place them in a boiling water-bath for 15 minutes. Cover tubes loosely.

Cool the tubes to room temperature and add 100 µl of the β-lactoglobulin binder to all tubes except NSB.

Vortex and incubate the tubes for 45 minutes at room temperature.

At the end of the incubation period add 400 µl of the dextran-coated charcoal to each tube and vortex for at least 10 s.

Incubate the tubes at room temperature for 10 min, but not longer than 20 min.

Centrifuge all tubes 10 min at 3000 *g*.

Decant the supernatants or put an aliquot from each tube into appropriately labelled vials for counting.

Count the tubes for 1 min in a gamma counter.

(c) Calculation

First calculate for each pair of tubes the average NSB-corrected counts per minute.

$$\text{Net count} = \text{Average CPM} - \text{Average NSB-CPM}$$

Next determine the binding of each pair of tubes as a percentage of the NSB-corrected maximum binding (MB) (=100%).

$$\text{Percent bound} = \frac{\text{Net counts}}{\text{Net MB counts}} \cdot 100$$

Plot the percent bound of the folate standards on the vertical axis of a semilogarithmic paper versus the folate concentration on the horizontal axis and draw the best fitting curve.

Folic acid concentration for the unknown samples may then be estimated from this curve by interpolation. The most modern gamma counters will perform this calculation by special software.

7.10.6 Performance characteristics

(a) Range of linearity

The range of linearity is within 0.5 and 24 ng/ml.

(b) Detection limit

The smallest single value that can be distinguished from 0 with the Diagnostic Products test kit is 0.2 ng/ml.

(c) Reproducibility

Intra-assay statistics were calculated for each of three different samples from the results of 20 pairs of tubes in a single assay:

Sample	Mean	SD	CV%
1	0.96 ng/ml	0.07	7.3%
2	2.06 ng/ml	0.06	2.9%
3	12.00 ng/ml	0.28	2.3%

(data according to Diagnostic Products)

Interassay statistics were calculated for each of the three samples from the results of 20 different assays:

Sample	Mean	SD	CV%
1	0.99 ng/ml	0.09	9.1%
2	2.06 ng/ml	0.09	4.4%
3	11.90 ng/ml	0.39	3.3%

(data according to Diagnostic Products)

The reliability data will guarantee corresponding results in different laboratories if borderlines are set up on a biological basis as demonstrated above. The advantage of radioassay procedures over microbiological assays is the possibility of having more comparable results on an international basis.

(d) Validity   No true validity tests are available at the moment.

7.10.7   Reference values   The reference values are, in general, population specific. For example, the average folate levels in serum obtained from 420 obviously healthy individuals (industrial workers from different companies in Germany) was 6.52 ± 3.52 ng/ml. The cumulative frequency distribution is given in Table 7.21. No influence of sex on the folate levels in serum was observed.

Table 7.21   Cumulative frequency distribution of serum folate (ng/ml)

Percentile	Females + Males (N = 420)	Females (N = 270)	Males (N = 150)
Min	1.0	1.2	1.0
5	2.4	2.5	2.4
25	4.2	4.3	4.1
50	5.7	6.0	5.6
75	8.0	8.8	7.6
95	12.8	13.0	12.7
Max	32.0	22.0	32.0
Mean	6.52	6.81	6.37
SD	3.52	3.56	3.49

7.10.8   Interpretation   According to the literature the reported incidence of folate deficiency varies widely. On the one hand folate deficiency is regarded as the most common hypovitaminosis not only in developing countries but throughout the world [167, 168]. On the other hand there are numerous reports and reviews stating that the folate status of the population is acceptable and only deficient in some groups such as pregnant women [169] or alcoholics [170]. The reason for these differences is the lack of objective criteria for evaluation of folate status. Generally only serum folate concentrations are taken for estimation of vitamin status and the so-called reference values are based on the limits of the 95% confidence interval of healthy 'reference groups'. The downward deviations from these values should be diagnosed as deficient.

Moreover there is no generally accepted lowest limit for normal serum concentration. The lowest limit of the 'reference' range found in the literature is 7 nmol/l (3 ng/ml) and the highest about 14 nmol/l (6 ng/ml).We therefore created biologically based borderlines to assess folate status [171, 172]. We correlated the folate concentration in serum and erythrocytes measured by the Diagnostic Products test kit with the lobe average of the neutrophilic granulocytes. Folic acid is responsible for the structure and formation of cells. In the case of folate deficiency cell division is disturbed and many granulocytes with five and more lobes are found. No alteration in the lobe average was found in serum folate concentrations higher than 4.5 ng/ml, there being on average up to 3.2 segments, which is within the assumed normal range. On the other hand when serum concentration is below 3.5 ng/ml there is a highly significant increase (more than 3.5 segments) in the lobe average. In the case of lobe average increased above 3.5, one finds that erythrocytic folate concentrations are decreased to less than 250 ng/ml.

These biologically based criteria for estimating folate status refer to one commercial radioassay, that of Diagnostic Products. To set up biologically based borderlines for other commercial radioassays, we compared four different, commonly used test kits [173]. Besides Diagnostic Products test kit we checked the radioassays from Bio–Rad Laboratories, Amersham–Buchler and Clinical Assays. With each of these test kits we analysed the folate concentration in 89 blood samples.

When we took our borderlines for the evaluation of the serum folate concentration measured with the different assays, the frequency for folate deficiency was between 4.5 and 12.4% respectively, 11.4 to 34.8% in the case of the marginal (4.5 ng/ml) borderline. When we took the borderlines of the producers of the test kits we found no folate deficiency with one (Bio–Rad), and a 5.6% deficiency with the other (Clinical Assays) as shown in Fig. 7.7.

On the basis of these findings we made a mathematical regression calculation of the serum results with different test kits.

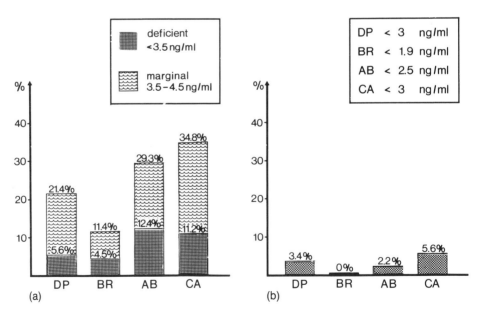

Fig. 7.7 Frequency of folate deficiency (serum concentration) depending on different methods (a) and different borderlines (b).

Depending on the specific regression function, we found borderlines for the deficiency status between 3.0 and 4.0 ng/ml and 4.0 and 5.0 ng/ml for the marginal state (see Table 7.22). Taking these mathematically corrected borderlines we have a nearly similar frequency in vitamin deficiency by different methods (see Fig. 7.8). If there is no possibility of performing the test with erythrocytes we propose taking these calculated borderlines for serum determination.

Table 7.22 Regression and correlation from different radioassays (in 89 blood samples: serum)

Method	Regression to Diagnostic Products $(y = a + bx)$	Correlation coefficient (r)	Borderline Biologically based (ng/ml) Marginal/deficient		Borderline acc. to kit producer (ng/ml)
Diagnostic Products	–	–	3.5–4.5	<3.5	3.0
Bio–Rad Laboratories	$Y_{BR} = 1.36 \cdot X_{DP}^{0.87}$	0.939	4.0–5.0	<4.0	1.9
Amersham–Buchler	$Y_{AB} = 0.82 \cdot X_{DP}^{1.03}$	0.902	3.0–4.0	<3.0	2.0
Clinical Assays	$Y_{CA} = 1.20 \cdot X_{DP}^{0.79}$	0.912	3.2–4.0	<3.2	3.0

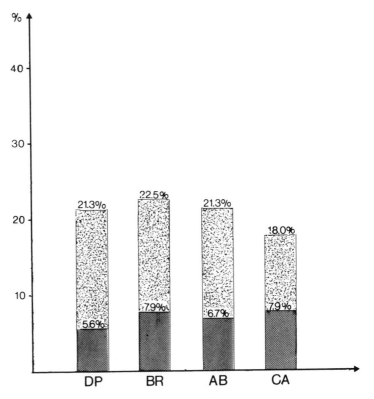

Fig. 7.8 Frequency of folate deficiency using mathematically adapted borderlines (89 samples).

Serum folate is not the characteristic for estimating folate status because serum concentration depends on actual food intake. Folate concentration in the erythrocytes represents the real body stores and reflects the nutritional status much better than serum concentration; therefore we also determined erythrocytic folate concentration.

Using the erythrocytic folate concentration to evaluate the folate status, differences between test kits are almost equalized. Data according to mathematical regression calculation are given in Table 7.23. The frequency is not very much affected either by the different methods and a fixed borderline of 250 ng/ml or by the different borderlines given by the manufacturers.

Table 7.23 Regression and correlation from different radioassays (in 80 blood samples: erythrocytes)

Method	Regression to Diagnostic Products ($y = a + bx$)	Correlation coefficient (r)	Borderline (manifest)	Borderline acc. to kit producer
Diagnostic Products	–	–	250 ng/ml	200 ng/ml
Bio–Rad Laboratories	$Y_{BR} = 0.81 \cdot X_{DP}^{1.05}$	0.915	265 ng/ml	200 ng/ml
Amersham–Buchler	$Y_{AB} = 0.58 \cdot X_{DP}^{1.09}$	0.972	220 ng/ml	235 ng/ml

The comparable results in erythrocytes depend on the biologically widespread distribution of erythrocytic folate concentration. In serum the opposite is true. Serum folate has a very small range and only small variations in the borderlines will result in great differences.

7.11 VITAMIN B$_{12}$ (TOTAL COBALAMINS) IN SERUM BY COMPETITIVE PROTEIN-BINDING ASSAY

7.11.1 Purpose and scope

Vitamin B$_{12}$ is a generic name for the group of cobalt-containing corrinoids with a biological activity in humans. Human serum not only contains the active cobalamins (mainly the hydroxy-, methyl- and 5′-deoxyadenosyl-cobalamins), but also a variable number of vitamin B$_{12}$ analogues which are biologically inactive non-cobalamin corrinoids [174]. Except as very small amounts in smokers, cyanocobalamin is normally not present in humans. However, as a result of its higher (heat-)stability, it is frequently used as standard in the analysis of vitamin B$_{12}$. Serum cobalamins can be determined by microbiological or radiodilution methods. The latter have become very popular as they are technically more simple, more easily standardized, and show a better precision. Radioassays using purified intrinsic factor (IF) as binder measure specifically cobalamins ('true vitamin B_{12}'). Radioassays, using 'R-binder' (or IF contaminated with R-binders), measure the sum of cobalamins and B_{12} analogues ('total vitamin B_{12}') [175]. There is still some discussion on what is the 'best' assay [176, 177].

Methylmalonate excretion (after oral valine loading) is considered as a functional but not very specific index of the the vitamin B_{12} status. The deoxyuridine (dU) suppression test has also proved to be of particular value in the biochemical assessment of the vitamin B_{12} status, but it is not very practical in large-scale analysis. For routine assessment of the vitamin B_{12} nutritional status of individuals, measurement of the serum vitamin B_{12} content is the first choice, but it cannot be used as the sole criterion in the diagnosis of vitamin B_{12} deficiency [177].

7.11.2 Principle of the method

Vitamin B_{12} in serum is extracted by heat-denaturation of the endogenous binding proteins (*trans*-cobalamins) in the presence of cyanide to convert the cobalamins into cyanocobalamin. The vitamin B_{12} content is quantified by competitive protein-binding assay using pure IF as binder. After incubation of the extract with ^{57}Co-labelled cyanocobalamin, the free and bound molecules are separated by BSA-coated charcoal precipitation. The amount of bound ^{57}Co-labelled cyanocobalamin, estimated by counting the radioactivity using a gamma-counter, is a measure of the vitamin B_{12} (cobalamin) content of serum.

Note 8.

The coated charcoal assay described here is based upon the original assay from Lau *et al.* [178], which is performed at low pH. The assay described here is carried out at pH 9.3 and is thereby suitable for simultaneous analysis of vitamin B_{12} and folate (see 7.11.5.(e)).

7.11.3 Chemicals and apparatus

(a) Chemicals

Boric acid p.a.
Cyanocobalamin, e.g. Merck, cat. No. 524950
Cyano[^{57}Co]cobalamin, specific radioactivity 180–300 Ci/g, e.g. Amersham, cat. No. CT 2
Cobinamide dicyanide, e.g. Sigma, cat. No. C-3021
Sodium azide (NaN_3) p.a.
Bovine serum albumin ('vitamin B_{12} free' BSA), e.g. Sigma, cat. No. A-3902
Norit A
Sodium hydroxide (NaOH) p.a.
Potassium cyanide (KCN), e.g. Merck, cat. No. 4967
Sodium chloride (NaCl) p.a.
Benzyl alcohol p.a.
Water: quartz-bidistilled every 2–3 days.

(b) Solutions

Buffer solutions of borate:
  Stock solution: 3.1 g boric acid (0.05 M), 8.5 g NaCl and 0.65 g NaN_3 are

dissolved in water to make about 900 ml. Adjust to pH 9.3 using 1 M NaOH and adjust volume to 1000 ml. Store at 4°C.

Working solution: Add 10 mg BSA and 5 mg KCN per 100 ml stock solution. Prepare fresh.

0.1% (w/v) BSA: 100 mg BSA (vitamin B_{12} free) is dissolved in water to make 100 ml.

0.5 M NaOH/0.5% (w/v) KCN: 2 g NaOH and 0.5 g KCN are dissolved in water to make 100 ml.

Intrinsic factor (IF) binder solutions:

Stock solution: Lyophilized IF (about 10 U) is dissolved in 10 ml 0.1% (w/v) BSA and stored in small aliquots at –20°C.

Working solution: Before each assay, an aliquot of the stock solution is diluted with 0.1% (w/v) BSA. The degree of dilution depends on the affinity of the IF preparation used and should be such that in the assay approximately 70% of the added undiluted [57]Co-cyanocobalamin tracer is bound (i.e. B_o/T = about 70%).

Note 9.

Each new batch of IF should be checked for the presence of contaminating R-binders by cross-reactivity studies with cobinamide.

Cyano[57Co]cobalamin tracer solution (15 pg/100 µl): For each assay an appropriate aliquot of the stock tracer (in 0.9% (v/v) benzyl alcohol) is diluted in working buffer to obtain a solution of 15 pg/ml.

Cyanocobalamin standard solutions:

Stock standard: About 30 mg cyanocobalamin is dissolved in water to make 1000 ml (solution A); 25 ml solution A is diluted to 100 ml with water (solution B). The concentration of B is measured spectrophotometrically by mixing 4 parts with 1 part of 0.5 M NaOH/0.5% KCN. The absorbance is measured at 368 nm against 0.5 M NaOH/0.5% KCN as the blank (molar absorption coefficient = 30 800; $E_{1\%, 1 \text{ cm}}^{368 \text{ nm}}$ = 227.3). Solution A is diluted 200 times with water and aliquots are stored at –20°C. Every six months a new stock standard is prepared.

Working standard: For each assay an aliquot of the stock standard solution is diluted 100 times (100 µl stock standard + 9.90 ml working buffer) and contains about 1500 ng/l. From this solution dilutions are prepared in working buffer containing 750, 375, 172.5, 86.8, 43.4, and 21.7 ng/l (the exact concentrations depend on the absorbance measured for the stock standard solution).

N.B.: Conversion factor: 100 ng/l = 73.8 pmol/l (MW: 1355)

Note 10.

Standards are preferentially prepared in '0' serum to eliminate matrix effects between serum and standard samples. Vitamin-B_{12}-free ('0') serum can be prepared by charcoal treatment or affinity chromatography using immobilized IF.

BSA-coated charcoal solution: 12.5 g Norit A is suspended in 500 ml water.

Dissolve 4 g BSA (not essential to be vitamin B$_{12}$-free, any BSA badge will do) in 40 ml water. The BSA solution is slowly added while stirring to the charcoal suspension. This solution is stored at 4°C for not more than one month. Before and during addition of the charcoal solution to the assay tubes, the suspension should be thoroughly mixed using a magnetic stirrer.

(c) Apparatus

Microlitre pipettes, 0–50 µl; 50–200 µl; 200–1000 µl (e.g. Eppendorf, Finn repeating pipettes) or repeating dispenser/diluter (e.g. Hamilton, Microlab 1000).

Liquid transfer system (e.g. Seripettor, Boehringer), 1–5 ml.

(Refrigerated) centrifuge.

Spectrophotometer.

Plastic tubes 11 × 70 mm (suitable for gamma-counter).

Borosilicate tubes, 16 × 100 mm.

(Multi-)vortex type mixer.

Boiling water-bath.

Gamma-scintillation counter.

7.11.4 Sample collection

Serum or plasma samples should be prepared by centrifugation of the blood samples. Serum samples can be stored for a maximum of 2 days at room temperature, for 3 days at 4°C and for 1 year at –20°C. Added ascorbate (to stabilize serum folates) may destroy endogeneous vitamin B$_{12}$ at room temperature.

7.11.5 Procedure

(a) Sample extraction

Aliquots of 100 µl standard (0–1500 ng/l), control and unknown samples are transferred in duplicate to borosilicate test tubes. For estimation of the non-specific binding (NSB) the highest and lowest standard concentrations, as well as two random serum samples are pipetted in duplicate in (extra) test tubes.

Add 500 µl working buffer to all tubes and mix vigorously using a multi-vortex.

After closing the tubes (e.g. by using a glass pearl), all tubes are heated on a boiling water-bath for 20 min.

(b) Competitive protein-binding assay

After cooling to room temperature, 100 µl working tracer solution is added to all tubes. For determination of the total radioactivity (total count), transfer in duplicate 100 µl working tracer to a plastic counting tube (set these TC tubes apart until counting).

Add 100 µl IF working solution to all tubes, except the NSB tubes. To the NSB tubes 100 µl 0.1% (w/v) BSA solution is added.

After mixing vigorously using a multivortex, all tubes are incubated for 1 h at room temperature.

After incubation, all tubes are transferred to a 'melting ice' bath and 500 µl of the cold charcoal suspension is added to all tubes.

After vortexing, the tubes are incubated for 15 min at 0°C (melting ice).

All tubes are centrifuged at 1500 *g* for 15 min at 4°C.

Transfer 1000 μl supernatant to a plastic counting vial and count the radio-activity of all tubes (including the TC tubes) using a gamma-counter.

(c) Calculation

The radioactivity of the standard and sample tubes is corrected for the non-specific binding by subtracting the NSB counts. The corrected counts are then expressed in percentage binding relative to the maximal bound counts ($B/B_0 \times 100$; B_0: i.e. the corrected counts for the '0' standard). The percentages of bound radioactivity ($B/B_o \times 100$) calculated for the standards are plotted against the vitamin B_{12} (cyanocobalamin) standard concentration. By reference to the standard curve the concentration of vitamin B_{12} in the serum and control samples can then be calculated, allowing for the serum volume assayed. Transformation of the standard data to fit straight standard curves, i.e. by plotting the logit of B/B_0 ($=\log[B/B_0]/(1-[B/B_0])$ against the log vitamin B_{12} concentration, is useful and offers increased speed. Automated data calculation programs for simple hand-held calculators up to sophisticated data processing packages to run on on-line (personal) computer systems are now easily available at relatively low cost.

(d) Calibration

Standards and control sera should be calibrated against reference preparations, e.g. the 1st British Standard Human serum Vitamin B-12 Code No. 81/563. This reference is available from the National Institute for Biological Standards and Control (NBSB, Holley Hill, London, UK). From the NBSB also an unclassified pernicious anaemia serum (Code No. 82/652) is available.

(e) Variations and modifications

The values obtained with radioassays for vitamin B_{12} may differ by the type of binder used as well as by the conditions used during extraction and the competitive protein binding assay [175, 178, 182]. Extraction of serum by boiling in diluted HCl [179], or glutamic acid buffer [180] also results in a clear extract, which permits the omission of the centrifugation step. Vitamin B_{12} is frequently assayed simultaneously with folate [178, 181]. Commercial reagent kits are available from various suppliers (e.g. Becton–Dickinson Immunodiagnostics; Diagnostic Products Corporation; Clinical Assays). In nearly all the simultaneous assays a pH of 9.3 is used to obtain an equal affinity for the oxidized (standard) pteroylglutamic acid and the reduced serum folates (mainly 5-methyl tetrahydrofolic acid). The affinity of cyanocobalamins to IF is slightly higher at lower pH values. Addition of antioxidants in the simultaneous assays for vitamin B_{12} and folate may slightly affect the vitamin B_{12} results [181]. 'No-boil' procedures, i.e. omission of the boiling step by extracting at high pH (= 11–12), have been described, but precision and recovery seem to be poor [182].

7.11.6 Performance characteristics

(a) Range of linearity

Within the range of the standard curve good parallelism was established after serial sample dilution. Extracts of samples with concentrations outside the standard range should be appropriately diluted with working buffer.

(b) Detection limit

The detection limit (defined as the amount of cyanocobalamin for 10% displacement of the tracer, i.e. $B/B_0 = 90\%$) amounts to about 1 pg/tube. This corresponds to a serum concentration of about 7 pmol/l.

(c) Recovery

In standard addition experiments recoveries between 95 and 105% were obtained.

(d) Reproducibility

In our laboratory the precision of the method is determined in each series by the analysis of three aliquots of pooled human serum. The within-assay coefficient of variation (CV) is about 3–5%, between-assay CV 3–7% (average pool level: 189, 321 and 1048 pmol/l serum, respectively).

(e) Validity

A good correlation has been obtained between vitamin B$_{12}$ levels in serum analysed by the competitive protein-binding assay and the microbiological assay with *L. leichmannii*. However, absolute levels are generally higher with the *L. leichmannii* method as this organism also grows on B$_{12}$ analogues (See also Purpose and scope, above.)

7.11.7 Reference values

Reference values are, in general, population specific. For example the average vitamin B$_{12}$ level for 207 healthy volunteers (blood donors from the centre of the Netherlands) with an average age of 37 ± 11.2 years (range 18–64 years) was 305 ± 113 pmol/l serum. The cumulative frequency distribution is given in Table 7.24. An effect of gender or oral contraceptive use was not observed [30]. Ageing results in a slight decrease of the serum vitamin B$_{12}$ content. This effect was especially seen for males.

Table 7.24 Cumulative frequency distribution of serum vitamin B$_{12}$ (N = 207 volunteers)

Percentile	B$_{12}$ pmol/l
Min	114
5	150
25	230
50	287
75	360
95	519
Max	916
Mean	306
SD	113

For 124 apparently healthy Dutch free-living elderly people with an average age of 72 ± 3.8 years (range: 65–89 years) [31], the vitamin B$_{12}$ level (331 ± 111 pmol/l plasma) was not significantly different from that of the groups of blood donors.

7.11.8 Interpretation

A serum vitamin B$_{12}$ level below 75 pmol/l (100 pg/ml) is considered diagnostic for vitamin B$_{12}$ deficiency [174]. The WHO Scientific Group on

Nutritional Anaemias (1968) adopted a level of 150 pmol/l (200 pg/ml) as the lowest acceptable level (as measured by microbiological assays). (See also Purpose and scope, above.)

7.12   BIOTIN

7.12.1   Purpose and scope

SECTION I   BIOTIN IN WHOLE BLOOD BY MICROBIOLOGICAL ASSAY

D(+)biotin (vitamin H or B_7) serves as the prosthetic group in a number of enzymes in which the biotin moiety functions as a mobile carboxyl carrier. The most common cause of biotin deficiency is the consumption of raw egg-white, which contains avidin, a glycoprotein binding biotin almost irreversibly, thereby rendering the vitamin biologically inactive. Furthermore, biotin deficiency is involved in some diseases and genetic defects [183]. Its nutritional status may be evaluated by analysis of biotin in biological fluids like blood, plasma, and urine.

At present the microbiological assay is still one of the practical means to measure the biotin level in biological samples [133, 184–186]. However, protein-binding assays are being developed for biotin analysis [187, 188] as well as assays for certain biotin enzymes as possible indicators of the biotin status [189].

The method described here uses *Lactobacillus plantarum* (ATCC 8014, formerly known as *L. arabinosus*; Ref. [185]) as the test organism. If the growth response to D(+)biotin is set at 100, the response to oxybiotin is about 50%. Dethiobiotin, biotinsulphoxide, biotinsulphon, and biocytin would not influence the test [184, 185, 190].

7.12.2   Principle of the method

Biotin is extracted from blood, plasma, or any other biological fluid by sterilization in sulphuric acid. After pH adjustment and filtration, biotin in the extract is measured by its growth response towards *L. plantarum*.

7.12.3   Chemicals and apparatus

(a) Chemicals

Sulphuric acid (H_2SO_4), 95–97% p.a.
Sodium hydroxide (NaOH) p.a.
Sodium chloride (NaCl) p.a.
Hydrochloric acid (HCl) p.a.
Ethyl alcohol, 96% (v/v) p.a.
Glycerol, specific weight 1.26 p.a.
Liquid nitrogen (N_2)
Antifoam emulsion, e.g. Sigma, cat. No. A-5757
L. Plantarum (ATCC 8014) from Difco, cat. No. 3211–30–3
Stock culture medium for *L. plantarum*: Bacto Lactobacilli Agar AOAC, dehydrated, Difco, cat. No. 0900–15–4
Inocula medium for *L. plantarum*: Bacto Lactobacilli Broth AOAC, dehydrated, Difco, cat. No. 0901–15–3
Assay medium for *L. plantarum*: Bacto Biotin Assay Medium, dehydrated, Difco, cat. No. 0419–15–8

D(+)biotin, e.g. Sigma, cat. No. B-4501; molecular weight: 244.3

Water: quartz-bidistilled every 2–3 days.

(b) Solutions

1 M H_2SO_4: 55 ml 95–97% H_2SO_4 made up to 1000 ml with water.

10 M NaOH: 40 g NaOH dissolved in water to make 100 ml.

2% (v/v) antifoam emulsion: 2 ml antifoam in water to make 100 ml.

Sterile 0.85% (w/v) NaCl: 8.5 g NaCl dissolved in water to make 1000 ml, divided in glass bottles and sterilized (15 min, 121°C). The sterilized solution is stored in the refrigerator for not more than one week.

Sterile 20% (v/v) glycerol: 30 ml glycerol is mixed with 120 ml 0.85% (w/v) NaCl and sterilized (15 min, 121°C). This solution is stored in the refrigerator for not more than one week.

For general information/procedures in microbiology, see Refs [133, 186].

Bacto Lactobacilli Agar AOAC: used for carrying stock cultures.

An amount of 48 g is suspended in 1 l water and heated to boiling (2–3 min) to dissolve completely. The agar is divided in glass culture tubes (diameter 16–20 mm; 10 ml each), sterilized (15 min, 121°C) and stored in the refrigerator for not more than one month.

Stock cultures are prepared by stab inoculation of one or more tubes of sterile medium. Cultures are incubated for 18–24 h at 37°C, held constant at ± 0.5°C. The cultures are stored at 2–8°C. Transplants are made at monthly intervals in triplicate.

(This procedure is not necessary if *L. plantarum* is stored as described under Preparation of the inoculum, below).

Bacto Lactobacilli Broth AOAC: used to prepare inocula.

An amount of 38 g is suspended in 1 l water and heated to boiling (2–3 min). After preparation, the pH of the medium is adjusted to 6.75 using diluted HCl or NaOH solutions. Divided in 10-ml aliquots in glass culture tubes (diameter 16–20 mm), the culture medium is sterilized (15 min, 121°C) before use and stored in the refrigerator for not more than one week.

Bacto Biotin Assay Medium: used in the assay of biotin.

An amount of 7.5 g is suspended in 100 ml water and heated to boiling (2–3 min). A slight precipitate is dispersed by agitation. The suspension is quickly cooled in running tap-water and the pH is adjusted to 6.75 using diluted HCl or NaOH solutions. The suspension is distributed in 2.5-ml amounts into test tubes. After addition of standard and test solutions, the volume is adjusted to 5 ml with water and the tubes are sterilized for 12 min at 121°C.

Preparation of the inoculum

Inocula are prepared by subculturing from the stock culture of *L. plantarum* to 10 ml of Bacto Lactobacilli Broth AOAC. After 18–20 h incubation at 37°C, 1 ml is diluted with 150 ml of the culture medium. This suspension is incubated at 37°C for a period (in general at least 20 h) till the increase of the absorption measured at 660 nm in a 1-cm cuvette is not more than 0.1 absorption unit per hour. Thereafter, the suspension is divided in tubes and centrifuged under aseptic conditions for 5 min at 2600 *g* and room temperature. The supernatant liquid is decanted and the cells are resuspended in

150 ml sterile NaCl solution and again centrifuged under aseptic conditions. The final inoculum suspension is prepared by suspending these cells in 150 ml sterile glycerol solution, followed by division in 1-ml aliquots into cryotubes and frozen in liquid nitrogen (−196°C). These samples can be stored in liquid nitrogen for years.

Standard solutions

D(+)biotin (molecular weight, 244.3) is dissolved in water to obtain solutions containing 0.1 ng/ml and 0.4 ng/ml. These solutions are used to construct the standard calibration curve (see Calibration, below).

(c) Apparatus

Glass culture tubes of 50 ml (18 × 150 mm), suited for centrifugation, e.g. Gibco Europe, cat. No. 3–42110; glass bottles of 30 ml (for sample extraction); glass assay tubes (18 × 120 mm); cryotubes of 3.8 ml, e.g. Nunc, cat. No. 3–66524.

Adjustable pipettes; dispensers; Vortex; filtration paper.

Sterilization equipment (autoclave); stove (incubation cabinet); inoculum cabinet provided with UV tubelight.

Water-bath; photometer provided with a 1-cm flow-through cuvette.

Hardware (e.g. glass tubes, pipettes etc) are sterilized after sealing in plastic bags by gamma-irradiation at 2.5 Mrad. After irradiation, sterility is assured for about 2 years.

Dewar container, e.g. L'Air Liquide, cat. No. BT 40; containing about 40 l liquid nitrogen for long-term storage of the inoculum samples of *L. plantarum*. The temperature of the liquid phase is −196°C and of the gas phase −140°C.

7.12.4 Sample preparation

If storage is required, samples can be stored in the refrigerator for several months or in the freezer for much longer periods. Samples can also be stored as extracts in 1 M H_2SO_4 in the freezer (see Sample extraction, below).

7.12.5 Procedure

(a) Sample extraction

At the day of analysis, samples are thawed in running tap water.

An amount of 3 ml of whole blood (plasma or urine) is extracted in 8 ml 1 M H_2SO_4 in a 30 ml glass bottle during 2 h at 121°C.

After cooling in running tap water, the pH is adjusted to 4.5 using 10 M NaOH and the volume is made up with water to 25 ml.

The solution is filtrated and adjusted to pH 6.75 using diluted HCl or NaOH solutions.

This final extract is used in the microbiological assay (see below).

(b) Calibration

A calibration curve is prepared from the 0.1 and 0.4 ng/ml standard solutions directly into incubation tubes containing 2.5 ml of the biotin assay medium. The total volume is made up with water to 5.0 ml. The D(+)biotin concentrations in these tubes range from 0 to 0.80 ng/5 ml (8 different levels). All standard incubations are carried out in triplicate. In general, an S-shaped curve is obtained when the observed absorptions are plotted against the concentrations.

Linearity hardly exists in microbiological assays. Therefore, sample extracts are assayed in duplicate and for three different volumes of the extracts (see Microbiological assay below) and read from the S-shaped calibration curve.

(c) Microbiological assay

Duplicate samples of 1.0, 1.5, and 2.5 ml of the final extract are brought into tubes containing 2.5 ml of the Bacto Biotin Assay Medium. The volume is adjusted to 5.0 ml using water.

Glass tubes containing the standard curve and those containing the samples are sterilized (12 min at 121°C).

After cooling, each tube (with the exception of a blank) is inoculated with 100 μl diluted inoculum (about 120 μl of inoculum is diluted with 25 ml sterile 0.85% (w/v) NaCl solution).

The tubes are incubated in the stove at 37°C for a period resulting in an absorption at 660 nm (1-cm cuvette) of the tube containing the highest standard concentration (0.80 ng/5 ml) of about 0.6 (i.e. normally after about 18–20 h).

The content of each tube is mixed with 100 μl 2% antifoam and the absorption at 660 nm is read against the blank tube.

(d) Calculation

The concentrations of the original samples are calculated on the basis of the absorption at 660 nm using the calibration curve and taking care of the proper dilution factors. (Readings from the calibration curve can be done by hand or by using a 6th degree orthogonal polynome for automatic calculations.)

7.12.6 Performance characteristics

(a) Range of linearity

Sample aliquots of blood, plasma or urine less than 3.0 ml (made up with 0.9% (w/v) NaCl to 3.00 ml) can be used with acceptable results provided the biotin levels are not too low.

(b) Detection limit

Based on the calibration curve, the detection limit of the microbiological assay for biotin in whole blood is about 0.5 nmol/l (about 25 ng/l).

(c) Recovery

Recovery is determined in each series by analysis of an aliquot of pooled whole blood and an aliquot of the same pooled whole blood to which biotin has been added. For that purpose, biotin is dissolved in the NaCl solution. To correct for volume changes, the same volume of the NaCl solution is added to pooled whole blood. For 57 series the analytical recovery of 1.02 nmol D(+)biotin added per litre whole blood was 97 ± 29%.

Pooled whole blood and recovery samples are stored as aliquots in the dark at −20°C for a period normally not exceeding six months. Similar procedures apply to other biological samples.

(d) Reproducibility

In our laboratory the precision of the method is determined in each series by analysis of pooled whole blood (see also Detection limit above). For a total of 57 series using the same pool (pool mean: 1.11 nmol biotin per litre whole blood) the overall CV of a single sample run in an arbitrary series amounted to 19%.

(e) Validity   Whether results obtained by the microbiological method match with those of other methods [187, 188] remains to be established.

7.12.7 Reference values   Reference values are, in general, population specific. For example, the average biotin level in whole blood obtained from 158 healthy volunteers (blood donors from the centre of the Netherlands) with an average age of 37 ± 11.2 years (range 18–64 years) was 1.31 ± 1.30 nmol/l [30]. The cumulative frequency distribution is given in Table 7.25. For this group of volunteers an influence of age, gender and/or oral contraceptive use on the level of biotin in whole blood was not observed.

Table 7.25 Cumulative frequency distribution of biotin in whole blood (N = 158 volunteers)

Percentile	Biotin nmol/l
Min	0.50
5	0.70
25	0.90
50	1.10
75	1.30
95	2.20
Max	15.00
Mean	1.31
SD	1.30

7.12.8 Interpretation   Deficiency is probable at whole blood levels below 0.5 nmol/l. Levels in red blood cells and plasma are comparable. Normal levels of urinary excretion are in the range of 30–60 µg/24 h.

SECTION II   BIOTIN IN PLASMA OR URINE BY RIA [187, 191, 193, 194]

7.12.9 Chemicals and apparatus

(a) Chemicals   Citric acid ($C_6H_8O_7$) p.a.
Disodium phosphate, dihydrate ($Na_2HPO_4 . 2H_2O$), e.g. Merck, cat. No. 6580
Ethylenediaminetetra-acetate, disodium salt, dihydrate (EDTA-$Na_2 . 2H_2O$) p.a.
Glutathione reduced (GSH), e.g. Merck, cat. No. 4090
Papain p.a., e.g. Merck, cat. No. 7144
Sulphuric acid (H_2SO_4) p.a.
Ammonium hydroxide ($NH_3 . aq.$) p.a.
Hydrochloric acid (HCl) 37% p.a.
Sodium chloride (NaCl) p.a.
D(+)biotin, biochemical grade, e.g. Merck, cat. No. 24514

2-mercaptoethanol p.a.

$[8,9,-^3H(N)]$- Biotin: 40 Ci/mmol–6.1 µg/mol, e.g. New England Nuclear Corporation (NEN), cat. No. NET-721

Avidin: 10–15 U/mg protein, e.g. Sigma Chemicals, cat. No. A9275

Gelatin from porcine skin, 175 Bloom, e.g. Sigma Chemicals, cat. No. G2625

Dextran T 70, MG (light scattering) 70 000 dalton, e.g. Pharmacia, cat. No. 17/028001

Charcoal p.a.

Biofluor, High Efficiency Cocktail, NEN, cat. No. NEF-961

Distilled and bidistilled water.

(b) Solutions

Buffer 0.1 mol/l, pH 5.7: citric acid 4.8 mmol (0.924 g) and $Na_2HPO_4 . 2H_2O$ 11.8 mmol (2.1 g) dissolved in 1000 ml bidistilled water. Fresh daily.

$EDTA-Na_2 . 2H_2O$ 26.8 mmol/l: 1 g dissolved in water to make 100 ml. Fresh daily.

GSH 32.5 mmol/l: 1 g dissolved in water to make 100 ml. Fresh daily.

2% Papain: 1 g papain is dissolved in buffer pH 5.7 to make 50 ml. The solution can be stored for 5 days at 4°C.

10% H_2SO_4: 60.6 ml made up to 1000 ml with water.

1% NH_3 . aq.: 46 ml made up to 1000 ml with water.

HCl 1 mol/l: 82.8 ml made up to 1000 ml with water.

0.9% NaCl.

Biotin stock standard: 25 mg D(+)-biotin are predissolved in 5 ml NH_3 1% and after addition of 2 ml HCl 1 mol/l, diluted with 0.9% NaCl to 250 ml. It can be stored at 4°C for 1 week.

Biotin working standard: Prepared by dilution of the stock standard with buffer pH 5.7 to a final concentration of 1 ng biotin/ml.

2-mercaptoethanol 10 mmol/l: 0.781 g dissolved in water to make 1000 ml.

^3H-biotin stock standard: $[8,9,-^3H(N)]$-biotin is dissolved 1:250 with 2-mercaptoethanol 10 mmol/l, divided in portions of 1.25 ml each and deep frozen in liquid nitrogen. It can be stored for at least 1 year without any loss of activity.

^3H-Biotin working standard: The stock standard is diluted 1:10 with bidistilled water. This working standard can be stored at 4°C for 3 days. Fifty microlitres of this working standard containing 20 nCi/0.122 ng of ^3H-biotin are used for the test.

Avidin solution: Avidin is dissolved in 0.9% NaCl solution to a final concentration of 1.1 mU/ml (1 U avidin binds 1 µg biotin). The specific activity of avidin is variable and has to be tested for every stock. It can be stored for 5 days at 4°C.

Dextran-coated charcoal: This is a modification of the original preparation of Rettenmaier [192]. 600 mg gelatin from porcine skin are dissolved in 65 ml bidistilled water at about 48°C, under gentle shaking. After recooling, 300 mg dextran T 70 and 6 g charcoal are added under intensive stirring. The suspension is made up with bidistilled water to 100 ml and stirring continued for another hour. The suspension can be stored at 4°C for 1 week.

(c) Apparatus

Automatic pipette device; centrifuge; glass test tubes of various dimensions; scintillation vials; ice-bath; Vortex.

Scintillation counter.

7.12.10 Sample collection

After collection of urine samples in clean containers and blood by venipuncture in heparin-lined vacutainers, followed by a centrifugation at low speed (to obtain plasma in this second case), the plasma and urine samples can be stored at −18°C for 1 year without any loss of biotin.

7.12.11 Procedure

(a) Sample preparation

In heat-stable test tubes with stopper, 1 ml freshly collected or thawed plasma or urine respectively is mixed with 1 ml buffer pH 5.7, EDTA 26.8 mmol/l and glutathione 32.5 mmol/l, 100 µl each, and 400 µl 2% papain. The tubes are stoppered and incubated at 57°C for 90 min in order to activate the rather heat-stable papain.

For the reduction of the non-specific binding (NSB) 1 drop H_2SO_4 10% is added to each sample followed by autoclaving at 120°C and 100 kPa (1 atm.) to inactivate an excess of papain. The NSB includes all biotin binding substances without avidin. It must be determined in each assay and it should be as low as possible to achieve high accuracy in the results.

(b) Technique

After recooling the samples are diluted with buffer (dependent on biotin content) 1:3 up to 1:5 before using. The assay is performed in duplicate in plastic centrifuge tubes as follows:

Test solution	MB† (µl)	Calibration curve (µl)	NSB‡ calibration (µl)	NSB‡ sample (µl)	Test sample (µl)
Buffer pH 5.7	2000	1900– 800	2100	2050–1100	1950–1000
Biotin working standard	–	100–1200	–	–	–
^{3}H-biotin working standard	50	50	50	50	50
Avidin solution	100	100	–	–	100
Sample volume	–	–	–	50–1000	50–1000

† MB = maximal binding
‡ NSB = non-specific binding
Final volume (each test vial) = 2150 µl

The test tubes are mixed well and kept for 20 min at room temperature under gentle shaking. Thereafter 250 µl charcoal suspension is added to each tube and kept in an ice-bath under continuous stirring. The samples are shaken thoroughly for 10 min (Vortex mixer) and finally centrifuged at 2500 g and 4°C for 10 min.

In disposable scintillation vials 2 ml of the supernatant are mixed with 15 ml Biofluor and the radioactivity measured in a liquid scintillation counter for 10 min (quench correction is not necessary, since the sample channel ratio is normally constant).

In addition for each duplicate, the total counts (TC) have to be determined. In a scintillation vial 2 ml buffer, 50μl ^{3}H-Biotin working standard and 15 ml Biofluor are mixed and the radioactivity measured as described.

Equivalence estimation of avidin: for each avidin solution the activity in relation to ^{3}H-Biotin must also be estimated. Fifty microlitres of ^{3}H-Biotin working standard are mixed with increasing volumes of avidin solution and buffer pH 5.7 to a final volume of 2150 μl and further treated as described. In this way the equivalence point is estimated, i.e. the minimal amount of avidin leading to the highest counting rate (c.p.m.). To calculate the avidin concentration needed for the solution, an amount corresponding to a value of about 10% below the equivalence point is employed (the tracer should be slightly in excess in relation to the binder).

(c) Calculation

To calculate the biotin content, the corresponding NSB must be subtracted from each calibration as well as sample value (mean value of duplicates). The NSB should not exceed 4% of the TC. The MB, on the other hand, should be 50% in excess of the TC, indicating a sufficient activity of the used avidin and ^{3}H-Biotin.

The calibration graph is established by plotting the counting rate of B/MB · 100 against the corresponding biotin concentration (B = measured counting rate of each concentration used diminished by NSB; MB = maximal binding). The biotin content of the sample is taken from the graph.

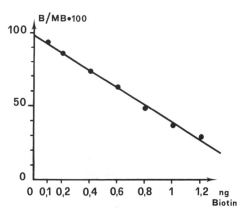

Fig. 7.9 Calibration curve for biotin protein binding assays.

The regression equation of the calibration graph (Figure 7.9) is as follows:

$$y = -59.27 \cdot x + 98.27$$

where: $y = B/MB \cdot 100$, $x = $ ng biotin.

7.12.12 Performance characteristics

(a) Range of linearity

Linearity of the graph is achieved in the range of 0.1 up to 1.2 ng biotin.

(b) Detection limit   This is 0.1 ng biotin (absolute amount in sample volume).

(c) Recovery   From 95% to 105%.

(d) Reproducibility   Within-day and day-to-day coefficient of variation amounted to 10%.

(e) Comparability   Comparing analyses using the conventional microbiological assay with *L. plantarum* resulted in slightly enhanced values, in plasma by 10.3% and in urine by 9.2%. There were good correlations with the RIA-test ($r = 0.926$ for plasma, $r = 0.934$ for urine).

7.12.13 Reference values   Less than 20 ng biotin/100 ml plasma = inadequate biotin status.

7.12.14 Interpretation   With the RIA test, as well as free biotin, all biotin derivatives with an intact ureido group are determined, such as biotin sulphoxide, norbiotin, etc. which are inactive. It is not known whether these are also excreted in human urine in small quantities, as is reported for some animals. Biocytin, the protein-bound form of biotin in plasma, is cleaved to free biotin by the preparation procedure.

7.13 PANTOTHENIC ACID IN WHOLE BLOOD BY MICROBIOLOGICAL ASSAY

7.13.1 Purpose and scope   D(+)pantothenic acid (vitamin B_5) is an essential part of the cofactor coenzyme A. The most important function of coenzyme A is to act as a carrier for carboxylic acids (e.g. acetyl-CoA) and thereby it plays a fundamental link between various food products (carbohydrates, fats, and proteins). As pantothenic acid is ubiquitously distributed ('panto' = ubiquitous) in natural foods, deficiency is seldom seen. A syndrome called 'burning feet syndrome' or 'nutritional melalgia' has been found to respond to treatment with pantothenic acid, although riboflavin and niacin seem to be involved as well [195].

Assessment of pantothenic acid nutritional status on the basis of dietary intake is difficult because reliable estimates of its daily requirement for man and sufficient information on contents in food products are not available. However, excretion in 24 h urine and blood levels of the vitamin have been found to reflect the dietary intake of pantothenic acid. For nutritional evaluation measurement of total blood pantothenic acid is recommended [196].

Urinary pantothenic acid has been found to be low in acute alcoholism but it is raised in chronic alcoholism; low, and occasionally increased blood pantothenic acid levels are found as well [197, 198]. Pantothenic acid deficiency seems not to be a widespread problem even in malnourished communities [199].

Pantothenic acid in blood, urine, and food can be analysed by microbiological methods (using *Saccharomyces uvarum*, *Lactobacillus casei* or *L. plantarum*) or by a radioimmunoassay [131, 133, 196, 200]. The sensitivity of both types of method is comparable and the correlation of the pantothenic acid levels obtained with these methods is high [201, 202]. Although the microbiological method can be expected to be replaced in the future by the radioimmunoassay, it is still the classical method for the analysis of pantothenic acid. The method described here uses *L. plantarum* (ATCC 8014, formerly known as *L. arabinosus*; Refs [131, 133, 200]) as the test organism. The growth response to D-pantothenic acid is maximal and to L-pantothenic acid and coenzyme A negligible. Pantothenic acid should therefore be released by hydrolysis before analysis.

7.13.2 Principle of the method	Pantothenic acid is liberated from its derivatives present in whole blood, plasma, or any other biological fluid by enzymatic hydrolysis using papain and Mylase-100. After sterilization, filtration and pH adjustment, pantothenic acid in the extract is measured by its growth response towards *L. plantarum*.

7.13.3 Chemicals and apparatus

(a) Chemicals

Sulphuric acid (H_2SO_4), 95–97% p.a.
Sodium hydroxide (NaOH) p.a.
Sodium chloride (NaCl) p.a.
Sodium acetate.3 H_2O p.a.
Hydrochloric acid (HCl) p.a.
Ethyl alcohol, 96% (v/v) p.a.
Glycerol, specific weight 1.26 p.a.
Liquid nitrogen (N_2)
Antifoam emulsion, e.g. Sigma, cat. No. A-5757
L. plantarum (ATCC 8014) from Difco, cat. No. 3211–30–3
Stock culture medium for *L. plantarum*: Bacto Lactobacilli Agar AOAC, dehydrated, Difco, cat. No. 0900–15–4
Inocula medium for *L. plantarum*: Bacto Lactobacilli Broth AOAC, dehydrated, Difco, cat. No. 0901–15–3
Assay medium for *L. plantarum*: Bacto Pantothenate Assay Medium, dehydrated, Difco, cat. No. 0604–15–3
Calcium-D(+)pantothenate, e.g. Sigma, cat. No. P-2250; molecular weight: 476.5 (molecular weight of pantothenic acid: 219.2)
Papain löslich, Merck, cat. No. 7147
Mylase-100, United States Biochemical Corporation (Cleveland, USA), cat. No. 19229
Water: quartz-bidistilled every 2–3 days.

(b) Solutions

1.5 M H_2SO_4: 83.2 ml 95–97% H_2SO_4 dissolved in water to make 1000 ml.
3 M Sodium acetate: 408 g sodium acetate.3 H_2O dissolved in water to make 1000 ml.
Sodium acetate buffer: 900 ml 3 M sodium acetate is mixed with 14 ml 1.5 M H_2SO_4. The pH is set at 4.50 using diluted H_2SO_4 or diluted NaOH solutions and the final volume is adjusted to 1000 ml.
Extraction buffer: 0.5 g Papain and 0.5 g Mylase-100 are dissolved in 100 ml of the sodium acetate buffer.

2% (v/v) antifoam emulsion: 2 ml antifoam in water to make 100 ml.

Sterile 0.85% (w/v) NaCl: 8.5 g NaCl dissolved in water to make 1000 ml and divided in glass bottles and sterilized (15 min, 121°C). The sterilized solution is stored in the refrigerator for not more than one week.

Sterile 20 % (v/v) glycerol: 30 ml glycerol is mixed with 120 ml 0.85% (w/v) NaCl and sterilized (15 min, 121°C). This solution is stored in the refrigerator for not more than one week.

For general information and procedures in microbiology, see Refs [131, 133].

Bacto Lactobacilli Agar AOAC: used for carrying stock cultures.

An amount of 48 g is suspended in 1 litre water and heated to boiling (2–3 min) to dissolve completely. The agar is divided in glass culture tubes (diameter 16–20 mm; 10 ml each), sterilized (15 min, 121°C) and stored in the refrigerator for not more than one month. Stock cultures are prepared by stab inoculation of one or more tubes of sterile medium. Cultures are incubated for 18–24 h at 37°C, held constant at ± 0.5°C. The cultures are stored at 2–8°C. Transplants are made at monthly intervals in triplicate. (This procedure is not necessary if *L. plantarum* is stored as described under Preparation of the inoculum, below).

Bacto Lactobacilli Broth AOAC: used to prepare inocula.

An amount of 38 g is suspended in 1 litre water and heated to boiling (2–3 min). After preparation, the pH of the medium is adjusted to 6.75 using diluted HCl or NaOH solutions. Divided in 10 ml aliquots in glass culture tubes (diameter 16–20 mm), the culture medium is sterilized (15 min, 121°C) before use and stored in the refrigerator for not more than one week.

Bacto Pantothenate Assay Medium: used in the assay of pantothenate.

An amount of 7.3 g is suspended in 100 ml water and heated to boiling (2–3 min). A slight precipitate is dispersed by agitation. The suspension is quickly cooled in running tap-water and the pH is adjusted to 6.75 using diluted HCl or NaOH solutions. The suspension is distributed in 2.5 ml amounts into test tubes. After addition of standard and test solutions, the volume is adjusted to 5 ml with water and the tubes are sterilized for 12 min at 121°C.

Preparation of the inoculum

Inocula are prepared by subculturing from the stock culture of *L. plantarum* (see above) to 10 ml of Bacto Lactobacilli Broth AOAC. After 18–20 h incubation at 37°C, 1 ml is diluted with 150 ml of the culture medium. This suspension is incubated at 37°C for a period (normally at least 20 h) till the increase of the absorption measured at 660 nm in a 1-cm cuvette is not more than 0.1 absorption unit per hour. Thereafter, the suspension is divided in tubes and centrifuged under aseptic conditions for 5 min at 2600 *g* and room temperature. The supernatant liquid is decanted and the cells are resuspended in 150 ml sterile NaCl solution and again centrifuged under aseptic conditions. The final inoculum suspension is prepared by suspending these cells in 150 ml sterile glycerol solution, followed by division in 1-ml aliquots into cryotubes and frozen in liquid nitrogen (–196°C). These samples can be stored in liquid nitrogen for years.

Standard solutions

Ca-D(+)pantothenate (molecular weight = 476.5) is dissolved in water to obtain solutions containing 20 ng/ml and 50 ng/ml. These solutions are used to construct the standard calibration curve (see Calibration, below).

(c) Apparatus

Glass culture tubes of 50 ml (18 × 150 mm) suited for centrifugation, e.g. Gibco Europe, cat. No. 3–42110; glass bottles of 30 ml (for sample extraction); glass assay tubes (18 × 120 mm); cryotubes of 3.8 ml, e.g. Nunc, cat. No. 3–66524.

Adjustable pipettes; dispensers; Vortex; filtration paper.

Sterilization equipment (autoclave); stove (incubation cabinet); inoculum cabinet provided with UV tubelight.

Water-bath; photometer provided with a 1-cm flow-through cuvette.

Hardware (e.g. glass tubes, pipettes etc) are sterilized after sealing in plastic bags by gamma-irradiation at 2.5 Mrad. After irradiation, sterility is assured for about 2 years.

Dewar container, e.g. L'Air Liquide, cat. No. BT 40; containing about 40 litres liquid nitrogen for long-term storage of the inoculum samples of *L. plantarum*. The temperature of the liquid phase is −196°C and of the gas phase −140°C.

7.13.4 Sample preparation

If storage is required, samples can be stored in the refrigerator for several months or in the freezer for much longer periods. Blood can also be stored frozen as 1-ml samples mixed with 19 ml sodium acetate buffer (see Sample extraction, below).

7.13.5 Procedure

(a) Sample extraction

On the day of analysis, samples are thawed in running tap-water.

An amount of 1 ml of whole blood (plasma or urine) is mixed with 19 ml sodium acetate buffer, followed by the addition of 5 ml of the extraction buffer.

This mixture is incubated for 2 h at 45°C and subsequently treated for 6 min at 121°C.

After cooling in running tap-water, the sample is filtrated and the pH is adjusted to 6.75 using diluted HCl or NaOH solutions.

This final extract is used in the microbiological assay (see below).

(b) Calibration

A calibration curve is prepared from the 20- and 50-ng/ml standard solutions directly into incubation tubes containing 2.5 ml of the pantothenic assay medium. The total volume is made up with water to 5.0 ml. The Ca-D(+)pantothenate concentrations in these tubes range from 0 to 100 ng/5 ml (8 different levels). All standard incubations are carried out in triplicate. In general, an S-shaped curve is obtained when the observed absorptions are plotted against the concentrations.

Linearity hardly exists in microbiological assays. Therefore, sample extracts are assayed in duplicate and for three different volumes of the extracts (see Microbiological assay) and read from the S-shaped calibration curve.

(c) Microbiological assay   Duplicate samples of 1.0, 1.5 and 2.5 ml of the final extract (see Sample extraction, above) are brought into tubes containing 2.5 ml of the Bacto Pantothenate Assay Medium. The volume is adjusted to 5.0 ml using water.

Glass tubes containing the standard curve and those containing the samples are sterilized (12 min at 121°C).

After cooling, each tube (with the exception of a blank) is inoculated with 100 μl diluted inoculum (about 120 μl of inoculum is diluted with 25 ml sterile 0.85% (w/v) NaCl solution).

The tubes are incubated in the stove at 37°C for a period resulting in an absorption at 660 nm (1-cm cuvette) of the tube containing the highest standard concentration (100 ng/5 ml) of about 0.6 (i.e. after about 18–20 h).

The content of each tube is mixed with 100 μl 2% antifoam and the absorption at 660 nm is read against the blank tube.

(d) Calculation   The concentrations of the original samples are calculated on the basis of the absorption at 660 nm using the calibration curve and taking care of the proper dilution factors. (Readings from the calibration curve can be done by hand or by using a 6th degree orthogonal polynome for automatic calculations.) One milligram of Ca-D(+)pantothenate is equivalent to 2.099 μmol Ca-D(+)pantothenate or 4.178 μmol D(+)pantothenic acid.

7.13.6   Performance characteristics

(a) Range of linearity   Sample aliquots of blood, plasma or urine less than 1.0 ml (made up with 0.9% (w/v) NaCl to 1.0 ml) can be used with acceptable results.

(b) Detection limit   Based on the calibration curve, the detection limit of the microbiological assay for D(+)pantothenic acid in whole blood is about 0.2 μmol/l (about 50 μg/l).

(c) Recovery   Recovery is determined in each series by analysis of an aliquot of pooled whole blood and an aliquot of the same pooled whole blood to which Ca-D(+)pantothenate has been added. For that purpose, Ca-D(+)pantothenate is dissolved in the NaCl solution.

To correct for volume changes, the same volume of the NaCl solution is added to pooled whole blood. Pooled whole blood and recovery samples are stored as aliquots in the dark at −20°C for a period normally not exceeding six months. Similar procedures apply to other biological samples. The analytical recovery of an amount of 0.527 μmol Ca-D(+)pantothenate (i.e. 1.05 μmol pantothenic acid) added per litre of pooled whole blood was 85 ± 12% (N = 59).

(d) Reproducibility   In our laboratory the precision of the method is determined in each series by analysis of pooled whole blood (see also Detection limit, above). For a total of 59 series using the same pool (pool mean: 1.33 μmol D(+)pantothenic acid per litre whole blood) the overall CV of a single sample run in an arbitrary series amounted to 17%.

(e) Validity

Levels of pantothenic acid in biological material obtained with the microbiological method show good correlation with those obtained by the radioimmunoassay [201].

7.13.7 Reference values

Reference values are, in general, population specific. For example, the average pantothenic acid level in whole blood obtained from 194 healthy volunteers (blood donors from the centre of the Netherlands) with an average age of 37 ± 11.2 years (range 19–64 years) was 1.18 ± 0.22 μmol/l [30]. The cumulative frequency distribution is given in Table 7.26.

Table 7.26 Cumulative frequency distribution of pantothenic acid in whole blood (N = 194 volunteers)

Percentile	Pantothenic acid μmol/l
Min	0.50
5	0.90
25	1.00
50	1.20
75	1.30
95	1.50
Max	2.20
Mean	1.18
SD	0.22

For this group of volunteers an influence of gender on the level of pantothenic acid in whole blood was not observed. A small but significant (P < 0.05) increase was seen with age, while women using oral contraceptives had a slightly higher (P < 0.05) level than those not using them [30].

7.13.8 Interpretation

No conclusive tests are available for the assessment of the pantothenic acid status; these tests should evaluate the coenzyme adequacy in the body. Urinary excretion of less than 1 mg/24 h is considered abnormally low. Suspicion of inadequate intake is further supported if whole blood values are well below 0.5 μmol/l.

7.14 VITAMIN C

SECTION I VITAMIN C IN PLASMA AND BUFFY COAT LAYER OF BLOOD BY DINITROPHENYL-HYDRAZINE ASSAY

7.14.1 Purpose and scope

Measurement of vitamin C in plasma provides an index of the circulating vitamin available for tissue use. It is the simpler of the two principal blood assays; it requires smaller amounts of blood and less complex and time-consuming initial work-up procedures than the alternative, buffy coat assay. Its main disadvantage is that plasma levels fluctuate according to recent intake, and are therefore less representative of long-term status than are buffy coat levels; moreover plasma levels decline to almost undetectable levels during severe dietary restrictions, long before the buffy coat and internal organs become severely depleted. Despite this however, the measurement of fasting plasma vitamin C can in the author's experience be a reasonably reliable index of vitamin C status for population studies, and it is quite efficient at identifying those individuals who have the lowest percentiles of habitual intakes.

Measurement of vitamin C in buffy coat concentrates provides an index of intracellular vitamin C, which has been found from experimental animal studies, and from some human observations, to change in parallel with the vitamin C content of many internal organs, so that it *can* provide a fairly accurate picture of body stores under certain circumstances, especially during acute (e.g. experimental) depletion, where body stores and buffy coat levels fall much more slowly than do plasma levels. Disadvantages of the assay, however, are firstly that it requires much more blood than the plasma assay; secondly that it requires a rather complex work-up procedure *immediately* after the blood is collected, which requires some specialized laboratory equipment (principally a Coulter counter), and thirdly that there may be difficulties of interpretation unless the numerical ratio of leukocytes to platelets lies within a fairly narrow range, or if leukocytosis has been recently induced, e.g. by infection. Thus, rapid fluctuations in buffy coat vitamin C levels following infections are more likely to represent redistribution, than real changes in overall tissue status.

Data on the rate of depletion of subjects on a near-zero intake are reported in the 'Sheffield' study [203]. In this study the plasma vitamin C fell to almost undetectable levels within a week of starting the very low intake, whereas buffy coat levels fell more gradually over a period of 2–3 months, and severe depletion coincided with the onset of clinical deficiency signs. During repletion, plasma levels responded very quickly, i.e. within an hour or two of oral dosing, whereas white cell levels increased more or less in parallel with the repletion of body stores. The rate of repletion will be greater the larger the doses given, and a subdivided-dose schedule is more effective than a single large dose.

7.14.2 Principle of the method

The assay procedure is based on the reaction of dehydroascorbate with 2,4-dinitrophenyl-hydrazine, as originally described by Roe and Kuether [204] and subsequently modified [205, 206].

The main reactions are oxidation of ascorbic acid to dehydroascorbate, reaction of the latter with 2,4-dinitrophenyl-hydrazine, to yield an orange osazone, and dissolution of the latter in sulphuric acid to permit measurement of its optical density and hence its concentration.

This requires a reasonably sensitive spectrophotometer and a centrifuge, plus an electronic cell counter if buffy coat vitamin C assay is included, but no other highly specialized laboratory equipment, and it is therefore suitable for fairly basic clinical laboratories.

7.14.3 Chemicals and apparatus

(a) Chemicals

Metaphosphoric acid flakes (HPO_3) p.a.
Ethanol (C_2H_5OH) p.a.
Methylcellulose, e.g. Koch Light, cat. No. 3768 H
Isoton and Zapoglobin (Coulter Electronics)
Boric acid (H_3BO_3) p.a.
2,6 Dichlorophenol-indophenol (phenolindo-2,6-dichlorophenol) p.a.
Dipotassium hydrogen orthophosphate (K_2HPO_4) p.a.

Homocysteine ($C_4H_9NO_2S$), e.g. Sigma, cat. No. H4628 (stored at 4°C)
Thiourea ($CS(NH_2)_2$) p.a.
Orthophosphoric acid (H_3PO_4) p.a.
2,4-Dinitrophenyl-hydrazine ($C_6H_6N_4O_4$) p.a.
Sulphuric acid (H_2SO_4) p.a.
L-ascorbic acid ($C_6H_8O_6$) crystals, for the calibration curve, e.g. Roche BP or Fluka, cat. No. 95209
Distilled water.

(b) Solutions

Metaphosphoric acid: 50% (w/v) in water; can be stored for not more than 3 weeks at 4°C, diluted to 6% and 2% (w/v) just before use.
Methylcellulose: 2% (w/v) in water; can be stored a few weeks at 4°C.
Boric acid: 0.81 mol/l in water, stored at room temperature.
2,6-Dichlorophenol-indophenol, 0.86 mmol/l in water, made fresh.
Dipotassium hydrogen orthophosphate, 2.58 mol/l in water, stored at room temperature.
Homocysteine, 46 mmol/l in water, made fresh.
Orthophosphoric acid, 64% (w/v) (12.2 M).
Thiourea, 0.66 mol/l, in 12.2 M orthophosphoric acid, made fresh.
Sulphuric acid, 25% (w/v) (9 N).
2,4-Dinitrophenyl-hydrazine: 0.20 mol/l in 9 N sulphuric acid; can be stored for a few weeks at 5°C, and filtered before use.
Sulphuric acid, 66% (w/v) (23.6 N).
Ethanol, 33% (v/v).
L-ascorbic acid standard: 5.6–112 μmol/l in 2% (w/v) metaphosphoric acid with 33% (v/v) ethanol, made up fresh just before use.

(c) Apparatus

Plastic tubes (ca. 15 ml) for buffy coat separation, centrifugation, and extraction; glass tubes with narrow (e.g. conical) ends for microaddition and incubation of reagents during assay, thus avoiding evaporation; cling-film to cover these; water-bath, set at 52°C; variable-volume automatic pipettes to cover the ranges: 0–0.02, 0–0.2 and 0–1.0 ml; Vortex mixer; refrigerated centrifuge, capable of running at 3000 r.p.m. (2300 *g*), at 4°C.
Coulter counter (electronic cell counter), if buffy coat ascorbate measurements are included.
Spectrophotometer capable of scale-expansion up to 0.2 OD units full scale, preferable double beam for stability. If small-scale operation is required, then microcuvettes are needed, and these can be 2 cm in path-length, in order to increase sensitivity. (The procedure given below provides a final volume of 0.99 ml, but this can be increased, e.g. to 2.97 ml, by using three times as much sample and reagents.)

7.14.4 Sample collection

Fasting blood samples (at least 2 ml for plasma assay and 10 ml for buffy coat assay) are collected into heparinized tubes and mixed.

7.14.5 Procedure

Remark
The biologically active forms of vitamin C are primarily: L-ascorbic acid and dehydroascorbate, which are interconvertible by oxidation and reduction.

Lactose ring-opening of dehydroascorbate yields biologically inactive diketo-gulonic acid, and the modified dinitrophenyl-hydrazine assay includes a blank subtraction procedure for each sample, which eliminates interference from diketogulonic acid and from most other potentially interfering compounds, except where the ascorbate level is extremely low and the contamination level is high.

(a) Sample preparation

Plasma vitamin C assay [205, 206]

Plasma is separated within 1–2 h by centrifuging at ca. 3000 r.p.m. (2300 *g*) at 4°C. The blood sample must not be haemolysed.

The separated plasma is stabilized immediately by addition of 1 vol. 6% metaphosphoric acid, and it can then be stored frozen (preferably at –70°, but –25°C is acceptable) for not more than 3 weeks. It must not be left in a bright light.

Just before carrying out the assay, 0.5 vol. ethanol is added to each unit volume of stabilized plasma, yielding a final concentration of 2% metaphosphoric acid and 33% ethanol. The mixture is thoroughly mixed and centrifuged to yield a clear supernate.

Buffy coat vitamin C assay [207]

To 9 ml heparinized blood is immediately added 1.0 ml 2% (w/v) methyl cellulose.

After mixing thoroughly by inversion, two equal aliquots are carefully trans-ferred to clean plastic tubes, without any material draining from above the meniscus down the sides of the tubes.

After 30 min standing on the bench, the upper layers are carefully removed, avoiding contamination with the lower layers of clumped red cells. This should yield a measured volume of around 2.0 ml buffy coat suspension from each tube.

The actual content of white cells should then be measured in an aliquot, by standard Coulter procedures for white cells; treating the sample as if it were whole blood.

After 1:500 dilution with Isoton, red cells are lysed with Zapoglobin before counting with instrument settings appropriate for white cells.

The remaining buffy coat suspension is centrifuged for at least 20 min at 4°C, at a speed of at least 3000 r.p.m. (2300 *g*). This should sediment all the white cells and platelets, together with the few remaining red cells (whose vitamin C content is relatively low and is usually disregarded).

The buffy coat pellet is resuspended by vortexing in 0.5 ml water, then 0.5 ml 0.6% metaphosphoric acid is added with mixing and the mixture is frozen (this will help to break up any remaining intact cells).

0.5 vol. ethanol is added to yield final concentrations of 2% metaphosphoric acid and 33% ethanol, as for the plasma samples.

The sample is then centrifuged to yield a clear supernate for assay.

(b) Technique

Work in glass tubes, and adjust volumes to those appropriate for the spectro-photometer cuvettes being used. The microprocedure described below (0.99 ml final volume) should be carried in narrow tubes, to minimize evaporation.

'Positive' (A) and 'Blank' (B) incubations are performed simultaneously on 2 aliquots of each sample extract (supernate).

Addition (at room temperature in order given):

A (positive)	*B (blank)*
0.20 ml supernate (sample)	0.20 ml supernate
0.05 ml boric acid	0.02 ml homocysteine
0.02 ml dichlorophenol-indophenol	0.02 ml water
0.05 ml K$_2$HPO$_4$	0.05 ml K$_2$HPO$_4$
0.02 ml homocysteine	

Leave 30 min on bench

0.1 ml thiourea/H$_3$PO$_4$	0.05 ml boric acid
	0.1 ml thiourea/H$_3$PO$_4$
0.05 ml dinitrophenyl-hydrazine/H$_2$SO$_4$	0.05 ml dinitrophenyl-hydrazine/H$_2$SO$_4$

Heat 80 min at 52°C; cool

0.5 ml 66% H$_2$SO$_4$	0.5 ml 66% H$_2$SO$_4$

Leave 45 min on bench

Read optical densities in cuvettes at 520 nm (spectrophotometer)

Note 11.

The order of addition of reagents differs between the blank (B) and the positive (A) samples, but by the end of the assay the two differ only in the replacement of the oxidant: 2,6-dichlorophenol-indophenol in the positive side, with water in the blank side. In the positive (A) side, boric acid is added to form a complex with dehydroascorbate when it is formed, followed by the oxidant, 2,6-dichlorophenol-indophenol in an amount sufficient to oxidize all the ascorbate (and other oxidizable substances) present. This is followed by dipotassium hydrogen phosphate, to raise the pH to 7–7.2 and then by homocysteine; but on this side the dehydroascorbate is already complexed with borate and is not therefore reducible by homocysteine. The dehydroascorbate–borate complex then reacts with 2,4-dinitrophenyl-hydrazine in a mildly reducing environment created by thiourea, and the precipitated osazone complex is finally dissolved in 23.6 N sulphuric acid for spectrophotometry.

   In the blank (B) side, homocysteine is added first, followed by water (replacing the oxidant dye) and then dipotassium hydrogen phosphate, to yield the pH (7–7.2) which is optimal for reduction of any dehydroascorbate present. Boric acid, which is added after this reduction step, complexes only with impurities, since all the biologically active vitamin C is in the reduced form.

   Likewise, the dinitrophenyl-hydrazine plus thiourea can only react with impurities, so that the optical density of the product in 23.6 N sulphuric acid represents the contribution of the impurities (including diketogulonic acid) only, and can be substracted from the A reading. The B readings obtained with the standard ascorbate acid calibration curve are very low.

'Zeros' (extractant only) and standards of ascorbic acid (5.6–120 µmol/l) are taken through the entire procedure, and the optical density of each sample and standard is read against the appropriate 'zero' (which will differ slightly between the A and B series). For the standards the B readings should be very low, whereas for the samples the B readings may be up to 50% of the A readings or perhaps even higher.

(c) Calculation

(A minus B) readings for the samples are related to the standard curve of (A minus B) readings in the usual way. Provided the standards were diluted in the same way as the samples (with metaphosphoric acid and ethanol), the computed concentration of vitamin C will not require correction for this dilution. For the buffy coat samples the total vitamin C in the entire extract obtained from the buffy coat button is calculated, then the white cell numbers are calculated for the same button, and the vitamin C content is expressed per 10^8 white cells (ignoring the platelet contribution).

7.14.6 Performance characteristics

(a) Range of linearity

The assay is linear over a range of vitamin C contents much greater than that encountered in plasma or buffy coat samples, but at very high contents a larger amount of dichlorophenol-indophenol oxidant is needed. This can be predicted if a very rapid oxidation (decolorization) occurs after the addition of this reagent to the sample during the assay.

(b) Detection limit

The detection limit is 2–3 µmol/l.

(c) Recovery

Recovery of internal standard vitamin C (added to plasma samples) is close to 100%.

(d) Reproducibility

The coefficient of variation observed was 4.5% (within assay) at vitamin C levels above 45 µmol/l, rising to 19.3% at levels less than 17 µmol/l.

7.14.7 Reference values

Reference values are population specific. In Table 7.27 are shown means and standard deviations of plasma vitamin C in some population groups.

Table 7.27 Means and standard deviations (SD) of plasma vitamin C in some population groups

Population group	Literature Reference	Plasma ascorbic acid (µmol/l)		
		Mean	SD	n
Pregnant Gambian women in early dry season				
(a) Urban (Bakau)	[208]	34	24	79
(b) Rural (West Kiang)	[208]	38	23	72
UK (Cambridge) pregnant women	[208]	43	20	22
UK (Cambridge) laboratory personnel	unpubl.	57	56	11
UK (Sunderland) elderly subjects	[209]	21	18	23

7.14.8 Interpretation

A limit of 0.2 mg/dl (11 μmol/l) in plasma or 0.10 μmol/10^8 cells in buffy coat is considered as rough indication for 'high-risk' cases backed by the 'classical' studies of induced vitamin C deficiency in human adults.

There are a number of influences, such as smoking [210], certain drugs (e.g. aspirin) [211], infections, stress, and other serious illness (e.g. cancer) [212], that are associated with lower-than-normal blood vitamin C levels, and in some instances there is evidence that the relationship between vitamin C intake and blood levels is altered, so that there may be an abnormal distribution or an increased turnover. Likewise, there is good evidence for a difference in blood levels between the sexes.

There is clearly a need for further research on the interpretation of these effects.

SECTION II TOTAL VITAMIN C IN WHOLE BLOOD AND PLASMA BY HPLC MICROMETHOD

7.14.9 Purpose and scope

Vitamin C is present as L-ascorbic acid and dehydro-L-ascorbic acid in practically all tissues and biological fluids [213, 214]. High levels are found especially in leukocytes and cerebrospinal fluid. The clinical manifestations of scurvy are well recognized [215], but the biochemical role of vitamin C is not yet fully understood. Ascorbic acid appears to be required as a reductant (e.g. in hydroxylation and iron utilization). Because of the limited knowledge of its metabolic functions, fully satisfactory and reliable biochemical procedures to identify a state of vitamin C deficiency or to assess its nutritional status have not been developed. Therefore, levels of vitamin C in biological fluids are used to obtain information on adequacy of this nutrient. Within a relatively limited range, serum (plasma) levels show a linear relationship with the intake of vitamin C. Leukocyte vitamin C levels more closely relate to tissue stores of the vitamin than serum levels. Urinary levels are probably prone to reflect the immediate dietary intake and subject to analytical problems.

Numerous methods have been described for the analysis of vitamin C as L-ascorbic acid, dehydro-L-ascorbic acid, or total vitamin C [216, 217]. Colorimetric and titrimetric methods are, however, not very specific. In recent years this drawback has resulted in the use of high-performance liquid chromatography (HPLC) with various methods of detection, depending on the compounds of interest.

In case a limited amount of biological material (e.g. leukocytes, or blood from prematures, etc.) is available, a micromethod should be used. A specific example using HPLC is described below.

7.14.10 Principle of the method

Vitamin C is extracted from whole blood or any other biological fluid by addition of metaphosphoric acid (MPA). After adjusting the pH, L-ascorbic acid is oxidized to dehydro-L-ascorbic acid using ascorbate oxidase. The latter is condensed with o-phenylene diamine to 3-(1,2-dihydroxyethyl) furo[3,4-b]quinoxaline-1-one (DFQ). After separation on a reversed-phase HPLC column, DFQ is detected fluorometrically. Total vitamin C is quantitated from peak area by integration using an external standard.

7.14.11   Chemicals and apparatus

(a) Chemicals

Metaphosphoric acid (MPA) p.a.
Glacial acetic acid (HAc, 100%) p.a.
Sodium chloride (NaCl) p.a.
Sodium hydroxide (NaOH) p.a.
Potassium hydroxide (KOH) p.a.
Potassium phosphate, monobasic (KH_2PO_4) p.a.
Methanol p.a.
o-Phenylene diamine (OPDA), e.g. Merck, cat. No. 7243
Ascorbate oxidase spatula, Boehringer Mannheim, cat. No. 736619
L-Ascorbic acid, crystalline pure, p.a. (Molecular weight = 176.13)
ODS Hypersil, 3 μm, Shandon Southern Products, cat. No. 58003010
Water: quartz-bidistilled every 2–3 days.

(b) Solutions

1% (w/v) MPA: 10 g MPA dissolved in water to make 1000 ml.
5% (w/v) MPA: 50 g MPA dissolved in water to make 1000 ml.
4.5 M Sodium acetate buffer solution, pH 6.1 ± 0.1: 160 g NaOH dissolved in water to make 500 ml; thereafter, 259 ml HAc is added under careful mixing and cooling. After cooling the volume is adjusted to 1000 ml.
0.1% (w/v) OPDA: 1 mg OPDA/ml water, prepared every day.
0.9% (w/v) NaCl: 9 g NaCl dissolved in water to make 1000 ml.
HPLC mobile phase, pH 7.8: this solution is prepared by dissolving 21.9 g KH_2PO_4 in 1600 ml water and setting the pH to about 7 using KOH pellets. Thereafter, 300 ml methanol is added and the pH is adjusted to 7.80 ± 0.02 using KOH pellets.
Vitamin C standard solution for HPLC: 40 mg of the vitamin C standard is dissolved in 100 ml 1% MPA. A portion of 1 ml of this solution is diluted to 50.0 ml with 5% MPA. Thereafter, 1.0 ml is mixed with 4.0 ml 5% MPA, 1.2 ml sodium acetate buffer, and one ascorbic acid spatulum and further treated as described for samples, but with the addition of 0.5 ml OPDA solution (see Sample extraction, below).

(c) Apparatus

Eppendorf tubes (of about 1.5 ml) suitable for centrifugation; adjustable pipettes; dispensers; Vortex.
Water-bath; refrigerated laboratory centrifuge.
HPLC apparatus consisting of:
Hyperchrome SC column, 125 × 4.6 mm diameter, filled with ODS Hypersil, 3 μm and provided with a 2-cm ODS Hypersil, 5 μm cartridge
Constant-flow pump
Automatic injector (or injection valve)
Fluorescence detector (e.g. Kratos Fluoromat filter fluorometer, model FS 950, provided with light source FSA 111 (365 nm), excitation band filter FS 403 (365 nm) emission cut-off filter FS 426 (418 nm), and a flow cell of 28 μl). Other fluorometers might be used if the instrument provides the correct excitation light and photomultiplier sensitivity.

Recorder

Integrator.

7.14.12 Sample collection

All procedures during sample treatment are carried out under subdued light conditions. The anticoagulant (citrate, EDTA, or heparin) used in the collection of whole blood or plasma does not influence the analytical procedures. Whole blood samples collected in vacuum tubes can be stored in the refrigerator (4°C) for about a week with a loss of vitamin C of less than 10% provided heparin is used as anticoagulant and the tube is kept closed during storage. At room temperature this period is only two days. Whole blood samples (with heparin as anticoagulant) can be stored for at least six months at –80°C if reduced glutathione (GSH) is added up to a concentration of 1 mg/ml whole blood. Heparin plasma (obtained from a heparin/GSH whole blood sample) can be stored at –80°C for not more than 10 days. For other conditions vitamin C should be analysed immediately after sample collection. There are indications that vitamin C in a metaphosphoric acid extract obtained from plasma within 15 min after blood collection (using freshly prepared MPA solution) and immediately stored at –70°C is stable for more than five years (F. Gey, Hoffman-La Roche, Basel, personal communication).

7.14.13   Procedure

(a) Sample extraction

An amount of 100 μl of well-mixed plasma or whole blood is brought into an Eppendorf tube containing 400 μl 5% (w/v) MPA. The tube is closed and vortexed thoroughly.

The tube is placed for 20 min in a refrigerator (4°C) and vortexed after about 10 min.

The tube is centrifuged for 10 min at 2000 *g* and 4°C.

An aliquot of 300 μl of the supernatant is brought into a second Eppendorf tube containing 40 μl 4.5 M sodium acetate buffer.

The top of an ascorbate oxidase spatulum is cut off and brought into the Eppendorf tube and mixed.

The tube is incubated for 5 min in a water-bath set at 37°C with mixing after 2 min.

Thereafter, 50 μl OPDA is added and mixed, and the tube is incubated in the water-bath for 30 min at 37°C.

The tube is cooled for 10 min at 4°C and then vortexed.

The metaphosphoric acid extract may be stored in the refrigerator for one day without appreciable loss of vitamin C.

The final solution is used for HPLC (derivatized samples should be kept at 4°C and subjected to HPLC analysis within 12 h).

Note 12.

As the sensitivity of the method described here is relatively high, an aliquot of only 10 μl sample would suffice for vitamin C analysis. In that case 10 μl sample is made up to 50 μl using 0.9% (w/v) NaCl. Thereafter, half the volumes mentioned above are used while 30 µl of the derivatized sample extract is subjected to HPLC analysis.

(b) Calibration

Before analysis a few aliquots of the derivatized external standard solution are injected to equilibrate the chromatographic system (constant peak height). In routine analysis, each series of five sample extracts is preceded by the external standard.

The linearity of the chromatographic system is controlled every month by a range of standard concentrations, corresponding to original levels of 0–200 µmol/l whole blood or plasma.

(c) HPLC

The entire chromatographic procedure is carried out at room temperature. Extracts in the HPLC injector are protected from UV light. Aliquots of 10 µl are subjected to reversed-phase HPLC. The flow rate of the mobile phase is 1.2 ± 0.3 ml/min. The retention time of DFQ is about 5 ± 0.5 min. DFQ fluorescence is detected using the optimal wavelength couple 355/425 nm (or suitable filters as indicated in the HPLC apparatus). The elution profiles are displayed on the recorder set at 10 mV full scale and a recording speed of 2 mm/min. The recorder as well as the integrator are connected directly to the fluorometer.

(d) Calculation

The concentration of vitamin C in the original sample is calculated from integration based on the peak area ratio sample/standard. In cases of failure of the integrator, peak heights are used. By the extraction method described, vitamin C is released quantitatively. Assuming the water content of whole blood is 85%, (of plasma 95%), the equation for calculation of the total vitamin C concentration in whole blood will be:

$$\text{total vitamin C (µmol/l)} = \frac{A_s \cdot C_{st} \cdot D}{A_{st}}$$

where A_s = peak area of the sample, A_{st} = peak area of standard, C_{st} = concentration of standard in µmol/l, and D = correction factor for dilution. For 100 µl whole blood, $D = \dfrac{390}{300} \cdot \dfrac{4.85}{6.7}$ and for 100 µl plasma, $D = \dfrac{390}{300} \cdot \dfrac{4.95}{6.7}$, where 6.7 is the dilution factor of the standard and the remainder the dilution/volume correction factor of blood and plasma, respectively.

7.14.14 Performance characteristics

(a) Range of linearity

Dilutions of blood samples (aliquots of 10–100 µl of sample made up to 50 or 100 µl with 0.9% (w/v) NaCl) result in comparable total vitamin C levels in the range up to about 200 µmol/l blood (see also Note 12).

(b) Detection limit

Assuming the signal-to-noise ratio is at least 3, the HPLC method described here shows a detection limit as low as 0.2 µmol/l (injected amount about 2 pmol or 350 pg vitamin C, respectively).

(c) Recovery

The recovery of L-ascorbic acid added to whole blood, plasma, or serum should be at least 95%.

(d) Reproducibility

In our laboratory the coefficient of variation (CV) of the within-assay analysis of vitamin C is about 4%. A reasonable stability of vitamin C in whole blood is obtained during storage at −80°C if reduced glutathione is added (see Sample collection). For a whole blood sample (average vitamin C level 62.5 µmol/l) stored under these conditions, an overall CV is obtained of about 6%. For plasma with an average total vitamin C concentration of 40 µmol/l stored in the proper way, an overall CV of a single sample run in an arbitrary series amounted to about 5%.

(e) Validity

There are no indications that the total vitamin C levels in blood obtained from healthy individuals using HPLC methods significantly deviate from those obtained with titrimetric or colorimetric methods.

7.14.15 Reference values

Reference values are, in general, population specific. For example, the average (± SD) total vitamin C level for 207 apparently healthy volunteers (blood donors from the centre of the Netherlands) with an average age (± SD) of 37 ± 11.2 years (range 18–64 years) was 40.5 ± 15.1 µmol/l whole blood [30]. The cumulative frequency distribution is given in Table 7.28. An influence of age or oral contraceptive use on the level of total vitamin C in whole blood was not observed. However, the vitamin C level of women was significantly (P < 0.001) higher than that of men (averages 47 and 33 µmol/l whole blood for women and men, respectively).

Table 7.28 Cumulative frequency distribution of total vitamin C in whole blood (N = 207 volunteers)

Percentile	Vitamin C µmol/l
Min	7.2
5	13.0
25	29.1
50	42.8
75	51.0
95	62.6
Max	77.2
Mean	40.5
SD	15.1

7.14.16 Interpretation

Whole blood levels of total vitamin C below 15 µmol/l most probably indicate a vitamin C deficiency.

REFERENCES

1. ICNND (1957) *Manual for Nutrition Surveys*, Interdepartmental Committee on Nutrition for National Defense, National Institute of Health, Bethesda.
2. ICNND (1963) *Manual for Nutrition Surveys*, 2nd edn, Interdepartmental Committee on Nutrition for National Defense, National Institute of Health, Bethesda.
3. Sebrell, W.H. and Harris, R.S. (eds) (1967–71) *The Vitamins. Chemistry, Physiology, Pathology, Methods*, Academic Press, New York.
4. Sauberlich, H.E., Dowdy, R.P. and Skala, J.H. (eds) (1974) *Laboratory Tests for the Assessment of Nutritional Status*, CRC Press, Cleveland (Ohio).
5. Brubacher, G.B. (1982) Are biochemical indicators available which reflect the intake of vitamins?, in *The Diet Factor in Epidemiological Research* (eds J.G.A.J. Hautvast and W. Klaver), EURO-NUT rep. 1, Wageningen, pp. 125–35.
6. Brubacher, G.B. (1988) Assessment of vitamin status in pregnant women, in *Vitamins and Minerals in Pregnancy and Lactation* (ed. H. Berger), Nestlè Nutrition Workshop Series Vol 16, Raven Press, New York, pp. 51–7.
7. Brubacher, G.B. and Schlettwein-Gisell, D. (1983) Vitamin nutriture in the elderly. *Bibl. Nutr. Dieta*, **33**, 142–51.
8. Amedee-Menesme, O., Luzeau, R., Wittpenn, J. *et al.* (1988) Impression cytology detects subclinical vitamin A deficiency. *Am. J. Clin. Nutr.*, **47**, 875–8.
9. Bamji, M.S. (1981) Laboratory tests for the assessment of vitamin nutritional status, in *Vitamins in Human Biology and Medicine* (ed. M.H. Briggs), CRC Press, Boca Raton (Florida), pp. 1–27.
10. Olson, J.A. (1984) Vitamin A, in *Handbook of Vitamins. Nutritional, Biochemical and Clinical Aspects* (ed. L.J. Machlin), Marcel Dekker, New York, pp. 1–43.
11. Smith, F.R. and Goodman De, W.S. (1976) Vitamin A transport in human vitamin A toxicity. *N. Engl. J. Med.*, **294**, 805–8.
12. International Vitamin A Consultative Group (IVACG) (1982) *Biochemical Methodology for the Assessment of the Vitamin A Status*, The Nutrition Foundation, Washington.
13. International Vitamin A Consultative Group (IVACG) (1982) Reprints of *Selected Methods for the Analysis of Vitamin A and Carotenoids in Nutrition Surveys*, The Nutrition Foundation, Washington.
14. Vuilleumier, J.P., Keller, H.E., Gysel, D. and Hunziker, F. (1983) Clinical chemical methods for the routine assessment of the vitamins status in human populations. *Int. J. Vit. Nutr. Res.*, **53**, 265–72.
15. Brubacher, G.B. and Vuilleumier, J.P. (1974) Vitamin A, in *Clinical Biochemistry, Principles and Methods* (eds H. Curtius and M. Roth), De Gruyter, Berlin, pp. 975–82.
16. Machlin, L.J. and Langseth, L. (1988) Vitamin–Vitamin Interactions, in *Nutrient Interactions* (eds C.E. Bodwell and J.W. Erdman), Marcel Dekker, New York, pp. 287–311.
17. Sauberlich, H.E., Dowdy, R.P. and Skala, J.H. (1974) Vitamin A (Retinol), in *Laboratory Tests for the Assessment of Nutritional Status* (eds H.E. Sauberlich, R.P. Dowdy and J.H. Skala), CRC Press, Cleveland (Ohio), pp. 4–13.
18. DeLuca, L.M., Glover, J., Heller, J. *et al.* (1981) *Recent Advances in the Metabolism of Vitamin A and their Relationship to Applied Nutrition*. A Report of the International Vitamin A Consultative Group (IVACG). The Nutrition Foundation, New York.
19. Olson, J.A. (1987) The storage and metabolism of vitamin A. *Chemica Scripta*, **27**, 179–83.
20. Sklan, D. (1987) Vitamin A in human nutrition. *Prog. Food Nutr. Sci.*, **11**, 39–55.
21. Bauernfeind, J.C. (ed.) (1986) *Vitamin A Deficiency and its Control*, Academic Press, Orlando.
22. Olson, J.A. (1982) New approaches to methods for the assessment of nutritional status of the individual. *Am. J. Clin. Nutr.*, **35**, 1166–8.

23 Speek, A.J., Van Agtmaal, E.J., Saowakontha, S. *et al.* (1986) Fluorometric determination of retinol in human tear fluid using high-performance liquid chromatography. *Curr. Eye Res.*, **5**, 841–5.

24. Natadisastra, G., Wittpenn, J.R., Muhilal, H. *et al.* (1988) Impression cytology: a practical index of vitamin A status. *Am. J. Clin. Nutr.*, **48**, 695–701.

25. Mobarham, S., Russell, R.M., Underwood, B.A. *et al.* (1981) Evaluation of the relative dose response test for vitamin A nutriture in cirrhotics. *Am. J. Clin. Nutr.*, **34**, 2264–70.

26. Ovesen, L. (1979) Drugs and vitamin deficiency. *Drugs*, **18**, 278–98.

27. Basu, T.K. (1988) *Drug-Nutrient Interactions*, Croom Helm, London.

28. Speek, A.J., Wongkham, C., Limratana, N. and Saowakontha, S. (1986) Microdetermination of vitamin A in human plasma using high-performance liquid chromatography with fluorescence detection. *J. Chromatogr.*, **382**, 284–9.

29. Dawson, R.M.C., Elliott, D.C., Elliot, W.H. and Jones, K.M. (1986) Vitamins and coenzymes, in *Data for Biochemical Research*, 3rd edn (eds R.M.C. Dawson, D.C. Elliott, W.H. Elliot and K.M. Jones), Clarendon Press, Oxford, pp. 115–39.

30. Knijff, J.H. (1987) Influence of age, gender and oral contraceptives on variables of the vitamin status and ferritin in apparently healthy adults. Zeist: CIVO-TNO report V 87.005 (available upon request).

31. Schrijver, J., Van Veelen, W.C. and Schreurs, W.H.P. (1985) Biochemical evaluation of the vitamin and iron status of an apparently healthy Dutch free-living elderly population. Comparison with younger adults. *Int. J. Vit. Nutr. Res.*, **55**, 337–49.

32. Menkes, M.S., Comstock, G.W., Vuilleumier, J.P. *et al.* (1986) Serum β-carotene, vitamins A and E, selenium, and the risk of lung cancer. *N. Engl. J. Med.*, **315**, 1250–4.

33. Orfanos, C.E., Braun-Falco, O., Farber, E.M. *et al.* (eds) (1980) *Retinoids*, Springer Verlag, New York.

34. Olson, J.A. (1986) Carotenoids, vitamin A and cancer. *J. Nutr.*, **116**, 1127–30.

35. Burton, G.W. and Ingold, K.U. (1984) β-carotene: an unusual type of liquid antioxidant. *Science*, **224**, 569–73.

36. Vuilleumier, J.P., Keller, H.E., Gysel, D. and Hunziker, F. (1983) Clinical chemical methods for the routine assessment of the vitamin status in human populations. Part I: The fat-soluble vitamins A and E, and β-carotene. *Int. J. Vit. Nutr. Res.*, **53**, 265–72.

37. Bieri, J.G., Brown, E.D. and Smith, J.C. (1985) Determination of individual carotenoids in human plasma by high performance liquid chromatography. *J. Liquid Chromatogr.*, **8**, 473–84.

38. Tangney, C.C. (1984) Individual carotenoid determinations in human plasma by high-performance liquid chromatography. *J. Liquid Chromatogr.*, **7**, 2611–30.

39. Van den Berg, H. and Schreurs, W.H.P. (1984) Methods for the assessment of the vitamin status in population groups, in *Proceedings of the GEN Workshop on Nutritional Status Assessment of Individuals and Population Groups* (ed. F. Fidanza), Group of European Nutritionists, Perugia, pp. 59–68.

40. Bouillon, R. (1983) Radiochemical assays for vitamin D metabolites: Technical possibilities and clinical applications. *J. Steroid Biochem.*, **19**, 921–7.

41. Seamark, D.A., Trafford, D.J.H. and Makin, H.J.L. (1981) The estimation of vitamin D and its metabolites in human plasma. *J. Steroid Biochem.*, **14**, 111–23.

42. Van den Berg, H., Boshuis, P.G. and Schreurs, W.H.P. (1986) Assessment of the vitamin D status by serum or plasma 25-hydroxyvitamin D analysis, in *Proceedings of the GEN Workshop on Nutritional Status Assessment of Individuals and Population Groups* (ed. F. Fidanza), Group of European Nutritionists, Perugia, pp. 191–201.

43. Lissner, D., Mason, R.S. and Posen, S. (1981) Stability of vitamin D metabolites in human blood serum and plasma. *Clin. Chem.*, **27**, 773–4.

44. Rodgers, R.P.C. (1982) Automated assay data processing and quality control: A review and recommendations, in *Radioimmunoassay and Related Procedures in Medicine*, IAEA, Vienna, pp. 383–410.

45. Bouillon, R., Van Herck, E., Keng Tan, B. *et al.* (1984) Two direct (nonchromatographic) assays for 25-hydroxyvitamin D. *Clin. Chem.*, **30**, 1731–6.

46. Mason, R.S. and Posen, S. (1977) Some problems associated with assay of 25-hydroxycholecalciferol in human serum. *Clin. Chem.*, **30**, 806–10.

47. Skinner, R.K. and Wills, M.R. (1977) Serum 25-hydroxyvitamin D assay: evaluation of chromatographic and non-chromatographic procedures. *Clin. Chim. Acta*, **80**, 543–54.

48. Mayer, E. and Schmidt-Gayk, H. (1984) Interlaboratory comparison of 25-hydroxyvitamin D determination. *Clin. Chem.*, **30**, 1199–204.

49. Jongen, M.J.M., van der Vijgh, W.J.F., van Beresteyn, E.C.H. *et al.* (1982) Interlaboratory variation of vitamin D metabolite measurements. *J. Clin. Chem. Clin. Biochem.*, **20**, 753–6.

50. Proszynska, K., Lukaszkiewicz, J., Jarocewicz, N. *et al.* (1985) Rapid method for measuring physiological concentrations of 25-hydroxyvitamin D levels in blood serum. *Clin. Chim. Acta*, **153**, 85–92.

51. Rhodes, C.J., Claridge, P.A., Trafford, D.J.H. *et al.* (1983) An evaluation of the use of Sep-Pak C18 cartridges for the extraction of vitamin D, and some of its metabolites from plasma and urine. *J. Steroid Biochem.*, **19**, 1349–54.

52. Markestadt, T. (1983) Plasma concentrations of 1,25-dihydroxyvitamin D, 24, 25-dihydroxyvitamin D, and 25,26-dihydroxyvitamin D in the first year of life. *J. Clin. Endocrinol. Metab.*, **57**, 755–9.

53. Machlin, L.J. (1984) Vitamin E, in *Handbook of Vitamins. Nutritional, Biochemical, and Clinical Aspects* (ed. L.J. Machlin), Marcel Dekker, New York, pp. 1–43.

54. Gey, K.F., Brubacher, G.B. and Stähelin, H.B. (1987) Cancer mortality inversely related to plasma levels of antioxidant vitamins, in *Anticarcinogenesis and Radiation Protection* (eds P.A. Cerutti, O.F. Mygaard and M.G. Simic), Plenum Press, New York, pp. 259–67.

55. Gey, K.F. (1989) Inverse correlation of vitamin E and ischemic heart disease, in *Elevated Dosages of Vitamins* (eds P. Walter, G.B. Brubacher and H.B. Stähelin) *Int. J. Vit. Nutr. Res.*, [Suppl. 30], 224–31.

56. Hashim, S.A. and Schuttringer, G.R. (1966) Rapid determination of tocopherol in macro- and microquantities of plasma. *Am. J. Clin. Nutr.*, **19**, 137–45.

57. Horwitt, M.K., Harvey, C.C., Dahm, C.H. and Searcy, M.T. (1972) Relationship between tocopherol and serum lipid levels for determination of nutritional adequacy. *Ann. N.Y. Acad. Sci.*, **203**, 223–36.

58. Brubacher, G., Stähelin, H. and Vuilluemier, J.P. (1974) Beriehung zwischen Lipoproteidgehalt des Serums und Plasma-Vitamin-E-Gehalt. *Int. J. Vit. Nutr. Res.*, **44**, 521–6.

59. Lehmann, J. (1981) Comparative sensitivities of tocopherol level of platelets, red blood cells, and plasma for estimating vitamin E nutritional status in the rat. *Am. J. Clin. Nutr.*, **34**, 2104–10.

60. Suttie, J.W., Mummah-Schendel, L.L., Shah, D.V. *et al.* (1988) Vitamin K deficiency from dietary vitamin K restriction in humans. *Am. J. Clin. Nutr.*, **47**, 475–80.

61. Shearer, M.J., McCarthy, P.T., Crampton, O.E. and Mattock, M.B. (1988) The assessment of human vitamin K status from tissue measurements, in *Current Advances in Vitamin K Research* (ed. J.W. Suttie), Elsevier Science, New York, pp. 437–52.

62. Shearer, M.J. (1983) High-performance liquid chromatography of K vitamins and their antagonists. *Adv. Chromatogr.*, **21**, 243–301.
63. Hart, J.P., Shearer, M.J. and McCarthy, P.T. (1985) Enhanced sensitivity for the determination of endogenous phylloquinone (vitamin K_1) in plasma using high-performance liquid chromatography with dual-electrode electrochemical detection. *Analyst*, **110**, 1181–4.
64. Shearer, M.J. (1986) Vitamins, in *HPLC of Small Molecules, A Practical Approach* (ed. C.K. Lim), IRL Press, Oxford, pp. 157–219.
65. Reed, A.H. and Henry, R.J. (1974) Accuracy, precision, quality control, and miscellaneous statistics, in *Clinical Chemistry, Principles and Technics*, 2nd edn (eds R.J. Henry, D.C. Cannon and J.W. Winkelman), Harper and Row, Hagerstown, pp. 287–341.
66. Suttie, J.W. (1984) Vitamin K, in *Handbook of Vitamins. Nutritional, Biochemical, and Clinical Aspects* (ed. L.J. Machlin), Marcel Dekker, New York, pp. 147–98.
67. Bjornsson, T.D., Meffin, P.J., Swezey, S.E. and Blaschke, T.F. (1980) in *Vitamin K: Metabolism and Vitamin K-Dependent Proteins* (ed. J.W. Suttie), University Press, Baltimore, pp. 328–32.
68. Olson, R.E. (1980) Vitamin K, in *Human Nutrition. A comprehensive treatise*, vol 3B (eds R.B. Alfin-Slater and D. Kritchesky), Plenum Press, New York, pp. 267–86.
69. Price, P.A. (1988) Role of vitamin-K-dependent proteins in bone metabolism. *Ann. Rev. Nutr.*, **8**, 565–83.
70. Vermeer, C., Soute, B.A.M., Ulrich, M. *et al.* (1984) The vitamin K-dependent carboxylation of proteins. *Biochem. Soc. Trans.*, **12**, 922–4.
71. Langenberg, J.P. (1985) *Bioanalsis of ultra-trace levels of K vitamins using electro-fluorometric detection in HPLC* [Thesis], State University, Leiden (The Netherlands).
72. Hiraike, H., Kimura, M. and Itokawa, Y. (1988) Distribution of K vitamins (phylloquinone and menaquinones) in human placenta and maternal and umbilical cord plasma. *Am. J. Obstet. Gynecol.*, **158**, 564–9.
73. Shearer, M.J. and McCarthy, P. (1987) The assessment of human vitamin K status from tissue measurements. Steenbok Symposium, abstract T41.
74. Pietersma-de Bruyn, A.L.J.M., van Haard, P.M.M., Beunis, M.H. *et al.* (1990) Vitamin K_1 levels and coagulation factors in healthy term newborns till 4 weeks after birth. *Haemostasis*, **20**, 8–14.
75. De Leenheer, A.P., Nelis, H.J., Lambert, W.E. and Bauwens, R.M. (1988) Chromatography of fat-soluble vitamins in clinical chemistry – Review. *J. Chromatogr. Biomed. Applns.*, **429**, 3–58.
76. Friedrich, W. (1988) Vitamin K, in *Vitamins* (ed. W. Friedrich), De Gruyter, Berlin, New York, pp. 285–338.
77. Van Haard, P.M.M., Engel, R. and Pietersma-de Bruyn, A.L.J.M. (1986) Quantitation of trans-vitamin K_1 in small serum samples by off-line multidimensional liquid chromatography. *Clin. Chim. Acta*, **157**, 221–30.
78. Van Haard, P.M.M., Engel, R. and Postma, T. (1987) Routine clinical determination of carotene, vitamin E, vitamin A, 25-hydroxy vitamin D_3 and trans-vitamins K_1 in human serum by straight phase HPLC. *Biomed. Chromatogr.*, **2**, 79–88.
79. Israels, L.G., Friesen, E., Jansen, A. and Israels, E.D. (1987) Vitamin K_1 increases system chromatic exchange in vitro in human leucocytes and in vivo in fetal sheep cells: a possible role for 'vitamin K deficiency' in the fetus. *Pediatric Res.*, **22**, 405–8.
80. Brin, M. (1967) Functional Evaluation of Nutritional Status: Thiamine, in *Newer Methods of Nutritional Biochemistry* (ed. A.A. Albanese), Academic Press, London, pp. 407–45.
81. Gubler, C.J. (1984) Thiamin, in *Handbook of Vitamins. Nutritional, Biochemical, and Clinical Aspects* (ed. L.J. Machlin), Marcel Dekker, New York, pp. 245–97.

82. Brin, M., Shohet, S.S. and Davidson, C.S. (1958) The effect of thiamine deficiency on the glucose oxidative pathway of rat erythrocytes. *J. Biol. Chem.*, **230**, 319–26.

83. Brin, M., Tai, M., Ostashever, A.S. and Kalinsky, H. (1960) The effect of thiamine deficiency on the activity of erythrocyte hemolysate transketolase. *J. Nutr.*, **71**, 273–7.

84. Schouten, H., Statius Van Eps, L.W. and Struyker-Boudier, A.M. (1964) Transketolase in blood. *Clin. Chim. Acta*, **10**, 474–6.

85. Dreyfuss, P.M. (1962) Clinical application of blood transketolase determination. *N. Engl. J. Med.*, **267**, 596–8.

86. Massod, M.F., McGuire, S.L. and Werner, K.R. (1971) Analysis of blood transketolase activity. *Am. J. Clin. Path.*, **55**, 465–70.

87. Kunovits, G. (1971) Die Farbereaktion der kohlenhydrate und aldehyde mit cystein und thioglykolsäure in schwefelsäure. *Anal. Chim. Acta.*, **55**, 221–9.

88. Brubacher, G.B., Haenel, A. and Ritzel, G. (1972) Transketolaseaktivität, Thiaminausschiedung und Blutthiamingehalt beim Menschen zur Beurteilung der Vitamin-B_1-Versorgung. *Int. J. Vit. Nutr. Res.*, **42**, 190–6.

89. Brubacher, G.B. (1982) Erythrocyte enzymes as an indicator for the assessment of vitamin and oligoelement supply, in *XI International Congress of Clinical Chemistry* (eds E. Kaïser, F. Gabl, M.M. Müller and M. Bayer), de Gruyter, Berlin, pp. 311–22.

90. Bamji, M.S. (1970) Transketolase activity and urinary excretion of thiamin in the assessment of thiamin-nutrition status of Indians. *Am. J. Clin. Nutr.*, **23**, 52–8.

91. Vuilleumier, J.P., Keller, H.E., Rettenmaier, R. and Hunziker, F. (1983) Clinical chemical methods for the routine assessment of the vitamin status in human populations. Part II: The water-soluble vitamins B_1, B_2 and B_6. *Int. J. Vit. Nutr. Res.*, **53**, 359–70.

92. Leevy, C.M. (1982) Thiamine deficiency and alcoholism. *Ann. N.Y. Acad. Sci.*, **378**, 316–26.

93. Hötzel, D. and Bitsch, R. (1976) Thiamine status of human subjects, estimated by biochemical methods. *J. Nutr. Sci. Vitaminol.*, **22** [suppl.], 41–5.

94. Becker, D.P. and Bitsch, R. (1979) Das Experiment-Enzymatische Ermittlung des Thiaminversorgungszustands. *Biologie in unserer Zeit (BIUZ)*, **9**, 187–9.

95. Bitsch, R. and Hötzel, D. (1981) Untersuchungen zur Objektivierung der Thiaminversorgung von Industriearbeitern. *Akt Ernähr*, **6**, 148–51.

96. Schrijver, J., Speek, A.J., Klosse, J.A. *et al.* (1982) A reliable semiautomated method for the determination of total thiamine in whole blood by the thiochrome method with high-performance liquid chromatography. *Ann. Clin. Biochem.*, **19**, 52–6.

97. Gubler, C.J., Fujiwara, M. and Dreyfus, P.M. (eds) (1976) *Thiamine*, John Wiley, New York.

98. Warnock, L.G. (1970) A new approach to erythrocyte transketolase measurement. *J. Nutr.*, **100**, 1057–62.

99. Buttery, J.E., Milner, C.R. and Chamberlain, B.R. (1982) The NADH-dependent transketolase assay: a note of caution. *Clin. Chem.*, **28**, 2184–5.

100. Kjosen, B. and Seim, S.H. (1977) The transketolase assay of thiamine in some diseases. *Am. J. Clin. Nutr.*, **30**, 1591–6.

101. Blass, J.P. and Gibson, G.E. (1977) Abnormality of a thiamine-requiring enzyme in patients with Wernicke–Korsakoff syndrome. *N. Engl. J. Med.*, **297**, 1367–70.

102. Kaczmarek, M.J. and Nixon, P.F. (1983) Variants of transketolase from human erythrocytes. *Clin. Chim. Acta*, **130**, 349–56.

103. Horwitt, M.K. (1986) Interpretations of requirements for thiamin, riboflavin, niacin-tryptophan, and vitamin E plus comments on balance studies and vitamin B_6. *Am. J. Clin. Nutr.*, **44**, 973–85.

104. Mawson, E.H. and Thompson, S.Y. (1948) A note on the estimation of vitamin B_1 in urine. *Biochem. J.*, **43**, 2–5.

105. Glatzle, D. (1970) Dependency of glutathione reductase activity on the riboflavin status, in 7th Int. Congr. Clin. Chem., Geneva/Evian. Vol. 2 *Clin. Enzymology*, Karger, Basel, pp. 89–94.

106. Glatzle, D., Körner, W.F., Christeller, S. and Wiss, O. (1970) Method for the detection of a biochemical riboflavin deficiency stimulation of $NADPH_2$. Dependent glutathione reductase from human erythrocytes by FAD in vitro. Investigations on the vitamin B_2 status in healthy people and geriatric patients. *Int. J. Vit. Res.*, **40**, 166–83.

107. Garry, P.J. and Owen, G.M. (1976) An automated flavin adenine dinucleotide dependent glutathione reductase assay for assessing riboflavin nutriture. *Am. J. Clin. Nutr.*, **29**, 663–74.

108. Thurnham, D.I. and Rathakette, P. (1982) Incubation of $NAD(P)H_2$: glutathione oxidoreductase (EC 1.6.4.2.) with flavin adenin dinucleotide for maximal stimulation in the measurement of riboflavin status. *Br. J. Nutr.*, **48**, 459–66.

109. Tillotson, J.A. and Baker, E.M. (1972) An enzymatic measurement of the riboflavin status in man. *Am. J. Clin. Nutr.*, **25**, 425–31.

110. Bates, C.J., Prentice, A.M. and Watkinson, M. (1982) Riboflavin requirement of lactating Gambian women: a controlled supplementation trial. *Am. J. Clin. Nutr.*, **35**, 701–9.

111. Bates, C.J., Powers, H.J. and Prentice, A.M. (1986) Measurement of riboflavin status by activation coefficient of erythrocyte glutathione reductase, and its automation with a Cobas Bio centrifugal analyser, in *Nutritional Status Methodology for Individuals and Population Groups* (ed. F. Fidanza), Group of European Nutritionists, Perugia, pp. 173–83.

112. Prentice, A.M. and Bates, C.J. (1981) A biochemical evaluation of the erythrocyte glutathione reductase (EC 1.6.4.2.) test for riboflavin status. 2. Dose-response relationships in chronic marginal deficiency. *Br. J. Nutr.*, **45**, 53–65.

113. Prentice, A.M. and Bates, C.J. (1981) A biochemical evaluation of the erythrocyte glutathione reductase (EC 1.6.4.2.) test for riboflavin status. 1. Rate and specificity of response in acute deficiency. *Br. J. Nutr.*, **45**, 37–52.

114. Cooperman, J.M. (1984) Riboflavin, in *Handbook of Vitamins. Nutritional, Biochemical and Clinical Aspects* (ed. J.L. Machlin), Marcel Dekker, New York, pp. 299–327.

115. Prentice, A.M., Bates, C.J., Prentice, A. *et al.* (1981) The influence of G-6-PD activity on the response of erythrocyte glutathione reductase to riboflavin deficiency. *Int. J. Vit. Nutr. Res.*, **51**, 211–15.

116. Carrigan, P.J., Machinist, J. and Kerhner, R.P. (1979) Riboflavin nutritional status and absorption in oral contraceptive users and non users. *Am. J. Clin. Nutr.*, **32**, 2047–51.

117. Sharada, D. and Bamji, M.S. (1972) Erythrocyte glutathione reductase activity and riboflavin concentration in experimental deficiency of some water soluble vitamins. *Int. J. Vit. Nutr. Res.*, **42**, 43–9.

118. Clements, J.E. and Anderson, B.B. (1980) Glutathione reductase activity and pyridoxine (pyridoxamine) phosphate oxidase activity in the red cell. *Biochem. Biophys. Acta*, **632**, 159–63.

119. Krämer, U. (1976) Beitrag zur Ermittlung des Riboflavin/status beim Menschen [Thesis], University Agricultural Faculty, Bonn (FRG).

120. Krämer, U., Bitsch, R. and Hötzel, D. (1977) Applicability of blood and urine analysis for the determination of nutritional status of riboflavin. *Nutr. Metabol.*, **21** [suppl. 1], 22–3.

121. Krämer, U., Bitsch, R. and Hötzel, D. (1977) Dünnschichtchromatographische Bestimmung von Riboflavin im Harn. *Klin. Wochenschr.*, **55**, 243–4.
122. Speek, A.J., Van Schaik, F., Schrijver, J. and Schreurs, W.H.P. (1982) Determination of the B_2 vitamer flavin-adenine dinucleotide in whole blood by high-performance liquid chromatography with fluorometric detection. *J. Chromatogr.*, **228**, 311–16.
123. Rivlin, R.S. (ed.) (1975) *Riboflavin*, Plenum Press, New York.
124. Yawata, Y. and Tanaka, K.R. (1977) Effect of metabolic stress on activation of glutathione reductase by FAD in human red blood cells. *Experientia*, **27**, 1214–21.
125. Ramachandaran, M. and Iyer, G.V.N. (1974) Erythrocyte glutathione reductase in iron deficiency anaemia. *Clin. Chim. Acta*, **52**, 225–30.
126. Komindr, S. and Nicholalds, G.E. (1980) Clinical significance of riboflavin deficiency, in *Nutritional Elements and Clinical Biochemistry* (eds M.A. Brewster and H.K. Naito), Plenum Press, New York, pp. 15–47.
127. Gatautis, V.J. and Naito, H.K. (1981) Liquid-chromatographic determination of urinary riboflavin. *Clin. Chem.*, **27**, 1672–5.
128. Sauberlich, H.E., Dowdy, R.P. and Skala, J.H. (1974) *Laboratory Tests for the Assessment of Nutritional Status*, CRC Press, Cleveland (Ohio), pp. 70–4.
129. Sauberlich, H.E. (1984) Newer laboratory methods for assessing nutriture of selected B-complex vitamins. *Ann. Rev. Nutr.*, **4**, 377–407.
130. Bonjour, J.P. (1980) Vitamins and alcoholism. VI. Niacin. *Int. J. Vit. Nutr. Res.*, **50**, 430–5.
131. Williams, S. (ed.) (1984) Official methods of analysis of the Association of Official Analytical Chemists. 14th edn, AOAC Arlington, pp. 862–73.
132. Difco Manual. (1984) *Dehydrated Culture Media and Reagents for Microbiology*, 10th edn, Detroit: Difco Laboratories, 1066–7 (Bacto Lactobacilli Agar AOAC), 1072–3 (Bacto Lactobacilli Broth AOAC) and 1096–8 (Bacto Niacin Assay Medium).
133. Kirsop, B.E. and Snel, J.J.S. (eds) (1984) *Maintenance of Microorganisms*, Academic Press, New York.
134. Joubert, C.O. and de Lange, D.J. (1962) A modification of the method for the determination of N′-methyl-2-pyridone-5-carboxylamide in human urine and its application in the evaluation of nicotinic acid status. *Proc. Nutr. Soc. S. Africa*, **3**, 60–5.
135. Sandhu, J.S. and Fraser, D.R. (1981) Measurement of niacin metabolites in urine by high pressure liquid chromatography. A simple, sensitive assay of niacin nutritional status. *Int. J. Vit. Nutr. Res.*, **51**, 139–44.
136. Pullman, M.E. and Colowick, S.P. (1954) Preparation of 2-and 6-pyridones of N′-methyl nicotinamide. *J. Biol. Chem.*, **206**, 121–7.
137. Bender, D.A. (1980), in *Vitamins in Medicine* (eds B.M. Barker and D.A. Bender), Heinemann, London, pp. 315–47.
138. Shaik, B., Pontzer, N.J., Huang, S.S. and Zielinski, W.L. (1980) Determination of N′-methyl nicotinamide in urine by high pressure liquid chromatography. *J. Chromatogr. Sci.*, **15**, 215–17.
139. Carter, E.G.A. (1982) Quantitation of urinary niacin metabolites by phase liquid chromatography. *Am. J. Clin. Nutr.*, **36**, 926–30.
140. McKee, R.W., Kang-Lee, Y.A., Panaqua, M. and Swendseid, M.E. (1982) Determination of nicotinamide and metabolic products in urine by high-performance liquid chromatography. *J. Chromatogr.*, **230**, 309–17.
141. Shibata, K., Kawada, T. and Iwai, K. (1987) Microdetermination of N′-methyl-2-pyridone-5-carboxamide, a major metabolite of nicotinic acid and nicotinamide, in urine by high performance liquid chromatography. *J. Chromatogr.*, **417**, 173–7.
142. Shibata, K. and Matsuo, H. (1989) Correlation between niacin equivalent intake and urinary excretion of its metabolites, N′-methylnicotinamide, N′-methyl-2-

pyridone-5-carboxamide, and N'-methyl-4-pyridone-3-carboxamide, in humans consuming a self-selected food. *Am. J. Clin. Nutr.*, **50**, 114–19.

143. Sauberlich, H.E., Dowdy, R.P. and Skala, J.H. (1974) *Laboratory Tests for the Assessment of Nutritional Status*, CRC Press, Cleveland (Ohio), pp. 37–49.

144. Coursin, D.B. (1964) Recommendations for standardization of the tryptophan load test. *Am. J. Clin. Nutr.*, **14**, 56–61.

145. Driskell, J.A. (1984) Vitamin B_6, in *Handbook of Vitamins* (ed. L.J. Machlin), Marcel Dekker, New York, pp. 379–401.

146. Skala, J.H., Waring, P.P., Lyons, M.F. *et al.* (1981) Methodology for determination of blood aminotransferases, in *Methods in Vitamin B_6 Nutrition: Analysis and Status Assessment* (eds J.E. Leklem and R.D. Reynolds), Plenum Press, New York, pp. 171–202.

147. Weber, H. and Wegmann, T. (1968) *Atlas der Klinischen Enzymologie* – Appendix: Methoden und Arbeitsvorschriften. Thieme, Stuttgart, pp. 6–9.

148. Stanulovic, M., Miletic, D. and Stock, A. (1967) The diagnosis of pyridoxine deficiency based on the estimation of the erythrocytic aspartate aminotransferase and its stimulation in vitro with pyridoxal-5'-phosphate. *Clin. Chim. Acta*, **7**, 353–62.

149. Leklem, J.E. and Reynolds, R.D. (eds) (1981) *Methods in Vitamin B_6 Nutrition. Analysis and Status Assessment*, Plenum Press, New York.

150. Schrijver, J., Speek, A.J. and Schreurs, W.H.P. (1981) Semi-automated fluorometric determination of pyridoxal-5'-phosphate (vitamin B_6) in whole blood by high-performance liquid chromatography (HPLC). *Int. J. Vit. Nutr. Res.*, **51**, 216–22.

151. Reynolds, R.D. and Leklem, J.E. (eds) (1985) *Vitamin B_6: Its Role in Health and Disease*, Alan R. Liss, New York.

152. Leklem, J.E. and Reynolds, R.D. (eds) (1988) *Clinical and physiological applications of vitamin B_6*, Alan R. Liss, New York.

153. Lumeng, L., Ryan, M.P. and Li, T.K. (1978) Validation of the diagnostic value of plasma pyridoxal 5'-phosphate measurements in vitamin B_6 nutrition of the rat. *J. Nutr.*, **108**, 545–53.

154. Lumeng, L., Cleary, R.E., Wagner, R. *et al.* (1976) Adequacy of vitamin B_6 supplementation during pregnancy. A prospective study. *Am. J. Clin. Nutr.*, **29**, 1376–83.

155. Coburn, S.P., Mahuren, J.D. and Guillarte, T.R. (1984) Vitamin B_6 content of plasma of domestic animals determined by HPLC, enzymatic and radiometric microbiological methods. *J. Nutr.*, **114**, 2269–73.

156. Chabner, B. and Livingstone, D. (1970) A simple and enzymic assay for pyridoxal phosphate. *Anal. Biochem.*, **30**, 413–23.

157. Van den Berg, H., Bogaards, J.J.P., Sinkeldam, E.J. and Schreurs, W.H.P. (1982) Effects of different levels of Vitamin B_6 in the diets of rats on the content of pyridoxamine-5'-phosphate and pyridoxal-5'-phosphate in the liver. *Int. J. Vit. Nutr. Res.*, **52**, 407–16.

158. Van den Berg, H. and Bruinse, H.W. (1988) Vitamin requirements in normal human pregnancy. *Wrld. Rev. Nutr. Diet.*, **53**, 1–27.

159. Gregory III, F.J. and Kirk, J.R. (1979) Determination of urinary 4-pyridoxic acid using high performance liquid chromatography. *Am. J. Clin. Nutr.*, **32**, 879–83.

160. Herbert, V. (1962) Experimental nutritional folate deficiency in man. *Trans. Assoc. Am. Physic.*, **75**, 307–20.

161. Waxman, S., Schreiber, C. and Herbert, V. (1971) Radioisotopic assay for measurement of serum folate status. *Blood*, **38**, 219–28.

162. Rothenberg, S.P., DaCosta, M. and Rosenberg, Z. (1972) A radioassay for serum

folate: use of a two-phase sequential-incubation, ligand binding system. *N. Engl. J. Med.*, **286**, 1335–9.

163. Waxman, S. and Schreiber, C. (1973) Measurement of serum folate levels and serum folate acid-binding protein by ^{3}H-PGA-radioassay. *Blood*, **42**, 281–90.

164. Longo, D.L. and Herbert, V. (1976) Radioassay for serum and red cell folate. *J. Lab. Clin. Med.*, **87**, 138–51.

165. Jones, P., Grace, C.S. and Rosenberg, M.C. (1979) Interpretation of serum and red cell folate results. A comparison of a microbiological and radioisotopic methods. *Pathology*, **11**, 45–52.

166. Givas, J.K. and Gutcho, S. (1975) pH dependence of the binding of folates to milk binder in radioassay of folates. *Clin. Chem.*, **21**, 427–8.

167. Brisson, M., Guay, A., Lamoureux, A. *et al.* (1974) L'apport alimentaire de l'acide folique chez les adolescents. *Union. Med. Can.*, **103**, 1385–9.

168. Urban, G. (1980) Die Beurteilung der Folatversorgung verschiedener Bevölkerungsgruppen anhand biochemischer und hämatologischer Messgrössen unter gleichzeitiger Berücksichtigung der Cobalamin-und Eisenversorgung [Dissertation], University of Bonn.

169. Kitay, D.Z. (1969) Folic acid deficiency in pregnancy. On the recognition, pathogenesis, consequences and therapy of the deficiency state in human reproduction. *Am. J. Obstet. Gynecol.*, **104**, 1067–107.

170. Wu, A., Chanarin, I., Slavin, G. and Levi, A.J. (1975) Folate deficiency in the alcoholic – its relationship to clinical and haematological abnormalities, liver disease and folate status. *Br. J. Haematol.*, **29**, 469–77.

171. Pietrzik, K., Urban, G. and Hötzel, D. (1978) Biochemische und hämatologische Massstässe zur Beurteilung des Folatstatus beim Menschen. 1. Mitteilung: Beziehung zwischen Serumfolat und neutrophilen Granulozyten. *Int. J. Vit. Nutr. Res.*, **48**, 391–6.

172. Pietrzik, K., Urban, G. and Hötzel, D. (1978) Biochemische und hämatologische Massstässe zur Beurteilung des Folatstatus beim Menschen. 2. Mitteilung: Vergleichende Messungen von Folat im Serum und in Erythrozyten. *Int. J. Vit. Nutr. Res.*, **48**, 397–401.

173. Pietrzik, K. and Hages, M. (1987) Folsäuremangel: Definition, Nachweis und Beurteilung der Versorgungslage, in *Folsäuremangel* (ed. K. Pietrzik), Zuckschwerdt Verlag, München.

174. Herbert, V. (1984) Vitamin B$_{12}$, in *Nutrition Reviews; Present Knowledge in Nutrition*, The Nutrition Foundation Inc., Washington (DC), pp. 347–64.

175. Kolhouse, J.F., Kondo, H., Allen, N.C. *et al.* (1978) Cobalamin analogues are present in human plasma and can mask cobalamin deficiency because current radioisotope dilution assays are not specific for true cobalamin. *N. Engl. J. Med.*, **299**, 785–92.

176. Herbert, V., Colman, N., Palat, D. *et al.* (1984) Is there a 'gold standard' for human serum vitamin B-12 assay? *J. Lab. Clin. Med.*, **104**, 829–41.

177. England, J.M. and Linnell, J.C. (1982) Problems with the serum vitamin B-12 assay. *Lancet*, **ii**, 1072–4.

178. Lau, K.S., Gottlieb, C.W., Wasserman, L.R. and Herbert, V. (1965) Measurement of serum vitamin B$_{12}$ level using radioisotope dilution and coated charcoal. *Blood*, **26**, 202–14.

179. Kubasik, N.P., Ricotta, M. and Sine, H.E. (1980) Commercially-supplied binders for plasma Cobalamin (vitamin B$_{12}$) analysis-'purified' intrinsic factor, 'cobinamide'-blocked R-protein binder, and non-purified intrinsic factor-R-binder compared to microbiological assay. *Clin. Chem.*, **26**, 598–600.

180. Ceska, M. and Lundkvist, U. (1971) Use of solid phase intrinsic factor for radiosorbent assay of vitamin B$_{12}$. *Clin. Chim. Acta*, **32**, 339–54.

181. Lindemans, J. and Van Kapel, J. (1981) The effect of oxidation state of the folate standard on the results of the simultaneous radioassay of serum folate and cobalamin. *Clin. Chim. Acta*, **114**, 315–20.

182. Lee, D.S.C. and Griffiths, B.W. (1985) Human serum vitamin B_{12} assay methods: A review. *Clin. Biochem.*, **18**, 261–6.

183. Sauberlich, H.E., Dowdy, R.P. and Skala, J.H. (1974) Biotin, in *Laboratory Tests for the Assessment of Nutritional Status* (eds H.E. Sauberlich, R.P. Dowdy and J.H. Skala), CRC Press Inc., Ohio, pp. 91–2.

184. Williams, S. (ed.) (1984) *Official Methods of Analysis of the Association of Official Analytical Chemists*, 14th edn, AOAC Arlington, pp. 862–73.

185. Difco Manual (1984) *Dehydrated Culture Media and Reagents for Microbiology*, 10th edn, Detroit: Difco Laboratories, 1066–7 (Bacto Lactobacilli Agar AOAC), 1072–3 (Bacto Lactobacilli Broth AOAC) and 1076–7 (Bacto Biotin Assay Medium).

186. Skeggs, H.R. (1963) Biotin, in *Analytical Microbiology* (ed. F. Kavanagh), Academic Press, New York, pp. 421–30.

187. Bitsch, R., Salz, I. and Hötzel, D. (1986) Bestimmung des Biotingehalts in *Lebensmitteln mit Hilfe eines Proteinbindungsassays*, Dtsch Lebensm Rundschau, **82**, 80–3.

188. Hood, R.L. (1975) A radiochemical assay for biotin in biological material. *J. Sci. Food Agric.*, **26**, 1847–52.

189. Bitsch, R., Tôth-Dersi, A. and Hötzel, D. (1985) Biotin deficiency and biotin supply. *Ann. N.Y. Acad. Sci.*, **447**, 133–9.

190. Ohsugi, M. and Imanishi, Y. (1985) Microbiological activity of biotin-vitamers. *J. Nutr. Sci. Vitaminol.*, **31**, 563–72.

191. Salz, I. (1986) Studien zum Biotinstatus des Menschen anhand versorgungsabhängiger Parameter [Thesis], University Agricultural Faculty, Bonn, (FRG).

192. Rettenmaier, R. (1980) Biotinbestimmung in Lebergewebe nach dem Prinzipder Isotopenverdünnungsmethode. *Anal. Chim. Acta*, **113**, 107–20.

193. Bitsch, R., Salz, I. and Hötzel, D. (1989) Biotin assessment in foods and body fluids by a protein binding assay (PBA). *Int. J. Vit. Nutr. Res.*, **59**, 59–64.

194. Bitsch, R., Salz, I. and Hötzel, D. (1989) Studies on bioavailability of oral biotin doses for humans. *Int. J. Vit. Nutr. Res.*, **59**, 65–71.

195. Gopalan, C. (1946) The 'burning feet' syndrome. *Indian Med. Gaz.*, **81**, 22–35.

196. Sauberlich, H.E., Dowdy, R.P. and Skala, J.H. (1974) Pantothenic acid, in *Laboratory Tests for the Assessment of Nutritional Status* (eds H.E. Sauberlich, R.P. Dowdy and J.H. Skala), CRC Press, Cleveland (Ohio), pp. 88–91.

197. Bonjour, J.P. (1980) Vitamins and alcoholism. V. Riboflavin. VI. Niacin. VII. Pantothenic acid. VIII. Biotin. *Int. J. Vit. Nutr. Res.*, **50**, 425–40.

198. Tao, H. and Fox, H.M. (1976) Measurements of urinary pantothenic acid excretions of alcoholic patients. *J. Nutr. Sci. Vitaminol.*, **22**, 333–7.

199. Srinivasan, V. and Belavady, B. (1976) Nutritional status of pantothenic acid in Indian pregnant and nursing women. *Int. J. Vit. Nutr. Res.*, **46**, 433–8.

200. Difco Manual (1984) *Dehydrated Culture Media and Reagents for Microbiology*, 10th edn, Detroit: Difco Laboratories, 1066–7 (Bacto Lactobacilli Agar AOAC), 1072–3 (Bacto Lactobacilli Broth AOAC) and 1100–2 (Bacto Pantothenate Assay Medium).

201. Wyse, B.W., Wittwer, C.W. and Hansen, R.G. (1979) Radioimmunoassay for pantothenic acid in blood and other tissues. *Clin. Chem.*, **25**, 108–15.

202. Walsh, J.H. (1979) Estimation of the pantothenic acid content of foods using a microbiological assay and a radioimmunoassay [Dissertation], Utah State University, Utah.

203. Bartley, W., Krebs, H.A. and O'Brien, J.R.P. (1953) *Vitamin C Requirement of Human Adults.* A Report by the Vitamin C Subcommittee of the Accessory Food Factors Committee. HMSO, London, Medical Research Council, Special Report Series No. 280.

204. Roe, J.H. and Kuether, C.A. (1943) The determination of ascorbic acid in whole blood and urine through the 2, 4-dinitrophenyl-hydrazine derivative of ascorbic acid. *J. Biol. Chem.*, **147**, 399–407.

205. Pelletier, O. (1968) Determination of vitamin C in serum, urine and other biological materials. *J. Lab. Clin. Med.*, **72**, 674–9.

206. Bates, C.J. (1977) Proline and hydroxyproline excretion and vitamin C status in elderly human subjects. *Clin. Sci. Mol. Med.*, **52**, 535–43.

207. Marchand, C.M. and Pelletier, O. (1977) Studies with an improved white cell isolation method to assess the vitamin C status in surveys. *Int. J. Vit. Nutr. Res.*, **47**, 236–47.

208. Reddy, V.A.P., Bates, C.J., Goh, S.G.J. *et al.* (1987) Riboflavin, folate and vitamin C status of Gambian women during pregnancy: a comparison between urban and rural communities. *Trans. Roy. Soc. Trop. Med. Hyg.*, **81**, 1033–7.

209. Bates, C.J., Rutishanser, I.H.E., Black, A.E. and Paul, A.A. (1977) Long-term vitamin status and dietary intake of healthy elderly subjects. 2. Vitamin C. *Br. J. Nutr.*, **42**, 43–56.

210. Smith, J.L. and Hodges, R.E. (1987) Serum levels of vitamin C in relation to dietary and supplemental intake of vitamin C in smokers and nonsmokers. *Ann. N.Y. Acad. Sci.*, **498**, 144–52.

211. Basu, T.K. (1981) The influence of drugs with particular reference to aspirin on the bioavailability of vitamin C, in *Vitamin C, Ascorbic Acid* (eds J.N. Counsell and B.H. Hornig), Applied Science Publishers, London, pp. 273–82.

212. Dickerson, J.W.T. (1981) Vitamin C and cancer, in *Vitamin C, Ascorbic Acid* (eds J.N. Counsell and B.H. Hornig), Applied Science Publishers, London, pp. 349–58.

213. Sauberlich, H.E., Dowdy, R.P. and Skala J.H. (1974) Vitamin C, in *Laboratory Tests for the Assessment of Nutritional Status* (eds H.E. Sauberlich, R.P. Dowdy and J.H. Skala), CRC Press Inc, Cleveland (Ohio), pp. 13–18.

214. Counsell, J.N. and Hornig D.H. (1982) *Vitamin C (Ascorbic acid)*, Applied Science Publishers, London.

215. Carpenter, K.J. (1986) *The History of Scurvy and Vitamin C*, Cambridge University Press, Cambridge.

216. Speek, A.J., Schrijver, J. and Schreurs, W.H.P. (1984) Fluorometric determination of total vitamin C in whole blood by high-performance liquid chromatography with pre-column derivatization. *J. Chromatogr.*, **305**, 53–60.

217. Pelletier, O. (1985) Vitamin C (L-ascorbic and dehydro-L-ascorbic acids), in *Methods of Vitamin Assay*, 4th edn (eds J. Augustin, B.P. Klein, D. Becker and P.B. Venugopal), Wiley-Interscience Publishers, New York, pp. 303–47.

8 Essential mineral and trace element nutriture methodology

8.1 Introduction   *P.J. Aggett*   332
8.2 Sodium   *W.P.T. James and A. Ralph*   335
8.3 Potassium   *W.P.T. James and A. Ralph*   340
8.4 Calcium   *D.M. Reid*   342
    Section I   Total serum/plasma calcium   344
    Section II   Ionized calcium   345
    Section III   Metacarpal indices   346
    Section IV   Urinary hydroxyproline   348
    Section V   Serum osteocalcin   349
8.5 Phosphorus   *P.J. Aggett*   350
8.6 Magnesium   *P.J. Aggett*   353
    Section I   Serum and urinary magnesium   353
    Section II   Serum magnesium by colorimetric method   354
8.7 Iron   *S. Hercberg, P. Galan and A. Dhur*   355
    Methods for assessing iron deficiency   355
    Section I   Methods for evaluating the risks of iron
                   deficiency (pre-pathogenic period)   356
    Section II   Methods for assessing iron status (pathogenic
                   period)   357
      Section IIA Indicators for evaluating the size of body
                   iron stores   357
      Section IIB Indicators of the adequacy of iron supply to
                   the erythroid marrow   362
      Section IIC Indicators of anaemia   372
                   Choice of indicators for assessing iron
                   deficiency in a population   376
                   Interpretation of iron status measurements   382
8.8 Zinc   *P.J. Aggett*   385
    Section I   Zinc in plasma or serum by atomic absorption
                   spectrophotometry   385
    Section II   Plasma or urine zinc   386
    Section III   Serum/plasma zinc – alternative method   387
    Section IV   Zinc in leukocyte and leukocyte subsets   388
    Section V   Hair zinc   391
    Section VI   Alkaline phosphatase   392

8.9   Copper   *P.J. Aggett*   395
    Section I   Plasma or serum copper by AAS   395
    Section II   Serum/plasma copper by colorimetric method   396
    Section III Measurement of human serum caeruloplasmin   396
    Section IV   Erythrocyte superoxide dismutase   398
8.10 Selenium   *G. Testolin, S. Ciappellano and J. Arthur*   401
    Section I   Blood selenium by spectrometry   402
    Section II   Blood selenium by fluorometric technique   404
    Section III Glutathione peroxidase activity   406
8.11 Chromium   *P.J. Aggett*   408
8.12 Manganese   *P.J. Aggett*   410

8.1   INTRODUCTION

Nutritional status is an imprecise term. One's approach to assessing 'status' should address whether or not one is wishing to discover if the individual or population under study is at risk of a deficiency or at risk of toxicity of the element in question. Except in the most extreme states few determinations, if any, can be used to answer both questions.

The selection of measurements and approaches to assess risks of deficiency or of toxicity depends on an understanding of the systemic metabolism and homeostatic regulation of any particular element.

Unlike organic nutrients, minerals cannot be transformed. They may alter their oxidation state, they may form complexes with other biological molecules as they are processed systemically, but their essential integrity is constant. Homeostasis is effected by regulation of absorption, hepatointestinal secretion, urinary excretion, or by sequestration of the element in either a specific systemic pool or relatively non-specific tissue pools (e.g. bone) with a very slow biological turnover. These factors are reflected by alterations in the elemental content of the various metabolic pools involved in body tissues and fluids. However, as yet the crucial susceptible metabolic pools that could provide warning of impending deficiency or toxicity of many minerals have not been identified.

This variation in composition or responses to deficiencies and excesses needs to be appreciated, and compositional analysis of tissues and fluids should always be interpreted in a physiological context. Furthermore, it should be appreciated that compositional analysis of many tissues may be too crude and insensitive to detect any altered concentrations in small but vital functional and sequestratory pools.

It is important that one does not overinterpret or become too reliant on physiologically senseless assays. To avoid this, functional parameters are being sought for many elements, the most promising of these are based on biochemical processes which are unequivocably dependent on the element being studied.

The spectrum of clinical response and systemic metabolic adaptation to elemental deficiencies and excesses is summarized in Table 8.1. It can be seen from this schema that deficiencies or excesses of a mineral stimulate different responses. Unfortunately the particular susceptible pools of the elements which initiate and regulate these homeostatic responses have not been identified and therefore they cannot be assessed either compositionally or functionally. Additionally the identity of the metabolic or anatomical pools involved in these responses probably differ according to whether the individual is at risk of deficiency or toxicity.

Table 8.1   The spectrum of mineral status and its associated pathophysiological phenomena

Death	
Toxicity:	Homeostatic excretion and tissue sequestration inadequate; clinical biochemical and pathological features
Compensatory homeostasis:	Homeostasis and sequestration adequate; no clinical disease
Initial excess:	Homeostatic storage and excretion
Adequacy	
Initial deprivation:	Homeostasis protects vital functional pools; no alterations in tissue and fluid concentrations; mobilization of stores; no clinical disease
Compensated metabolic phase:	Homeostasis becoming inadequate, 'early' functional defects; metabolism of other nutrients disrupted; health effects may occur
Decompensated metabolic phase:	Extensive specific and non-specific functional defects.
Gross clinical phase	
Death	

With extreme deficits or excesses of elements biochemical and compositional changes are more obvious and are accessible for analysis; such gross changes are those most frequently monitored by the current approaches used to assess the risk of deficiency or excess states. However, here again the usefulness of these assays depends on the selection and identification of the most appropriate functional and compositional pools for analysis.

The scope for doing this is improving as better analytical techniques are developed and more insight is acquired into possible susceptible functional pools.

Techniques developed from investigations of healthy individuals or animal models may not be applicable to clinical situations, since the systemic distribution of some minerals and their homeostatic mechanisms are deranged secondary to disease.

Approaches to determining individual's or population's 'status' based on measurements of mediators of homeostasis or of the homeostatic mechanisms themselves have not been fully developed, although such an approach is conceivable currently for some of the major elements, in particular calcium, and in the foreseeable future for zinc. However, in any event these approaches will be tedious and expensive and may therefore be best suited only in systematic studies of individual nutrient requirements, or for validating other assays of 'status', rather than in extensive nutritional surveys. Thus the following sections refer predominantly to compositional and functional analyses. In using these analyses it must always be remembered that these assays do not necessarily represent the biological ideal; such ideal measurements will only become established as knowledge is improved of the metabolism and biochemical roles of the nutrients in question.

The ultimate test of a pre-existent deficiency state for many minerals (e.g. Fe, Zn, Cu, and Se) is still that of monitoring the biochemical responses of one or, ideally, more relevant compositional, functional, or homeostatic parameters after supplementation of the element in question.

In the past three decades considerable progress has been made in inorganic analysis. A variety of techniques are now available for the determination of mineral concentrations in tissues and fluids. These include atomic absorption spectrophotometry (AAS), emission spectroscopy (ES), mass spectrometry (MS), neutron activation analysis (NAA), X-ray fluorescence spectrometry (XRF), and classic chemical methods such as colorimetry. The specificity, sensitivity, and detection limits of these methods vary from element to element and valuable overviews of these points as they relate to biochemistry are available [1–3].

Methods based on NAA, MS, and XR require expensive equipment and considerable analytical expertise [2, 3], and they are not outlined here. Even so, methods for determining the trace element concentration of biological material need adequate sensitivity at the low concentrations at which these micro-nutrients exist. In the absence of suitable sensitivity, appropriate precision and accuracy cannot be achieved [4, 5].

Throughout this section it should be remembered that rigorous effort is needed to avoid contamination during processing of samples for mineral analysis. This applies to the collection of material, separation and preparation of subsamples for analysis, the storage of material during which water losses as well as contamination may lead to spurious results, contamination from haemolysis and from needles and knives, analytical interferences, and contamination from prolonged storage [2, 6].

The use of external quality control material can go a long way towards improving inorganic analysis. The National Bureau of Standards provides Standard Reference Materials that are defined as 'well characterised materials produced in quantity and certified for one or more physical and chemical properties'. The theory and application of the use of the SRM to ensure good laboratory procedure and to monitor laboratory precision and accuracy has been well described [7–9] and details of such materials can be obtained from the National Institute of Standards and Technology, Gaithersberg, Maryland, USA, MD20899; the Analytical Quality Control Services, International Atomic Energy Agency, P.O. Box 100, A1400, Vienna, Austria; and, in Europe, the Community Bureau of Reference – BCR., Rue de la Loi 200, B1049 Brussels, Belgium.

An International Directory of Certified Reference Materials is available from

Society for REMCO, International Organization for Standardization 1, Rue de Varembe, Case Postale 56, 1211 Geneva 20, Switzerland.

The following outlines are not comprehensive and more extensive reviews of standard laboratory techniques merit consultation before establishing analyses [1–6, 10].

8.2   SODIUM

8.2.1   Purpose and scope

Sodium status is usually taken to relate to the concentration of Na in the blood. Yet so many mechanisms ensure that fluctuations in plasma Na concentration are minimized, that only in unusual pathological circumstances does hypo- or hypernatraemia occur. The measurements of plasma Na concentrations are therefore of little consequence in nutritional terms.

The hormonal regulation of sodium metabolism is also part of the explanation for sodium homeostasis so it is not easy to identify different levels of hormonal response as an index of the state of adaptation to sodium intake. Total body Na is of greater interest than serum Na concentration but is technically difficult to measure.

Total body sodium (or more accurately total exchangeable Na measured with radioisotopes) is increased in malnutrition because of a change in the distribution of Na between extra- and intracellular fluid. These measurements are not easy to make and are only appropriate to a few specialized research establishments. The changes in sodium distribution in malnutrition are illustrated in Table 8.2 derived from Shizgal's data on malnourished adult patients in Canada [11]. Here it is evident that the chronic effects of malnutrition lead to a rise in total body sodium. Since plasma Na tends to fall, this signifies a marked increase in intracellular Na as indicated for example by the rise in erythrocyte Na concentration. Although these increases may be considered to reflect a reduction in renal plasma flow and glomerular filtration rate, the evidence is against this factor as a primary cause [12] and a change in membrane transport is much more likely.

In malnourished adults there is an 18% increase in total body Na and associated with this a rise in total body water when this is expressed on a weight basis, so a distinction between an apparent and a real rise in body sodium demands independent measurements of total body fat, which have not yet been undertaken. Nevertheless a 7.5 kg loss of body fat in malnutrition is accompanied by a fall in body water of only 1 kg despite a concomitant drop in lean body mass of 3.8 kg (Table 8.2). Thus these data imply an increase in tissue hydration in malnutrition. Despite the estimated increase in intracellular Na, however, the main increase in body water seems to affect the extracellular volume, for reasons which are unclear.

Stress also leads to a rise in total body sodium as shown by Shizgal in measurements of postoperative patients (Table 8.2). This again reflects both a rise in intracellular sodium concentrations and an expansion of the extracellular fluid volume. The effects therefore seem to be a common response to stress. These measurements have been extended to studies on hypertension but no consistent increase in TB sodium has been found.

Table 8.2 Body composition in malnutrition and after major elective surgery

	Normal	Malnourished	Difference in malnutrition	Preoperative	Postoperative	Postoperative difference
Body weight (kg)	70.4 ± 2.5	58.9 ± 1.8	0.001	66.2 ± 1.9	65.3 ± 1.8	0.001
% Fat	28.7	21.6	0.01	27.5	25.8	–
Lean body mass	50.3 ± 1.9	46.5 ± 1.3	–	48.0 ± 1.8	47.2 ± 1.6	–
TBW l/kg body-wt	64.9	75.0	–	65.1	68.7	–
ICW/TBW %	57.5 ± 1.1	49.1 ± 0.9	0.001	55.7 ± 1.9	53.5 ± 1.6	–
ECW/TBW %	42.5 ± 1.1	50.0 ± 0.9	0.001	44.3 ± 1.9	46.5 ± 1.6	–
Na_e/TBW mmol/l	77.4 ± 0.9	94.7 ± 0.9	0.001	77.3 ± 2.1	82.5 ± 2.2	0.01
K_e/TBW mmol/l	80.0 ± 1.0	51.8 ± 1.2	0.001	78.2 ± 2.8	68.3 ± 3.1	0.05
Na_e/K_e	0.98 ± 0.02	1.95 ± 0.08	0.001	1.04 ± 0.08	1.29 ± 0.11	0.01

Compiled and recalculated from Shizgal [11].

TBW = total body water
ICW = intracellular water
ECW = extracellular water

8.2.2 Principle of methods

Total body sodium is measured as total exchangeable Na measured with dilution of radioisotopes ^{22}Na or ^{24}Na [13, 14], and is similar to the method in Section 2.3 for ^{42}K.

8.2.3 Procedure

The full description of this method, which requires specialized equipment, and the calculation is reported in Moore [14] and in section 2.3.

8.2.4 Interpretation

Sodium status has rarely been measured on a population level. More data are available on measures of nutrient intake and excretion. But so many homeostatic mechanisms sustain mineral balance that only at extreme ranges of intake is the monitoring of mineral intake likely to be of much significance as an indication of body stores, or indeed of metabolic function. The scepticism about the value of measures of mineral intake must, however, now be revised if it proves true that a high intake of NaCl or a low intake of Ca promote the development of hypertension. In this condition the metabolic response of the body to a particular nutrient ingested may be more important than the inflow of the mineral *per se*. Thus, if a natriuretic factor proves to be significant in the development of hypertension, Ca intake may be found to dampen the stimulation of the hormone induced by sodium ingestion. One might also theorize that Ca:Na ratios and Cl/P interactions might be found; they may all affect the distribution of intracellular Ca in arteriolar cells by a common hormonal pathway. In view of these highly speculative ideas in conjunction with the re-emerging interest in Ca, K, and Na intakes, some assessment of the measurements of mineral intake is warranted.

We have summarized elsewhere [15] the problem that emerges when attempts are made to establish the individual's habitual intake of a particular mineral. Not only are there problems because people change their intake when under study but there is also the question of how one ensures that an assessment of intake during one period is relevant to the habitual intake of the same person.

Table 8.3 shows data on total daily Na and K excretion and its variability. The assumption has been made that Na and K intake can best be monitored by measuring output in urine. This is because it is very difficult to be sure of the amount of salt in different foods, particularly when they are cooked at home with variable amounts of cooking and with table salt being added. Cooking also tends to leach out the potassium, so this problem of cooking affects both elements. The data are taken from a Cambridgeshire study where 12 consecutive 24-h urines were collected [16]. This was considered necessary because of possible substantial intraindividual variations in intakes when considered on a daily basis. The problem of within-person variability in epidemiological studies and its consequences when subjects may be incorrectly classified was first emphasized by Gardner and Heady [17]. From a detailed statistical analysis they showed how the minimum number (n) of repeated measurements which must be made to achieve any desired degree of correlation between the observed mean values and the 'correct' values for each subject could be calculated from measurements of intraindividual variation. The assumption is that the errors between different individuals and within individuals are independent of the level of each other and of the true value of the

Table 8.3   Intra- and inter-individual variability in the first March study
(Based on 48 subjects, including both men and women)

Variable	Mean value	Residual* variance	Intraindividual variance (σ_a^2)	SD (σ_a)	No. of repeats (k)	Interindividual variance** (σ_r^2)	SD (σ_r)	Ratio σ_a^2/σ_r^2
Urine vol. (l/day)	1.62	0.384	0.303	0.55	12	0.359	0.60	0.84
K excretion (mmol/day)	70.50	172.000	215.000	14.70	12	154.000	12.40	1.40
Na excretion (mmol/day)	148.000	900.000	1694.000	41.20	12	759.000	27.50	2.23
Creatinine (mmol/day)	13.00	1.490	1.670	1.29	12	1.35	1.16	1.24
Urea (mmol/day)	635.00	9025.000	11760.000	108.00	12	8045.000	89.70	1.46
K/Creatinine	5.52	0.940	1.570	1.25	12	0.810	0.90	1.94
Na/Creatinine	11.60	4.280	10.810	3.29	12	3.380	1.84	3.20
Systolic BP	119.00	92.000	50.400	7.10	13	88.100	9.40	0.57
Diastolic BP	69.70	45.400	38.600	6.22	13	42.400	6.50	0.91
Mean BP	86.00	46.500	32.900	5.73	13	44.000	6.60	0.75

* Variance between mean values for individuals after excluding any components associated with differences in parental BP group, sex, age, and body-weight.
** Obtained from the above by subtracting the intraindividual contribution (σ_a^2/k).

intake. The within-person variability is also assumed to be the same for all individuals.

Similar statistical methods and assumptions were applied by Liu *et al.* [18] who went on to consider the effect of intraindividual and interindividual variability in one variable (for example, Na excretion) on the estimation of the interindividual correlation with a second variable (for example blood pressure). They showed that the estimated correlation coefficient would be reduced by a factor $f = \sqrt{[k/(k+r)]}$, where k was the number of measurements (of Na excretion) made on each individual subject and r was the ratio of the intra- to interindividual variance component. Clearly the reduction in correlation is most serious for high values of the ratio r, but can be ameliorated by compensating increases in the number of observations of k. The value of k required to limit the reduction to a value f can be calculated from the equation $k = rf^2/(1-f^2)$, where $0 < f < 1$. For example, the correlation will only be reduced by 10% of its true value if f is taken as 0.9, when k must be at least 4.2 r (Table 8.4).

Table 8.3 shows that the ratios of variances (r) were surprisingly small for Na excretion in the Cambridgeshire study compared with a ratio of 3.2 found in Chicago business personnel by Liu *et al.* [19]. On the basis of the Chicago data 14 collections of 24-h urine would have been necessary to limit the weakening of the correlation of the apparent with the true sodium excretion to less than 10%. The data in Table 8.3 suggest that a 5% limit on the reduction in correlation requires 7 and 7 days in men and 12 and 6 days in women for Na and K excretion respectively. For any large-scale study it would be desirable to

Table 8.4 Attenuation factors for correlation coefficients

The correlation coefficients between two variables, each measured on a number of individuals, will be reduced by the factor f when measurements of one of the variables are affected by intraindividual variation. Let σ_a^2 and σ_r^2 be the *intra-* and *inter*-individual components of variance and let the variable affected be estimated as the mean of k independent measurements on each individual:

$$\text{then } f = \sqrt{[1/(1+\sigma_a^2/k\sigma_r^2)]} = \sqrt{[k/(k+r)]} \text{ where } r = \sigma_a^2/\sigma_r^2$$

r	k						
	1	*2*	*3*	*5*	*10*	*15*	*20*
	Attenuation factor						
0.1	0.95	0.98	0.98	0.99	1.00	1.00	1.00
0.2	0.91	0.95	0.97	0.98	0.99	0.99	1.00
0.4	0.85	0.91	0.94	0.96	0.98	0.99	0.99
0.8	0.75	0.85	0.89	0.93	0.96	0.97	0.98
1.0	0.71	0.82	0.87	0.91	0.95	0.97	0.98
1.5	0.63	0.76	0.82	0.88	0.93	0.95	0.96
2.0	0.58	0.71	0.77	0.85	0.91	0.94	0.95
3.0	0.50	0.63	0.71	0.79	0.88	0.91	0.93
4.0	0.45	0.58	0.65	0.75	0.85	0.89	0.91
8.0	0.33	0.45	0.52	0.62	0.75	0.81	0.85

Liu *et al.* [18].

establish by a preliminary survey the number of observations that might be required for an accurate assessment of the usual excretory rate of these minerals.

For estimating Na intake the assumption has been made that urinary output is a good reflection of intake. This was assessed in a metabolic study [20] and found urinary Na to be 93% of intake (Table 8.5). This supports the concept of urinary Na excretion as an index of intake but assumes that sweat losses of Na are small in all climates and conditions. It is likely that a similar approach could be taken for potassium, since 5–10% of K loss occurs in the faeces, with even smaller sweat losses.

Simple approaches to assessing the proportion of ingested Na excreted via the urine have unfortunately failed. Originally it was hoped that the use of lithium would be helpful. Thus in metabolic studies it was shown that there was a remarkable concordance of Na and lithium handling in man. An oral dose of Li, e.g. 250 mmol, could then perhaps be used to assess the proportions of Li (or Na) being excreted in the urine by a particular population group [21]. For example, it might be found that a group of miners working at the coal-face are losing half their Na via sweat and that in these individuals any analysis of urinary Na excretion and blood pressure would be invalid. This could be overcome by providing the miners with a standard dose (or doses) of Li while the 24-h urine collections were being made for monitoring the habitual rate of Na excretion.

Unfortunately new studies show that under conditions of high sweat rates sodium but not lithium is lost in the sweat, and no simple validation is available. Lithium can in these circumstances only be used as a check on urinary collections. If some urine is lost, then Na and Li excretion will be underestimated. A more useful rapid check on urine collections, however, involves the use of another marker, para-aminobenzoic acid (PABA) [22], which with its measurable metabolites is almost completely excreted in urine.

A scheme for validating Na intakes by a combination of these methods is shown in Table 8.6. This scheme is the most rigorous that one could apply. In the absence of PABA one has to assume completeness of the collection. Any loss in urinary Na will be accompanied by the loss of urinary Li, which can only be used as a long-term urinary marker rather than as a correlation factor to derive Na intake. The same approach with Li marking could be applied to chloride output or to K or P measurements, but again sweat and faecal losses of K and P are very unlikely to be paralleled by equivalent Li losses, particularly under conditions where considerable sweat loss is occurring.

Table 8.5   The routes of excretion of ingested sodium and lithium

	Urine (% total output)	*Faeces* (% total output)	*Sweat* (% total output)
Sodium	93.2 ± 3.4	1.4 ± 1.2	2.0 ± 0.5
Lithium	93.2 ± 1.4	1.7 ± 0.9	1.7 ± 0.9

Data from Sanchez-Castillo *et al.* [21].

Table 8.6   Theoretical approaches to validating dietary sodium intakes

1   Repeated urine collection, e.g. 13 days

2   Give 250 mmol lithium carbonate daily, orally for long term collections

3   Give para-aminobenzoic acid (PABA) in capsules twice daily for short term, i.e. 1–2 day collections

Measure urinary lithium (Li), sodium and para-aminohippuric acid and other metabolites of PABA in urine.

If PABA metabolites are equivalent to >85% intake, or Li excretion is >90% then consider the collection complete.

The number of days chosen for collection will depend on the precise nature of the study and the intra-individual and inter-individual variation of the excretion of Na in the urine. This can be estimated in a pilot survey. Whereas PABA can be used for short term studies the build up and slower excretion of Li from body pools only makes it useful for collections lasting 1–2 weeks.

8.3   POTASSIUM

8.3.1   Purpose and scope

Potassium status is assessed by considering two principal components: the circulating plasma concentration of K and total body potassium (TBK). Ninety-eight per cent of TBK is intracellular but the ratio of extra- to intracellular K is a critical determinant of the membrane potential of excitable tissues so the control of the free K is very important.

Dietary K intake commonly varies from 80 to 150 mmol daily with the kidney being the principal route of excretion; only 5–15 mmol K is lost by the faecal route each day. The external balance is controlled by the kidney, perhaps primarily by aldosterone, which increases K output while stimulating the distal renal tubule to retain Na. The internal balance of K ions across membranes is complex and poorly understood. Normally intracellular K amounts to 180 mmol/l but some of this is bound to intracellular anions e.g. proteins. Much of the intracellular K is located in muscle so as muscle depletion occurs in malnutrition, K is lost with the protein. This is a loss of K capacity rather than a fall due to true cellular depletion of K in terms of intracellular water.

This distinction between a fall in TBK from a fall in tissue capacity for K and a fall due to cellular depletion of K is important. In the former an increase in TBK depends on the laying down of new intracellular components such as protein, which increases the intracellular mass and K binding capacity; this process is therefore slow, whereas a true K-depleted state can readily be corrected over a short time.

8.3.2 Principle of methods

Total body potassium may be measured by referring to the total mass of protein by measuring total body nitrogen (TBN) by neutron activation analysis [23]. In whole body terms there is a close relationship between TBN and TBK but the intercept of a graph of fat-free mass (estimated from skinfold thickness) suggests that there is a component of the fat-free mass (FFM) which is free of both N and K. Once this is allowed for, the K concentration in FFM can be derived as described in Chapter 2, section 2.4. Studies on whole body nitrogen require facilities available at very few centres in the world, therefore this approach is for the present, a research tool rather than a method for the repeated monitoring of patients or for population studies. The method is described in Chapter 2, section 2.4.

Total body potassium is usually measured by ^{42}K dilution or by whole body counting of the naturally abundant ^{40}K to determine the amount of lean tissue [24]. Although this technique is of limited availability, facilities may be built into a mobile van as at the East Kilbride Nuclear Reactor Centre in Scotland, where some important studies have been completed. These methods are described in Chapter 2, section 2.3 and in [13] and [14].

More direct measures of K depletion in tissues require muscle biopsies [25]. It is necessary to be cautious about the frame of reference since loss of N by tissues is accompanied by a fall in K. The reference value in a tissue may be taken to be the collagen protein content, since this seems to be maintained in malnutrition.

8.3.3 Procedure

A description of measurement of total body K by radioisotope dilution and whole body counting is given in Chapter 2, sections 2.3 and 2.4.

8.3.4 Performance characteristics

(a) Reproducibility   Refer to Chapter 2, section 2.3.

(b) Validity   Refer to Chapter 2, section 2.3.

8.3.5 Reference values   Refer to Chapter 2, section 2.3 and Moore *et al.* [14].

8.3.6 Interpretation   Refer to Chapter 2, section 2.3.

8.4 CALCIUM

8.4.1 Purpose and scope

Calcium, as the fifth most abundant element in the body, has many differing and indispensable functions. Ninety nine per cent of the element in the body is to be found in the bones [26] where it is largely in the form of calcium phosphate crystals, which give rigidity and strength to the collagen and proteoglycan matrix. At the cellular level it is responsible for the maintenance and regulation of many biochemical processes, for the integrity and permeability of cell membranes, as a coupling factor between excitation and contraction in muscle, as a regulator of nerve excitability and as regulator of secretions from exocrine and endocrine glands [27].

Calcium in blood is found in the plasma compartment in diffusible and non-diffusible forms. The latter is bound principally to albumin, is un-ionized and non-filtratable. About 40% of calcium is in the protein-bound form, with approximately 10% complexed to phosphate, citrate, and bicarbonate, and the remaining 50% appearing in an ionized form [28]. The ionized form of the element is responsible for many of the physiological properties of calcium, and in particular in the bloodstream, for one of its most important functions, the regulation of the blood coagulation cascade.

Assessment of calcium status in the body depends on considering which function or pool of calcium is the most appropriate for the investigator. Measurement of calcium for assessment of its physiological function is best carried out by plasma ionized calcium [29], whereas some indication of its bone function can be obtained by measuring total plasma calcium (for example in osteomalacia and hyperparathyroidism). Measurement of bone mass or bone density can be used to assess the size of the major calcium reservoir, while assessment of calcium kinetics require, at the very least, an accurate measurement of calcium absorption, bone turnover (bone resorption and bone formation) and urinary calcium loss. Assessment of calcium homeostasis includes measurements of the calciotrophic hormones parathyroid hormone, calcitonin, and the various vitamin D metabolites.

8.4.2 Principles of methods

Ionized calcium is measured directly in the plasma by means of a calcium selective electrode, but can be calculated indirectly by 'correcting' total calcium concentrations for the variations in the plasma proteins, albumin, and globulin and for alterations in blood pH [30].

Total plasma calcium is usually measured by means of autoanalysers using colorimetric techniques, but can be measured manually, usually by atomic absorption spectrometry. Again a variety of methods have been described to 'correct' the total calcium measurements for variations in serum albumin [31].

Measurement of bone mass and bone density is a rapidly expanding field in which new methods are described frequently. Measurement of total body calcium can be carried out directly by means of neutron activation analysis [32] or by total body bone mineral content using dual-photon absorptiometry [33]. The two methods are extremely well correlated ($r > 0.99$), although the radiation dose with the former method is much greater [34]. Both these methods are expensive, the former relying on a source of neutrons and a lead-shielded whole-body counter and the latter requiring a commercially available dual-photon absorptiometer such as the Novo BMC-Lab 23 or the Lunar DPA 4. Other densitometry methods are available, most relying on dedicated densitometers using photon absorptiometry [35]. Newer dedicated machines based on dual energy X-ray absorption (DXA) are only now being developed and may have considerable benefits over photon absorptiometric methods with respect to speed of operation, radiation dose, and precision [36].

Quantitative computed tomography (CT) can be used to measure the vertebral mineral density and has the advantage of giving a measurement of pure trabecular bone. It can be carried out with most whole-body CT scanners but usually requires the purchase of a dedicated software package and a specially designed phantom [37]. None of these methods of bone mineral assessment is freely available, and for extensive population-based study of bone density, the use of radiographs of the hand to measure cortical indices, and radiographs of the pelvis to measure trabecular patterns still have to be considered.

The measurement of cortical indices is particularly useful as compared to other measurements of bone density or mass in not requiring specialist equipment and yet having the potential for computer-assisted calculation. It is therefore useful for community-based studies provided there is an available radiology department to undertake the radiographs.

Measurement of calcium kinetics should include measurement of calcium absorption by single or dual-isotope methodology, *in-vivo* non-invasive assessment of bone turnover by measurement of urinary hydroxyproline to estimate bone resorption and breakdown, and serum osteocalcin to evaluate bone formation. In the past, serum alkaline phosphatase was used for this latter purpose, but it is rather non-specific in site of origin, also arising from liver amongst other organs.

Measurement of total urinary hydroxyproline is used as an indicator of bone resorption, although as a collagen breakdown product it may arise from many other sites including skin, tendon, cartilage, etc. An elevated level cannot therefore be taken necessarily to indicate increased bone resorption. It can be influenced strongly by dietary factors, especially those containing collagen, e.g. gelatin.

Osteocalcin, also known as bone GLA protein, is a vitamin-K-dependent protein whose exact physiological function is currently unknown, although it is believed to play a part in calcium binding [38]. It also inhibits hydroxyapatite precipitation *in vitro* [39] and is a chemoattractant for bone resorbing cells [40]. It is clear from many *in vitro* and *in vivo* studies that osteocalcin derives largely from osteoblasts and accordingly can be used as a marker of bone formation [41]. Osteocalcin is elevated when there is excess new bone formation, such as after a fracture [42], and reduced when bone formation is depressed, such as in patients treated with corticosteroid therapy [43].

Calcium loss should be measured by urinary calcium excretion, because much of the calcium in faeces arises from unabsorbed calcium in the diet.

SECTION I   TOTAL SERUM/PLASMA CALCIUM

8.4.3 Principle of the method

The automated technique is based on a colorimetric method [44] which makes use of a calcium complexing dye, cresolphthalein complexone, in an alkaline medium. The product of the interaction is a pink-coloured calcium dye complex with a maximum absorption at 570 nm.

8.4.4 Chemicals and apparatus

(a) Chemicals

For the Technicon autoanalyser the following reagents are available:

8-Hydroxyquinoline containing water, 8-hydroxyquinoline 2.5 g/l and HCl 0.3 N (Technicon product No. T01-0708).

Cresolphthalein complexone, each litre containing water, hydrochloric acid 7.03 g, 8-hydroxyquinoline 2.5 g, cresolphthalein complexone 0.07 g, and surfactant (Technicon product No. T01-0709).

Diethylamine reagent, each litre containing water and diethylamine 26.7 g (Technicon product No. T01-0867).

(b) Apparatus

Technicon autoanalyser or equivalent.

8.4.5 Sample collection

Analysis can be carried out on either serum or plasma samples; however, since heparin complexes some of the calcium present in plasma, serum is preferable. Ideally, to avoid interference of binding proteins, the samples should be taken without tourniquet assistance, and prolonged venous stasis should be avoided. Samples should be taken while the subject is in the recumbent position because higher levels are found when subjects are upright [45]. Serum samples should be separated from red cells and analysed promptly.

8.4.6 Procedure

Neat or prediluted serum is added to diluted HCl containing 8-hydroxyquinoline. The HCl releases the protein-bound calcium and 8-hydroxyquinoline binds free magnesium ions, which would otherwise interfere with the assay. The free, ionized calcium ions are dialysed across a semipermeable type H membrane into the analytical stream of cresolphthalein complexone. Upon the addition of diethylamine to the analytical stream, a coloured complex is formed at 37°C between the calcium and the dye. The absorbance of the reaction product is measured at 570 nm in a flowcell that has a 10-mm light path and an inside diameter of 0.5 mm.

8.4.7 Performance characteristics

(a) Reproducibility

The day-to-day coefficient of variation is 3.2–3.4%, and 2.1–2.7% within a run, across a normal range.

(b) Validity

Several substances can interfere with the method. Calcium salts in distilled water or in ordinary filter paper as well as contaminating bromsulphthalein or hydralazine can produce increased calcium values, while oxalates and fluorides can precipitate calcium, artificially decreasing the values [46].

8.4.8 Reference values

Most automated methods quote normal values of 2.20–2.60 mmol/l (8.5–10.5 mg/dl) but it is recommended that each laboratory should establish its own reference values.

8.4.9 Interpretation

The correlation between the colorimetric method described and methods based on atomic absorption spectrometry [47] is extremely good, $r = 0.980$ [48]. A number of formulae have been constructed to correct total calcium concentrations for variations in serum proteins, particularly albumin [49]. One of the most commonly used formulae is to adjust for serum albumin by subtracting 0.025 mmol/l from serum calcium for every 1 g/l by which serum albumin exceeds 40 g/l, with the reverse procedure for albumin values below 40 g/l. There may be a need for adjustment of total serum calcium, especially where urgent serum calcium has been measured [50].

SECTION II   IONIZED CALCIUM

8.4.10 Chemicals and apparatus

(a) Chemicals

Reagents and calibrator solutions as supplied with the apparatus.

(b) Apparatus

An ion-selective calcium electrode (ISE) is required. Examples of these are the Radiometer ICA1 (Radiometer A/S, Copenhagen) and the Nova 8 (Nova Biomedical Inc., Waltham, Massachusetts). These have been termed second-generation ISEs as they simultaneously measure not only Ca^{2+}, but also pH. These improvements are achieved by using two types of liquid-membrane sensors namely organophosphate and neutral carrier.

8.4.11 Sample collection

Ionized calcium can be measured in whole blood, plasma, or serum. Anticoagulants should be avoided or, if used, calcium titrated sodium heparin used. Haemolysis of samples should be avoided and samples analysed within 4 h, with specimens stored at 0–4°C between sampling and analysis. To avoid any effects of posture, diurnal variation, or recent food ingestion, some authorities recommend sampling in the morning after an overnight fast while the subject remains supine.

8.4.12 Procedure

Details of the technique have recently been published [51]. Samples of serum or equivalent are measured directly in the commercial apparatus, with the result being available at around 90 s.

8.4.13 Performance characteristics

Reproducibility

The precision of the technique expressed as the coefficient of variation of repeated measurements of external controls varies from 1.0% to 1.4%.

8.4.14 Reference values

The $Ca^{2+}_{7.4}$ limits for adults under basal conditions using the Radiometer ICA 1 are from 1.17 to 1.29 mmol/l [51].

8.4.15 Interpretation

Ionized calcium can be falsely elevated in venous stasis, but can show markedly reduced levels when total serum calcium levels remain at or near normal, such as after cardiac arrest [52], or when large volumes of citrated blood have been infused [53]. *In vitro* Ca^{2+} is artificially lowered at high pH and vice versa. Hence ionized calcium values are frequently corrected to pH 7.4, i.e. $Ca^{2+}_{7.4}$. Samples taken in ambulant patients can be elevated by up to 0.04 mmol/l. Measurements of free or ionized calcium are still not widely used but may soon be included on large autoanalysers [54]. While corrected total calcium values correlate well with ionized calcium values in most situations, this is not always the case in critically ill individuals [55, 56]. Albumin may not be the only factor influencing the relationship, as globulin and pH may also play a part [57].

SECTION III   METACARPAL INDICES

This technique has the advantage over most other measurements of bone density or mass in not requiring specialized equipment.

8.4.16 Apparatus

A standard X-ray tube is all that is required to obtain the radiographs. Assessment of metacarpal indices from the resultant radiographs also requires the use of a set of Vernier callipers with a scale reading to 0.1 mm.

8.4.17 Procedure

(a) Technique

The technique is based on a single posteroanterior X-ray of the hands taken on non-screen film with the film 1 m from the source. The exposure should be standardized to 52 mA for 0.04 s [58].

The various metacarpal indices described are all derived from basic geometrical measurements obtained directly from the radiographs. The length (L) of the second, third, and fourth metacarpals, usually of both hands, are measured with a millimetre rule. At the mid-point of each metacarpal the external diameter (D) and the internal diameter (d) are measured with the Vernier scale calliper.

(b) Calculation

From these measurements are derived the following indices:

Cortical width	$D - d$
Per cent cortical width	$D - d/D$
Cortical area	$D^2 - d^2$
Per cent cortical area	$D^2 - d^2/D^2$
Cortical area per unit length	$D^2 - d^2/L$
Cortical area/total area	$D^2 - d^2/DL$

Most of these indices have their supporters, but the indices using some measurement of metacarpal length or external diameter have the advantage of 'correcting' for skeletal size, at least in part.

When the technique was initially used a single metacarpal was measured (usually the second right) but reproducibility was poor and this was improved by using the middle three metacarpals in the right hand and then by including the middle metacarpals of the left hand as well. The final result is achieved by dividing the total value of the index chosen by the number of metacarpals included in the measurement. The first and fifth metacarpals are excluded because of irregularity of shape.

8.4.18 Performance characteristics

(a) Reproducibility

The precision expressed as the coefficient of variation of measurements repeated in normal controls over a short time period is 1–2% depending on the index used [59]. The intra-observer variation is, as expected, less than the inter-observer variation [60]. Precision may be improved by the use of computer-assisted measurement using a digitizer and a microcomputer [61].

(b) Validity

The technique is valid for cortical bone in the periphery only and it cannot be considered to be a technique for diagnosing osteoporosis, a disorder which affects principally trabecular bone in the axial skeleton. For example, patients with exogenous corticosteroid-induced osteoporosis who have reduced total bone mass have normal metacarpal indices [62], and patients with endogenous Cushing's syndrome can have markedly reduced vertebral trabecular bone density with high normal metacarpal indices [63].

8.4.19 Reference values

These vary dramatically throughout life and between the sexes. Although using the correction factors described above allows for differing skeletal size, the differences between men and women do not become apparent until after the menopause [64]. Metacarpal indices fall with age in both sexes although there is controversy as to when the bone loss commences, and also the mathematical function that the rate of loss follows. Most authorities agree that cortical bone loss is linear in men, probably starting in the fifth decade, and many now believe that cortical bone loss in women also follows a linear function, perhaps starting in the fourth decade. There are racial differences between populations studied and hence it is usually necessary for reference ranges to be derived locally, although data for European [65] and American [66] populations are published.

8.4.20 Interpretation

Metacarpal indices correlate well with other more sophisticated measurements of bone density, especially where measured sites contain a major proportion of cortical bone. Hence the correlations between metacarpal indices and total body calcium (the total skeleton containing 80% of cortical bone) are better ($r = 0.6$–0.9) [67] than between metacarpal indices and vertebral bone mineral density measured by dual-photon absorptiometry. The major disadvantage with metacarpal indices are that they only give a measurement of cortical bone in the peripheral part of the skeleton.

SECTION IV URINARY HYDROXYPROLINE

8.4.21 Apparatus

Samples must be assessed photometrically usually by a colorimeter equipped with a narrow band interference filter of about 560 nm. Alternatively a spectrophotometer can be used at 560 nm wavelength.

8.4.22 Sample collection

This is critical. It is recommended that estimations be carried out on urine samples collected over a 24-h period while patients are established on a collagen-free diet containing no meat, soup, gravy, ice cream, candy, or other products containing gelatin. This diet is highly restrictive and as dietary collagen is cleared from the extracellular fluid within 12 h of eating [68], a 2-h specimen of urine collected after an overnight fast is usually acceptable. The subject is asked to empty the bladder at 8 a.m. and urine is collected over the subsequent 2-h period. The urine sample should contain no preservative and should not be acidified. A 10-ml aliquot of the sample can be kept cool for up to 24 h prior to the determination, but if longer storage is required the sample should be stored at −20°C.

8.4.23 Procedure

(a) Technique

Commercial kits are available to carry out the analysis. That described here involves the use of the Hypronosticon kit (Organon Teknika). Each determination is performed in duplicate. As the technique is designed to measure total hydroxyproline, it is necessary to hydrolyse the urine by adding a resin tablet to each tube followed by vigorous shaking by hand, centrifugation for 5 min at 1500 g and incubation of the supernatant overnight (16 h) in a heating bath at 102 ± 2°C. The bath should preferably be filled with glycerol or silicone oil.

After incubation the tubes are cooled to room temperature, 1% phenolphthalein added, and the tubes again centrifuged. After removal of the supernatant, buffer and oxidant solutions are added and the solution allowed to stand for at least 4 min before colour reagent is added and the resultant reaction measured photometrically.

(b) Calculation

The resultant urinary excretions are expressed as ratios to creatinine, which avoids errors in the timed urine samples and allows comparison between individuals, correcting for differences in body weight [69].

Alternatively, if 24-h samples of urine have been collected the values should be corrected for body surface area (A) using the formula:

$$A = H^{0.725} \cdot W^{0.425} \cdot 71.84 \cdot 10^{-4}$$

where H = the height in cm and W = the weight in kg.

8.4.24 Performance characteristics

(a) Reproducibility

The precision expressed as the coefficient of variation between paired samples can be as low as 5.3% with some methods [69].

(b) Validity

Dietary uncertainties and the difficulty of measurement have led to a search for alternative methods of assessing collagen breakdown. The assessment of collagen cross-links (pyridinium) in the urine appears to be such a method [70] and these can now be measured by high-performance liquid chromatography [71]. One of the cross-link products, deoxypyridinoline appears to arise specifically from bone [72] and has recently been shown to correlate extremely well with urinary hydroxyproline [73].

8.4.25 Reference values

These are affected by the age of the subject as shown below.

Age	mg hydroxyproline/24 h/m^2
1 week to 1 year	55–220
1–13 years	25– 80
22–65 years	6– 22
over 66 years	5– 17

It is recommended that each laboratory should establish its own reference values.

8.4.26 Interpretation

The technique as described shows good agreement with values found using other methods [74]. The values obtained can be useful in assessing disease activity in various metabolic disorders, especially Paget's disease [75], and in assessing rapid bone loss in osteoporosis [76].

SECTION V   SERUM OSTEOCALCIN

8.4.27 Chemicals and apparatus

(a) Chemicals

Commercial kits are generally based on rabbit antibodies directed against ^{125}I bovine osteocalcin. Bound and free fractions are separated with goat anti-rabbit anti-serum.

(b) Apparatus

Osteocalcin is measured by radioimmunoassay and a scintillation counter is all that is required.

8.4.28 Sample collection

Osteocalcin concentrations show substantial diurnal variation, with the levels being lowest in the morning, rising to a maximum around 4.00 a.m. [77]. Samples should therefore be collected at a standard time of day, for example in the morning, although as there appears to be no dietary effect, fasting samples are not required.

Blood samples should be processed within 2–3 h, centrifuged cold if possible, and then serum stored at −70°C.

8.4.29 Procedure

The measurements are usually carried out by radioimmunoassay, but enzyme immunoassay can also be used. Commercial kits are currently available from Immuno Nuclear Stillwater (Minnesota, USA) and CEAORIS Industrie, Sacley (France), amongst other suppliers. The assays are based on the use of polyclonal antibodies and many laboratories have made or are developing their own. In summary 50-μl aliquots of unknown serum sample or standards are mixed with 200 μl of rabbit anti-bovine osteocalcin and ^{125}I bovine osteocalcin. After overnight incubation at room temperature with constant shaking, the bound and free fractions are separated with goat anti-rabbit anti-serum. The total counts in the supernatant are measured in a scintillation counter.

8.4.30 Performance characteristics

(a) Detection limit

Assays are sensitive to at least 0.1 mg/ml.

(b) Reproducibility

Inter- and intra-assay variations are less than 15% and 10% respectively with all available kits.

8.4.31 Reference values

Values are at their highest during first year of life (25–40 mg/ml), fall back in childhood, only to peak again in adolescence (2–12 mg/ml). In adult life the values fall back again, the levels being slightly higher in men (6.8 ± 0.5 mg/ml) than in women (5.8 ± 0.5 mg/ml). It is recommended that each laboratory should establish its own reference values.

8.4.32 Interpretation

Repeated freeze-thawing considerably reduces osteocalcin values, as will haemolysis of the samples [41]. The biphosphonates, specifically etidronate, and lead may displace osteocalcin from bone, resulting in falsely elevated levels [41].

High values are found after menopause [78], in thyrotoxicosis [79], Paget's disease [80] and in early life [81].

8.5 PHOSPHORUS

8.5.1 Purpose and scope

The human adult contains 17–20 mol (530–620 g) of phosphorus as phosphate. The skeleton embodies 85% to 95% of this in the form of hydroxyapatite. The rest is distributed about the body in roughly equal proportions between extracellular and intracellular compartments. Phosphate in the extracellular fluid is in equilibrium with the skeletal and cellular inorganic phosphate pools and with a large number of organic phosphate compounds involved with cellular metabolism. Intracellularly, phosphate is an important component of structural molecules such as phospholipids and phosphoproteins. There is additionally within the cells an important 'inorganic' phosphate pool, which participates in high-energy transfer reactions involving bi-phosphorylated and tri-phosphorylated nucleotides; the major form of which is adenosine triphosphate (ATP) formed by mitochondrial oxidative phosphorylation. Inorganic phosphate (Pi), by virtue of transitions between HPO_4^{2-}; $H_2PO_4^-$ is an important component for acid–base balance.

The humoral control of systemic homeostasis of phosphorus is imperfectly understood. Parathormone, calcitonin, and calcitriol are all involved, probably indirectly via their influence on calcium metabolism. Plasma phosphate concentrations are regulated principally by renal excretion of phosphate, which is influenced directly by parathormone which reduces the renal tubular reabsorption of the anion.

8.5.2 Principle of the method

After precipitation of protein and the concomitant release of bound Pi by trichloroacetic acid the determination of Pi depends on the formation of a hexavalent complex between the phosphate ion and molybdate usually as an ammonium phosphomolybdate salt $[(NH_4)_3(PO_4(MoO_3)_2)]$, which can be reduced to a pentavalent form and determined spectrophotometrically at approximately 700 nm [82].

8.5.3 Chemicals and apparatus

(a) Chemicals

Trichloroacetic acid ($C_2HCl_3O_2$) p.a.
Ammonium molybdate $[(NH_4)_6Mo_7O_{24} . 4H_2O]$ p.a.
Sodium bisulphite ($NaHSO_3$) p.a.
Semidine hydrochloride (N-phenyl-p-phenylenediamine hydrochloride) ($C_6H_5NHC_6H_4NH_2 . HCl$) p.a.
Ethanol, absolute (C_2H_5OH) p.a.
Potassium dihydrogen phosphate (KH_2PO_4) p.a.
De-ionized water.

(b) Solutions

Trichloracetic acid, 0.61 mol/l: 100 g of trichloroacetic acid is added to approximately 800 ml of de-ionized water in a 1-litre volumetric flask. The solution is mixed thoroughly and made up to volume. When prepared, it is stable at room temperature for four weeks and at 4°C for six months.

Ammonium molybdate, 8 mmol/l: 9.887 g of ammonium molybdate are dissolved in 700–750 ml of de-ionized water in a 1-litre volumetric flask. The mixture is stirred thoroughly and then made up to 1000 ml. This can be stored in a polyethylene bottle at room temperature and is stable for four weeks.

Sodium bisulphite, 96 mmol/l: 10 g of sodium bisulphite are dissolved in de-ionized water to make 1000 ml.

Semidine hydrochloride, 2.76 mmol/l, is prepared by weighing out 250 mg of semidine HCl in a polystyrene weighing boat and adding 0.5 ml of absolute ethanol. The semidine is washed with the previously prepared sodium bisulphite solution into a 500-ml volumetric flask, mixed well, and made up to volume with residual bisulphite solution. This preparation should be filtered through a glass wool plug into a dark borosilicate container and stored in the dark at room temperature. At the first evidence of any discoloration, the solution should be discarded.

Phosphorus standard solutions:

Stock standard, 20 mmol/l: 1.36 g potassium dihydrogen phosphate is dissolved in 200–300 ml de-ionized water and made up to 500 ml.

Working standards, range 0.1–0.2 mmol/l. These should be prepared by appropriate dilutions of the stock standard.

(c) Apparatus

Automatic pipette device; glass test tubes of various dimensions. All glassware should be acid washed and free of detergents.

Centrifuge

Spectrophotometer.

8.5.4   Sample collection

Blood should be collected without venous stasis (cf. sampling for Ca), and preferably after a fast. Plasma/serum Pi are reduced postprandially. Serum or heparinized plasma should be separated from the cells within 30 min of withdrawing the blood, because prolonged standing increases the hydrolysis of erythrocyte and platelet organic phosphates, thereby releasing inorganic phosphate and spuriously elevating the plasma or serum Pi concentrations. Since haemoglobin spoils the assay, haemolysed samples should not be used; chelating anticoagulants (e.g. citrate, oxalate, EDTA, EGTA) impair the formation of phosphomolybdate and should not be used.

8.5.5   Procedure

The assay may be performed on either serum or heparinized plasma. Clean and washed tubes are prepared and appropriately labelled for standards, controls, and unknown samples. Into each, pipette 1.8 ml of trichloroacetic acid, and then add 0.2 ml of sample.

The mixture(s) is allowed to stand for 45 min and mixed gently, after which the tubes are centrifuged at 1200 *g* for 10 min at room temperature, and the contents are again mixed, left to settle for 10 min, and re-centrifuged for 10 min. If any supernatant contains any obvious particles it should be transferred to another tube and again centrifuged.

1 ml of supernatant is transferred to a 5-ml tube, to which 2.0 ml of the semidine-HCl reagent is added, and mixed thoroughly.

0.2 ml of ammonium molybdate solution is then added and the contents again mixed. The tubes are left to stand for 10 min. Absorbance is then read at 740 nm against a water blank. Alternatively, a setting between 650 and 700 nm (usually 680 nm) can be used.

A calibration curve for absorbance against concentration of standards is prepared simultaneously and the values in the samples can be determined from this.

It is important to perform the assay in the sequence outlined. This method has been adapted to automatic analysis.

8.5.6 Performance characteristics

Reproducibility

The intra-batch coefficient of variation is approximately 1%.

8.5.7 Reference values

These vary with age, sex, and physiological maturity. In neonates 1.2–2.78 mmol/l, young children 1.29–1.78 mmol/l, falling thereafter to 0.9–1.3 mmol/l after puberty; a detailed range is available [83]. However it is recommended that each laboratory should establish its own reference values.

8.6 MAGNESIUM

SECTION I SERUM AND URINARY MAGNESIUM [47]

8.6.1 Purpose and scope

The adult contains approximately 25 g of magnesium, most (55%) is in the skeleton and approximately 30% is in muscle. In human magnesium deficiency serum concentrations of magnesium are an earlier indicator of depletion than are erythrocyte concentrations. However, serum magnesium concentrations below 0.5 mmol/l do not occur until some 25% of intracellular magnesium has been lost. It is at this stage that systemic features of magnesium deficiency first appear. Since renal conservation plays a major part in the homeostasis of magnesium, urinary excretion of magnesium may also be a useful index of magnesium deprivation. The assays of serum and urinary magnesium concentrations are similar in principle.

8.6.2 Principle of the method

Serum specimens are diluted 50-fold with acidic lanthanum chloride or oxide and analysed by direct aspiration into an AAS at a wavelength of 258.2 nm. Serum or plasma magnesium concentrations are determined from a calibration curve prepared with an identical lanthanum diluent containing sodium and potassium in concentrations close to those present in 1 + 49 diluted plasma or serum. The use of sodium and potassium salts in standard solutions compensate for spectral interferences which these elements may induce when the diluted serum or plasma samples are aspirated. Lanthanum (or strontium) is added to the sample diluent to bind with phosphates which would otherwise complex magnesium in the AAS flame and cause spuriously low absorbance readings. Urinary magnesium concentration can be determined similarly.

8.6.3 Chemicals and apparatus

(a) Chemicals

Lanthanum oxide (La_2O_3) p.a. (high grade)
Hydrochloric acid (HCl) p.a.
Sodium chloride (NaCl) p.a.
Potassium chloride (KCl) p.a.
De-ionized water.

(b) Solutions	Lanthanum oxide diluent, 0.43 g La (III)/l (i.e. 0.5 g La_2O_3/dl), is prepared by adding 10 ml concentrated HCl to 800 ml of de-ionized water, this is added to 5 g of La_2O_3, mixed, and the solution is then made up with de-ionized water to 1 litre.

Standard solutions of Mg:

Working standards are made up by diluting commercially available Mg atomic absorption standard solutions with the lanthanum oxide diluent containing 164 mg NaCl (2.8 mmol Na^+/l) and 7.5 mg KCl (0.1 mmol K^+/l). The lanthanum oxide salt serves as the zero standard for the calibration curve and for zeroing the AAS instrument.

Working standards should be prepared to the concentration range of 0–0.04 mmol Mg(II)/l final concentration, i.e. equivalent to plasma or serum concentration of 2.0 mmol/l. Standards can be stored in polypropylene or polyethylene containers and are stable at room conditions.

(c) Apparatus	Polypropylene or polyethylene containers; adjustable pipettes. Atomic absorption spectrometer.

8.6.4 Sample collection

Whole blood should be collected without venous stasis, and since erythrocytic magnesium concentrations are higher than those in serum, haemolysed samples should not be used. The serum or plasma should be separated immediately. Once separated, serum magnesium concentrations are relatively stable for up to ten days if the sample is stored at –4°C or less.

8.6.5 Procedure

The AAS instrument is zeroed using a magnesium-free lanthanum salt diluent (i.e. a blank standard). The standard curve is then constructed using the prepared standards and samples are then aspirated. It is advisable to aspirate further standards after five or six samples. A suitable approach would be to spray two standards which approximate to the absorbances of the test solutions. This confirms of the stability of operating conditions.

Each pair of standards should contain at least one of the standards sprayed in the previous pair. This is a useful standard practice which is still important even if one is using modern AAS instruments with automatic recalibration facilities. The concentration of magnesium in the aspirated samples can be determined by appropriate comparisons with the calibration curve.

8.6.6 Reference values

Serum magnesium: 0.6–1.1 mmol/l. Serum levels in neonates are lower: 0.5–0.9 mmol/l. Adult levels are achieved after five months of age. No appreciable diurnal variation has been reported but in women serum values may be higher at menstruation. It is recommended that each laboratory should establish its own reference values.

SECTION II   SERUM MAGNESIUM BY COLORIMETRIC METHOD

8.6.7 Principle of the method

For laboratories that do not have access to AAS, manual and automated colorimetric methods are available. The most convenient uses the complex Calmagite. The coloured Calmagite–Mg complex is formed by mixing the reagent with 50 µl of plasma. Plasma magnesium is determined by measuring the absorbance at 520 nm and comparing it with the absorbancies of Calmagite–Mg standards [84].

8.6.8 Procedure and performance characteristics

For the procedure and performance characteristics we refer to the method of Abernethy and Fowler [84].

8.7 IRON

The history of iron deficiency and its treatment is as old as our civilized world. Four thousand years ago, Melampos cured the son of King Argos with rust from the sacrifice sword. Greeks and Romans used iron in numerous medical preparations to restore the health of the sick. For European alchemists in the Middle Ages, iron was the universal remedy; in the seventeenth century, Sydenham considered it as the correct treatment for chlorosis. First known as 'cachexy' or 'chlorosis', iron deficiency was described as anaemia only at the end of the nineteenth century. Since then, technical advances in haematology and a better understanding of iron metabolism have enabled the use of new and accurate indicators for assessing iron status.

Iron deficiency was identified long ago but is still a major public health problem. It affects 10–20% of the world population, particularly in developing countries [85]. However, industrialized countries are also affected by the disease. Reliable methods for assessing iron status are essential in order to develop effective public health policies for combating iron deficiency. The correct choice of reliable indicators of iron deficiency is mandatory. In the present report, the various indicators for assessing iron deficiency are described. Their significance, use, and limitations in epidemiological studies are also discussed. Most of the described techniques of reference are taken from the International Nutritional Anemia Consultative Group report* on measurement of iron status [86].

For more details on techniques and particularly on practical aspects, the INACG manual is recommended as a reference.

METHODS FOR ASSESSING IRON DEFICIENCY

Iron deficiency is represented by diminished total body iron content [87]. Nutritional iron deficiency appears when the iron requirements are not met by the diet [85, 88, 89] and/or when there is an increase in iron loss from the body. The human body reacts to this imbalance by drawing from iron storage sites and also by increasing the absorption of dietary iron. If the imbalance cannot be corrected, iron stores will become exhausted and metabolic functions involving iron compounds will be disturbed [90, 91], including restriction of erythropoiesis leading to anaemia, deficiencies in tissue iron compounds, etc.

Nutritional iron deficiency appears gradually. The various indicators of iron status reflect a change in different body iron compartmentalizations and are affected at different levels of iron depletion. The natural history of iron

---

* With the authorization of the International Nutritional Anemia Consultative Group (INACG) Secretariat (Contributors: Cook, J.D., Bothwell, T.H., Covell, A.M., Dallman, P.R., Lynch, S.R., Worwood, M.A. and Reusser, M.E). The Nutrition Foundation, Washington, DC, 1985.

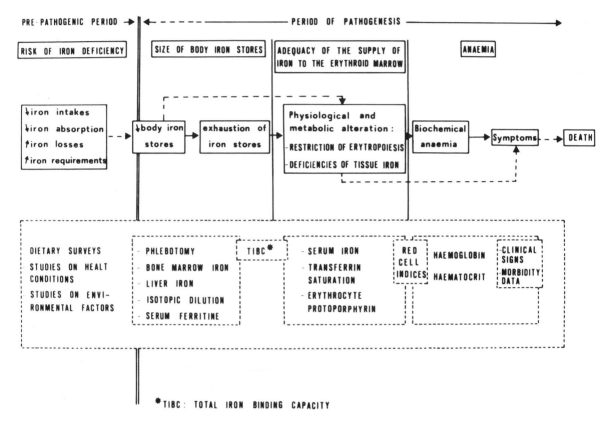

Fig. 8.1 Natural history of iron deficiency and the chronological use of indicators of iron status in the progression of the deficiency.

deficiency, from the pre-pathological stage to anaemia and the chronological use of the various indicators to assess the progression of the deficiency are shown in Figure 8.1.

SECTION I METHODS FOR EVALUATING THE RISKS OF IRON DEFICIENCY (PRE-PATHOGENIC PERIOD)

Using these methods, information can only be provided on factors facilitating the development of iron deficiency. These factors represent a risk of iron deficiency, but do not in themselves constitute the iron deficiency, owing to compensatory physiological mechanisms. The greater the number of risk factors involved and combined, the greater the chance of developing iron deficiency.

8.7.1 Dietary surveys

Dietary surveys provide information on the inadequacy of iron supply with regard to quantity and quality of iron [92–94]. Surveys measure food iron concentration of normal diet, level of haem iron (higher bioavailability) and non-haem iron (lower bioavailability), the presence of enhancers of iron absorption (meat, ascorbic acid, etc.), and inhibitors (tea, coffee, dairy products, etc.), and highlight specific dietary habits. Techniques such as the dietary history [95], which characterizes eating habits, appear to be valuable for investigating the dietary determinants of iron stores. These techniques seem more relevant in this case than quantitative techniques applied to very short observation periods.

8.7.2   Studies of health conditions

These provide information on:

The specific iron requirements of individuals of a particular population [87, 89]: age, sex, physiological circumstances (pregnancy, lactation, etc.). Such studies permit recognition of individuals with a high risk of iron requirements: children during periods of rapid growth, menstruating women, and particularly pregnant and lactating women.

The existence of additional iron loss in relation to pathologies or customs [89, 96]: parasitosis (hookworm, etc.); chronic bleeding (haemorrhoids, gastro-intestinal cancers, etc.); use of drugs capable of producing minor haemor-rhages (aspirin, anticoagulants); blood donations; or use of intrauterine devices.

An eventual reduction in iron absorption: use of antacids, malabsorption pathologies.

8.7.3   Studies on environmental factors

These studies essentially provide information on the socioeconomic level of populations and also on habits or practices likely to influence iron status [97].

SECTION II   METHODS FOR ASSESSING IRON STATUS (PATHOGENIC PERIOD)

SECTION IIA   INDICATORS FOR EVALUATING THE SIZE OF BODY IRON STORES

(a) Phlebotomy

The most quantitative means for assessing body iron storage levels is to determine the amount of storage iron mobilized by phlebotomy. Bleeding is repeated at weekly intervals until anaemia appears. The initial iron stores are calculated by determining the total amount of haemoglobin removed, and the induced deficit in circulating haemoglobin iron [98].

(b) Determination of reticuloendothelial storage iron in bone marrow or in liver

The histological evaluation of haemosiderin content of bone marrow smears or sections accurately reflects reticuloendothelial iron stores [85, 99, 100]. Specimens should be examined both unstained and after staining with potassium ferrocyanide. Usually results are classified into absent, reduced, normal, or increased levels of iron.

It is also possible to predict storage iron concentration in the liver by histological examination of a biopsy specimen.

(c) Determination of non-haem iron concentration in various organs

Non-haem iron concentrations can be quantitatively determined on a necropsy sample or on biopsies by biochemical methods [85, 99]. A calculation of storage iron content from the known or estimated organ mass is then performed. The liver contains about one-third of the total body iron stores and is therefore the organ of choice. However, this method can also be applied to bone marrow, spleen, and skeletal muscle.

(d) Isotopic dilution techniques [101]

A trace quantity of ^{55}Fe is introduced into the plasma to label haemoglobin in circulating red cells. During phagocytosis of the red cells by the reticuloendothelial system, the radioiron mixes with the iron in the tissues, and as a result there is a relatively sharp decline in the specific activity of haemoglobin iron. After complete mixing it is possible to calculate the total miscible tissue iron.

(e) Measurement of serum ferritin

In 1972 the use of a sensitive immunoradiometric assay demonstrated that small amounts of ferritin were present in normal serum and that the circulating ferritin concentration was directly proportional to the body level of iron stores [102, 103]. Since then many studies with normal subjects and in patients with iron deficiency and iron overload have confirmed this finding. An impressive correlation was found between serum ferritin concentration and iron stores as determined by phlebotomy, iron absorption, and histological or biochemical determinations [104, 109]. All of these studies showed that in adults having a normal serum ferritin concentration (range 12–250 µg/l) 1 µg/l was equivalent to 8–10 mg of storage iron (in children, 1 µg/l serum ferritin was equivalent to approximately 120 µg/kg [90]). Values lower than 10–12 µg/l indicate virtual exhaustion of body iron stores. Many laboratory methods are available [85, 100, 110], including immunoradiometric assays (IRMA) using radiolabelled antibody, radioimmunoassays (RIA) using radiolabelled antigen, and more recently enzyme-linked immunosorbent assays (ELISA), which eliminate the need for radioisotopes.

The original assay for serum ferritin described by Addison and co-workers [102] in 1972 was an immunoradiometric assay (IRMA) in which horse ferritin was used to prepare radiolabelled antiferritin antibody. In the routine assay, a solution containing ferritin standard or unknown was incubated with this antibody and the unreacted ferritin was then removed by adding an excess of immunoadsorbent (horse ferritin coupled to diazocellulose particles). The amount of radioactivity remaining in solution after centrifugation was related to the concentration of ferritin in the original solution. This method was followed by the development of a two-site IRMA in which ferritin in serum was reacted with a plastic surface that had been coated with antiferritin. In a second reaction the ferritin which had become bound to the wall of the tube was incubated with radiolabelled antihuman ferritin and the unreacted antibody then removed by washing. This technique is often referred to as the 'sandwich' technique because the ferritin is sandwiched between antiferritin serum on the solid phase and ^{125}I-labelled antiferritin globulin.

The above assays, in which the antibody is labelled, are referred to as immunoradiometric assays. The other main radioisotopic technique for serum ferritin measurement is a radioimmunoassay (RIA), in which the antigen rather than the antibody is tagged. In this assay a known quantity of radiolabelled ferritin is added to ferritin standard or unknown serum followed by the addition of antiferritin antibody, in an amount insufficient for complete binding of the labelled and unlabelled ferritin. The degree of displacement of a labelled ferritin from antigen–antibody complexes isolated in a subsequent step in the assay provides a measure of the amount of ferritin present in the original sample. Early RIA techniques were less sensitive than IRMA, but with refinements in techniques for iodinating human ferritin, the sensitivity of the two approaches for assaying serum ferritin has become roughly comparable.

The most important subsequent innovation in serum ferritin measurements was the introduction of an enzyme-linked immunoassay, or ELISA. This assay is based on exactly the same principle as the two-site IRMA, except that antiferritin is tagged with an enzyme rather than an isotope. In eliminating the need for radionuclides, this method offers several important advantages, particularly for non-specialized laboratories. The need for specialized isotopic facilities and costly automated counting equipment is eliminated, and the potential hazards of handling radioisotopes in the laboratory are avoided. Furthermore, because there is no isotopic decay of the enzyme label, it is not necessary to perform repeated iodinations of antibody, which represent the most troublesome aspect of the IRMA. Conjugation of antiferritin was usually done with horseradish peroxidase. Horseradish peroxidase is more advantageous than alkaline phosphatase because of its lower cost, greater sensitivity, and enhanced stability.

The ELISA method for serum ferritin is of particular interest for assessing iron status in population surveys. The volume of sample required for the assay has been reduced to 10 µl of serum in order to permit measurements on capillary samples. In designing the technique, every effort was made to achieve maximal sensitivity in the iron-deficient range of serum ferritin levels. As a result, samples with serum ferritin above 100 µg/l must be diluted to obtain readings within the working range of the standard curve. Enhanced sensitivity and reproducibility at low ferritin levels have been achieved by using monoclonal antibodies. The use of polyclonal rather than monoclonal reagents reduced sensitivity by a factor of 4, to 2 µg/l. However, an even more important advantage in using monoclonal reagents was the sharp reduction in background absorbance values. The ELISA procedure employs microtitre plates permitting efficient processing of large numbers of samples when an automatic plate reader is available. Satisfactory measurements can also be obtained by transferring the contents of each well from the plate to a cuvette for individual readings in a spectrophotometer.

Although experience with the ELISA method described below is still limited, there appear to be several advantages over the two-site IRMA apart from the avoidance of radioisotopes. The 'high-dose hook effect' is largely eliminated in the two-site ELISA, and some laboratories have found lower day-to-day variability. The precision of ELISA is at least comparable to the two-site IRMA and the time required to obtain a result is less.

SECTION IIA(i)   SERUM FERRITIN BY ELISA TECHNIQUE

8.7.4   Principle of the method

Polystyrene microtitre plates are coated with antiserum to human ferritin (capture or solid-phase antibody) and thoroughly rinsed on the day of assay. Ferritin standards or unknown sera are then added and allowed to incubate at room temperature for 2 h, during which time ferritin binds to the solid phase. After rinsing the wells, antiferritin immunoglobulin which has been previously conjugated with horseradish peroxidase (HRP) is added and allowed to incubate for 2 h at room temperature. During this stage the ferritin being assayed becomes sandwiched between the solid phase and the indicator antibody. The wells are then washed, and in the final step the amount of enzyme retained in each well is measured by adding the substrate o-phenylenediamine dihydrochloride (OPDD). After 30 min, the reaction is stopped by adding sulphuric acid; the absorbance in each well, which is proportional to the amount of unsolubilized antigen, is measured spectrophotometrically.

8.7.5   Chemicals and apparatus

(a) Chemicals

Sodium carbonate (Na_2CO_3) p.a.
Sodium bicarbonate ($NaHCO_3$) p.a.
Bovine serum albumin (BSA; globulin-free, e.g. Sigma cat. No. A7030)
Potassium chloride (KCl) p.a.
Sodium chloride (NaCl) p.a.
Disodium hydrogen phosphate (Na_2HPO_4) p.a.
Potassium dihydrogen phosphate (KH_2PO_4) p.a.
Tween 20 (polyoxyethylene sorbitan monolaurate, e.g. Sigma)
Citric acid monohydrate ($C_2H_8O_7.H_2O$) p.a.
Hydrogen peroxide (H_2O_2, 30%) p.a.
o-Phenylenediamine dihydrochloride (OPDD, e.g. Sigma cat. No. P1526)
Sulphuric acid (H_2SO_4) p.a.
Antiferritin serum: rabbit anti-human ferritin antisera; at least 1:16 titre
Conjugated antiferritin: purified polyclonal rabbit IgG.

(b) Solutions

Phosphate-buffered saline (PBS), 0.15 M, pH 7.2:
   Stock solution (1.5 M): dissolve in distilled water 80 g sodium chloride, 2 g potassium chloride, 11.5 g disodium hydrogen phosphate, and 2 g potassium dihydrogen phosphate. Dilute to 1 litre with distilled water.
   Working PBS–Tween (PBST) buffer (0.15 M): dilute 100 ml concentrated PBS to 1 litre with distilled water and add 0.5 ml Tween 20. A pH of 7.2 is not achieved until this stock solution is diluted.
Phosphate-buffered saline containing 0.5% BSA (PBST/BSA): add 0.5 g BSA to 100 ml working PBST.
Carbonate buffer, 0.05 M, pH 9.6: dissolve 1.59 g sodium carbonate and 2.93 g sodium bicarbonate, in 1 litre distilled water.
Citrate phosphate buffer, 0.15 M, pH 5.0:
   Stock solution A: Dissolve 21 g citric acid monohydrate in 1 litre distilled water.

Stock solution B: Dissolve 28.4 g disodium hydrogen phosphate in 1 litre distilled water.

Fresh buffer is prepared on the day of each assay by mixing 49 ml solution A with 51 ml solution B.

Blocking solution: add 0.5 g BSA to 100 ml carbonate buffer.

Coating reagent:

Prepare the plate-coating reagent by diluting whole ferritin antiserum in carbonate buffer. A 25-ml coating reagent is required for each plate. The optimal dilution should be predetermined for each lot of antiserum by coating plates with dilutions ranging from 1:1000 to 1:30 000. To ensure an excess of solid-phase antibody, employ twice the concentration of the maximal dilution of antiserum, which results in no fall-off in dose response. The usual dilution for antiferritin serum with a titre of 1:32 is approximately 1:5000.

Purified IgG may also be used for the coating procedure. The optimal concentration must be determined by coating plates with dilutions of IgG ranging from 0.05 to 10 µg/ml in carbonate buffer. A satisfactory concentration of purified IgG for coating is approximately 2 µg/ml.

A high-affinity monoclonal antibody may be employed in a concentration of approximately 1 µg/ml in carbonate buffer. The diluted antibody should be used immediately for coating.

Antiferritin enzyme conjugate:

The conjugate is diluted in PBST containing 1% BSA to a concentration that gives an absorbance reading of approximately 1.2–1.3 for the 100-µg/ litre ferritin standard under the conditions of the assay. If the absorbance of the zero standard is greater than 0.05 at this concentration of conjugate, the antibody–enzyme conjugation procedure should be repeated.

Working ferritin standards are prepared each week from this material by diluting to concentrations of 20, 50, and 100 µg/l ferritin in 0.15 M phosphate-buffered saline (PBS), pH 7.2, containing 0.05% (v/v) Tween 20 (PBST) and 0.5% (w/v) BSA (PBST/BSA). Each of these is further diluted 1:10 in PBST/BSA to obtain working standards containing 0, 2, 5, 10, 20, 50, and 100 µg/l.

Substrate solution:

This must be prepared immediately before the assay. Add 35 µl hydrogen peroxide, 30%, to 100 ml citrate phosphate buffer and mix well. Add 34 mg OPDD to this solution and mix.

Stopping solution (sulphuric acid, 25%):

Place several hundred ml distilled water in a 1-litre volumetric flask. Carefully add 250 ml concentrated sulphuric acid and make up to volume with distilled water. May be stored at room temperature.

(c) Apparatus

Microtitre plates, 96-well (it is essential to use polystyrene plates specifically designed for immunoassays and specially treated to achieve optimal protein-binding characteristics).

Plate sealer

Multichannel pipettor, 8–12 channels, 50–250 µl

Plate washer
Automatic plate reader.

8.7.6   Procedure   Add 200 µl PBST/BSA to each well of an antiferritin-coated microtitre plate.
Add 10 µl standard or unknown serum to individual wells.
Incubate at room temperature for 120 min. Empty plate and wash three times
    with PBST.
Add 200 µl HRP conjugate to each well.
Repeat incubation step.
Add 200 µl OPDD substrate and incubate for 30 min.
Add 50 µl 25% H_2SO_4.
Read optical density within 30 min at 492 nm.

Calculation   Ferritin concentrations of the unknown samples can be determined graphically
by plotting the mean absorbance of the ferritin standard against the ferritin
concentrations on log-log paper. A standard curve is drawn and used to
determine the ferritin concentrations.

SECTION IIB   INDICATORS OF THE ADEQUACY OF IRON SUPPLY TO THE ERYTHROID MARROW

The serum iron concentration refers to iron in the plasma bound to its specific
plasma transport protein, transferrin. Transferrin may be assayed immunologically as protein and the concentration expressed as the amount of protein
per litre; but serum transferrin is more often assayed by its capacity to bind iron
and is referred to as total iron-binding capacity (TIBC). Transferrin saturation
is calculated by dividing the concentration of serum iron by the TIBC and
multiplying by 100 to express the result as a percentage.

The iron transport parameters usually do not change until storage iron is
completely exhausted. Only TIBC may begin to increase as iron stores are
depleted (but it is less sensitive to changes in iron stores than serum ferritin). A
wide variety of techniques are available for the determination of serum iron
using atomic absorption spectroscopy or colorimetric techniques [85, 111].
These methods can be automated. An even greater spectrum of methods is
available for the determination of plasma transferrin. Measurement is possible
by the same methods used for serum iron. Immunological measurement of
transferrin can be used and TIBC may subsequently be calculated.

Methods for measuring the concentration of iron present in the plasma were
first described more than half a century ago. Since then, many techniques for
determining the concentration of iron in the plasma have been described. No
single method has yet proven to be clearly superior. Indeed, all existing
techniques have certain limitations or pitfalls, and current methods will almost
certainly undergo further refinements.

SERUM IRON

Colorimetric and AAS methods   **Techniques involving deproteinization [86].** The plasma iron (or serum)
concentration methods generally considered most accurate are those involving

deproteinization. They have in common three basic steps: plasma or serum is acidified to dissociate the iron–transferrin complex, plasma proteins are then precipitated with trichloroacetic acid or heating and removed by centrifugation, and finally a sensitive iron chromogen is added to the supernatant to determine the iron concentration colorimetrically. An important variable in these methods is the way in which the iron is released from transferrin. In the majority of earlier techniques hydrochloric acid alone was used. Although this approach is apparently adequate for measurements performed on fresh plasma, a significant loss of iron may occur with the precipitated protein when analyses are performed on frozen or lyophilized specimens. But it has been shown that complete recoveries can be obtained by adding a reducing agent such as thioglycolic acid or ascorbic acid to the plasma prior to protein precipitation.

There is a second problem relating to the recovery of iron in methods involving deproteinization. While complete recovery of plasma iron can be ensured by wet ashing with concentrated acid and heating in the presence of an oxidizing agent, falsely high values for transferrin iron are obtained with this method. This is due to the iron contained in plasma haemoglobin. In addition, methods in which complete release of transferrin iron is ensured by early addition of a strong reducing agent also suffer from the drawback that significant amounts of haemoglobin iron may be released. In systematic studies of this problem by the Iron Panel of the ICSH, it was observed that the release of iron from haemoglobin present in the plasma could be avoided by adding the reducing agent after acidification and not before, as was originally proposed. (Release of haemoglobin iron has also been observed with lyophilized samples, but this is a matter of concern only in programmes concerned with the interlaboratory standardization of plasma iron concentration measurements.)

Techniques omitting deproteinization [86]. In these techniques, an acid buffer and a reducing agent are first added to release the iron from transferrin. A ferrous chromogen is then added directly without protein precipitation. The background optical density of the plasma is determined either in a second tube or in the same tube prior to adding the chromogen. The majority of the techniques published in recent years have used this approach because of its greater simplicity. Other advantages include the low volume of plasma required for the measurement, as compared with deproteinization methods, and the possible reduction in the risk of iron contamination as a result of fewer manipulations of the sample. However, a serious disadvantage of direct measurements is the fact that the background optical density of the plasma is often high in relation to the colour developed with the iron chromogen. This is due to the presence of substances such as bilirubin, haemoglobin, and plasma lipids, all of which are removed in the deproteinization methods.

Importance of iron chromogen. There has been a steady and continuing improvement in the sensitivity of the colour reagents used in plasma iron methods over the past two decades. The first major advance was the introduction of bathophenanthroline, which led to a more than two-fold increase in sensitivity over the then currently available agents such as thiocyanate, bipyridyl and 0-phenanthroline. Bathophenanthroline is insoluble in water, which meant that the colour complex had to be extracted into alcohol. However, it was subsequently found that the disodium salt of the sulphonated derivative of bathophenanthroline was highly soluble in water, and this compound has been the most extensively used chromogen to date.

An important colour reagent, ferrozine, has recently been introduced and has now replaced both bathophenanthroline and TPTZ (2, 4, 6-tripyridyl-1, 3, 5-triazine) in a number of published methods. Ferrozine, which is highly soluble in water and reacts rapidly with ferrous but not with ferric iron to form a purple complex at 562 nm, has an exceptionally wide pH range of 4–9. Ferrozine has the major advantage of being 25% more sensitive than TPTZ or bathophenanthroline, and in addition it can be obtained at a small fraction of the cost of the latter. The only disadvantage of this chromogen is that it reacts with copper, and a significant error in plasma iron concentration determinations may therefore be introduced in patients having a high plasma copper concentration and a low plasma iron concentration. The problem has been largely solved by adding the agent neocuprin, which reacts with copper and thereby makes it more than 95% unavailable to ferrozine. Ferrozine may therefore well be the chromogen of choice for plasma iron concentration determinations.

Techniques employing atomic absorption spectroscopy [86]. Several methods have been described for measuring the plasma iron concentration by atomic absorption spectroscopy. While the ability to measure the 'total iron' in plasma may appear superficially attractive, atomic absorption spectroscopy has the serious disadvantage of including any haemoglobin iron present in the plasma or serum. As a result, values obtained by wet digestion or by atomic absorption spectroscopy are consistently higher than those obtained by colorimetric determinations, and when such methods are used, it is necessary to carry out parallel plasma haemoglobin concentration estimations so that suitable corrections can be made. Atomic absorption spectroscopy is associated with another systematic error. This is due to matrix interference, which is caused by plasma protein or other plasma constituents. The problem can be circumvented either by extracting iron chelated with bathophenanthroline into an organic solvent, or by deproteinization of the plasma with trichloroacetic acid. However, if it is necessary to use these approaches, then atomic absorption spectroscopy offers little or no advantages over traditional colorimetric measurements.

Other forms of iron in plasma. While the term 'plasma iron' is usually regarded as synonymous with 'transferrin iron', there exist clinical situations in which significant amounts of iron not bound to transferrin may be measured by conventional techniques. There are several examples. An important one is haemoglobin iron, already mentioned. Another group includes parenteral medicinal iron compounds such as iron dextran, which may circulate for prolonged periods in the plasma and thus introduce significant errors in the estimation of the plasma iron concentration. Finally, there is evidence that other endogenous forms of non-transferrin iron may exist in plasma, although the extent to which they interfere with plasma iron determinations is not entirely clear. Recent studies have shown that a substantial quantity of ferritin may be contained in the plasma in certain clinical disorders, such as transfusional siderosis, haemochromatosis and liver disease. In such situations, concentrations between 10 and 20 µg ferritin protein/dl have been recorded, and were this protein fully saturated with iron, and were it measured quantitatively by conventional plasma iron techniques, errors on the order of 100 to 200 µg iron/dl could result. However, it is unlikely that this would occur. Firstly, in a conventional deproteinization method such as the ICSH reference technique, only 20–25% of ferritin in patients with iron overload has a very low iron content. It is therefore likely that errors in plasma iron determinations as a result of circulating ferritin do not exceed 5–10 µg/dl, even in the presence of severe iron overload.

Finally, for the determination of the plasma iron concentration, it is clear that there is no perfect method. Optimal precision and accuracy can be obtained with manual deproteinization techniques, and these should be used for reference purposes, as has been proposed by the Iron Panel of the ICSH. This method should also be used when reliability is essential, as in ferrokinetic measurements and in certain other clinical investigations. The status of the various direct colorimetric assays that have appeared in the more recent literature is unclear, and is likely to remain so until an interlaboratory evaluation is undertaken, of the type performed by the ICSH for deproteinization techniques. In the majority of hospital laboratories, the large number of determinations required for routine clinical purposes justifies using one of the automated methods, which are probably more reproducible and certainly more efficient. Additional advantages are the smaller volumes of plasma or serum required, and the greater precision (coefficient of variation 2–4%) as compared with manual methods. Nevertheless, automated methods are by no means free of systematic errors. The volume of plasma or serum required by different methods varies widely, from as high as 2.0 ml with the International Committee for Standardization in Haematology (ICSH) technique to as little as 0.1 ml with certain automated ones. The loss in precision with these techniques is often justified in health screening or in nutrition surveys, particularly in the paediatric age group.

SECTION IIB(i)   IRON IN PLASMA OR SERUM BY THE IRON PANEL OF THE ICSH [86]

8.7.7 Principle of the method

Acid extraction of serum or plasma with hydrochloric acid and trichloroacetic acid liberates the iron from transferrin and precipitates the proteins. The acid reagent also contains thioglycolic acid, which reduces the iron to the ferrous state. The iron is measured by adding ferrozine in sodium acetate solution and measuring the absorbance of the lilac colour formed at 562 nm [96, 97]. The function of the sodium acetate is to buffer the solution to the correct pH for maximal absorbance of the iron chromogen. The recommended method is based on that described by the Iron Panel of the ICSH. However, ferrozine has been used as the chromogen instead of sulphonated bathophenanthroline because it is less expensive and has greater sensitivity.

8.7.8 Chemicals and apparatus

(a) Chemicals

All the following reagents must be of analytical grade with the lowest obtainable iron content.

Trichloroacetic acid ($C_2HCl_3O_2$) p.a.
Hydrochloric acid (HCl) p.a.
Thioglycolic (mercaptoacetic) acid ($C_2H_4O_2H_2S$) p.a.
Sodium acetate ($C_2H_3NaO_2$) p.a.
Ferrozine, 3-(2-pyridyl)-5, 6-bis(4-phenylsulphonic acid)-1, 2, 4-triazine
Electrolytic iron wire, purity greater than 99.5%
Iron-free water. (Water used to rinse glassware and for the preparation of reagent solutions should be iron free, as defined by a concentration below 1 μg/dl).
Iron-free glassware. (All glassware used for the preparation of reagents and performance of the method must be rendered iron free. After thorough washing with a laboratory detergent, glassware should be soaked in 50% nitric or 25% hydrochloric acid overnight and then rinsed with distilled and finally iron-free water).

(b) Solutions

Protein precipitant solution:
  Add to 200–300 ml iron-free water, 50 g trichloroacetic acid, 0.5 moles hydrochloric acid and 15 ml concentrated thioglycolic acid. Dissolve and make up to 500 ml with iron-free water. The iron content of the trichloroacetic acid should be lower than 0.3 p.p.m.
Chromogen solution (1.5 M sodium acetate containing 0.025% ferrozine):
  Add 102 g sodium acetate and 125 mg ferrozine in 200–300 ml iron-free water. Dissolve and make up to 500 ml with iron-free water. The iron content of the sodium acetate should be less than 0.2 p.p.m.
Iron standards:
  Stock iron standard solution (1 mg/ml): place 100 mg of dry, polished, certified electrolytic iron wire in a 100-ml volumetric flask containing 2 ml concentrated hydrochloric acid. After dissolving the wire by allowing it to stand overnight or by placing the flask in a boiling water bath, make the solution up to volume with iron-free water. Alternatively, iron standards can be purchased from commercial sources.
  Working iron standard solution (2 μg/ml): place 2 ml of the stock iron standard and 0.4 ml concentrated hydrochloric acid in a 1-litre volumetric flask and make up to volume with iron-free water.
  ICSH iron standards: each batch of stock iron standard solution should be compared to what is available from the National Institute for Biological Standards and Control (NIBSC, London).

(c) Apparatus

Vortex mixer (optional)
Centrifuge
Spectrophotometer with microcuvettes, sample capacity 1–1.5 ml. (If a spectrophotometer is not available, a filter photometer can be used, with the filter having a peak at approximately 562 nm.)

8.7.9   Procedure

To an iron-free test tube containing 1 ml plasma or serum, add 1 ml of the protein precipitant solution and mix thoroughly for 45 s either by hand or with a vortex mixer. Allow to stand for at least 5 min and centrifuge at 1500 *g* for 15 min. At the end of this time, the supernatant should be optically clear.

To 1 ml of the working iron standard solution, add 1 ml of the protein precipitant solution. Mix thoroughly and allow to stand for at least 5 min.

Prepare a reagent blank by substituting iron-free water for plasma in the first step.

Transfer 1 ml of the supernatant solution described in the first step and the solutions in the second and third steps to separate iron-free test tubes. Add 1 ml of the chromogen solution to each, mix well and allow the tubes to stand for at least 10 min.

Measure the absorbance of the solution in the fourth step in a spectrophotometer with the wavelength set at 562 nm against distilled water.

Calculation

$$\text{Plasma iron concentration } (\mu g/dl) = \frac{A_{unk} - A_{blk}}{A_{std} - A_{blk}} \cdot 200$$

where A_{unk}, A_{blk} and A_{std} are the absorbance of the plasma unknown, blank, and iron standard respectively.

IRON BINDING CAPACITY

Earlier *in vitro* techniques for measuring the iron-binding capacity of plasma were based on the fact that, when colourless apotransferrin complexes with iron, it takes on a salmon pink colour which can be read at 470 nm, the peak absorbance of the complex. Therefore, if known increments of iron are added to plasma or serum, a progressive increase in absorbance is observed until the point of complete saturation of transferrin with iron is reached. Thereafter, no further change in absorbance occurs with further iron additions. In this approach, transferrin is saturated by adding a large excess of iron. The UIBC (unsaturated iron-binding capacity) is then determined by measuring the change in absorbance and relating it to a calibration curve. However, techniques based on this principle suffer from the drawback of low sensitivity.

Because of the low absorbance of iron-transferrin, a number of techniques have been introduced in which the sensitivity has been increased by using iron chromogens. In such techniques, a measured quantity of iron is added to plasma or serum in an amount which is sufficient to saturate all the unbound transferrin. An iron chromogen is then added which reacts only with the unbound excess of iron. The UIBC is calculated by subtracting the amount of iron bound to chromogen from that which was initially added to the plasma [86, 112, 113]. The major disadvantage of the many methods that have used this approach is the fact that absorbance readings must be performed against the high background absorbance caused by plasma proteins and pigments. While such techniques are probably adequate for routine clinical measurements, they lack the precision required for a primary reference standard.

The most popular methods for determining the iron-binding capacity of plasma or serum are those in which iron in excess of the binding capacity of transferrin is added. The unbound iron is then physically removed from the sample prior to analysis. The usual approach is to add an insoluble material which complexes with unbound iron and which can then be removed by centrifugation. Methods of this type are conveniently classified according to the nature of the iron adsorbent. In the first such techniques, the iron was added as ferric ammonium citrate and the excess was removed by an iron exchange resin, Amberlite IRA 410, which binds citrate in exchange for chloride [114]. In a second method, the iron was added in the form of ferric chloride and the excess was adsorbed onto magnesium carbonate [115]; ferrous ammonium sulphate was used to saturate the transferrin in a third method and the unbound excess iron was removed by adding charcoal particles coated with haemoglobin [116].

Two approaches have been used to estimate the iron content of the supernatant after the removal of excess iron by adsorption. With both the resin and magnesium carbonate methods, colorimetric TIBC determinations have been carried out on the supernatant in order to obtain the TIBC. Such a technique cannot, however, be applied when coated charcoal is used as the adsorbent because of contamination of the supernatant with iron present in the charcoal [116].

Magnesium carbonate is probably the most satisfactory of the adsorbents currently available and the recommended method described in this section is therefore one in which magnesium carbonate is used.

SECTION IIB(ii)   IRON BINDING CAPACITY OF PLASMA OR SERUM

8.7.10   Principle of the method

A solution containing iron in excess of the binding capacity of transferrin is added to a plasma or serum sample. The unbound iron is then removed from the sample by adsorption onto magnesium carbonate [117]. There are then two possible approaches to the measurement of the iron-binding capacity of the serum. In the first, an aliquot of the supernatant is removed after centrifugation and a colorimetric iron estimation is carried out on it using the method described in the previous section. In this way, a measurement is made of the iron present in the sample when the transferrin is totally saturated (i.e. TIBC). In the second approach, the saturating iron solution is a radioactive one of known specific activity and, by measuring the radioactivity present in the supernatant after treatment with magnesium carbonate, it is possible to estimate the amount of iron taken up by the free transferrin in the sample (i.e. UIBC).

The choice between the colorimetric and radioactive methods depends on the facilities available in a particular laboratory. Unless the laboratory has easy access to radioisotopes, good counting facilities, and some expertise in their use, it is advisable to limit binding capacity measurements to the colorimetric method. It is this method which is described below.

8.7.11   Chemicals and apparatus

(a) Chemicals

Iron-free water and glassware are required as described in the method for the measurement of plasma iron.

Basic magnesium carbonate ($MgCO_3$) 'light' grade
Ferric chloride ($FeCl_3.6H_2O$) p.a.
Hydrochloric acid (HCl) p.a.

(b) Solutions

Saturating iron solution:
  Stock iron solution (containing approximately 60 µg iron/ml in 0.05 M HCl) place 300 mg ferric chloride and 4 ml concentrated HCl in a 1-litre volumetric flask. Make up to volume with iron-free water.
  Working solution of saturating iron is prepared daily by diluting the stock solution 1:10 with iron-free water.

(c) Apparatus

Rotating turntable
Centrifuge
Spectrophotometer.

8.7.12 Procedure

Place 1 ml plasma or serum in an iron-free tube and add 1 ml saturating iron solution. Mix carefully by hand and leave at room temperature for at least 15 min.

Add 200 mg ($\pm$ 25 mg) light magnesium carbonate and cap the tube with a rubber stopper covered with parafilm. Shake it vigorously and place it on a rotating turntable for 30 min. (Sufficient accuracy for dispensing magnesium carbonate can be obtained by using an appropriate size plastic scoop or by filling a glass tube marked at a level corresponding to 200 mg magnesium carbonate).

Centrifuge at 3000 *g* for 15 min. Carefully transfer the supernatant with a Pasteur pipette to a clean, iron-free tube and repeat centrifugation.

Transfer 1 ml of the supernatant to an iron-free tube and measure the iron concentration in 1 ml of the supernatant colorimetrically as described for the plasma iron determination (fourth step).

Prepare a supernatant blank by substituting 1 ml water for plasma in first step and proceed as outlined in second and third steps. Measure the iron concentration in 1 ml of the supernatant as described for the plasma iron measurement.

Calculation

$$\text{TIBC (µg/dl)} = \frac{A_{unk} - A_{blk}}{A_{std} - A_{blk}} \cdot 400$$

Transferrin may be measured by the nephelometric method and transferrin iron binding may be calculated by multiplying the transferrin concentration by 25.

ERYTHROCYTE PROTOPORPHYRIN (EP)

Protoporphyrin is the complex that combines with iron to form haemoglobin. A lack of iron supply to the developing red cell impairs haem synthesis and results in an accumulation of protoporphyrin IX in circulating red cells. Usually, the EP increases after several weeks of iron-deficient erythropoiesis [100, 118]. In epidemiological surveys, values greater than 700 µg/l whole blood or 3 µg/g of haemoglobin indicate that the iron supply to the erythroid marrow is suboptimal [119].

Extraction techniques are the reference for measurement of EP, but EP concentration can be determined more rapidly by a simple fluorescence assay. This can be done either by using a fluorometer or an instrument especially designed for directly determining red cell protoporphyrin by the fluorescence of a thin film of blood [120].

Of the two types of method for the analysis of EP, the simpler, more convenient haematofluorometer is used in many clinics. This is because such instruments require little technician time or training and provide results immediately, making it possible to detect and initiate treatment for iron deficiency during a single visit to the clinic. However, there are unsolved problems with respect to standardization and instrument stability. Although the extraction methods are used less widely than the haematofluorometer, they may be useful for standardization.

SECTION IIB(iii)   HAEMATOFLUOROMETRIC METHOD [121]

8.7.13 Principle of the method

Porphyrin compounds fluorescence in the red portion of the spectrum (approximately 600 nm) when excited by light at a wavelength corresponding to their Soret absorption maximum (approximately 400 nm). The intensity of this fluorescence is proportional to the concentration of porphyrin in the blood sample.

Haematofluorometers are designed specifically for the measurement of zinc protoporphyrin (ZP). The instrument can be factory calibrated to read out total EP, based on the assumption that ZP accounts for 95% of total EP in the red blood cell.

Excitation light at a wavelength of 415 nm is focused on the lower surface of a horizontal slide covered with a thin film of blood. The intensity of the light emitted from the sample is proportional to µg ZP/g haemoglobin (Hb). Because ZP is measured in relation to haemoglobin, the amount of blood placed on the slide does not have to be measured.

Haematofluorometer methods have certain advantages. The volume of the blood sample need not be measured, no processing of anticoagulated blood is necessary, the instruments are portable and results can be obtained in less than a minute. However, as mentioned previously, there are still unresolved questions in relation to standardization and long-term instrument stability.

8.7.14 Chemicals and apparatus

(a) Chemicals

No reagents (with AVIV models) or factors for oxygenation of blood (with HELENA models) are necessary.

(b) Apparatus

Haematofluorometers are single-channel front-face fluorometers of the filter type: AVIV (Lakewood, New Jersey, USA), HELENA Laboratories (Beaumont, Texas, USA).

8.7.15 Procedure

With the AVIV model, place a single drop of blood (20–40 µl) from the finger or from a heparinized capillary tube on a coverslip over the target area in the instrument well. The sample must be large enough to prevent drying before completion of the analysis. Stir the sample to oxygenate it with an implement that will not scratch the cover slip, such as a plastic micropipette tip. Then press the button. The instrument then calibrates itself against the internal Kapton reference slide and automatically transports the cover slip into the measuring compartment for the ZP determination. The result is displayed digitally and the cover slip is returned for disposal.

With the HELENA model, the blank is first measured by inserting the empty sample holder (no coverslip) into the instrument. Calibration is assured with two calibrators (high and low). A drop of sample is mixed with two drops of oxygenation factor on a coverslip. The sample holder is inserted into the instrument and the result is displayed digitally.

Expression of results

In the haematofluorometer designed for measuring ZP in whole blood, the fluorescent material is ZP while the absorbing material is primarily haemoglobin (Hb). Thus, the 'natural' unit of the haematofluorometer is µg ZP/g haemoglobin, which is the way in which results are displayed in some instruments (like AVIV model 5). However, other haematofluorometers have been factory-set to read out a calculated EP value per 100 ml blood based on an assumed haematocrit of 35% for children or 42% for adults. If the haematocrit (PCV) has been measured, the value for EP/dl whole blood can be corrected as follows:

$$\text{corrected EP} = \text{observed EP} \cdot \frac{\text{actual PCV}}{\text{assumed PCV}}$$

EP values can be converted to µg EP/dl RBC or µg EP/g Hb as follows:

$$\mu g\ EP/dl\ RBC = \frac{\mu g\ EP/dl\ \text{whole blood}}{PCV}$$

$$\mu g\ EP/g\ Hb = \frac{\mu g\ EP/dl\ \text{whole blood}}{\mu g\ Hb/dl\ \text{whole blood}}$$

With HELENA models results are expressed by µmol ZP/mol haem. To obtain results in µg EP/g Hb, it is necessary to divide the measurement by 28.68.

SECTION IIB(iv)   EXTRACTION METHOD

The method described by INACG [86] is that of Piomelli [122] with minor modifications. Fluorometer wavelength and slit width settings were modified to retain sensitivity (permitting low sample volume) while decreasing the risk of error due to non-porphyrin fluorescence. Extraction losses may average 10 to 15% but tend to be consistent, resulting in acceptable precision. No correction for extraction losses is made in this method.

A measured sample of anticoagulated blood is extracted with ethylacetate–

acetic acid. This procedure releases protoporphyrin from its zinc complex and extracts this freed EP, as well as a small quantity of already free EP (FEP), from the red blood cell. The total EP is then back-extracted from the ethylacetate–acetic acid into 1.5 M HCl. Although the haem that is a component of the haemoglobin molecule is present in vast excess over EP in the red blood cell, it is only very weakly fluorescent and, in any case, remains unextracted in the ethylacetate phase.

The primary standard is protoporphyrin IX, but since it is photodegradable, especially in daylight, the more stable coproporphyrin is often used as a secondary working standard. Working standards are checked against the primary standard on a regular basis. However, protoporphyrin IX is satisfactory as the sole standard, provided it is kept in the dark at 4°C.

A spectrofluorometer can be used with a xenon light source and a red-sensitive photomultiplier tube. The excitation wavelength is 405 nm and the emission wavelength is 620 nm. Alternatively, a less expensive filter fluorometer with appropriate interference filters can be used.

SECTION IIC   INDICATORS OF ANAEMIA

SECTION IIC(i)   HAEMOGLOBIN

8.7.16   Purpose and scope

The advanced stage of iron deficiency is associated with a significant decrease in circulating haemoglobin. Usually, only when the haemoglobin level (or haematocrit) has decreased below a cut-off level according to sex, age, or other physiological circumstances can subjects be considered anaemic. The arbitrary limits of normal haemoglobin concentration defined by WHO [87, 88] are often challenged, but many surveys have used the following values, which can be considered as rough guidelines (at sea level):

Children from 6 months to 6 years	11 g/100 ml
Children from 6 to 14 years	12 g/100 ml
Adult males	13 g/100 ml
Adult females	12 g/100 ml
Pregnant adult females	11 g/100 ml

Haemoglobin is measured after dilution of the blood sample in a solution that converts haemoglobin to cyanmethaemoglobin, which is then quantitated spectrophotometrically [123]. The analysis may be performed automatically on an electronic counter.

8.7.17   Principle of the method

In solution, the ferrous ions (Fe-II) of the haemoglobins are oxidized to the ferric state (Fe-III) by potassium ferricyanide to form haemiglobin (methaemoglobin or ferrihaemoglobin). In turn, haemiglobin reacts with the cyanide ions (CN-) provided by potassium cyanide to form HiCN. The time necessary for full colour development is shortened to 3 min if dihydrogen potassium phosphate is substituted for sodium bicarbonate in classic Drabkin's reagent. The addition of a non-ionic detergent enhances erythrocytic lysis and minimizes turbidity resulting from lipoprotein precipitation.

Because the absorbance of HiCN at 540 nm is proportional to its concentration (Lambert-Beer's law), an HiCN standard can be used to calibrate the measuring instrument (spectrophotometer or colorimeter). The haemoglobin concentration in the sample is then calculated from the measured absorbance in a calibrated spectrophotometer or from reading against a standard curve with a photometer.

In certain field situations, the transport of a large number of samples may be facilitated by placing a measured volume of blood (e.g. 20 µl) on a piece of filter paper. The stained section of the paper can then later be cut out and placed directly into the reagent vial. Errors with this approach may occur if the haemoglobin is not completely eluted from the paper, if some of the blood remains on the side of the pipettor, or if blood has migrated beyond the cut section of the filter paper.

8.7.18   Chemicals and apparatus

(a) Chemicals

Potassium cyanide (KCN) p.a.
Potassium ferricyanide ($K_3Fe(CN)_6$) p.a.
Dihydrogen potassium phosphate (KH_2PO_4) p.a.
Non-ionic detergent.

(b) Solutions

Cyanmethaemoglobin solution: dissolve 0.050 g potassium cyanide (see Precaution below), 0.200 g potassium ferricyanide and 0.140 g dihydrogen potassium phosphate in a 1-litre volumetric flask containing 200–300 ml water. Add 1 ml non-ionic detergent and dilute with water to 1 litre.

PRECAUTION:
Potassium cyanide is highly toxic, and particular caution should be taken when handling the solid material. Gloves should be worn when preparing the reagent, and hands should be washed thoroughly immediately thereafter. Solutions and samples should be discarded into running water in the sink, avoiding any contact with acid.

(c) Apparatus

The most reliable instrument is a dual-beam spectrophotometer, since it is least subject to error from fluctuations in line voltage. Single-beam spectrophotometers are much less expensive and also give satisfactory results provided the stability is carefully monitored by performing repeated measurements of the blank and standard. Spectrophotometers allow calculations of the haemoglobin content in an unknown sample from absorbances measured at 540 nm. Haemoglobin content can be determined using a colorimeter with a yellow-green filter covering the range of 530–555 nm, by comparison with a standard curve or measurement of a reference solution. While more susceptible to voltage fluctuation errors, colorimeters are less expensive than spectrophotometers, and voltage problems can be diminished by the use of a voltage regulator.

8.7.19   Procedure

Draw the blood sample slowly into a pipette designed to contain 0.02 ml and fill to not more than 5 mm beyond the mark.

Wipe the outside of the distal portion of the pipette with damp gauze while taking care not to draw the specimen from the pipette. Adjust the amount of blood in the pipette to the mark by touching the pipette tip with tissue paper or damp gauze.

Place the pipette into a tube containing 5.0 ml of reagent so that the tip of the pipette is below the surface of the solution. Slowly expel the blood from the pipette and then rinse the pipette several times with the reagent from top of the tube.

Cap the tube and mix 5–6 times by inversion.

Allow diluted haemoglobin solution to stand for at least 5 min to achieve full colour development.

Measure the absorbance of the unknown sample (A_{unk}) and that of a standard of known haemoglobin content (A_{std}) as described below.

(a) Calculation

$$\text{Haemoglobin unknown (g/litre)} = \frac{A_{unk}}{A_{std}} \cdot \text{haemoglobin standard (g/litre)}$$

(b) Standardization

Certified HiCN calibration standards conforming to the specifications of the ICSH are commercially available (Sigma). The equivalent haemoglobin content of the HiCN calibration standard is obtained by multiplying the stated HiCN content with the dilution factor used in processing the blood sample.

SECTION IIC(ii)   HAEMATOCRIT

The packed cell volume(PCV) is a measure of the ratio of the volume occupied by red cells to the volume of whole blood in a sample of capillary or venous blood. This ratio is determined after centrifugation and should be expressed as a decimal fraction. The terms PCV and haematocrit are often regarded as synonymous, although originally the haematocrit referred to the apparatus or procedure used to determine the volume occupied by red cells in whole blood.

Haematocrit can also be calculated with the electronic counter. In addition the haematocrit can be measured directly after centrifugation of the whole blood by comparing the height of the entire column of packed red cells with the height of the entire column of red cells and plasma.

The PCV provides a convenient and rapid measure of the degree of anaemia and, from a nutritional standpoint, provides information comparable to the haemoglobin concentration. One of the major advantages of PCV measurement by the microhaematocrit procedure is that a small volume of plasma can be recovered following centrifugation for microdeterminations such as serum ferritin levels. The micromethod requires only about 50 μl blood for each measurement. Either venous or capillary blood is drawn into a heparinized capillary tube, which is sealed at one end and centrifuged.

8.7.20 Apparatus

Apparatus

Capillary tubes. The microhaematocrit method requires special disposable capillary tubes (length 75 mm; internal diameter, 1.16 mm; wall thickness, 0.20 mm).

Tube Sealant. Capillary tubes must be sealed with a clay-type sealing compound, which is usually dispensed in small trays 5–7 mm in depth.

Centrifuge. The microhaematocrit procedure requires a specially designed centrifuge which normally holds up to 24 capillary samples in numbered positions. The centrifuge should be capable of maintaining a centrifugal force above 10 000 *g* at the periphery for 5 min without exceeding a temperature of 45°C.

Reading device. Several instruments are available to determine the ratio of the column of packed cells to the length of the column of red cells and plasma.

8.7.21 Procedure

Fill two capillary tubes with blood to between 5.5 and 6 cm of the total 7.5 cm length. Close off the dry end of the tube bore with the tip of the finger.

Taking care to hold the capillary tube in a horizontal position, remove the finger and place the dry end into the tray containing sealing compound at a 90° angle. Rotate the capillary tube slightly and remove it from the tray. The sealant plug should be 4–6 mm long.

Place the filled, sealed capillary tube in the centrifuge with the sealed end toward the periphery. Record the position numbers.

Centrifuge for 5 min.

Remove the tubes one at a time and read the results using a special reading device. The difference in duplicate determinations should not exceed 0.015 (two standard deviations). When taking readings, ensure that the bottom of the packed cell column is lined up correctly with the zero mark. Also ensure that the buffy coat (greyish-red layer of leukocytes at the interface between the red cells and the plasma) is excluded from the red cell column measurement.

The results should be read within 10 min after the centrifuge has come to a stop; leaving the tubes in a horizontal position will, in time, produce slanting of the cells/plasma interface.

Calculation

The PCV is calculated from measurements of the red cell and plasma columns as follows:

$$PCV = \frac{\text{length of red cell column (mm)}}{\text{length of cells + plasma column (mm)}}$$

SECTION IIC(iii)   RED CELL INDICES

Morphological characteristics of the red cells provide information on the severity of anaemia. The most useful indices are mean corpuscular volume (MCV) and mean corpuscular haemoglobin (MCH). The finding of anaemia together with low MCV (< 85 fl in adults) and low MCH (< 27 pg in adults) usually implies that haemoglobin synthesis has been inhibited by a curtailment in the supply of iron to the erythroid marrow.

Reference values according to age exist for red cell indices [124]. MCV is directly measured by electronic counters. Other red cell indices can also be obtained by electronic counter but they are not directly measured: MCH is derived by dividing haemoglobin concentration by red cell count.

SECTION IIC(iv)   THERAPEUTIC IRON TRIAL

The most conclusive evidence of iron deficiency anaemia is the haemoglobin rise following oral or parenteral therapy [100, 125]. An increase of 1 g/l is often considered significant, but a 2-g increase is much more reliable.

SECTION IIC(v)   CLINICAL SYMPTOMS

Decreased haemoglobin concentration leads to a lowered capacity of carrying oxygen to body tissue and, as a consequence, deprivation of parenchymal tissue, in particular heart and brain needing a great quantity of oxygen. There are a number of symptoms observed in anaemia: these include dyspnoea, pallor, lethargy, lipothymia, etc. As anaemia becomes more severe subjects may experience disturbances in respiratory, cardiovascular, renal, neuromuscular, and gastrointestinal functions. Most symptoms are not consistent and results are not easy to interpret. Severe anaemia is also associated with an increase in fetal, neonatal and maternal morbidity and mortality [126, 127], and a reduction in physical work capacity [128] and resistance to infections [129].

These deleterious effects of anaemia are difficult to evaluate and to quantitate. Parameters such as duration and frequency of pregnancy, birth-weight, frequency of infections, and work capacity may be used as indirect indicators of the consequences of iron deficiency, but there are too many factors involved in their determinants.

CHOICE OF INDICATORS FOR ASSESSING IRON DEFICIENCY IN A POPULATION

The choice of indicators is determined by the following parameters:

The objectives of the survey
The characteristics of the study population
The feasibility of the chosen tests
The quality of the tests.

8.7.22 Objectives of the survey

The first and most important consideration in the planning of a nutritional survey to assess the iron deficiency of a population is to define its objectives as clearly and precisely as possible. This definition should serve as the basis for deciding on the sampling of the population, on the methodology to be used, the choice of the indicators and the utilization of the information obtained.

The objectives may vary widely; for example the assessment of nutritional status of a population, determination of the prevalence of iron deficiency (at every stage or at a specific stage), identification of groups at high risk, evaluation of risk factor, determination of aetiological factors, evaluation of the severity of the deficiency and of consequences of the iron deficiency on public health, experimental works, supervision of a population, measurement of the impact of a given intervention (supplementation and/or fortification).

8.7.23 Characteristics of the study population

The choice of indicators for assessing iron deficiency is closely linked to the characteristics of the population considered. Such characteristics include age, sex, race, existing pathological state (infections, parasitosis, haemoglobino-pathies, etc.). The presence of a pathological condition could modify the validity of the chosen tests.

In the same way initial information regarding the possible prevalence of iron deficiency (high, moderate, low) will lead to the choice of indicators for testing either the early or advanced stage of the condition.

8.7.24 Feasibility of the tests

Feasibility of the tests is linked to the compliance of the population, the cost and complexity of the tests, the qualifications and experience of available staff, and the practical organization of the survey.

Certain techniques such as bone marrow or liver biopsy, phlebotomy, and isotopic dilution, cannot be used with a population because of their traumatic or invasive character. Therapeutic iron trials are possible, but in practice are difficult to perform on populations, especially over a long period of time. In a theoretically healthy population, only blood sampling is acceptable. As far as compliance is concerned, it is necessary to draw the smallest quantity of blood in a non-traumatic manner. For this reason, serum ferritin, transferrin, erythrocyte protoporphyrin and haemoglobin/haematocrit measurements can easily be carried out with less than 500 µl of blood. Usually, serum iron measurements require more blood and are not readily obtained, except by venepuncture. This introduces a problem in the sampling of children under 3 or 4 years of age.

Both fingerprick and heelprick blood (in children below 1 year) can easily be obtained by health workers after minor training. The use of automatic blood drawing equipment is less traumatic and more acceptable. It is necessary to standardize sampling techniques prior to analysis and to use the same technique within each defined group.

Difficulties are directly related to the test itself, qualifications of the staff, laboratory equipment storage or transport of samples and working conditions in the field. At present, automatic analysers exist for haemoglobin, red cell indices, serum iron, and erythrocyte protoporphyrin, greatly facilitating the tests. The great advantage with automated equipment, in addition to its rapidity and ease of usage, is the reduction in experimental error. Serum ferritin measurements are relatively difficult to perform and require skilled personnel. The availability of commercial kits has improved the situation, but running costs may be high.

A haematofluorometer for the assay of erythrocyte protoporphyrin is convenient and quick to use (around 10 s/sample) and does not require qualified staff. It can be operated 'in the field'.

For each analytical test, it is absolutely essential to have well-calibrated instruments. In addition, quality control samples should frequently be assayed so that variability within and between laboratories can be determined.

When working directly in the field, it is essential to retain blood samples in good condition (away from heat and light). This restraint imposes a time limit of a few hours between the collection of blood and the assay. Blood for serum iron, total iron binding capacity, and serum ferritin can, after centrifugation, be frozen and stored for up to two years before assay.

8.7.25 Quality of the indicators for assessment of iron deficiency

The main qualities of iron deficiency indicators can be established from what is known of their sensitivity, specificity, and variability. The most useful indicators, from an epidemiological point of view, are those which in the working conditions of the study have the highest sensitivity, the highest specificity, and the lowest variability.

(a) Sensitivity of indicators of iron deficiency

Sensitivity of an indicator of iron deficiency may be defined by the probability that an iron-deficient subject can be identified as such by the use of the indicator. As far as iron deficiency indicators are concerned, two levels of sensitivity can be distinguished: 'diagnostic sensitivity' and 'biochemical sensitivity'. Figure 8.1 (p. 356) shows the relation between the different physiological stages of iron deficiency and the application of each different indicator, thus allowing a deduction of the 'diagnostic sensitivity' of indicators of iron deficiency, i.e. their capacity to detect the earliest stage of iron deficiency.

Decreases in haemoglobin, haematocrit and/or the expression of clinical symptoms of anaemia correspond to a delayed stage of the deficiency. They indicate severe iron deficiency and can be considered, from a diagnostic point of view, to have low sensitivity. They are less sensitive than those that indicate the iron supply to the marrow (such as serum iron, TIBC, erythrocyte protoporphyrin). The latter are, however, less sensitive than the indicators measuring the size of the iron stores (such as serum ferritin). Depletion of the iron stores (reduction of serum ferritin) reveal the inadequacy existing between iron supply and iron requirements. Therefore, the serum ferritin measurement appears to be the most sensitive indicator for assessing iron status in a population.

In addition to 'diagnostic sensitivity', we must take into consideration 'biochemical sensitivity', that is, sensitivity reflecting every stage of the deficiency. In certain circumstances, biochemical sensitivity is reduced, thereby decreasing the value of a particular indicator. Such circumstances include various pathological conditions and therapeutic regimes. In Table 8.6 are shown the main causes of false negative cases of iron deficiency. These tend to underestimate iron deficiency in epidemiological surveys. A knowledge of the presence of such factors in a population implies a discussion of the choice of tests to be considered.

(b) Specificity of indicators of iron deficiency

We can define the specificity of an indicator of iron deficiency by the probability that a non-iron-deficient subject will not be identified as a deficient subject.

Clinical symptoms of anaemia are not very specific. They can be observed in many pathological situations other than iron deficiency.

Table 8.6 Confusing factors which may interfere with the significance of iron status indicators

	False negatives (Iron-deficient subjects not classified as deficient)	*False positives* (Non iron-deficient subjects classified as deficient)
Serum ferritin	Inflammatory syndromes, infection [108, 130–132] Liver disease [108, 133] Malignant disease [110, 133, 134] Acute leukaemia [135, 136] Hodgkin's disease [136] Rheumatoid arthritis [137] Thalassaemia major [85]	
Serum iron	Chronic alcoholism [138] Oral contraceptive use [139, 140] Folates and vit. B_{12} deficiencies [85] Haemoglobinopathies with chronic haemolysis [141] Acute viral hepatitis [142, 143] Acute leukaemia [144] Pyridoxine deficiency [145]	Inflammatory syndromes, infection [119, 131, 136, 147, 148] Ascorbic acid deficiency [148] Malignancy [149, 150] Chronic skin disorders [151] Rheumatoid arthritis [152] Shock (acute myocardial infarction [153] Physical trauma [111]
Total iron-binding capacity	Protein malnutrition [154–156] Chronic infections [146] Alcoholic cirrhosis [138] Malignant disease [157] Nephrotic syndromes [158] Enteropathy [159]	Oral contraceptive use [160, 162, 163] Pregnancy [161] Acute viral hepatitis [110]
Erythrocyte Protoporphyrin		Inflammatory syndromes, infection [124, 162, 163] Lead poisoning [164, 165] Porphyrin disorders [157]
Mean cell volume	Folate and vit. B_{12} deficiency [96]	Thalassaemia minor [100, 126] Chronic disease [112]
Haemoglobin		Folate and vit. B_{12} deficiencies [87, 88, 96] Haemoglobinopathies [87, 166] Parasitosis [87, 166] Chronic infection [139, 167]

As for biochemical indicators, certain confounding factors can also modify their significance and be responsible for false positive cases (Table 8.6). In these conditions there is a risk of overestimating the prevalence of iron deficiency. Serum ferritin measurement has excellent specificity: a value of serum ferritin < 12 µg/l always denotes exhaustion of iron stores (however, serum ferritin concentrations may be underestimated due to the technical phenomenon of the 'high-dose hook effect', encountered in many immuno-assays [168, 169].

Confounding factors (pathological and/or therapeutic) may be more or less recognized in a particular population and taken into account. But a major factor intervening in the sensitivity and specificity of the indicators for assessing iron deficiency is more difficult to avoid: the total variability of the indicators.

(c) Total variability of indicators of iron deficiency

Total variability of a test results in the combination of analytic variability (linked to the method of measurement) and biological variability (linked to the subject).

Analytical variability. Analytical variability can be divided into several categories.

Instrumental variability: This can be assessed in most laboratory tests by determining, over a short period, the 'within-assay' reproducibility (multiple analysis of an identical sample on the same day) and, over a longer period, the day-to-day reproducibility (multiple analysis on sequential days) [170].

Haemoglobin, haematocrit and MCV have low instrumental variability (1–3%) [165, 166]. Instrumental errors are decreased with the use of electronic counters.

Serum iron measurements present considerable instrumental variability linked to environmental contamination. Instrumental error is 9% using the manual technique [170, 171], but it can be lowered considerably by using automatic equipment, which reduces the risk of contamination [172, 173].

Instrumental variability for the TIBC [173, 175] is more or less equivalent to that of serum iron (5–6%). For the erythrocyte protoporphyrin assay, the instrumental error is between 1.5% and 2.5% using haematofluorometer methods, and 5% using extraction techniques [176, 177]. Instrumental variability is about 3.5% for serum ferritin one-day assays and twice that for sequential day assays [178], whatever method is used (ELISA, IRMA, RIA).

Pre-instrumental variability: This precedes the assay itself, and the causes may be the following: blood drawing technique, left or right arm collection, use of a tourniquet, subject's position, or physical activity before sampling.

Very little information exists on the importance of the pre-instrumental variability of most tests, but it can be minimized in epidemiological surveys by standardizing as much as possible the sampling technique (i.e. use of the same conditions, same arm, same position) etc.

Biological variability. The biological variability can be divided into several categories.

Intraindividual variability: This is due to variations in each individual observed over a period of time, and includes biological rhythms (diurnal, menstrual, etc.). It can be evaluated by repeating a measurement in the same person over a short period (within a day, between days, weeks) or for a longer period.

Intraindividual variability for haemoglobin and haematocrit within a short time in 'healthy' subjects is similar to analytical variability (1–3%) [179]. For serum iron measurements, there is pronounced diurnal variation, from 13 to 20% [108, 173, 180, 181]. Even when blood is collected within the same hour in the same subject, day-to-day variability is 30–50% [173, 174, 180, 182].

Moreover, serum iron levels in women usually drop prior to the onset of menstruation and may not return to normal for several days [183, 184]. For TIBC, intraindividual variability is lower than for serum iron and remains similar to that of analytical error [174, 180]. Erythrocyte protoporphyrin measurement by the haematofluorometer reveals day-to-day variations lower than with extraction methods [170].

Intraindividual variability for serum ferritin is of the order of 6–10% for within-day variation and is lower than 15% for between-day variation [185, 186]. There appears to be no variation during the menstrual cycle. The magnitude of intraindividual variability of indicators of iron status in subjects with decreased iron stores is not as great as that seen in subjects with normal body iron stores [173].

Interindividual variability: This involves variability observed over a given population. It represents a major problem in our understanding of the significance of biological tests for assessing the iron status of individuals and populations.

There is an 'overlap' in the distribution values observed in 'normal' subjects and in iron-deficient subjects, especially when deficiency is mild. This is true particularly for haemoglobin. The use of a cut-off of 'normality' for haemoglobin may be responsible for a large number of false negatives and false positives. The problem was demonstrated by Garby *et al.* [125], who defined anaemia in the population by the response or lack of response to oral iron therapy. Using a simple cut-off point, they found that 17% of truly anaemic women were classified as normal, while 35% of normal women were classified as anaemic. Similar results were obtained by frequency distribution analysis of haemoglobin in pregnant women. One quarter of both anaemic and normal women were misclassified when a single cut-off of 11 g/dl of haemoglobin was used [187].

Results of population studies indicate that the distribution of haemoglobin values is Gaussian, with a standard deviation of about 7% when subjects with iron deficiency are rigorously excluded [188]. The distribution curve is skewed to the left in apparently normal population by the presence of anaemic individuals within such population. It is difficult to find a clear-cut dividing line between normal and anaemic subjects. By administering iron and then repeating haematological measurements, it is possible to obtain a more precise definition of the lower limits of 'normality'. Garby *et al.* [125] were able to show that only 2% of women with an initial haematocrit of 36% or higher responded to supplementation. In other words, a woman with a haematocrit of 36% or higher has a 98% chance of not being anaemic.

Another approach to improving the quality of the limit of 'normality' is the use of a lower value of 95% of a reference range. The reference range must be defined on a representative sample of subjects, excluding all subjects with haemoglobinopathy, inflammation, or laboratory evidence of iron deficiency.

Reference values must be determined for various age or sex groups [189, 190]. Recently some authors have proposed a mathematical approach using the mixed distribution analysis of haemoglobin to reveal the true prevalence of anaemias [191, 192]. This model also permits assessment of the contribution of iron deficiency to the determining of anaemia.

INTERPRETATION OF IRON STATUS MEASUREMENTS

Despite the widespread use and established validity of the measurements described above, the optimal method for employing them to characterize the iron status of a population remains uncertain. Most information published on the interpretation of iron measurements deals with clinical diagnosis in individual patients rather than epidemiological evaluation of a population. Newer techniques for statistical evaluation of survey data are only now emerging, and much further work will be required before the optimal approaches have been identified.

8.7.26   Criteria for iron deficiency

(a) Single criterion

The simplest way to define the prevalence of iron deficiency is to use a single cut-off level for a given measurement of iron status. When used as a single criterion, haemoglobin defines iron deficiency anaemia; transferrin saturation

Table 8.7   Deficiency criteria for parameters of iron status

	Cut-off
Haemoglobin	
0.5–10 years	<110 g/l
11–15 years – males	<120 g/l
– females	<115 g/l
>15 years – males	<130 g/l
– females	<120 g/l
Pregnancy	<110 g/l
Haematocrit	
0.5–4 years	<32%
5–10 years	<33%
11–15 years – males	<35%
– females	<34%
>15 years – males	<40%
– females	<36%
Serum iron	<60 μg/dl
Total iron-binding capacity	>400 μg/dl
Transferrin saturation	
0.5–4 years	<0.12
5–10 years	<0.14
>10 years	<0.16
Eryhthrocyte protoporphyrin	
0.5–4 years	>80 μg/dl RBC
>4 years	>70 μg/dl RBC
Serum ferritin	
0.5–15 years	<10 μg/l
>15 years	<12 μg/l

or erythrocyte protoporphyrin defines iron-deficient erythropoiesis; and serum ferritin defines iron storage depletion. Criteria widely used for clinical purposes are listed in Table 8.7.

The limitation in using the haemoglobin or haematocrit level alone as a single criterion of iron deficiency is now well recognized. The major difficulty arises from the fact that there is a marked overlap in haemoglobin levels between normal and anaemic individuals. This limitation of haemoglobin determinations was first recognized by Garby *et al.* [125], who administered oral iron to adult women and defined as anaemic those who showed a significant increase in haematocrit. They observed that with a single criterion, roughly 20% of normal women were incorrectly classified as anaemic on the basis of initial haematocrit, whereas an equal number of anaemic women had been incorrectly classified as normal. Haemoglobin determination should therefore be regarded as a screening measurement useful in defining only severe degrees of iron deficiency. The major advantage of haemoglobin determination is its use in monitoring the response to an iron intervention programme in a population with a relatively high prevalence of anaemia. The haemoglobin measurement is used extensively for this purpose, since the primary objective of most intervention programmes is to reduce the prevalence of anaemia rather than iron deficiency.

In some studies iron deficiency has also been defined on the basis of a single cut-off level for serum ferritin, transferrin saturation, or erythrocyte protoporphyrin. However, the problem of overlapping values between normal and abnormal populations applies to these parameters as well. The serum ferritin level may be of some value in defining the frequency of storage iron depletion, especially in populations where anaemia is uncommon. However, because abnormalities in erythrocyte protoporphyrin and transferrin saturation are less specific, these measurements provide only a rough guide to the prevalence of iron deficiency.

(b) Multiple criteria

Many of the limitations in defining the prevalence of iron deficiency using isolated measurements can be circumvented by using combinations of two or more independent variables. When this approach was used in a prevalence survey of relatively replete individuals [193], it was observed that when only one index of iron status was in the abnormal range (serum ferritin, transferrin saturation, or erythrocyte protoporphyrin), the prevalence of anaemia increased only slightly, from 8.3 to 10.9%. However, when two of these parameters were abnormal, the prevalence of anaemia rose to 28%, and when all three were abnormal it averaged 63%. This indicates that two or three abnormal indicators of iron status are more commonly associated with iron deficiency of increasing severity than is a single abnormal value. It has become apparent from subsequent studies that the most reliable approach to characterizing iron deficiency in a population is to use a combination of laboratory measurements to detect iron deficiency. For example, this approach was the basis for estimating the prevalence of iron deficiency in the US population in the second National Health and Nutrition Examination Survey (NHANES II), 1976–1980 [194] and in large-scale epidemiological surveys performed in Africa [195, 196].

8.7.27 Quantitative body iron estimates

One of the important questions involved in characterizing the iron status of a population is whether total body iron or iron stores are continuously distributed in the population, or whether there are two discrete populations of iron-deficient and normal individuals. In certain geographical areas, conditions may exist which lead to separate frequency distributions of body iron, as, for example, when a particular segment of the population has heavy hookworm infestation. On the other hand, in most populations, there are a large number of determinants of body iron stores such as rate of body growth, iron intake, nature of the diet, menstrual blood loss, gastrointestinal blood loss, inflammatory disease, and malnutrition. The end result may therefore be a single normal distribution of body iron stores in the population, rather than separate populations of iron-deficient and normal individuals.

The assumption of a single frequency distribution of iron stores is the basis for another approach for evaluating the iron status of a population. This method uses a combination of iron measurements to obtain a quantitative estimate of body iron stores. The two measurements described in this section which are quantitatively related to body iron are serum ferritin in iron-replete individuals and haemoglobin in those with advanced iron deficiency. It is therefore possible to fix the two ends of the frequency distribution of iron stores in a population. Additional points along the frequency distribution can be obtained by employing various combinations of erythrocyte protoporphyrin and transferrin saturation. Preliminary studies with this model in an iron-depleted population have demonstrated its feasibility. One problem in estimating the prevalence of iron deficiency is that there is no general agreement as to what constitutes iron deficiency. An advantage of estimating body iron stores quantitatively is that *a priori* definitions of iron deficiency are not required.

8.7.28 Conclusion

The choice of indicators for assessing iron deficiency in populations depends on each particular situation. The diagnosis of iron deficiency must, of course, begin with an acknowledged definition. According to this definition each indicator has its own significance and is subject to different errors. The limits of each indicator of iron deficiency have to be determined by its specificity and its sensitivity in the working conditions of the survey. Prior knowledge of the characteristics of a given study population (age, sex, basal iron status, infection, lead poisoning, thalassaemia minor, etc.) must be taken into account when choosing a suitable indicator. No single iron parameter monitors the entire spectrum of iron deficiency. The best combination of indicators will depend on the objectives of the survey and the required sensitivity or specificity. The use of several indicators, effective at different levels of iron depletion, enables an estimate of the distribution of iron within the body and an evaluation of the iron status of a population.

Strict standardization of techniques, centralized laboratory facilities, the validation of methods of assay (particularly in accordance with the INACG* recommendations), the application of quality control samples, the use of international standards, all help to decrease the variability linked to measurements,

* International Nutritional Anemia Consultative Group

and improve the reliability of collected data, allowing comparisons between the different surveys.

In addition the use of reference biochemical indicators based on supplementation trials or studies of randomized populations (excluding subjects with laboratory evidence of iron deficiency and/or inflammation), will make it possible to more accurately classify a larger proportion of subjects for each stage of iron deficiency. With such information, it then becomes possible to choose and measure the impact of the intervention.

A new indicator of iron status has recently been proposed, based on the same immunoenzymological principle as that of serum ferritin but using antibodies derived from the placenta: the measure of circulating transferrin receptors. In addition to other iron status parameters, the evaluation of serum transferrin receptors (needing a very small blood volume) could be of value in the assessment of iron status.

8.8 ZINC

SECTION I ZINC IN PLASMA OR SERUM BY ATOMIC ABSORPTION SPECTROPHOTOMETRY [197]

8.8.1 Principle of the method

Plasma or serum samples diluted $1 + 4$ aspirated into the atomic absorption flame. The concentration of zinc is determined by comparing the signal from the diluted plasma with that from aqueous standards which are prepared in a diluted glycerol matrix (50 ml/l) to simulate the viscosity of the diluted plasma.

8.8.2 Chemicals and apparatus

(a) Chemicals

Glycerol ($C_3H_8O_3$) p.a.
De-ionized water.

(b) Solutions

Glycerol diluent is prepared by adding 50 ml of reagent grade glycerol to 1000 ml of de-ionized water.
Standard solutions of zinc:
Working standards are prepared using commercially available atomic absorption standard solutions. Since the linear range for zinc determination by AAS is up to about 16 µmol/l, standard dilutions up to 80 µmol/l may be prepared. They will subsequently be diluted $1 + 4$ for the preparation of working standards.

These standards are stable in polypropylene bottles at room temperature and do not need to be freshly prepared with each test run, but fresh standards should be prepared, checked and replaced monthly.

(c) Apparatus

Polypropylene bottles; plastic test tubes; adjustable pipettes.
The atomic absorption spectrometer should be set up according to the manufacturer's instructions. Absorbance is measured at 213.8 nm, with a slit width of 0.7 nm. An air–acetylene flame is used. The instrument conditions, burner height, gas pressures, flow rate, sample aspiration rate, and lamp current should be adjusted to achieve optimum sensitivity.

8.8.3 Sample collection

Venous blood is collected ideally without any venous stasis, from a recumbent subject at a standardized time of day.

Precautions must be taken to avoid haemolysis and contamination of the samples and reagents with rubber or other potential sources of zinc. Samples collected after fasting give higher zinc concentrations than those collected after meals.

8.8.4 Procedure

(a) Technique

Plasma or serum is allowed to come to room temperature and is then mixed by inversion; 0.5 ml specimen is added to a suitable sized plastic test tube, 2.0 ml of de-ionized water is added and the solutions are mixed thoroughly. The spectrometer is set to maximum sensitivity and minimum background noise. It should be zeroed using the baseline glycerol diluent. This procedure should be repeated during the analytical sequence to correct for any baseline drift and to reset the baseline to zero if necessary. Working standards are aspirated and used to establish the standard curve. The specimens are then aspirated and, during the analytical run, repeat determinations of pairs of standards should be performed approximately every six samples.

(b) Calculation

The concentration of zinc in the samples is determined from their absorbance reading by interpolation from the standard curve.

8.8.5 Performance characteristics

Reproducibility

This method gives an initial interbatch CV of about 5%.

8.8.6 Reference values

Plasma zinc ranges from 9 to 22 µmol/l. It is, however, recommended that each laboratory should establish its own reference values.

8.8.7 Interpretation

Levels are reduced with infection, stress, pregnancy, and use of oral contraceptive agents. Plasma and serum levels are similar; discrepancies between serum and plasma values probably arise from delay in separating the plasma or serum from cells, and from the use of citrate rather than de-ionized heparin anticoagulant for plasma collection [198].

SECTION II PLASMA OR URINE ZINC [199]

8.8.8 Principle of the method

Plasma or serum samples are diluted with de-ionized, distilled water at $1 + 9$ dilutions. The zinc concentration is determined by comparing the AAS absorbance with that from similarly diluted aqueous standards. This method can also be used for urine.

8.8.9 Chemicals and apparatus

(a) Chemicals

N-butyl alcohol ($C_4H_{10}O$) p.a.
Sodium chloride (NaCl) p.a.
De-ionized water (resistivity >16 ohm).

(b) Solutions

N-butyl alcohol, 1 mol/l: 60 ml of N-butyl alcohol is made up to 1000 ml with water (diluent).
NaCl, 1.5 mmol/l: 87.6 mg of NaCl are dissolved in water to make 1000 ml.
Standard solutions of zinc are prepared from commercially available atomic absorption standard solutions.
Standard dilutions are prepared by adding appropriate volumes of the standard solution and 10 ml of NaCl 1.5 mmol/l to de-ionized water to achieve total volumes of 100 ml.
Working standards are prepared by adding 1 part of each standard dilution to 9 parts of N-butyl alcohol 1 mol/l. Classically this involves taking 0.5 ml of each stock standard and adding 4.5 ml of N-butyl alcohol 1 mol/l. These are then thoroughly mixed and the solutions are used to calibrate the instrument.

(c) Apparatus

Polypropylene bottles and tubes; adjustable pipettes.
Atomic absorption spectrometer.

8.8.10 Procedure

The specimens for analysis are diluted 1 + 9 with the diluent. More usually 0.5 ml of each sample of serum or plasma is added to 4.5 ml of diluent. However, with experience or if limited volumes of sample are available, smaller volumes may be used. The zinc concentrations of the diluted specimens are then determined under optimum instrument conditions using the approach outlined above (8.8.4).

8.8.11 Performance characteristics

(a) Detection limit

The lowest reliably measured concentrations of biological fluid involving this technique is reported at 0.1 µg/l.

(b) Reproducibility

This technique is reported to give interbatch and intrabatch coefficients of variation of 1.8% and 1% respectively.

8.8.12 Reference values

See 8.8.6.

SECTION III   SERUM/PLASMA ZINC – ALTERNATIVE METHOD [200]

Another means of preparing plasma and serum samples for aspiration has been reported in which serum or plasma samples are deproteinated by the addition of trichloroacetic acid. In this method volumes of samples are diluted either 1 + 1 or 1 + 2 with 10% (w/v) or 15% (w/v) trichloroacetic acid (high-purity grade), mixed thoroughly and allowed to stand for 10 min. The samples are then centrifuged at 1000 *g* for 10 min. The supernatants are transferred to another set of clean plastic or glass containers for determination of their zinc content by atomic absorption spectroscopy.

SECTION IV   ZINC IN LEUKOCYTE AND LEUKOCYTE SUBSETS

8.8.13   Purpose and scope

Since leukocytes, as a tissue, have a rapid turnover it is possible that with increasing risk of zinc deficiency, leukocytes or some leukocyte subsets will display compositional and functional features of zinc deficiency sooner than other tissues.

Assays on mixed leukocytes are less easily interpreted than on white cell subsets because these have differing zinc content and half-lives which, since the relative proportions of white cell subsets alters with physiological and pathological processes, could result in misleading assessments of zinc content if these were based on the entire cellular population. For example, the reduced mixed leukocyte zinc content that occurs in pregnancy probably reflects the varying degree of neutrophilia that develops during pregnancy and labour.

There are many approaches to isolating white cells and their subsets and to determining their respective zinc content. In clinical studies it is important to remember that alterations in red cell and other blood cell characteristics may dictate the method used to separate cells and, certainly, whatever isolation procedure is used it should be thoroughly validated before it is applied on a routine basis [201, 202]. However, the method outlined below has been used in both health and disease states [203].

8.8.14   Principle of the method

White cells are separated from whole blood and are then subdivided further to provide separate samples of total leukocytes, polymorphonuclear leukocytes, and mononuclear leukocytes, which can be further separated into monocytes and lymphocytes. The cells are then lysed, and the protein and zinc content of the supernatant is determined.

8.8.15   Chemicals and apparatus

(a) Chemicals

Nitric acid (HNO_3) Aristar grade (trace-element free), e.g. BDH Ltd., cat. No. 45004

Preservative and trace-element free heparin, e.g. Plasmagel, Uniscience Ltd., London (UK)

RPMI 1640 tissue culture medium, e.g. Flow Labs Ltd.

Phosphate-buffered saline, e.g. Flow Labs Ltd.

Lymphoprep density gradient, e.g. Nycomed Ltd., Birmingham (UK)

De-ionized water.

(b) Solutions

50% (v/v) nitric acid
4% (v/v) nitric acid.

(c) Apparatus

Acid-washed glassware; sterile polystyrene containers; test tubes; pipette tips; adjustable pipettes.

Atomic absorption spectrophotometer.

8.8.16 Sample collection

Haemolysis-free blood (10–20 ml) is collected and transferred immediately to a trace-element free de-ionized tube containing 100 units of preservative-free heparin.

8.8.17 Procedure

Technique

All items of glassware used should be prepared by soaking for at least 12 hours in 50% trace-element free nitric acid with subsequent rinsing in de-ionized water. Similarly sterile polystyrene containers, all tubes, and pipette tips should be washed thoroughly at least 3 times in de-ionized water.

Separation of leukocytes. The freshly collected blood sample (10 ml) is centrifuged at 750 g for 10 min. The plasma supernatant is removed and is replaced with RPMI 1640 tissue culture medium containing 7.5% (v/v) autologous plasma. An equal volume of Plasmagel is added, the solutions are mixed gently and then incubated at 37°C for 30 min. During this time the red blood cells sediment. The leukocyte-rich supernatant is then removed and centrifuged at 750 g for 5 min. De-ionized water (5 ml) is added for 15 s after which 5 ml of phosphate-buffered saline is added. The mixture is centrifuged at 200 g for 10 min and the supernatant containing lysed residual red cells and platelets is discarded. This treatment is repeated with a further 5 ml of phosphate-buffered saline and then with 10 ml phosphate-buffered saline. The mixed white cell pellet is then washed twice in RPMI 1640, and then twice more in phosphate-buffered saline. At each stage the white cell pellet is re-precipitated by centrifugation at 400 g for 10 min. To the final pellet 1 ml of de-ionized water is added for the preparation of the cell lysate (see below).

Separation of mononuclear and polymorphonuclear cells. The leukocyte-rich supernatant collected after plasma gel sedimentation is resuspended in 5 ml of RPMI 1640 and layered onto 3 ml Lymphoprep density gradient in a round-bottomed centrifuge tube and centrifuged at 250 g for 15 min at 20°C. The pellet contains polymorphonuclear cells and residual red cells. The mononuclear cells containing lymphocytes and monocytes accumulate at the interface between the RPMI 1640 and the basal Lymphoprep. The poly-morphonuclear leukocytes can then be washed, separated from residual red cells and platelets, and prepared for analysis in the same way as has been described for mixed leukocytes.

Isolation of monocytes and lymphocytes. The mononuclear cell suspension can be prepared for analysis in the same way as described for the poly-morphonuclear leukocytes, alternatively it can be further separated into mono-cyte and lymphocyte fractions. This is done by first washing the mononuclear cell suspension in RPMI 1640 (1 ml), twice at 400 g and once at 200 g for 10 min each. Cells are then resuspended in 1 ml of RPMI 1640 and incubated at 37°C for 1 h in a Petri dish which has been previously treated with autologous plasma. At the end of incubation the non-adherent cells are washed from the dish using 3×1 ml aliquots of RPMI 1640 at 37°C. The washings were pooled. The non-adherent cells contain approximately 90% lymphocytes. This lymphocyte-rich fraction is washed at $400\,g$ for 10 min, twice in RPMI 1640, and then twice in phosphate-buffered saline. To the final cell pellet 1 ml of de-ionized water is added for the preparation of the cell lysate.

In the Petri dish the adherent cells are 90% enriched with monocytes. These are detached by gently scraping the surface of the dish with a siliconized plastic bung. The cells are then removed by adding 1 ml of ice cold RPMI 1640 and incubating the mixture and dish on ice for 5 min before removing the resuspended monocytes. This is repeated once more. The monocyte-rich suspensions are pooled and treated the same way as has been described for the lymphocyte-enriched fraction.

Cell lysis. Each leukocyte subset is resuspended in 1 ml of de-ionized water. Each preparation is then disrupted by sonification for at least 1 min. After centrifugation at $1000\,g$ for 5 min, 0.5 ml of supernatant is taken for protein assay and the remainder is transferred to tubes containing 12.5 μl of 4% (v/v) HNO_3. This mixture can be stored for up to two months at $-20°C$ for subsequent analysis.

The zinc and possible other trace element content of the lysates is determined by graphite furnace atomic absorption spectroscopy.

8.8.18 Performance characteristics

Reproducibility

Intra-batch and inter-batch coefficient of variation of analyses of 3.8 and 9.8% respectively have been reported. In the original description of this method the coefficient of variation for the analyses were 8.9%, 9.6% and 10.1% for neutrophils, lymphocytes, and monocytes respectively.

8.8.19 Reference values

In a cohort of 12 individuals the mean (SD) zinc concentration in monocytes was 2.58 (0.65) nmol/mg protein, that in lymphocytes was 1.85 (0.32) nmol/mg protein, and that in polymorphoneutrophils was 1.26 (0.27) nmol/mg protein [203]. The intracellular zinc content can be altered by isolation and separation procedure [201].

This is a difficult assay and there are no universally accepted reference ranges. Each unit using this assay should determine its own reference values and also decide whether or not it wishes to express these values in terms of cell number, or cellular DNA and/or protein content.

An alternative technique for the separation of mononuclear and polymorpho-nuclear leukocytes offers the advantage of using a smaller volume of whole blood (about 5 ml) and analysis by flame atomic absorption spectrophotometry [204].

8.8.20 Interpretation

The purity of cell preparations and the yield of the viable cells should be determined by appropriate white cell counts, and cytochemical and biochemical assays of the subset fractions.

In samples collected from fasting individuals concentrations of zinc in neutrophils and lymphocytes were approximately 25% and 23% lower respectively than in samples collected after breakfast. By contrast, concentrations in monocytes were generally higher in the fasted than non-fasted state.

SECTION V   HAIR ZINC

8.8.21 Purpose and scope

Although analysis of the zinc and other trace-element content of hair has proved popular in epidemiological studies, these results are of little use for individuals or for studies of acute deficiency or excess. Furthermore, with the exception of toxicity and probably moderate zinc deficiency, the trace-element content of hair bears little relationship to the amount that is available for physiological functions in the body. This is because hair is an immobile pool of zinc.

The trace-element content of hair is very much dependent on the growth rate of the hair. Even short periods of protein deprivation can produce changes in bulb morphology indicative of whether or not the hair is growing (anagen), stationary (telogen), or in an intermediate state (catagen). In malnutrition, particularly marasmus, the proportion of hairs in telogen is greatly increased, and as a consequence the growth rate of hair is less than the rate of deposition of trace-elements; hence the mineral content may be normal or increased. However, in mild zinc deficiency hair zinc may be decreased when growth rate exceeds the rate of elemental deposition. Thus in some circumstances an inverse correlation between 'nutritional status' and hair mineral content can be observed [205, 206].

8.8.22 Principle of the method

Hair is collected in a standardized way. It is washed thoroughly, digested, and the elemental content determined by atomic absorption spectrophotometry.

8.8.23 Chemicals and apparatus

(a) Chemicals

Non-ionic detergent G Decon 75 p.a.
Ionic detergent, e.g. sodium lauryl sulphate p.a.
Ethylenediaminetetra-acetic acid (EDTA), disodium salt dihydrate p.a.
Nitric acid (HNO_3), concentrated, Aristar grade, e.g. BDH Ltd., cat. No. 45004
Perchloric acid ($HClO_4$), concentrated, Aristar grade, e.g. BDH Ltd., cat. No. 45005
Carborundum chips
De-ionized or trace-element free water.

(b) Solutions

G Decon 75 solution: 10 ml of G Decon 75 are made up to 1000 ml with de-ionized water.
Sodium lauryl sulphate, 34.6 mmol/l: 10 g are dissolved in water to make 1000 ml.
Ethylenediaminetetra-acetic acid, 0.1 mol/l: 37.22 g are dissolved in water to make 1000 ml.

8.8.24   Sample collection   Samples should be collected from the nape and should be from the most proximal 2 cm of hair. With increasing distance from the scalp, obtained values are higher and show much greater variability. Trace metals in pubic hair correlate poorly with those derived from scalp hair.

Contamination of hair leading to invalid results is caused by sweat, shampoos, hair spray, soap, perfumes, dust, and other cosmetics.

8.8.25   Procedure   Between 0.2 and 1 g hair is cut into short (i.e. 0.5–1 cm) lengths and shaken for 30 min in 10–20 ml of 1% non-ionic detergent. It is rinsed thoroughly in de-ionized water and then treated similarly for 15 min in a cold solution (5–10 ml) 0.1 mol/l EDTA. The sample is then further rinsed in de-ionized water and is dried at 60°C for 18 h. Care should be taken to prevent clumping.

The dried hair (0.2 g) is then transferred to an appropriate tube and treated with 30 ml concentrated HNO_3 and 1 ml 70% $HClO_4$; carborundum chips are added. The hair is digested at 160°C. Digestion is assumed to be complete when 0.5 ml clear liquid remains. The digest solution is transferred quantitatively to standard flasks and the mineral content of the remaining solution is assessed by standard means.

8.8.26   Performance characteristics

(a) Reproducibility   This should be determined locally.

(b) Validity   This should be determined locally.

8.8.27   Reference values   These should be determined locally. Published values [207] in children are 2.07 (SD = 0.73) μmol/g.

SECTION VI   ALKALINE PHOSPHATASE

8.8.28   Purpose and scope   The isoenzymes of alkaline phosphatase activity operate optimally at a pH of about 10 *in vitro*. Magnesium activates the enzyme *in vivo*, and *in vitro* this activity can be replaced by cobalt and manganese. Alkaline phosphatase is a zinc metalloenzyme. Isolated determinations of alkaline phosphatase activity are of doubtful value in enabling one to assess the possibility that a patient is zinc deficient. However, monitoring changes in alkaline phosphatase activity after zinc supplementation is of possible but not certain value [208].

8.8.29   Principle of the method   There are many methods determining alkaline phosphatase activity. The method outlined below depends on the enzymatic hydrolysis of phosphate from 4-nitrophenyl phosphate (4-NPP; PNPP), which is colourless, to form 3, 4-nitrophenol; under alkaline conditions this is converted to 4-nitrophenoxide ion, which assumes a quinonoid form, simultaneously developing an intense yellow colour. The rate of formation of 4-nitrophenol by the action of the enzyme on 4-nitrophenyl phosphate at 30°C can be followed with a recording spectrophotometer. If necessary a two-point analysis can be undertaken by determining the 4-nitrophenoxide production at a known time interval, the final point of which can be made more accurate by adding 10 ml NaOH (0.05 mol/l) to a 1-ml reaction mixture to stop the reaction. The added NaOH raises the pH to about 12, inactivates the enzyme, ensures that all the phenoxide is converted to the quinonoid form, and dilutes the colour to a determinable intensity [209, 210].

8.8.30 Chemicals and apparatus

(a) Chemicals

2-amino-2-methyl-1-propanol (AMP), ($C_4H_{11}NO$) p.a.
Hydrochloric acid (HCl) concentrated 37% (fuming) p.a.
Magnesium chloride hexahydrate, 59% ($MgCl_2 . 6H_2O$)
4-nitrophenylphosphate disodium salt hexahydrate (PNPP), ($C_6H_4NO_6PNa_2 . 6H_2O$), high purity
4-nitrophenol (4-NP), ($C_6H_5NO_3$), 99% p.a., high purity
Sodium hydroxide (NaOH) p.a.
Distilled and carbon-dioxide-free water.

(b) Solutions

Hydrochloric acid, 1 mol/l: 83.3 ml of concentrated HCl are made up to 1000 ml with water.

Sodium hydroxide, 0.05 mol/l: 2 g of NaOH are dissolved in water to make 1000 ml.

Buffer, AMP, 0.84 mol/l, pH 10.3 at 30°C. This is prepared in a 2 litre volumetric flask by mixing 300 ml of HCL 1 mol/l and 150 g of AMP dissolved in 1 litre of H_2O and making to volume with additional water. The pH is adjusted to 10.3 ($\pm$ 0.02) at 30°C. Carbon-dioxide-free water should be used in preparing the buffer, and care should be taken to avoid contact with air during preparation and storage. In these circumstances the buffer is stable at room temperature for 60 days.

Stock $MgCl_2$ solution, 150 mmol/l: 3.0 g of $MgCl_2 . 6H_2O$ is dissolved in water to make 100 ml; this is stable at room temperature for 30 days.

Working $MgCl_2$ solution, 1.5 mmol/l. This is prepared fresh for each analysis by diluting 1 ml of the stock $MgCl_2$ solution to 100 ml.

Substrate solution of 215 mmol/l of 4-NPP in 1.5 mmol/l $MgCl_2$ solution. 800 mg of PNPP is dissolved in 10 ml of the working magnesium chloride solution. If necessary this substrate solution can be kept without negligible decomposition for about seven days at 4°C in the dark.

Standard solutions of 4-NP:

Stock standard, 1 mmol/l: 139.1 mg of 4-NP dissolved in water to make 1000 ml. This solution is stable if kept in the dark. If high purity 4-NP is not available commercially it can be purified by recrystallizing 4-NP from hot water and drying overnight in a vacuum dessicator.

4-NP working standard, 40 µmol/l in 0.84 mol/l AMP buffer: 10 ml of stock standard is pipetted into 250 ml volumetric flask and diluted to volume with the AMP buffer. The standard solution is mixed thoroughly. The absorbance of this should be checked by measuring its value in a narrow beam spectrophotometer at 400 nm in standard 1-cm cell at 30°C. Ideally the reading should be 0.75 ± 0.002. A similar dilution of the stock 4-NP in NaOH, 0.05 mol/l measured at 401 nm at 25°C should give a value of 0.735.

(c) Apparatus

Adjustable pipettes; test tubes; cuvettes; pippette tips.

Centrifuge; water bath.

A spectrophotometer with thermostated cell compartment and connected to a recorder is needed. Alternatively an automatic analyser capable of repeated timed absorbance readings and with suitable rate of valuation programme can be used.

8.8.31 Sample collection   Haemolysis-free serum or heparinized plasma should be used.

8.8.32 Procedure

(a) Technique

The wavelength is pre-set at 404 nm. The temperature of the cell compartment is adjusted to 30 ± 0.1°C. The cuvettes are pre-warmed to 30°C in the compartment or in an incubator. 2.7 ml of buffer is pipetted into a 10-ml volume test tube. 100 µl of serum or plasma is then added using disposable polyethylene pipette tips. The tubes containing buffer and serum are then placed for at least 5 min in a water-bath at 30°C. A tube containing an aliquot of substrate is placed in a water-bath; simultaneously the reaction is initiated by adding 200 µl of the warm substrate to the tube containing the buffer and serum. The mixture is then transferred immediately to a pre-warmed cuvette and placed in the cell compartment of the spectrophotometer. The changes in the solution absorbance are measured at 404 nm and are recorded for 2–5 min. The observed changes in absorbance over time should comprise a straight line for at least 2–3 minutes' duration. The rate of change of absorbance with time can then be calculated.

(b) Calculation

If the molar extinction of 4-NP is 18 750, then the absorbance of a 1 mmol 4-NP/l would be 18.75 and the measured change in absorbance per minute would correspond to $\dfrac{A/min}{18.75} \cdot$ mol 4-NP/ml.

This quantity of 4-NP is contained in 3 ml when the serum plasma volume used is 0.1 ml. Therefore alkaline phosphatase activity (U/l) =

$$\frac{A/min}{18.75} \cdot 1 \cdot 3 \cdot \frac{1000}{0.1} = (\text{change in absorbance/min}) \cdot 1600$$

where 1 = mmol 4-NP/ml; 3.0 = total volume in cuvette; 0.1 = volume of serum or plasma in cuvette; 1000 converts mmol to µmol.

8.8.33 Performance characteristics

(a) Reproducibility

Inter- and intra-batch coefficients of variation are about 5%.

(b) Validity

Each laboratory should validate its own method and establish reference values.

8.8.34 Reference values These vary with age and sex; cited values are: adults 25–100 U/l. Values in children vary with growth rate and pubertal stage, and may be as high as 500 U/l. It is recommended that each laboratory should establish its own reference values.

8.8.35 Interpretation Alkaline phosphatase activity is subject to many physiological influences, and levels are raised during rapid growth. The best way to use alkaline phosphatase activity is to monitor its response to zinc supplementation.

8.9 COPPER **SECTION I PLASMA OR SERUM COPPER BY AAS**

8.9.1 Purpose and scope The procedures described for the determination of plasma/serum zinc concentrations can be used for copper (see sections 8.8.1–8.8.3).

8.9.2 Principle of the method See Zinc, Section I to Section III.

8.9.3 Chemicals and apparatus

(a) Chemicals See Zinc, Section I to Section III.

(b) Solutions See Zinc, Section I to Section III.

(c) Apparatus Atomic absorption spectrophotometer set up according to the manufacturer's instructions.

8.9.4 Sample collection Venous blood collected as recommended for zinc analysis; although haemolysis is less problematical for copper determination than for that of zinc, haemolysed samples are best avoided.

8.9.5 Procedure See Zinc, Section I to Section III.
 The absorbance is measured at 324.7 nm, and in most flame AAS the response is linear up to approximately 60 µmol/l (i.e. 3.8 mg/l).

8.9.6 Performance characteristics See Zinc, Section I to Section III.

8.9.7 Reference values This is 10–22 µmol/l. It is recommended that each laboratory should establish its own reference values.

8.9.8 Interpretation Plasma and serum copper concentrations are increased by stress, oral contraceptive agents, liver disease, and infections. Levels are low with inborn errors of metabolism (e.g. Wilson disease and Menkes syndrome).

References See [197–200].

SECTION II SERUM/PLASMA COPPER BY COLORIMETRIC METHOD [211]

A colorimetric technique for the determination of serum copper has been developed using 4-(3,5-dibromo-2-pyridylazo)-N-ethyl-N-sulphopropylaniline (DiBr-PAESA). 0.1 ml of serum is mixed with 1.5 ml reagent comprising 1 mg DiBr-PAESA dissolved in 100 ml acetate buffer (0.2 mol/l; pH 5.0) and incubated for 5 min at 37°C. Absorbance of the chelate-Cu complex is measured at 580 nm. The molar absorptivity of the complex is $80\ 000\ l \cdot mol^{-1} \cdot cm^{-1}$. The lower limit of detection is 1.6 μmol/l and the reaction is reported to be linear to approximately 75 μmol/l. The intra-batch coefficient of variation at 11 μmol/l is 3.3%; inter-batch variation is 2.8%.

SECTION III MEASUREMENT OF HUMAN SERUM CAERULOPLASMIN

8.9.9 Purpose and scope

Caeruloplasmin is an α_2-macroglobulin (MW $\approx$ 135 000), which possesses numerous oxidase activities.It contains 0.335% by weight of copper, that is 6–7 atoms of copper per mole. Between 90 and 95% of plasma or serum copper is bound to caeruloplasmin. Methods for the quantitative determination of caeruloplasmin have depended on its colour, which has a maximum absorbance at 605 nm with a specific absorbance of $0.068 \cdot g^{-1} \cdot cm^{-1}$. Immunoassay techniques are available but these are independent of the constituent copper and, albeit rarely, determinations of what is essentially immunoreactive apocaeruloplasmin can yield values in the absence of any functional activity.

Therefore one should be cautious in using immunoassay rather than functional assessments of caeruloplasmin even though the former are more precise.

Most functional estimations of caeruloplasmin activity are based on the oxidase activity. The most common procedures use as substrates, p-phenylenediamine (PPD), N, N-dimethyl-p-phenylene diamine, and o-dianisidine dihydrochloride.

8.9.10 Principle of the method

At pH 5.4 caeruloplasmin catalyses the oxidation of PPD to yield a coloured product the production of which is proportional to the concentration of serum caeruloplasmin, provided a correction is made for spontaneous oxidation of the substrate. Non-enzymatic production of the PPD oxidation product is monitored in controlled systems containing sodium azide, which dissociates copper from the caeruloplasmin molecule, thereby inhibiting its enzymatic activity [212].

8.9.11 Chemicals and apparatus

(a) Chemicals

Sodium acetate (CH_3COONa) p.a.
Acetic acid (CH_3COOH) p.a.
Sodium azide (NaN_3) p.a.
Phenylenediamine (PPD) dihydrochloride ($C_6H_{10}Cl_2N_2$), e.g. BDH cat. No. 29503

Sodium hydroxide (NaOH) p.a.
De-ionized water.

(b) Solutions   Sodium acetate, 0.2 mol/l: 16.4 g of sodium acetate are dissolved in water to make 1000 ml.

Acetic acid, 0.2 mol/l: 12.01 ml of acetic acid are made up to 1000 ml with distilled water.

Acetate buffer, 0.1 mol/l, pH 5.45 at 37°C is prepared by adding 430 ml of sodium acetate 0.2 mol/l to 70 ml of acetic acid 0.2 mol/l. The mixture is warmed to 37°C in a water bath and the pH is adjusted to 5.4–5.5 by addition of sodium acetate or acetic acid. Contents of the flask are then made up to 1000 ml with de-ionized water.

Sodium azide, 1.5 mol/l: 97.5 g of sodium azide are dissolved in de-ionized water to make 1000 ml.

Sodium hydroxide, 1 mol/l: 40 g of NaOH are dissolved in water to make 1000 ml.

Buffered PPD solution, 27.6 mmol/l is prepared by adding 0.5 g phenylenediamine dihydrochloride to a 100 ml volumetric flask and dissolved in approximately 75 ml of the prewarmed acetate buffer to pH 5.45. The contents of the flask are readjusted to pH 5.45 by dropwise addition of sodium hydroxide 1 mol/l and made up to 100 ml with the acetate buffer. This solution is stable for 3 h.

(c) Apparatus   Adjustable pipettes; test tubes; cuvettes.
Laboratory centrifuge; water-bath.
Spectrophotometer.

8.9.12 Sample collection

The oxidase activity of serum or plasma that has been stored at room temperature is variable. Samples are best preserved at 4°C or −20°C.

8.9.13 Procedure

(a) Technique   Into two test tubes (12 × 75 mm) are pipetted 2 ml of acetate buffer. One test tube will serve as a reaction system (R) the other as the blank (B); 0.1 ml of serum or plasma is added to each tube, and the tubes are placed in a water-bath at 37°C. A flask containing the buffered PPD is similarly prewarmed.

Warmed, buffered PPD solution (1 ml) is added to both tubes. The contents of the tubes are mixed thoroughly and they are kept unstoppered in a water-bath. The water-bath is covered to avoid exposure to light.

After 5 min, 50 μl of sodium azide 1.5 mol/l is added to the blank system and the contents are mixed, the tube is replaced in the water bath, and the water bath is again covered.

30 min later, 50 μl of sodium azide 1.5 mol/l is added to the reaction tube and the contents mixed.

The reaction and blank samples are transferred to spectrophotometer cuvettes (1-cm light path) and their absorbance at 530 nm is measured. The colour of the samples remains stable for 6 h.

(b) Standardization

The PPD oxidase assay can be standardized against solutions containing crystalline human caeruloplasmin. Immediately before PPD oxidase assays the concentration of caeruloplasmin in sodium phosphate buffer 0.1 mol/l, pH 7.0, can be assessed by measuring the differences in the absorbance at 605 nm before and after adding ascorbic acid to the solution (sodium azide is a suitable alternative), and dividing the observed changes in absorbance by the extinction coefficient of human caeruloplasmin (at a concentration of 1 g/l in a 1-cm light path the extinction coefficient at 605 nm of caeruloplasmin is 0.68). The concentrated caeruloplasmin solution can then be used to standardize the PPD oxidase assay. In the description of this technique this approach yielded a mean calibration factor of 0.752 (SE = 0.004). The concentrated caeruloplasmin solutions in sodium phosphate buffer were stable at 4°C for 6 months.

(c) Calculation

Caeruloplasmin (g/l) = 0.752 (A_R − A_B), where A_R is the absorbance of sample R and A_B is the absorbance of sample B. Absorbance activity at 530 nm can be calibrated against caeruloplasmin standards prepared from commercial sources.

Another approach using PPD in acetate buffer is performed at pH 6.0 in 1-cm cuvettes at 37°C. The reaction is read at 30 min and the result reported in absorbance units. This is more convenient for large batches in busy laboratories. Caeruloplasmin oxidase activity in this system has a sharp optimum pH 6.0. Since photo catalysis of PPD occurs it is always important to use an activated blank and to allow the reaction to proceed in the dark. An assay using o-dianisidine dihydrochloride has also been described.

8.9.14 Performance characteristics

Reproducibility

Intra-batch coefficient of variation was reported as 1.25%, that for inter-batch variability was 2.8%.

8.9.15 Reference values

This should be determined locally. Values approximate 315 (SD = 49) mg/l; 1.2–2.9 µmol/l.

8.9.16 Interpretation

Serum/plasma caeruloplasmin levels are increased with stress, exercise, pregnancy, oestrogen administration, infections, trauma, malignancy, and with biliary obstruction. Levels are reduced with malnutrition, protein-losing enteropathies, nephrosis, and advanced hepatic disease.

SECTION IV   ERYTHROCYTE SUPEROXIDE DISMUTASE

8.9.17 Purpose and scope

Erythrocyte superoxide dismutase is a cytosolic metalloprotein containing zinc at its structural site and copper at the catalytic site. It catalyses reduction of superoxide to hydrogen peroxide and oxygen and it can be distinguished from the similar activity of mitochondrial superoxide dismutase, which is a manganoenzyme, by the inhibition of its action by cyanide [213, 214]. Cu, Zn-SOD activity is probably a better indicator of reduced copper 'status' than circulating levels of copper or caeruloplasmin. ·

8.9.18 Principle of the method

Superoxide is generated by the aerobic activity of xanthine oxidase on xanthine. The superoxide can be detected by its ability to reduce reagents such as cytochrome C, which can be followed spectrometrically at 550 nm, or nitroblue tetrazolium, which can be measured at 560 nm. The inhibition of this reaction by superoxide dismutase can be used as an indicator of the enzyme activity.

Other substrates such as adrenaline (epinephrine) or pyrogallol have been used.

8.9.19 Chemicals and apparatus

(a) Chemicals

Sodium chloride (NaCl) p.a.
Chloroform ($CHCl_3$) p.a.
Ethanol (C_2H_5OH) 100% p.a.
Ammonium sulphate ((NH_4)$_2SO_4$) p.a.
Xanthine oxidase
Ethylenediaminetetra-acetic acid (EDTA) ($C_{10}H_{16}N_2O_3$) p.a., e.g. BDH Ltd., cat. No. 10424
Nitroblue tetrazolium (NBT) ($C_{40}H_{30}Cl_2N_{10}O_5$), e.g. BDH cat. No. 34060
Sodium carbonate (Na_2CO_3) p.a.
Superoxide dismutase (Cu, Zn-SOD) from bovine liver or from bovine erythrocytes
Copper chloride ($CuCl_2$) p.a.
De-ionized water.

(b) Solutions

0.9% saline: 9 g of NaCl are dissolved in water to make 1000 ml.
Ammonium sulphate, 2 mol/l: 264.28 g are dissolved in water to make 1000 ml.
Xanthine oxidase, 167 U/l is available with specific activity of 1 kU/g as 20 U per 1.2 ml of the enzyme supplied. 20 µl of this is diluted to 2 ml with freshly prepared ice-cold 2 mol/l ammonium sulphate, giving a final concentration of xanthine oxidase of 167 U/l.
EDTA, 0.6 mmol/l: 175 mg of EDTA are dissolved in water to make 1000 ml.
Nitroblue tetrazolium solution, 150 µmol/l: 122.6 mg of NBT are dissolved in water to make 1000 ml.
Na_2CO_3, 400 mmol/l: 42.3 g of Na_2CO_3 are dissolved in water to make 1000 ml.
Bovine serum albumin 1 g/l.
Superoxide dismutase assay reagent: to a 200-ml beaker are added:
> 40 ml of 0.3 mmol/l xanthine
> 20 ml of 0.6 mmol/l EDTA
> 20 ml of 150 µmol/l NBT
> 12 ml of 400 mmol/l Na_2CO_3, and
> 6 ml of 1 g/l bovine serum albumin.

Superoxide dismutase standards: these can be prepared from commercially available bovine liver or erythrocyte Cu, Zn-SOD material.
$CuCl_2$, 0.8 mmol/l: 107.5 mg of $CuCl_2$ are dissolved in water to make 1000 ml.

(c) Apparatus Adjustable pipettes; test tubes; cuvettes.
Centrifuge; ice-bath.
Spectrophotometer.

8.9.20 Sample collection Erythrocytes are separated from whole blood by centrifugation at 1000 g for 10–15 min at 4°C, washed at 1000 g for 10 min and then resuspended three times with 0.9% saline.

After the final centrifugation they are lysed in 3.0 ml of water and placed in an ice-bath for 15 min.

Chloroform (0.6 ml) and ethanol (1.0 ml) are added, and the mixture is mixed thoroughly before being centrifuged at 5000 g at 4°C for 20 min. The supernatant is diluted 1/49 before being used immediately for the superoxide dismutase assay.

8.9.21 Procedure

(a) Technique The superoxide dismutase assay reagent prepared as above is enough for 40 assays.

Assay reagent (2.45 ml) is added to each of 40 tubes and to each is then added 0.5 ml of pure Cu, Zn-SOD (0–270 ng), or sample for assay. This provides a final assay volume of about 3.0 ml containing, per litre, 0.1 mmol of xanthine, 0.1 mmol of EDTA, 50 mg of bovine serum albumin, 25 μmol of NBT, 9.9 nmol of xanthine oxidase, and 40 mmol of Na_2CO_3 (pH 10.2). The tubes are then placed in a water-bath at 25°C and to each tube 50 μl of xanthine oxidase solution is added (bringing the actual volume to 3.0 ml). The tubes are incubated for 20 min and the reaction is terminated by adding 1 ml of 0.8 mmol/l $CuCl_2$. The spectrometric absorbance is determined at 560 nm.

(b) Calculation The percentage inhibition is calculated as:

$$\frac{(A_{blank} - A_{sample})}{A_{blank}} \cdot 100\%$$

The standard and addition curve is prepared by plotting the percentage inhibition of activity on the y axis (ordinate) and the enzyme protein concentration on the x axis (abscissa).

A separate standard curve should be prepared for each assay run using pure Cu, Zn-SOD.

8.9.22 Performance characteristics

Reliability There is as yet no uniformly standardized assay of superoxide dismutase. As a consequence the values from different laboratories cannot be compared easily. Thus when this assay is established it should be independently and completely evaluated.

8.9.23 Reference values

In the paper describing the above method the following Cu, Zn-SOD concentrations were derived from healthy adults and are expressed in term of whole blood volume:

Erythrocytes 242 ± 4 mg/l (N = 44)
Serum 548 ± 20 μg/l (N = 38)
Plasma 173 ± 11 μg/l (N = 44)

All values are mean $\pm$ the standard error of the mean and the number of specimens analysed is indicated in parentheses. The best way to express SOD has not been established.

Other reference values include 4.059 (SD = 0.34) nmol/g red cells; in adult females [215] and 1461 (SD = 451) U/g Hb in young children [216].

8.9.24 Interpretation

Increased erythrocyte superoxide dismutase activity has been described in animal models with severe oxidant stress or iron deficiency anaemia and in humans with Down's syndrome or uraemia. Levels are reduced in leukaemia and lymphoproliferative disorders [213]. Otherwise activities appear to be better indicators of reduced copper 'status' than circulating levels of copper or caeruloplasmin [215, 216].

8.10 SELENIUM

8.10.1 Purpose and scope

The methods actually used for assessment of selenium nutritional status, as described below, are Se content and GSHpx activity; these variables are tested in whole blood or plasma or lysate erythrocytes. Blood Se content is certainly an index that can be correlated to Se nutritional status, but is influenced by different factors and sometimes it is not possible to find any correlation between Se content and Se nutritional status. In low Se intake, an increase in its amount in the diet on previous days influences appreciably the whole blood Se content, and consequently this value is not a representative index for individual nutritional status, as Se is not yet utilized in biological mechanisms. In adequate Se intake, a lower Se diet in previous days influences not so much the Se content in erythrocytes as in plasma. Se assay in blood can be an acceptable index of nutritional status for populations only if they have a uniform and continuous intake of food produced in the same area. The activity of GSHpx, at present the main enzyme for which Se is an essential cofactor, is a parameter widely utilized to assess nutritional Se status. Plasma can be used for this test as plasma GSHpx, which appears to be of hepatic origin, changes with dietary Se level; so this variable is reliable in assessing short-term responses to dietary Se in animals and humans. Erythrocytes and whole blood are not a good index for assessing nutritional Se status because their changes are related to the Se content in erythropoiesis time. Platelets may be a useful material [217, 218]; in fact they are rich in GSHpx and respond to changes in Se diet intake in time corresponding to that of liver.

SECTION I   BLOOD SELENIUM BY SPECTROMETRY

8.10.2 Principle of the method

Selenium content in whole blood, plasma or lysed erythrocytes is determined using an electrothermal atomic spectrometric method.

8.10.3 Chemicals and apparatus

(a) Chemicals

Palladium atomic absorption standard solution 1000 µg/ml, e.g. Sigma cat. No. P–4400
Triton X–100, e.g. Baker cat. No. 49855
Selenium atomic absorption standard solution 1 mg/ml, e.g. Carlo Erba cat. No. 497621.

(b) Solutions

1.0 g of Triton X–100 made up to 1000 ml with distilled water.
Matrix modifier solution: 10 ml of palladium (1000 µg/l) made up to 100 ml with Triton X–100 solution (0.1 g/100 ml).

(c) Apparatus

A Perkin–Elmer model 3030 atomic absorption spectrometer equipped with an HGA–600 graphite furnace and Zeeman background correction can be used. A Perkin–Elmer electrodeless discharge lamp (Se) serves as line source. This is run at manufacturer's recommended current (7 mA). A spectral band pass of 0.7 nm is used.

8.10.4 Sample collection

Whole blood (5–10 ml) is taken with a heparinized syringe and used to prepare plasma and washed erythrocytes.

8.10.5 Procedure

(a) Technique

Samples are diluted, adding distilled water and Triton X–100 (0.1%), 1 + 7 times for whole blood and erythrocytes and 1 + 3 for plasma, obtaining a final Se concentration between 10 and 20 p.p.b. Diluted samples are drawn automatically and mixed with solution containing matrix modifier (palladium) and dispensed in L'vov platform. To minimize the matrix effect the technique of standard addition has been used.

Programming mode HGA–600 (example of electrothermal atomic absorption spectrometric method)

Wavelength (nm): 196.0
Slit   (nm):   0.7
Pyrocoated tube with platform
Pretreatment temperature: 1200°C
Atomize temperature: 2100°C

Step number	Furnace temperature (°C)	Time Rampe (s)	Time Hold (s)	Internal Gas flow (ml/min)
1	90	20	5	300
2	120	50	20	300
3	530	20	50	300
4	1200	10	20	300
5	2100	0	5	0 (read)
6	2650	1	6	300
7	20	1	6	300
8	–	1	–	300

(b) Calculation

The sample and the samples plus additions are analysed to determine the slope of the calibration curve, thus allowing the concentration in the sample to be calculated.

Example, whole blood:

Sample	Dilution	Signal
Sample + water	(1:1)	0.011–0.010
Sample + 12.5 p.p.b. Se	(1:1)	0.022–0.023
Sample + 25.0 p.p.b. Se	(1:1)	0.034–0.036

from linear regression: $y = 0.96 \cdot 10^{-3}x + 0.01$ $(r = 0.997)$
$$y = 10.63 \cdot 8 \text{ (dilution)} = 85.04 \text{ p.p.b. Se}$$

8.10.6 Performance characteristics

(a) Detection limit

The detection limit is about 15–20 µg/l.

(b) Reproducibility

The precision, expressed as the coefficient of variation (CV%), is 5.2% and 5.1% for plasma and erythrocytes respectively. The correlation between the hydride evolution technique and the method based on atomic absorption spectrometry is extremely good, in fact the means ± SD are 92.1 ± 1.8 µg/l and 93.5 ± 1.8 µg/l respectively.

8.10.7 Reference values

Reference values vary with geographical area, depending on soil Se content; values are not influenced by age and sex in adults. Values found in plasma and erythrocytes of a group of males and females of North Italy are 109 ± 23 and 99 ± 24 (mean ± SD) respectively. Our findings are comparable with other population groups of Europe [219, 220].

8.10.8 Interpretation

Selenium determination with deuterium background correction is influenced by the presence of Fe and/or P in samples; Zeeman effect eliminates this interference and permits Se evaluation also in erythrocytes.

SECTION II   BLOOD SELENIUM BY FLUOROMETRIC TECHNIQUE

8.10.9 Principle of the method

This method uses a low-temperature perchlorate digestion of serum which can be applied equally to other biological tissues and fluids. The advantage of the method is its relative sensitivity and its lack of dependence on the rather complicated atomic absorption methodologies. It has a disadvantage of needing appropriate laboratory facilities for perchlorate digestion.

8.10.10 Chemical and apparatus

(a) Chemicals

Nitric acid (HNO_3) concentrated p.a.
Perchloric acid ($HClO_4$) 60% p.a.
Hydrochloric acid (HCl) concentrated p.a.
Hydroxylamine chloride (H_4ClNO) p.a.
EDTA ($C_{10}H_{14}N_2Na_2O_8.2H_2O$) p.a.
Ammonia (NH_4OH) 40% p.a.
Cresol red indicator p.a.
2,3-diaminonaphthalene ($C_{10}H_{10}N_2$) p.a.
Cyclohexane ($CH_2(CH_2)_4CH_2$) p.a.
Distilled water.

(b) Solutions

0.1 N HCl: 8.3–8.5 ml 36% (w/v) HCl made up to 1000 ml with distilled water.

10% HCl: 277.8 ml 36% (w/v) HCl made up to 1000 ml with water.

Hydroxylamine/EDTA solution: 9 g of EDTA dissolved in 900 ml of distilled water, 25 g hydroxylamine chloride added and mixed to dissolve, then made up to 1000 ml with water.

Cresol red solution: 0.05 g cresol red dissolved in 1 ml distilled water plus a drop of NH_4OH, and diluted up to 250 ml.

DAN solution: 500 mg 2,3-diaminonaphthalene is dissolved in 0.1 N HCl to make 1000 ml. Grind DAN with a small volume of the HCl in a glass pestle and mortar to make it dissolve more easily. The DAN solution is then extracted with 60 ml cyclohexane and the cyclohexane discarded. The DAN is stored in a foil-covered bottle in a cupboard and is stable for at least one month.

Working standards: 0.01–0.2 µg/l in 0.1 ml distilled water, prepared from a commercial standard solution.

(c) Apparatus

Quickfit boiling tubes with stoppers; boiling chips; glassware (soaked in 50:50 concentrated nitric acid and de-ionized water for 30 min before rinsing with de-ionized then distilled water).
Digestion rack
Heating platform
Fluorometric spectrophotometer

8.10.11 Sample collection

Whole blood (5–10 ml) is taken with a heparinized syringe and used to prepare plasma and washed erythrocytes.

Biological tissues, after grinding, are weighed and treated as plasma or blood.

8.10.12 Procedure

Digestions are carried out in 75 ml Quickfit boiling tubes which will take B24 stoppers. Known weights of tissues <1 g in weight or blood samples <1 ml are placed with a few BDH boiling chips. Nitric acid (8 ml) is added and the samples left overnight.

The samples are then heated gently on a digestion rack until violent frothing subsides, 2.5 ml of 60% perchloric acid is then added to the digestions which are first allowed to cool for 1–2 min. The heat is then reapplied to the digestions and the nitric acid boiled off (time 2–3 h). When all nitric acid has been removed, dense white fumes of perchloric acid appear. The heat is then turned down so the perchloric acid is not boiled off but just refluxes in the boiling tubes. This heating is continued for 30 min.

At this stage 2.5 ml 10% HCl is added very carefully to the digests. This drives off excess nitric acid and ensures any of the selenium as selenate is converted to selenite. There is no need to heat the digest in a water-bath at this stage, as suggested by the published method [221].

Five millilitres of hydroxylamine/EDTA [222] is added to each digest followed by 2 or 3 drops of cresol red solution; 40% ammonia is added till the indicator turns yellow; 10% HCl is then added dropwise till the indicator starts to turn pink/orange. This brings the digest to pH 1.5–2.5, optimal for diaminonaphthalene (DAN) complex formation with selenium. The digests are then diluted to 50 ml with distilled water.

Five millilitres of DAN solution is then added to digests and the mixture stoppered and heated at 50°C for 30 min in a covered water-bath. DAN is light sensitive and precipitate will appear on exposure to direct sunlight. There is no need, however, to use a darkened room.

The reaction mixture is cooled to room temperature and 6 ml cyclohexane are added, shaking for 20 s to extract the DAN/Se complex.

After the mixture has been allowed to separate for at least 10 min the cyclohexane layer is removed using a pipette. The fluorescence of the DAN/Se complex in the cyclohexane is then measured (excitation 366 nm, emission 525 nm) and compared to that produced by standards.

There is no need to digest the standards. We add 2.5 ml of 60% perchloric acid to standards in 0.1 ml distilled water and then continue from hydroxylamine/EDTA addition.

8.10.13 Performance characteristics

(a) Detection limits

Detection limits are 10–100 ng.

(b) Reproducibility

Comparison between the described method, the hydride evolution technique, and the method based on atomic absorption spectrometry is extremely good; above concentrations of 100 ng/g, coefficient of variation should be less than 8%.

8.10.14 Reference values   These vary geographically. For this reason each laboratory should establish its own reference values. Significant risk of selenium deficiency is present at plasma concentrations less than 15 µg/l.

8.10.15 Interpretation   The fluorometric method is cheap, but it has the disadvantage of requiring a lot of attention and labour and of using perchloric acid for digestion; it therefore needs appropriate fume covers and ventilation. Furthermore, care must be taken with the digestion to avoid the loss of selenium due to its volatility. A digestion procedure, using nitric acid/phosphoric acid, has been developed as an alternative to the use of perchloric acid [223]. Spuriously high results can be gained from the enhanced fluorescence induced by samples with a high lipid content and by contaminants on glassware.

Selenium determination by atomic absorption spectrometry with deuterium or Zeeman background correction is influenced by the matrix effect of samples, while the fluorescence method eliminates this interference and permits Se evaluation also in diet samples.

SECTION III   GLUTATHIONE PEROXIDASE ACTIVITY

8.10.16 Principle of the method   The Se-dependent enzyme glutathione peroxidase (GSHpx) catalyses with high specificity the detoxification of hydrogen peroxide by the oxidation of reduced glutathione according to the following reaction:

$$2GSH + H_2O_2 \xrightarrow{\text{GSHpx}} GSSG + 2H_2O$$

Rather than measuring the loss of GSH, we maintain this substrate at constant concentration by the addition of glutathione reductase (GR) and NADPH [224]. This converts the produced GSSG to the reduced form:

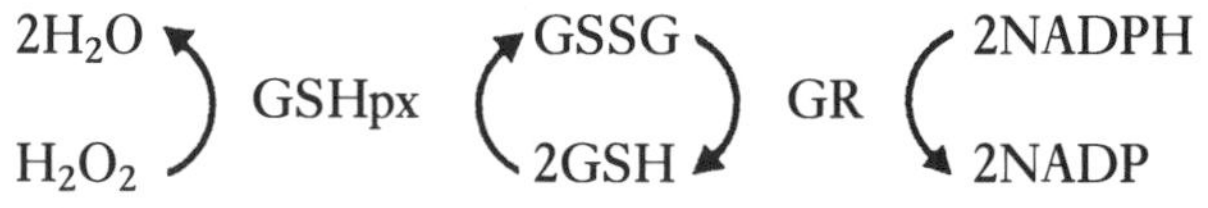

$$
\begin{array}{ccc}
2H_2O & GSSG & 2NADPH \\
\Big) \; GSHpx \; \Big(& \Big) \; GR \; \Big(& \\
H_2O_2 & 2GSH & 2NADP
\end{array}
$$

The activity of GSHpx is directly related to the rate of change of NADPH to NADP, which is followed at 340 nm. This method can be used for the GSHpx assay in whole blood, plasma, lysate erythrocytes and platelets [225].

8.10.17 Chemical and apparatus

(a) Chemicals   Dipotassium phosphate (K_2HPO_4) p.a.
Glutathione reductase (GR), e.g. Sigma cat. No. G–4751
Glutathione reduced form ($C_{10}H_{17}N_3O_6S$), e.g. Sigma cat. No. G–4251
NADPH, e.g. Sigma cat. No. N–2385
Hydrogen peroxide solution 35% (H_2O_2) p.a., e.g. Carlo Erba
EDTA ($C_{10}H_{14}N_2Na_2O_8 \cdot 2H_2O$) p.a., e.g. BDH Ltd. cat. No. 28025
Sodium azide (NaN_3) p.a., e.g. BDH Ltd. cat. No. 10369

Potassium hexacyanoferrate (III) ($K_3Fe(CN)_6$) p.a., e.g. Fluka cat. No. 60299
Potassium cyanide (KCN) p.a., e.g. Fluka cat. No. 60178
Potassium dihydrogen phosphate (KH_2PO_4) p.a., e.g. Fluka cat. No. 60219.

(b) Solutions

Phosphate buffer: 2.09 g K_2HPO_4 dissolved in 50 ml distilled water; 22.33 g EDTA and 1.30 g NaN_3 are added and pH is adjusted to 7; finally make to 100 ml.

Drabbkin's reagent: 0.068 g KH_2PO_4, 0.099 g $K_3Fe(CN)_6$ and 0.198 g KCN are dissolved in distilled water and diluted to make 500 ml.

GR solution, 120 U/ml: 1 ml GR (500 units) made up to 4.1 ml with phosphate buffer.

GSH solution, 0.1 mmol/l: 0.307 g GSH dissolved in distilled water to make 100 ml.

NADPH, 2 mmol/l: 0.015 g NADPH dissolved in distilled water to make 10 ml.

H_2O_2, 8.8 mmol/l: 0.7 ml H_2O_2 made to 1000 ml with distilled water.

(c) Apparatus

Adjustable pipettes; test tubes; cuvettes.
Centrifuge.
Spectrophotometer (e.g. Cary 219) equipped with recorder and temperature controller.

8.10.18 Sample collection

Venous blood (5–10 ml) is taken with a heparinized syringe and used to prepare washed erythrocytes, plasma, and platelets.

8.10.19 Procedure

(a) Erythrocytes lysis

Washed erythrocytes (0.200 ml) are collected and added to 1.8 ml of haemolysing solution (Drabbkin's reagent). After 3 min incubation at room temperature, the lysate is centrifuged at 9000 g for 15 min to eliminate cellular membranes, and the supernatant is collected for GSHpx assay.

(b) Technique

In the cuvette, phosphate buffer (2.1 ml), a known volume of sample (0.1 ml) (plasma, lysate erythrocytes, or platelets), GR solution (0.025 ml) and GSH solution (0.025 ml) are added and left to stand for about 5 min to equilibrate at 30°C. Then NADPH solution (0.250 ml) is added, and NADPH decrease is followed on the recorder (at 340 nm) to determine the hydroperoxide-independent NADPH consumption (blank sample).

Afterwards H_2O_2 8.8 mmol/l (0.020 ml) is added and the OD decrease is followed (sample test). Furthermore, each time new solutions are prepared, and sometimes during GSHpx assay, blank of reagents is measured. In this case the cuvette contains all reagent mixture, in which the sample is substituted by distilled water or diluted Drabbkin's reagent; then H_2O_2 8.8 mmol/l is added and the OD decrease at 340 nm is recorded (blank reagent). The blanks are tested to measure the non-enzymatic NADPH consumption coming from samples or reagents.

(c) Calculation

A unit of GSHpx is defined as µmole of NADPH oxidized per minute, calculated on the basis of the molar extinction of NADPH at 340 nm.

ΔOD/min (sample)$-(\Delta$OD/min (blank reagent)$-\Delta$OD/min (blank sample)) = correct ΔOD/min

$$\frac{\text{correct } \Delta\text{OD/min} \cdot 2.5 \cdot 1000}{6.22 \cdot 0.1} = \text{U/l (plasma)}$$

$$\frac{\text{correct } \Delta\text{OD/min} \cdot 2.5 \cdot 1000}{6.22 \cdot 0.1 \cdot \text{g/l (Hb)}} = \text{U/g (erythrocytes)}$$

where 2.5 = test tube volume (ml); 6.22 = µmolar extinction of NADPH at 340 nm; 0.1 = sample volume (ml); 1000 = reference volume.

8.10.20 Performance characteristics

(a) Reproducibility

The coefficient of variation (CV%) determined from ten repeated analyses is about 5%.

(b) Validity

Each laboratory should validate its own method.

8.10.21 Reference values

These vary geographically and should be determined locally.

8.10.22 Interpretation

High results can be gained from the enhanced decrease of NADPH due to contamination of reagents and samples. Values obtained are representative of true nutritional status if it is known that erythrocytes are an index of Se nutritional status of previous months, and plasma reflects very short time changes of Se intake with diet.

8.11 CHROMIUM

8.11.1 Purpose and scope [226–228]

The assay of chromium is notoriously difficult. Nonetheless the determination of chromium in biological materials is likely to remain of appreciable interest because of the role that the element appears to play in the metabolism of carbohydrates and lipids. Such compositional assays have as yet no clear role in assessing 'status' other than excessive levels. Similarly, since the precise function of chromium is unknown, there is as yet no good functional assay suitable for the determination of any risk of chromium deficiency. Valuable reviews of these problems have been published [5, 226].

8.11.2 Principle of the method

Chromium can be determined by neutron-activation analysis, mass spectrometry, and graphite furnace atomic absorption spectroscopy. The latter technique is more appropriately described in a text of this nature. The major difficulty with the determination of chromium, once scrupulous cleanliness has been achieved, arises from the need to correct for matrix interference and background absorption.

8.11.3 Chemicals and apparatus

(a) Chemicals

Hydrochloric acid (HCl) concentrated 37% (fuming) p.a.
Magnesium nitrate hexahydrate ($Mg(NO_3)_2.6H_2O$) p.a.
Dichlorodimethylsilane (DCDMS), (CH_4Cl_2Si) p.a.
Toluene ($C_6H_5CH_3$) p.a.
Methanol (CH_3OH) p.a.
De-ionized water.

(b) Solutions

Chromium standard solutions:
   Working standards are prepared by appropriate dilution of a commercial atomic absorption standard solution.
   5% DCDMS in toluene: 5 ml of dichloromethylsilane are made up to 100 ml with toluene.
   $Mg(NO_3)_2$, 0.07 mol/l: 18.6 g dissolved in water to make 1000 ml.
   HCl, 0.1 mol/l: 8.26 ml of concentrated HCl are made up to 1000 ml with water.

(c) Apparatus

Quartz glass test tubes should be used. They should be thoroughly acid-washed and dried. They are then silanised by soaking in 5% DCDMS in toluene, and rinsed in methanol once and in water six times.
Polypropylene/polyethylene tubes; polyethylene pipettes; quartz glass beakers.
Centrifuge.
Laminar-flow cabinet.
Acid-washed utensils free of chromium should be used.
Muffle furnace.
Graphite furnace atomic spectrometer: it is essential that the graphite furnace atomic spectrometer (electrothermal atomic absorption spectrometer) has capable background correction facilities; Zeeman is preferable. The operating system should be totally free of stainless steel components. Standard operating conditions should be used as recommended by the manufacturer and as determined within the laboratory.

8.11.4 Sample collection

It is exceedingly important to collect samples and to store them without contamination. Plastic syringes should be used and needles for venepuncture, if made of stainless steel, can cause significant contamination. It may be best to collect specimens through intravenous polyethylene or polypropylene cannulae. However, short siliconized needles of the butterfly type (e.g. Abbott or equivalent) with an attached length of polyvinylchloride tubing do not cause contamination.

The blood should be centrifuged immediately and the serum removed with sterile polyethylene pipettes and aliquots stored in similar sterile polypropylene/polyethylene tubes, at −20°C.

8.11.5 Procedure

Laminar-flow cabinets and clean room conditions should, ideally, be used throughout the preparation of equipment and of samples. Serum samples

(1–2 ml) are weighed into the silanised tubes and $Mg(NO_3)_2$ added (10 µl per ml of serum/plasma); a similar volume of water is used as a blank.

Samples and blanks are freeze dried in a stainless steel free instrument and then ashed in a muffle furnace at 100°C for 1 h, 150°C for 4 h, 200°C for 4 h then 250°C for 1 h before being increased to 480°C for a 8-h ashing. Throughout this procedure the sample should be protected from environmental contamination; the reference cited uses quartz glass beakers to do this.

The cool ash is dissolved in 0.1 mol/l HCl in a volume equal to the original serum volume, and 25 µl aliquots of this are pipetted into the graphite furnace for analysis.

8.11.6   Reference values

A range of 0.08–0.20 µg/l by AAS has been reported [227]. It is recommended that each laboratory should establish its own reference values.

8.11.7   Interpretation

Since this is a difficult method there is still a need for considerable development in its evaluation and application.

8.12   MANGANESE

8.12.1   Purpose and scope [5, 229–231]

The reliable determination of manganese in biological tissues and fluids especially plasma/serum is only marginally less problematical than that of chromium. Extraneous contamination of manganese is difficult to control and as with other assays of trace elements, ultra-pure chemicals, and clean room conditions favour the best results.

8.12.2   Principle of the method

Manganese can be determined in plasma and serum, in whole blood (which has the advantage of giving higher recordings because of the manganese present in erythrocytes), and in hair, which is of particular relevance when assessing manganese toxicity. However, a reliable method for determining low manganese status has only been developed with difficulty [229], and human manganese deficiency has not been recognized. An additional approach to detecting reduced manganese status may be developed by assaying the activity of cyanide insensitive superoxide dismutase (see section IV, p. 398).

8.12.3   Sample collection (whole blood, plasma, urine or hair)

The use of stainless steel needles to collect blood creates a significant risk of contamination. This can be minimized by allowing the first flow of blood to wash out the tube and then collecting the latter flow of blood for analysis. Non-metallic cannulae are preferred but, as with chromium, siliconized butterfly type needles can be suitable. However, each set should be assessed before use.

Heparin is a significant source of manganese contamination. If this is used as an anticoagulant, it should be first treated with a chelator. Haemolysed samples should not be used. Plasma or serum should be separated from the red cells within an hour of collection.

Urine can be collected, and after addition of HCl stored at –20°C in suitably sized polypropylene containers.

Hair should be collected from the occiput. It should be washed sequentially with non-ionic detergent (e.g. Triton X–100) and rinsed several times in de-ionized water, before being washed in 95% ethanol and rinsed again in de-ionized water; then dried at 60°C. Chelating agents should not be used in preparing hair.

8.12.4 Chemicals and apparatus

(a) Chemicals

Iso-Octylphenoxypolyethoxyethanol (Triton X–100), e.g. BDH Ltd. cat. No. 30632
Ethanol (C_2H_5OH) 95% p.a.
Nitric acid (HNO_3) p.a.
De-ionized water.

(b) Solutions

HNO_3, 30 mmol/l: 1.2 ml HNO_3 made up to 1000 ml with water.
Standard solutions of manganese:
  Working standards: 0, 0.2, 0.4, 0.6 µg/l in 30 mmol/l HNO_3, prepared from a commercial atomic absorption standard solution.

(c) Apparatus

Adjustable pipettes; polyethylene tubes; polypropylene containers.
Laboratory centrifuge.
Graphite furnace atomic absorption spectrophotometer.

8.12.5 Procedure

Analysis is by graphite furnace atomic absorption spectroscopy, at a wavelength of 279.5 nm with a manganese monochromator source, and the smallest slit width. Argon produces a sensitive and more reliable assay than does nitrogen as a carrier gas.

Continuum source background correction is needed, and whereas a dueterium arc may be suitable, Zeeman background correction is preferable. Pyrolytically coated tubes are most effective.

Charring is normally conduced at 1100°C, and atomization at 2400–2600°C with rapid heating produces better and more consistent peaks.

Glass tubes can contaminate samples and may additionally adsorb manganese; decontaminated polyethylene tubes are most appropriate for storage.

Usually 20–50 µl volumes are assayed, but modified techniques are available to enable determination of manganese in volumes as small as 5 µl.

50 µl of plasma sample is placed into each of the four auto-analyser cups with 200 µl of one of the working standards. The furnace programme should be determined for each laboratory. The following programme was developed on a Perkin–Elmer 500 and HGA 500 graphite furnace (Perkin–Elmer Corporation) [230].

8.12.6 Performance characteristics

(a) Range of linearity and detection limit

See reference [229].

Graphite furnace programme

Step	Temperature (°C)	Ramp (s)	Hold (s)
1	90	10	60
2	120	20	20
3	1000	10	30
4	2500	0	4 with recorder and read-out on
5	2700	2	3
6	20	2	18

On this cycle the graphite tubes last approximately 120 cycles.

(b) Reproducibility

Reported precisions vary. Great variability arises from inadequate background correction and from inadequate dilution of the samples. Better intra-batch precision is obtained when the concentration of manganese is high. At levels about 0.1 mmol/l, reported CV is 12.5%, and that for the method described above was 16%.

8.12.7 Reference values

Reliable electrothermal AAS assays suggest a reference range of 6.55–17.47 nmol/l [231] which corresponds to values determined by other methods [5]. It is recommended that each laboratory should establish its own reference values.

8.12.8 Interpretation

More extensive work with reliable analyses is needed before the value of these assays can be interpreted reliably in detecting deficiency status. Plasma levels are elevated with toxic exposure and in liver disease.

REFERENCES

1. Stika, K.M. and Morrison, G.H. (1981) Analytical methods for the mineral content of human tissues. *Fed. Proc.,* **40**, 2115–20.
2. *Elemental Analysis of Biological Materials.* (1980) Current problems and techniques with special reference to trace elements. International Atomic Energy Agency (IAEA), Vienna, Tech. Rept. Series No. 197.
3. Riordan, J.F. and Vallee, B.L. (1988) Metallobiochemistry, in *Methods in Enzymology* (eds J.N. Abelson and M.I. Simon), Vol. 158, Academic Press, New York.
4. Versieck, J. and Cornelis, R. (1980) Normal levels of trace elements in human plasma or serum. *Anal. Chim. Acta,* **116**, 217–54.
5. Versieck, J. (1985) Trace elements in human body fluids and tissues. *CRC Crit. Rev. Clin. Lab. Sci.,* **22**, 97–184.
6. Thiers, R.E. (1957) Contamination in trace element analysis and its control. *Methods Biochem. Anal.,* **5**, 273–335.
7. Kosta, K. (1980) Reference samples for trace elements in biological materials and associated analytical problems, in *Elemental Analysis of Biological Materials*, IAEA, Vienna, Tech. Rept. Series No. 197, 317–67.
8. Taylor, J.K. (1985) *Handbook for SRM Users*, National Bureau of Standards, NBS special publication, Gaithersburg (Maryland), 260–100.

9. Versieck, J. *et al.* (1988) Certification of a second-generation biological reference material (freeze-dried serum) for trace element determinations. *Anal. Chim. Acta*, **204**, 63–75.

10. Tietz, N.W. (ed.) (1986) *Textbook of Clinical Biochemistry*, W.B. Saunders, London, Philadelphia.

11. Shizgal, H.M. (1978) Symposium on nutritional requirements of the surgical patient. I. Nutrition and body composition. *Can. J. Surg.*, **21**, 483–8.

12. Coward, W.A. and Lunn, P.G. (1981) The biochemistry and physiology of kwashiorkor and marasmus. *Br. Med. Bull.*, **37**, 19–24.

13. Shizgal, H.M., Spanier, A.H., Humes, J. and Wood, C.D. (1977) Indirect measurement of total exchangeable potassium. *Am. J. Physiol.*, **233**, F253–9.

14. Moore, F.D., Oleson, K.H., McMurray, J.D. *et al.* (1963) The body cell mass and its supporting environment. Body composition in health and disease. Saunders, Philadelphia, pp. 13–42 and 519–35.

15. James, W.P.T., Bingham, S.A. and Cole, T.J. (1981) Epidemiological assessment of dietary intake. *Nutr. Cancer*, **2**, 203–12.

16. Schofield, E.C., Walker, C.A., Haraldsdottir, J. *et al.* (1986) Salt intake and blood pressure in young adults from hypertensive and normotensive families. *Hum. Nutr. Clin. Nutr.*, **40C**, 333–43.

17. Gardner, M.J. and Heady, J.A. (1973) Some effects of within-person variability in epidemiological studies. *J. Chron. Dis.*, **26**, 781–95.

18. Liu, K., Stamler, J., Syer, A. *et al.* (1978) Statistical methods to assess and minimize the role of intra-individual variability in obscuring the relationship between dietary lipids and serum cholesterol. *J. Chron. Dis.*, **31**, 399–418.

19. Liu, K., Cooper, R., McKeever, J. *et al.* (1979) Assessment of the association between habitual salt intake and high blood pressure: methodological problems. *Am. J. Epidemiol.*, **110**, 219–26.

20. Sanchez-Castillo, C.P., Branch, W.J. and James, W.P.T. (1987) A test of the validity of the lithium marker technique for monitoring dietary sources of salt in man. *Clin. Sci.*, **72**, 87–94.

21. Sanchez-Castillo, C.P., Seidell, J. and James, W.P.T. (1987) The potential use of lithium as a marker for the assessment of the sources of dietary salt: cooking studies and physiological experiments in men. *Clin. Sci.*, **72**, 81–6.

22. Bingham, S. and Cummings, J.H. (1983) The use of 4-para-amino-benzoic acid as a marker to validate the completeness of 24 h urine collections in man. *Clin. Sci.*, **64**, 629–35.

23. Morgan, D.B. and Burkinshaw, L. (1983) Estimation of non-fat body tissues from measurement of skinfold thickness, total body potassium and total body nitrogen. *Clin. Sci.*, **65**, 407–14.

24. Womersley, J., Boddy, K., King, P.C. and Durnin, J.V.G.A. (1972) A comparison of fat free mass of young adults estimated by anthropometry, body density and total potassium content. *Clin. Sci.*, **43**, 469–75.

25. Edwards, R.H. (1984) New techniques for studying human muscle function, metabolism and fatigue. *Muscle & Nerve*, **7**(8), 599–609.

26. Fourman, P. and Royer, P. (1968) *Calcium Metabolism and the Bone*, Blackwell Scientific Publications, Oxford, p. 20.

27. Robertson, W.G. (1976) Cellular calcium and calcium transport, in *Calcium, Phosphate and Magnesium Metabolism* (ed. B.E.C. Nordin), Churchill Livingstone, Edinburgh, pp. 230–56.

28. Marshall, H.D. (1976) Plasma fractions, in *Calcium, Phosphate and Magnesium Metabolism* (ed. B.E.C. Nordin), Churchill Livingstone, Edinburgh, pp. 162–85.

29. McLean, F.C. and Hastings, A.B. (1934) A biological method for the estimation of calcium ion concentration. *J. Biol. Chem.*, **107**, 337–50.

30. White, T.F., Farndon, J.R., Conceiaco, S.C. *et al.* (1986) Serum calcium in health and disease: a comparison of measured and derived parameters. *Clin. Chim. Acta*, **157**, 199–214.

31. Editorial. (1977) Correcting the calcium. *Br. Med. J.*, i, 598.

32. Reid, D.M. (1986) Measurement of total bone mass by total body calcium: a review. *J. R. Soc. Med.*, **79**, 33–7.

33. Peppler, W.W. and Mazess, R.B. (1981) Total body mineral and lean body mass by dual photon absorbtiometry. *Calcif. Tissue Int.*, **33**, 353–9.

34. Mazess, R.B., Peppler, W.W., Chestnut, C.H. *et al.* (1981) Total body bone mineral and lean body mass by dual-photon absorbtiometry: II. Comparison with total body calcium by neutron activation analysis. *Calcif. Tissue Int.*, **33**, 361–3.

35. Cummings, S.R. (1987) Position paper. Bone mineral densitometry. *Ann. Intern. Med.*, **107**, 932–6.

36. Sartoris, D.J. and Resnick, D. (1988) *Digital radiography may spark renewal of bone densitometry*, Miller Freeman, New York, pp. 145–57.

37. Genant, H.K., Steiger, P., Black, J.E. *et al.* (1987) Quantitative computed tomography: update 1987. *Calcif. Tissue Int.*, **41**, 179–86.

38. Hauschka, P.V. (1986) Osteocalcin: The vitamin K-dependent Ca^{2+}–binding protein of bone matrix. *Haemostasis*, **16**, 258–72.

39. Price, P.A., Williamson, M.K., Hala, T. *et al.* (1982) Excessive mineralization with growth plate in chronic warfarin treatment. *Proc. Natl. Acad. Sci., USA*, **79**, 7734–8.

40. Mundy, G.R. and Poser, J.W. (1983) Chemotactic activity of the gamma-carboxyglutamic-acid-containing protein in bone. *Calcif. Tissue Int.*, **35**, 164–8.

41. Lian, J.B. and Gundberg, C.M. (1988) Osteocalcin. Biochemical considerations and clinical applications. *Clin. Orthop. Rel. Res.*, **226**, 267–91.

42. Slovik, R.M., Gundberg, C.M., Neer, R.M. and Lian, J.B. (1984) Clinical evaluation of bone turnover by serum osteocalcin measurements. *J. Clin. Endocrinol. Metab.*, **59**, 228–30.

43. Reid, I.R., Chapman, G.E., Franser, T.R.C. *et al.* (1986) Low serum osteocalcin levels in corticoid-treated asthmatics. *J. Clin. Endocrinol. Metab.*, **62**, 379–83.

44. Gitelman, H.J. (1967) An improved automated procedure for the determination of calcium in biochemical specimens. *Anal. Biochem.*, **18**, 521–31.

45. Renoe, B.W., Macdonald, J.M. and Ladenson, J.H. (1980) The effect of stasis with and without exercise on precalcium, various cations, and related parameters. *Clin. Chim. Acta*, **103**, 91–100.

46. Young, D.S., Pestaner, L.C. and Gibberman, V. (1975) Effect of drugs on clinical laboratory tests. *Clin. Chem.*, **21**, 1D–432D.

47. Bowers, G.N. and Pybus, J. (1972) Total calcium in serum by atomic absorption spectrophotometry, in *Standard Methods of Clinical Chemistry* Vol. 7 (ed. G.R. Cooper), Academic Press, New York, pp. 143–50.

48. Rush, R.J. and Nabb, D.P. (1977) Bringing it all together on three SMAC systems, in *Advances in Automated Analysis* (Technicon International Congress 1976. Vol 1), Mediad Inc., New York, pp. 197–203.

49. Payne, R.B., Carver, M.E. and Morgan, D.B. (1979) Interpretation of serum total calcium: effects of adjustment for albumin concentration on frequency of abnormal values and on detection of change in the individual. *J. Clin. Pathol.*, **32**, 56–60.

50. Iqbal, S.J., Giles, M., Ledger, S. *et al.* (1988) Need for albumin adjustments of urgent total serum calcium. *Lancet*, ii, 1477–8.

51. Bowers, G.N. Jr., Brassard, C. and Sena, S.F. (1986) Measurement of ionized

calcium in serum with ion selective electrodes: A mature technology that can meet the daily service needs. *Clin. Chem.*, **32**, 1437–47.

52. Urban, P., Scheidegger, D., Buchanan, D. and Barth, D. (1988) Cardiac arrest and blood ionized calcium levels. *Ann. Intern. Med.*, **109**, 110–13.

53. Gray, T.A., Buckley, B.M., Sealey, M. *et al.* (1986) Plasma ionized calcium during liver transplantation. *Transplantation*, **41**, 335–9.

54. Larrson, L. and Ohman, S. (1989) Correcting total serum calcium. *Lancet*, **i**, 326.

55. Gray, T.A. and Paterson, C.R. (1988) The clinical value of ionized calcium assays. *Ann. Clin. Biochem.*, **25**, 210–19.

56. Urban, P., Baeriswyl, G. and Bouillie, M. (1989) Correcting total serum calcium. *Lancet*, **i**, 326.

57. Kanis, J.A. and Yates, A.J. (1985) Measuring serum calcium. *Br. Med. J.*, **290**, 728–9.

58. Dequeker, J. (1976) Quantitative radiology: radiogrammetry of cortical bone. *Br. J. Radiol.*, **49**, 912–20.

59. Reid, D.M. (1984) Bone mass in rheumatic diseases [MD Thesis], University of Aberdeen, Aberdeen, (UK), pp. 95–107.

60. Dequeker, J. (1982) Precision of the radiogrammetric evaluation of bone mass at the metacarpal bone, in *Non-Invasive Bone Measurements* (eds J.V. Dequeker and C.C. Johnston Jr), IRL Press, London, pp. 27–32.

61. Kalla, A.A., Kotze, T.J.V.W., Meyers, O.L. and Parkyn, N.D. (1989) Screening for osteoporosis: An old method revisited, in *Osteoporosis and Bone Mineral Measurement* (eds E.J.F. Ring, W.D. Evans and A.S. Dixon), IPSM Publications, York, pp. 124–6.

62. Reid, D.M., Nicoll, J.J., Brown, N. *et al.* (1989) Measurement of hand bone mass by single photon absorptiometry in rheumatoid arthritis and asthma: comparison with metacarpal indices, in *Osteoporosis and Body Mineral Measurement* (eds E.J.F. Ring, W.D. Evans and A.S. Dixon), IPSM Publications, York, pp. 224–32.

63. Genant, H.K., Cann, C.E. and Faul, D.D. (1982) Quantitative computed tomography for assessing vertebral bone mineral, in *Non-Invasive Bone Measurements* (eds J.V. Dequeker and C.C. Johnston Jr), IRL Press, London, pp. 215–49.

64. Andresen, J. and Nielsen, H.E. (1982) Metacarpal bone mass in normal adults and in patients with renal failure, in *Non-Invasive Bone Measurements* (eds J.V. Dequeker and C.C. Johnston Jr), IRL Press, London, pp. 169–73.

65. Dequeker, J. (1972) *Bone Loss in Normal and Pathological Conditions*, University Press, Leuven.

66. Garn, S.M. (1972) The course of bone gain and the phases of bone loss. *Orthop. Clin. North Am.*, **3**, 503–20.

67. Cohn, S.H., Ellis, K.J., Wallach, S. *et al.* (1974) Absolute and relative deficit in total skeletal calcium and radial bone mineral in osteoporosis. *J. Nucl. Med.*, **1**, 428–35.

68. Hodgkinson, A. and Thompson, T. (1982) Measurement of the fasting urinary hydroxyproline/creatinine ratio in normal adults and its variation with age and sex. *J. Clin. Pathol.*, **35**, 807–11.

69. Seymour, G.C. and Jackson, M.J. (1974) Specific automated method for measurement of urinary hydroxyproline. *Clin. Chem.*, **20**, 544–6.

70. Robins, S.P. (1982) Turnover and crosslinking of collagen, in *Collagen in Health and Disease* (eds J.B. Weiss and M.I.V. Jayson), Churchill Livingstone, Edinburgh, pp. 160–78.

71. Black, D., Duncan, A. and Robins, S.P. (1988) Quantitative analysis of the pyridinium crosslinks of collagen in urine using ion-paired reversed-phase high-performance liquid chromatography. *Anal. Biochem.*, **169**, 197–203.

72. Robins, S.P. and Duncan, A. (1987) Pyridinium crosslinks of bone collagen and

their location in peptides isolated from rat femur. *Biochem. Biophys. Acta*, **914**, 233–9.

73. Teitsson, I., Black, D., Robins, S.P. and Reid, D.M. (1988) Urinary metabolites of pyridinium in a patient with Paget's disease: New markers of collagen breakdown. *Scott. Med. J.*, **33**, 317.

74. Prockop, D.J. and Kivirikko, K.I. (1967) Relationship of hydroxyproline excretion in urine to collagen metabolism. *Ann. Intern. Med.*, **66**, 1243–66.

75. O'Donoghue, D.J. and Hosking, D.J. (1987) Biochemical response to combination of disodium etidronate with calcitonin in Paget's disease. *Bone*, **8**, 219–25.

76. Christiansen, C., Riis, B.J. and Rodbro, P. (1987) Prediction of rapid bone loss in post menopausal women. *Lancet*, **i**, 1105–8.

77. Grunberg, C.M., Markowitz, M.E. Mizruchi, M. and Rosen, J.F. (1985) Osteocalcin in human serum: A circadian rhythm. *J. Clin. Endocrinol. Metab.*, **60**, 736–9.

78. Delmas, P.D., Stenner, D., Wahner, W.H. *et al.* (1983) Increase in serum bone gamma-carboxyglutamic acid protein with aging in women. *J. Clin. Invest.*, **71**, 1316–21.

79. Delmas, P.D. (1987) Clinical applications of serum bone GLA-protein (osteocalcin) assays in metabolic bone diseases, in *Osteoporosis* (eds C. Christiansen, J.S. Johansen and B.J. Riis), Osteopress ApS, Copenhagen, pp. 664–71.

80. Grundberg, C.M., Lian, J.B., Gallop, P.M. and Steinberg, J.J. (1983) Urinary gamma-carboxyglutamic acid and serum osteocalcin as bone markers: Studies in Osteoporosis and Paget's disease. *J. Clin. Endocrinol. Metab.*, **57**, 1221–5.

81. Grundberg, C.M., Lian, J.B. and Gallop, P.M. (1983) Measurements of gamma-carboxyglutamate and circulating osteocalcin in normal adults and children. *Clin. Chim. Acta*, **128**, 1–8.

82. Garber, C.C. and Miller, R.C. (1983) Revisions of the 1963 semidine HCl standard method for inorganic phosphorus. *Clin. Chem.*, **29**, 184–8.

83. Clayton, B.E., Jenkins, P. and Round, J.M. (1980) *Paediatric Chemical Pathology*, Blackwell Scientific, London.

84. Abernethy, M.H. and Fowler, R.T. (1982) Micellar improvement of the Calmagite compleximetric measurement of magnesium in plasma. *Clin. Chem.*, **28**, 520–2.

85. Bothwell, T.H., Charlton, R.W., Cook, J.D. and Finch, C.A. (1979) *Iron metabolism in man*, Blackwell Scientific, London, p. 576.

86. *INACG Measurements of iron status.* (1985) A report of the International Nutritional Anemia Consultative Group. The Nutrition Foundation Inc., Washington (DC), p. 78.

87. World Health Organization. (1968) *Nutrition Anaemia*, Techn. Rep. Series No. 405, WHO, Geneva.

88. World Health Organization. (1975) *Control of Nutritional Anemia With Special Reference to Iron Deficiency*, Techn. Rep. Series No. 580, WHO, Geneva, p. 60.

89. Demaeyer, E.M. (1980) Epidemiologie, traitement et prévention de la carence en fer et de l'anémie ferriprive. *Rev. Epidemiol. Santé Publique*, **28**, 235–49.

90. Finch, C.A. and Cook, J.D. (1984) Iron deficiency. *Am. J. Clin. Nutr.*, **39**, 471–7.

91. Galan, P., Hercberg, S. and Touitou, Y. (1984). The activity of tissue enzymes in iron-deficient rat and man: an overview. *Comp. Biochem. Physiol.*, **B77**, 647–53.

92. Hercberg, S., Soustre, Y., Galan, P. *et al.* (1984) Apports alimentaires en fer dans une population de femmes françaises en âge de procréer. *Ann. Nutr. Métab.*, **28**, 77–84.

93. Hallberg, L. (1981) Bioavailability of dietary iron in man. *Ann. Rev. Nutr.*, **1**, 123–47.

94. Cook, J.D. and Reusser, M.E. (1983). Food iron availability, in *Groupes à risque de carence en fer dans les pays industrialisés* (eds H. Dupin and S. Hercberg), INSERM, Paris, **113**, 179–90.

95. Cubeau, J. and Pequignot, G. (1980) La technique du questionnaire alimentaire quantitatif utilisée par la Section nutrition de l'INSERM. *Rev. Epidemiol. Santé Publique*, **28**, 367–72.

96. Baker, S.J. and Demaeyer, E.M. (1979) Nutritional anemia: its understanding and control with special reference to the work of the World Health Organization. *Am. J. Clin. Nutr.*, **32**, 368–417.

97. Andelman, M.B. and Sered, B.R. (1966) Utilization of dietary iron by term infants: a study of 1048 infants from a low socioeconomic population. *Am. J. Dis. Child.*, **3**, 45–55.

98. Haskins, D., Stevens, A.R. Jr, Finch, S.C. and Finch, C.A. (1952) Iron metabolism. Iron stores in man as measured by phlebotomy. *J. Clin. Invest.*, **31**, 543–7.

99. Torrance, J.D. and Bothwell, H. (1980) Tissue iron stores, in *Methods in Hematology: Iron* (ed. J.D. Cook), Churchill Livingstone, New York, pp. 90–113.

100. Cook, J.D. (1982) Clinical evaluation of iron deficiency. *Semin. Hematol.*, **19**, 6–18.

101. Green, R., Charlton, R.W., Seftel, H. *et al.* (1968) Body iron excretion in man. A collaborative study. *Am. J. Med.*, **45**, 336–53.

102. Addison, G.M., Beamish, M.R., Halcs, C.N. *et al.* (1972) An immunoradiometric assay for ferritin in the serum of normal subjects and patients with iron deficiency and iron overload. *J. Clin. Pathol.*, **25**, 326–9.

103. Jacobs, A., Miller, F., Worwood, M. *et al.* (1972) Ferritin in the serum of normal subjects and patients with iron deficiency and iron overload. *Br. Med. J.*, **4**, 206–8.

104. Walters, G.O., Miller, F. and Worwood, M. (1973) Serum ferritin concentration and iron stores in normal subjects. *J. Clin. Pathol.*, **26**, 770–2.

105. Bezwoda, W.R., Bothwell, T.H., Torrance, J.D. *et al.* (1979) The relation between marrow iron stores, plasma ferritin concentration and iron absorption. *Scand. J. Haematol.*, **22**, 113–20.

106. Magnusson, B., Björn-Rasmussen, E., Hallberg, L. and Rossander, L. (1981) Iron absorption in relation to iron status. Model proposed to express results of iron absorption measurements. *Scand. J. Haematol.*, **27**, 201–8.

107. Milman, N., Pedersen, S.N. and Visfeld, J. (1983) Serum ferritin in healthy Danes: relation to marrow haemosiderin iron stores. *Dan. Med. Bull.*, **30**, 115–20.

108. Lipschitz, D.A., Cook, J.D. and Finch, C.A. (1974) A clinical evaluation of serum ferritin. *N. Engl. J. Med.*, **290**, 1213–16.

109. Finch, C.A., Cook, J.D., Labbe, R.F. and Culala, M. (1977) Effect of blood donation on iron stores as evaluated by serum ferritin. *Blood*, **50**, 441–7.

110. Worwood, M. (1980) Serum ferritin, in *Methods in Hematology: Iron* (ed. J.D. Cook), Churchill Livingstone, New York, pp. 59–89.

111. Fielding, J. (1980) Serum iron and iron binding capacity, in *Methods in Hematology: iron* (ed. J.D. Cook), Churchill Livingstone, New York, pp. 15–43.

112. Williams, H.L. and Conrad, M.E. (1966) A one-tube method for measuring the serum iron concentration and unsaturated iron-binding capacity. *J. Clin. Med.*, **67**, 171–6.

113. Schade, A.L., Oyama, J., Reinhart, R.W. and Miller, J.R. (1954) Bound iron and unsaturated iron-binding capacity of serum: rapid and reliable quantitative determination. *Proc. Soc. Exp. Biol. Med.*, **87**, 443–8.

114. Peters, T., Giovanniello, T.J., Apt, L. and Ross, J.F. (1956) Laboratory methods: a new method for the determination of serum iron-binding capacity. *J. Lab. Clin. Med.*, **48**, 274–9.

115. Ramsay, W.N.M. (1957) The determination of iron in blood plasma or serum. *Clin. Chim. Acta*, **2**, 221–6.

116. Herbert, V., Gottlieb, C.W., Kam Seng, L. *et al.* (1966) Coated charcoal assay of unsaturated iron-binding capacity. *J. Lab. Clin. Med.*, **67**, 855–62.

117. International Committee for Standardization in Hematology. (1978) The measurement of total and unsaturated iron-binding capacity in serum. *Br. J. Haematol.*, **38**, 281–90.

118. Labbe, R.F. and Finch, C.A. (1980) Erythrocyte protoporphyrin: application in the diagnostic of the diagnosis of iron deficiency, in *Methods in Hematology: Iron* (ed. J.D. Cook), Churchill Livingstone, New York, pp. 44–58.

119. Cavill, I. (1982) Diagnostic methods. *Clin. Hematol.*, **11**, 259–73.

120. Blumberg, W.E., Eisinger, J., Lamola, A.A. *et al.* (1977) Zinc protoprophyrin level in blood determined by a portable hematofluorometer: a screening device for lead poisoning. *J. Lab. Clin. Med.*, **89**, 712–23.

121. Lamola, A.A., Eisinger, J. and Blumberg, W.E. (1980) Erythrocyte protoporphyrin/heme rate by hematofluorometry. *Clin. Chem.*, **26**, 677–8.

122. Piomelli, S. (1973) A micromethod for free erythrocyte porphyrins: the FEP test. *J. Lab. Clin. Med.*, **81**, 932–40.

123. Cartwright, G.E. (1968) *Diagnostic Laboratory Hematology*, 4th edn, Grune and Stratton, New York.

124. Dallman, P.R., Siimes, M.A. and Stekel, A. (1979) Iron deficiency in infancy and childhood. *Am. J. Clin. Nutr.*, **33**, 86–118.

125. Garby, L., Irnell, L. and Werner, I. (1969) Iron deficiency in women of fertile age in a Swedish community III. Estimation of prevalence based on response to iron supplementation. *Acta Med. Scand.*, **185**, 113–17.

126. MacGregor, M. (1963) Maternal anaemia as a factor in prematurity and perinatal mortality. *Scott. Med. J.*, **8**, 134–40.

127. Singla, P.N. and Agarwal, K.N. (1983) Effect of maternal anemia on the newborn infant and the placenta, in *Groupes à risque de carence en fer dans les pays industrialisés* (eds H. Dupin and S. Hercberg), INSERM, Paris, **113**, pp. 117–26.

128. International Nutritional Anemia Consultative Group (INACG). (1983) *Iron Deficiency and Work Performance,* The Nutrition Foundation, Washington (DC).

129. Pearson, H.A. and Robinson, J.E. (1976) The role of iron in host resistance. *Adv. Pediatr.*, **23**, 1–33.

130. Birgerard, G., Hällgren, R., Killander, A. *et al.* (1978) Serum ferritin during infection – a longitudinal study. *Scand. J. Haematol.*, **21**, 333–40.

131. Elin, R.J., Wolff, S.M. and Finch, C.A. (1977) Effect of induced fever on serum iron and ferritin concentrations in man. *Blood,* **49**, 147–53.

132. Konijn, A.M. and Hershko, C. (1977) Ferritin synthesis in inflammation. Pathogenesis of impaired iron release. *Br. J. Haematol.*, **13**, 924–33.

133. Prieto, J., Barry, M. and Sherlock, S. (1975) Serum ferritin in patients with iron overload and with acute and chronic liver disease. *Gastroenterology,* **68**, 525–33.

134. Hazard, J. and Drysdale, J.W. (1977) Ferritinaemia in cancer. *Nature,* **265**, 755–6.

135. Koller, M.E., Romslo, I.L., Finne, P.H. and Haneberg, B. (1979) Serial determinations of serum ferritin in children with acute lymphoblastic leukemia. *Acta Paediatr. Scand.*, **68**, 93–6.

136. Jones, P.A.A., Miller, F.M., Worwood, M. and Jacobs, A. (1973) Ferritinaemia in leukaemia and Hodgkin's disease. *Br. J. Cancer,* **27**, 212–17.

137. Smith, R.J., Davis, P., Thomson, A.B. *et al.* (1977) Serum ferritin levels in anemia of rheumatoid arthritis. *J. Rheumatol.*, **4**, 389–92.

138. Waller, H.D. and Benohr, H.C. (1978) Alcohol related disturbances in haematopoiesis. *Klin. Wochenschr.*, **56**, 259–65.

139. Burton, J.L. (1967) Effect of oral contraceptives on haemoglobin, packed cell volume, serum iron and total iron binding capacity. *Lancet,* **i**, 978–80.

140. Heilmann, E. and Risse, E. (1974) Effect of oral contraceptives on serum iron and total iron binding capacity. *Med. Welt.*, **25**, 767–8.

141. Herschko, C., Graham, G., Bates, G.W. and Rachmelewitz, E.A. (1978) Non-specific serum iron in thalassaemia: An abnormal serum iron fraction of potential toxicity. *Br. J. Haematol.*, **40**, 255–63.

142. Roeser, H.P. (1980) Iron metabolism in inflammation and malignant disease, in *Iron in Biochemistry and Medicine II* (eds A. Jacobs and M. Worwood), Academic Press, London and New York, pp. 605–40.

143. Ducci, H., Spoerer, A. and Katz, R. (1952) Serum iron in liver disease. *Gastroenterology*, **22**, 52–62.

144. Caroline, L., Rosner, F. and Kozinn, P.J. (1969) Elevated serum iron, low unbound transferrin and candidiasis in acute leukemia. *Blood*, **34**, 441–51.

145. Harris, J.W. (1958) Alterations in iron metabolism secondary to vitamin B_6 and vitamin B_{12} abnormalities, in *Iron in Clinical Medicine* (eds R.O. Wallerstein and S.R. Mettier), Univ. of California Press, Berkeley, pp. 227–50.

146. Cartwright, G.E. and Lee, G.R. (1971) The anaemia of chronic disorders. *Br. J. Haematol.*, **21**, 147–52.

147. Lipschitz, D.A., Simon, M.O., Lynch, S.R. *et al.* (1971) Some factors affecting the release of iron from reticuloendothelial cells. *Br. J. Haematol.*, **21**, 289–303.

148. Lipschitz, D.A., Bothwell, T.H., Seftel, H.C. *et al.* (1971) The role of ascorbic acid in the metabolism of storage iron. *Br. J. Haematol.*, **20**, 155–63.

149. Al-Ismail, S., Cavill, I., Evans, I.H. *et al.* (1979) Erythropoiesis and iron metabolism in Hodgkin's disease. *Br. J. Cancer*, **40**, 365–70.

150. Miller, A., Chodos, R.B., Emerson, C.P. and Ross, J.F. (1956) Studies of the anemia and iron metabolism in cancer. *J. Clin. Invest.*, **35**, 1248–62.

151. Marks, J. and Shuster, S. (1968) Iron metabolism in skin disease. *Arch. Dermatol.*, **98**, 469–75.

152. Mowot, A.G., Hothersall, T.E. and Aitchinson, W.R.C. (1969) Nature of anemia in rheumatoid arthritis and changes in iron metabolism reduced by administration of corticotrophin. *Ann. Rheum. Dis.*, **28**, 303–8.

153. Syrkis, I. and Machtey, I. (1973) Hypoferremia in acute myocardial infarction. *J. Am. Geriatric Soc.*, **21**, 28–30.

154. Lahey, M.E., Behar, M., Vitera, F. and Scrimshaw, N.S. (1958) Values for copper, iron and iron binding capacity in the serum in kwashiorkor. *Pediatrics*, **22**, 72–9.

155. McFarlane, H., Reddy, S. and Adcock, K.J. (1970) Immunity, transferrin and survival in kwashiorkor. *Br. Med. J.*, **4**, 268–70.

156. Reeds, P.J. and Laditan, A.A.O. (1976) Serum albumin and transferrin in protein energy malnutrition. Their use in the assessment of marginal undernutrition and the prognosis of severe undernutrition. *Br. J. Nutr.*, **36**, 255–63.

157. Griffin, A.C., Dale, S.C., Wellington, D. and Ward, V.C. (1965) Serum iron levels in patients with malignant disease. *Proc. Soc. Exp. Biol. Med.*, **118**, 741–5.

158. Handock, D.E., Oustad, J.W. and Woolf, I.L. (1976) Transferrin loss into the urine with hypochromic microcytic anemia. *Am. J. Clin. Pathol.*, **65**, 73–8.

159. Saito, H., Kato, Y., Susuki, T. and Kato, H. (1977) A case of atransferrinemia and 35 cases of hypotransferrinemia as detected by radioassay of total-iron binding capacity of the serum. *Jap. J. Med.*, **16**, 342–8.

160. Horne, C.H.W., Howie, P.W., Weir, R.J. and Goudie, R.B. (1970) Effect of combined oestrogen–progesterone oral contraceptives on serum levels of α_2-macroglobulin, transferrin, albumin and IgG. *Lancet*, **i**, 49–51.

161. Carr, M.C. (1974) The diagnostic of iron deficiency in pregnancy. *Obstet. Gynecol.*, **43**, 15–21.

162. McLaren, G.D., Carpentier, J.T. and Nino, H.V. (1975) Erythrocyte protoporphyrin in the detection of iron deficiency. *Clin. Chem.*, **21**, 1121–7.

163. Walsh, J.R. and Fredrichson, M. (1977) Serum ferritin, free erythrocyte

protoprophyrin and urinary iron excretion in patients with iron disorders. *Am. J. Med. Sci.*, **273**, 293–300.

164. Doss, M. (ed.) (1978) *Diagnosis and Therapy of Porphyrias and Lead Intoxication*, Springer-Verlag, New York.

165. Granick, J.L., Sassa, S. and Kappas, A. (1978) Some biochemical and clinical aspects of lead intoxication. *Adv. Clin. Chem.*, **20**, 287–339.

166. Woodruf, A.W. (1972) Recent work in anaemia in the tropics. *Br. Med. Bull.*, **28**, 92–5.

167. Douglas, S.W. and Adamson, J.W. (1975) The anemia of chronic disorders: studies of marrow regulation and iron metabolism. *Blood*, **45**, 55–65.

168. Revenant, M.C. and Beaudonnet, A. (1982) Serum ferritin determination by enzyme immunoassay: importance of sample dilution (the 'Hook Effect'). *Clin. Chem.*, **28**, 253–4.

169. Ng, R.H., Brown, B.A. and Valdes, R. (1983) Three commercial methods for serum ferritin compared and the high-dose 'Hook Effect' eliminated. *Clin. Chem.*, **20**, 1109–13.

170. Dallman, P.R. (1984) Diagnosis of anemia and iron deficiency: analytic and biological variations of laboratory tests. *Am. J. Clin. Nutr.*, **39**, 937–41.

171. Kaplow, L.S., Schauble, M.K. and Bechtel, J.P. (1979) Validity of hematologic data in Veterans Administration Hospital laboratories. *Am. J. Clin. Pathol.*, **71**, 291–300.

172. Koepke, J.A. (1975) Inter-laboratory trials: the quality control survey programme of the College of American Pathologists, in *Quality Control in Hematology* (eds S.M. Lewis and J.F. Coster), Academic Press, New York, pp. 57–67.

173. Statland, B.E. and Winkel, P. (1977) Relationship of day-to-day variation of serum iron concentration to iron-binding capacity in healthy young women. *Am. J. Clin. Pathol.*, **67**, 84–90.

174. Statland, B.E., Winkel, P. and Bokelund, H. (1976) Variation of serum iron concentration in healthy young men: within-day and day-to-day changes. *Clin. Biochem.*, **9**, 26–9.

175. Chilsholm, J.J. and Brown, D.H. (1975) Micro-scale photofluorometric determination of 'free erythrocyte protoporphyrin' (protoporphyrin IX). *Clin. Chem.*, **21**, 1669–82.

176. Schifman, R.B. and Finley, P.R. (1981) Measurement of near-normal concentrations of erythrocyte protoporphyrin with the hematofluorometer. Influence of plasma in 'front surface illumination' assay. *Clin. Chem.*, **27**, 153–6.

177. Pilon, V.A., Howanitz, P.J., Howanitz, J.H. and Domres, N. (1981) Day-to-day variation in serum ferritin concentration in healthy subjects. *Clin. Chem.*, **27**, 78–83.

178. Statland, B.E., Winkel, P., Harris, S.C. *et al.* (1977) Evaluation of biologic sources of variation of leukocyte counts and other hematologic quantities using very precise automated analysers. *Am. J. Clin. Pathol.*, **69**, 48–54.

179. Sinniah, R., Doggart, J.R. and Neill, D.W. (1969) Diurnal variations of the serum iron in normal subjects and in patients with haemochromatosis. *Br. J. Haematol.*, **17**, 351–8.

180. Cook, J.D. (1968) An evaluation of absorption methods for measurement of plasma iron-binding capacity. *J. Lab. Clin. Med.*, **76**, 497–506.

181. Tarquini, B., Torcia, M., Sensi, G. *et al.* (1983) Chronobiological aspects of iron metabolism (significant components in the circadian and infradian domain of serum iron and ferritin), in *Groupes à risques de carence en fer dans les pays industrialisés* (eds H. Dupin and S. Hercberg), INSERM, Paris, **113**, pp. 237–62.

182. Mardell, M. and Zilva, J.F. (1967) Effect of oral contraceptives and the variation in serum iron during the menstrual cycle. *Lancet*, **ii**, 1323–5.

183. Zilva, J.F. and Patston, V.J. (1966) Variations in serum-iron in healthy women. *Lancet*, **i**, 459–62.

184. Dawkins, S., Cavill, I., Ricketts, C. and Worwood, M. (1979) Variability of serum ferritin concentration in normal subjects. *Clin. Lab. Haematol.*, **1**, 41–6.

185. Birgegard, G. (1980) Serum ferritin physiological and methodological studies. *Clin. Chim. Acta*, **103**, 277–85.

186. Cook, J.D., Alvarado, J., Gutnisky, A. *et al.* (1971) Nutritional deficiency and anemia in Latin America: a collaborative study. *Blood*, **38**, 591–603.

187. Bothwell, T.H. and Chalton, R.W. (1981) Assessment of the iron nutritional status of a population, in *Nutrition in Health and Disease and International Development* (eds A.E. Harper and G.K. Davis), Symposia from the XII International Congress of Nutrition, A.R. Liss, New York, pp. 311–21.

188. Yip, R., Johnson C. and Dallman, P.R. (1984) Age-related changes in laboratory values used in the diagnosis of anemia and iron deficiency. *Am. J. Clin. Nutr.*, **39**, 427–36.

189. Dallman, P.R., Yip, R. and Johnson, C. (1984) Prevalence and causes of anemia in the United States, 1976 to 1980. *Am. J. Clin. Nutr.*, **39**, 437–45.

190. Cook, J.D. and Finch, C.A. (1979) Assessing iron status of a population. *Am. J. Clin. Nutr.*, **32**, 2115–19.

191. Meyers, L.D., Habicht, J.P., Johnson, C.L. and Brownie, C. (1983) Prevalence of anemia and iron-deficiency anemia in black and white women in the United States estimated by two methods. *Am. J. Publ. Health*, **73**, 1042–9.

192. Hercberg, S., Galan, P., Assami, M. and Assami, S. (1988) Evaluation of the frequency of anemia and iron deficiency anemia in a group of algerian menstruating women by mixed distribution analysis. Contribution of folate deficiency and inflammatory process in the determination of anemia. *Int. J. Epidemiol.*, **17**, 136–41.

193. Cook, J.D., Finch, C.A. and Smith, N.J. (1976) Evaluation of the iron status of a population. *Blood*, **48**, 449–55.

194. *Assessment of the Iron Nutritional Status of the US Population based on Data Collected in the Second NHANES 1976–1980.* Life Sciences Research Office, Federation of American Societies for Experimental Biology, Bethesda (MD), August 1984, pp. 1–66.

195. Hercberg, S., Chauliac, M., Galan, P. *et al.* (1986) Relationship between anaemia, iron and folacin deficiency, haemoglobinopathies and parasitic infestation. *Hum. Nutr. Clin. Nutr.*, **40C**, 371–9.

196. Hercberg, S., Galan, P., Chauliac, M. *et al.* (1987) Nutritional anaemia in Beninese pregnant women: consequence on haematological profile of newborn. *Br. J. Nutr.*, **57**, 185–93.

197. Smith, J.C. Jr, Butrimovitz, G.P. and Purdy, W.C. (1979) Direct measurement of zinc in plasma by atomic absorption spectroscopy. *Clin. Chem.*, **25**, 1487–92.

198. Smith, J.C. Jr, Lewis, S., Holbrock, J. *et al.* (1987) Effect of heparin and citrate on measured concentrations of various analytes in plasma. *Clin. Chem.*, **33**, 814–16.

199. Meret, S. and Henkin, R.I. (1971) Simultaneous direct estimation by atomic absorption spectrophotometry of copper and zinc in serum, urine and cerebrospinal fluid. *Clin. Chem.*, **17**, 369–73.

200. Davies, I.J.T., Musa, M. and Dormandy, T.L. Measurements of plasma zinc. *J. Clin. Pathol.*, **21**, 359–65.

201. Patrick, J. and Dervish, C. (1984) Leucocyte zinc in the assessment of zinc status. *CRC. Crit. Rev. Clin. Lab. Sci.*, **20**, 95–114.

202. Milne, D.B., Ralston, N.V.C. and Wallwork, S.C. (1985) Zinc content of cellular components of blood: methods of cells separation and analysis evaluated. *Clin. Chem.*, **31**, 65–9.

203. Goode, H.F., Kelleher, J. and Walker, B.E. (1989) Zinc concentrations in pure populations of peripheral blood neutrophils, lymphocytes and monocytes. *Ann. Clin. Biochem.*, **26**, 89–95.
204. Purcell, S.K., Hambidge, K.M. and Jacobs, M.A. (1986) Zinc concentrations in mononuclear and polymorphonuclear leucocytes. *Clin. Chim. Acta*, **155**, 179–84.
205. Dorea, J.G. and Paine, P.A. (1985) Hair zinc in children: its uses, limitations and relationship to plasma zinc and anthropometry. *Hum. Nutr. Clin. Nutr.*, **39**, 389–98.
206. Anttila, P. *et al.* (1984) Serum and hair zinc as predictors of clinical symptoms in acrodermatitis enteropathica. *J. Inherited Metab. Dis.*, **7**, 46–8.
207. Gibson, R.S., Vanderkooy, P.D.S., MacDonald, A.C. *et al.* (1989) A growth-limiting, mild zinc-deficiency syndrome in some Southern Ontario boys with low height percentiles. *Am. J. Clin. Nutr.*, **49**, 1266–73.
208. Weismann, K. and Hoyer, H. (1985) Serum alkaline phosphatase and serum zinc levels in the diagnosis and exclusion of zinc deficiency in man. *Am. J. Clin. Nutr.*, **41**, 1214–19.
209. Bowers, G.N. and McComb, R.B. (1966) A continuous spectrophotometric method for measuring the activity of serum alkaline phosphatase. *Clin. Chem.*, **12**, 70–89.
210. Bowers, G.N. and McComb, R.B. (1975) Measurement of total alkaline phosphatase activity in human serum. *Clin. Chem.*, **21**, 1988–95.
211. Abe, A., Yamashita, S. and Noma, A. (1989) Sensitive, direct colorimetric assay for copper in serum. *Clin. Chem.*, **35**, 552–4.
212. Sunderman, F.W. and Nomoto, S. (1970) Measurement of human serum caeruloplasmin by p-phenylenediamine oxidase reactivity. *Clin. Chem.*, **16**, 903–10.
213. Sun, Y., Oberley, L.W. and Li, Y. (1988) A simple method for clinical assay of superoxide dismutase. *Clin. Chem.*, **34**, 497–500.
214. Salin, M.L. and McCord, J.M. (1974) Superoxide dismutases in polymorphonuclear leukocytes. *J. Clin. Invest.*, **54**, 1005–9.
215. Yardrick, M.K., Kenney, M.A. and Winterfeldt, E.A. (1989) Iron, copper and zinc status: Response to supplementation with zinc or zinc and iron in adult females. *Am. J. Clin. Nutr.*, **49**, 145–50.
216. Uauy, R., Castillo-Duran, C., Finsberg, M. *et al.* (1985) Red cell superoxide dismutase activity in an index of human copper nutrition. *J. Nutr.*, **115**, 1650–5.
217. Levander, O.A., DeLoach, D.P., Morris, V.C. and Moser, P.B. (1983) Platelet glutathione peroxidase activity as an index of selenium status in rats. *J. Nutr.*, **113**, 55–63.
218. Lombeck, I., Kasparek, K., Iyengar, G.V. *et al.* (1982) Selenium in platelets of children with low selenium state, in *Trace Element Metabolism in Man and Animals* (eds J.M. Gawthorne, J.C. Howell and C.L. White), Springer-Verlag, Berlin, pp. 26–9.
219. Verlinden, M., Van Sprundel, M., Van der Auwera, J.C. and Eylenbosch, W.J. (1983) The selenium status of Belgian population groups, I. Healthy adults. *Biol. Trace Elem. Res.*, **5**, 91–102.
220. Verlinden, M., Van Sprundel, M., Van der Auwera, J.C. and Eylenbosch, W.J. (1983) The selenium status of Belgian population groups, II. Newborns, children and the aged. *Biol. Trace Elem. Res.*, **5**, 103–13.
221. Olson, O.E., Palmer, I.S. and Cary, E.E. (1975) Modification of the official fluorimetric method for selenium in plants. *JAOAC*, **58**, 117–21.
222. Shawky, M. and White, C.L. (1975) Fluorimetric determination of submicrogram concentration of selenium in sulfide samples. *Anal. Chem.*, **48**, 1484–6.
223. Reamer, D.C. and Veillon, C. (1983) Elimination of perchloric acid in digestion of

biological fluids for fluorimetric determination of selenium. *Anal. Chem.*, **54**, 1605–6.

224. Paglia, D.E. and Valentine, W.N. (1967) Studies on the quantitative and qualitative characterization of erythrocytes glutathione peroxidase. *J. Lab. Clin. Med.*, **70**, 158–69.

225. Levander, C.A., De Loach, D.P., Morris, V.C. and Moser, P.B. (1983) Platelet glutathione peroxidase activity as an index of selenium status in rats. *J. Nutr.*, **113**, 55–63.

226. Veillon, C. (1988) Chromium. *Methods Enzymol.*, **158**, 334–43.

227. Kumpulainen, J., Lehto, J., Koivistoinen, P. *et al.* (1983) Determination of chromium in human milk, serum and urine by electrothermal atomic absorption spectrometry without preliminary ashing. *Sci. Total Environ.*, **31**, 71–6.

228. Kayne, F.J., Komar, G., Laboda, H. and Vanderlinde, R.E. (1978) Atomic absorption spectrophotometry of chromium in serum and urine with a modified Perkin–Elmer 603 atomic absorption spectrophotometer. *Clin. Chem.*, **24**, 2151–4.

229. Baruthio, F., Guillard, O., Arnaud, J. *et al.* (1988) Determination of manganese in biological materials by electrothermal atomic absorption spectrometry: a review. *Clin. Chem.*, **34**, 227–34.

230. Casey, C.E., Jacobs, M.A. and Hambidge, K.M. (1987) Atomic absorption spectrometry of manganese in plasma. *Clin. Chem.*, **33**, 1253–4.

231. Halls, D.J. and Fell, G.S. (1981) Determination of manganese serum and urine by electrothermal atomic absorption spectrometry. *Anal. Chem. Acta*, **129**, 205–11.

9 Immunocompetence methodology

9.1 Introduction   *R.K. Chandra and P. Sarchielli*   425
9.2 Lymphocyte count   *P. Sarchielli and R.K. Chandra*   428
9.3 Delayed cutaneous hypersensitivity   *P. Sarchielli and R.K. Chandra*   429
9.4 Complement C3 and Factor B   *P. Sarchielli and R.K. Chandra*   432
9.5 Secretory IgA   *P. Sarchielli and R.K. Chandra*   434
9.6 T-Lymphocyte and subset percentage   *P. Sarchielli and R.K. Chandra*   436
9.7 Lymphocyte proliferation response   *P. Sarchielli and R.K. Chandra*   438

9.1 INTRODUCTION

One of the most frequent and sometimes life-threatening complications of malnutrition is infection. Since host immunity is an important protective mechanism against micro-organisms, an assessment of immunocompetence is a logical approach to evaluating nutritional status [1].

Immunocompetence has the advantage of being a sensitive functional index of nutrition [2]. This is because it precedes other better-recognized markers of malnutrition, and a correlation between impaired immune responses and risk of infection has been established on the basis of studies on primary immuno-deficiency disorders [3, 4]. For example, both thymic dysplasia and complement deficiencies enhance susceptibility to infection, and both cell-mediated immunity [5, 6] and the complement system [7] are impaired in malnutrition. In fact prospective studies in developing countries point to the significant reduction in T cell number and complement C3 levels early in the genesis of malnutrition, prior to growth failure in young children [1]. Another advantage is that some immuno-logical tests are relatively non-invasive and/or require very little blood.

One disadvantage of using immunocompetence in nutritional assessment is its non-specific nature. Abnormalities in immune responses can occur as a result of concurrent infections or of underlying diseases that can in themselves impair immunocompetence. Rarely, defects in immune function are due to primary immunodeficiency disorders. Secondly, for certain tests, a relatively large amount of blood is required. Thirdly, cellular studies require immediate processing of blood, although the alternative of freezing cells for subsequent testing has been used successfully in some cases. Finally, some techniques may require costly equipment and trained personnel.

The choice of methods is governed by several determinants, including the outcome variables being investigated, site of investigation (field or hospital), age group, prevalence of common infections in the community, presence of an underlying primary disorder, etc. For example, in field studies in most countries, obtaining repeated blood samples by venipuncture is not practical. It is interesting to note, on the other hand, that in some communities, anthropometry and skin tests are frowned upon and difficult to obtain, whereas blood samples may be permitted.

Many aspects of the immune function are susceptible to the influence of nutritional disorders. In PEM, the greatest impact is on the number and function of T cells and subsets [8] and cell-mediated immunity, but there are changes also in secretory IgA antibody response [9], the level and function of various components of the complement system [7], and phagocytic bactericidal activity [10].

This impairment of immunocompetence can contribute to an increased incidence and severity of bacterial, viral, fungal, and parasitic diseases in malnutrition.

In vitamin deficiency states, especially those of vitamins A, B$_6$, E, and folate, many immune functions are impaired. In some cases, high dosages of certain vitamins such as vitamin A may even have a negative effect on immunocompetence [11]. Deficiencies or excesses of trace elements (zinc, selenium, iron, copper) and minerals impair immune responses [12]. Evidence for this has been obtained in experimental animals as also in humans.

Specific nutrient deficiencies may complicate clinical problems observed in hospitalized patients and in those with chronic diseases and may contribute to immunodepression observed in these conditions [13].

The duration of malnutrition can influence the extent of impaired immunocompetence. Short periods of starvation have in fact only minimal effect on immune functions, and may include changes in lymphocyte response to mitogens, levels of complement C3, and an increase in suppressor cell number. Similar changes can also be observed for a few days in postoperative surgical patients [14].

In obese animals, there are well-documented changes in cell-mediated immunity. However, the influence of obesity on immunological functions in humans and on the risk of infectious disease is controversial [15, 16]. The quantitative influence of obesity on various aspects of host defences has not been determined.

The mechanisms leading to the impairment of immune functions in obesity remains obscure. Hyperlipidaemia and hyperglycaemia have been considered possible contributing factors. Alteration of the levels of hormones (adrenocorticoids, insulin, growth hormone) can have a substantial impact on immune responsiveness. Also, the high incidence of iron and zinc deficiencies seen in obese subjects can be considered another factor leading to immune dysfunction; in one study there was a good correlation between deficiency of these nutrients and immune depression [17].

Ageing is associated with many changes in immune functions [18]. These include thymic involution with resultant decrease in level of thymic hormones, lymphopenia, and an increase in the number of immature lymphocytes.

Changes in the proportion of helper T cells (CD4+) and suppressor T cells (CD8+) are variable. The number of B cells does not appear to be modified. The concentration of IgA and IgG increases while that of IgM decreases. Moreover, the decrease in antibody production to specific foreign antigens is associated with an increased incidence of autoantibodies and monoclonal immunoglobulins. This may be attributed to altered immunoregulation. Since almost one-third of subjects above 65 years of age retain immune responsiveness at levels seen in young individuals, immunological decline cannot be considered to be part of the normal ageing process [19].

Among other factors, malnutrition occurring in the elderly further compromises immune responses, but this can be diagnosed and is potentially reversible [20].

The use of immunocompetence to assess malnutrition during pregnancy is complicated by the fact that pregnancy is characterized by active immune suppression. This immune suppression has the principal aim of preventing the recognition of paternal alloantigens, particularly at the level of the placenta, but this is also reflected to some extent in the peripheral blood [21].

In pregnant women the presence of malnutrition can further confound immune function impairment. Furthermore malnutrition during pregnancy, particularly if severe, can lead to intrauterine fetal growth retardation that places the newborn infant at a considerable risk for increased mortality and morbidity: the latter includes poor physical growth, learning difficulties, and increased susceptibility to infections that can be considered a consequence of the impairment of the immune function [22, 23].

Recent investigations have demonstrated a consistent and significant depression of cell-mediated immunity that may persist for a long time – several months to years [24].

Finally, in assessment of immunocompetence, cyclic variation of immune responses should also be considered. The multi-frequency time rhythms of immunological function are important confounding factors. The circadian variation of circulating lymphocytes and subsets and of proliferative response to mitogens can in part be explained on the basis of the cortisol rhythm, but other environmental and life-style factors such as the daily routine, exercise, meal pattern, stress, and genetic factors may also need to be taken into account [25].

Based on the most consistent abnormalities in immune responses the following tests can be employed in the assessment of immunocompetence in nutritional deficiencies:

total lymphocyte count;
delayed hypersensitivity reactions;
complement C3, factor B;
T cell and subset number;
secretory IgA in saliva and/or nasopharyngeal secretions.

Other less satisfactory tests that can be used in selected specific instances or for research purposes include:

lymphocyte proliferation response to mitogens and antigens;

allogeneic T lymphocyte responses;
NK cell activity;
in vitro production of specific antibodies;
lymphokine production;
leukocyte terminal deoxynucleotidyl transferase activity.

The final choice of immunological tests to be used in nutritional assessment will depend upon the particular requirements of the study, technical facilities available, age of the subject, and economic resources. The main objective of nutritional assessment is to find out the risk of complications, especially infection, and final outcome, i.e. survival or death. In achieving this objective immunocompetence scores over other methods.

9.2 LYMPHOCYTE COUNT

9.2.1 Purpose and scope

Although lymphopenia is considered a hallmark of primary severe combined immunodeficiency, it can also occur in secondary immunodeficiency such as that due to malnutrition.

The number of lymphocytes in peripheral blood has been considered to be indicative of the degree of impairment of cell-mediated immune response in many nutritional disorders, in particular protein–energy malnutrition. In these cases lymphocyte count has been proposed as an important predictor of subsequent mortality [26–28].

In hospitalized people lymphocyte count has been recognized as a useful test for identifying patients at nutritional risk and at risk of postoperative septic complications. Dionigi *et al.* [29] proposed the use of this variable together with other anthropometric, biochemical, and immunological tests in a cluster analysis for monitoring increased susceptibility to postoperative infections and effectiveness of nutritional therapy. In this study, calculation of the risk of postoperative sepsis on the basis of lymphocyte count alone showed the inability of this test to stratify septic patients on the basis of the degree of malnutrition. Lymphocyte count showed a sensitivity of 36%, a specificity of 77%, and an accuracy of 44%.

Finally, in a study performed by Bowers *et al.* [30], patients with anorexia nervosa whose average weight was 63% of their ideal body weight presented not only a markedly low white blood cell (WBC) count but also a lower absolute count of lymphocytes.

9.2.2 Principle of method

The WBC count can be performed automatically by a computerized blood-cell counter. The lymphocyte count is derived from cell percentages obtained from the WBC formula. Automated equipment to perform them is now available in hospital practice. Alternatively, conventional methods of enumerating total white cells in a counting chamber and a stained blood smear for differential count can be used for calculating the number of lymphocytes.

9.2.3 Procedure

Refer to the Instructions of automated counter units, e.g. cc–720, Gelman, Gelaire.

9.2.4 Performance characteristics

Reproducibility and comparability are reported in the Instructions of automated counter units.

9.3 DELAYED CUTANEOUS HYPERSENSITIVITY

9.3.1 Purpose and scope

Delayed cutaneous hypersensitivity (DCH) to a panel of ubiquitous antigens can be considered one of the oldest, most useful, and simplest tests for assessing cell-mediated immune function *in vivo*. In fact the development of an erythematous and indurative reaction at the site of the antigen injection implies an intact (afferent, central, efferent) response, confirming the ability to mount an efficient inflammatory response.

More than twenty antigens have been used for skin testing in humans. The common useful ones include: Candida, mumps, tetanus toxoid, diphtheria toxoid, purified protein derivate (PPD), streptokinase streptodornase (SK–SD), Trichophyton. Phytohaemagglutinin can be used with advantage in individuals whose previous exposure to common antigen is doubtful.

Other antigens may be used for specific diagnostic purposes. The sensitization with a primary antigen, e.g. dinitrochlorobenzene (DNCB), was also proposed as another test of *in vivo* cell-mediated immunity, but it has the drawback of producing rather vigorous and painful responses in some individuals, leaving a nasty scar in those with normal immunity. Serial studies of DCH may be useful for demonstrating anergy which has predictive value in many clinical settings, even in malnutrition and in monitoring the effects of its treatment.

Delayed cutaneous hypersensitivity is impaired in many nutritional disorders. A depression of DCH to a large number of antigens has been observed in children affected by severe and moderate PEM [3].

The frequency of positive response to delayed cutaneous hypersensitivity tests has been investigated by Chandra *et al.* [31] in relation to the serum albumin levels in PEM, confirming the usefulness of the DCH as a functional index of altered visceral protein synthesis and of reduced LBM.

One explanation of this depression is a reduction in the number of T cells and in the inflammatory migration of cells. This is due in part to reduced clonal expansion.

In the course of self-induced semistarvation, as in anorexia nervosa, contrasting results concerning DCH have been obtained [32, 33].

The negative influence of obesity in humans on cell-mediated immunity *in vivo* has been investigated and confirmed by the depression of cutaneous DCH responsiveness to Candida, PPD, SK–SD, mumps and Tricophyton in many obese patients [17], although the extent of changes is less marked than in PEM.

An essential fatty acid-deficient diet resulted in a reduction of delayed-type hypersensitivity but it was demonstrated only in experimental animals. Zinc deficiency alone, as in patients with acrodermatitis enteropathica, causes a depression of DCH. This may be linked to the reduction of T helper cell function [34]. Moreover patients with zinc deficiency failed to develop positive reactions when sensitized with a primary antigen.

Animals deprived of copper and selenium showed a reduction of cell-mediated immunity *in vivo* as much as during magnesium deficiency.

Finally, iron deficiency is associated with a depression of cell-mediated immunity. In patients with iron deficiency (some of whom showed anaemia and/or concurrent infections) contrasting results concerning DCH impairment have been obtained [35, 36].

A depression of cell-mediated immunity *in vivo* was observed during vitamin deficiency in experimental animals. Vitamin A, biotin, vitamin B_6, and folic acid deficiency induce a DCH depression to many recall antigens. On the other hand the administration of an excess of retinoic acid resulted in a remarkable suppression of delayed-type hypersensitivity responses to diphtheric toxoid in complete Freund's adjuvant.

The above-reported data confirm the usefulness of the tests of DCH as a functional index of cell-mediated immunity in malnutrition, but there is no consensus on the best technique, the method, and the range of antigens that should be used.

According to Frazer *et al.* [37]:

Testing recall of DCH to a single antigen lacks sensitivity whereas the usual panel of antigens provides better discrimination of anergic subjects but is less convenient and requires the continued availability of the panel of standardized antigens suitable for *in vivo* use; some antigens, particularly mumps, SK–SD, and Trichophyton skin test antigens may be difficult to obtain.

A device, the Multitest, allows simultaneous intradermal application of seven standardized antigens and thus overcomes the inconvenience of seven separate injections of antigens and the technical difficulty of ensuring their intradermal rather than subcutaneous injection.

This test appears to give results which were reproducible and comparable with those obtained by the conventional panel of antigens.

However, the induration produced in response to each antigen in the Multitest is rather small, and 2 mm is considered a positive reaction. Occasionally it may be very difficult to classify a reaction as positive or negative. It must be emphasized that this device is very expensive (approximately US $10 per test) and will be beyond the economic reach of most studies, particularly in countries where nutritional deficiencies are rampant.

9.3.2 Principle of the method

The conventional method is based on intradermal injection of each of a panel of several recall antigens. An induration of more than 5 mm is considered a positive response. The Multitest device permits simultaneous application of a panel of six recall antigens (Candida, Tricophyton, tuberculin, diphtheric toxoid, tetanus toxoid, streptococcal antigen, Proteus). The induration diameters (mm) are read 48 h after application of both tests.

Note 1.

The Multitest is convenient to use and the smaller mean reaction size should increase its acceptability to test subjects without reducing the ability of the test to discriminate between anergic and normal response.

9.3.3 Procedure

For the conventional method, reference should be made to the procedure suggested by Frazer *et al.* [37], Urbaniak *et al.* [38], or WHO Scientific Group [39].

For the Multitest, reference should be made to the Instructions of the Multitest CMC (Institute Merieux, Lyon) [40].

For the DNCB skin test we recommend the method of Catalona *et al.* [41].

9.3.4 Performance characteristics

Reproducibility

For the Multitest, one study performed by Frazer *et al.* [37] showed inter-observer reproducibility to be high ($r = 0.89$) and the correlation between repeated tests was also high ($r = 0.88$). Similar data for conventional DCH tests is not available, but the correlation between the two tests was of the order of 0.65.

9.3.5 Reference values

There are no general reference values for skin test responses and there is very little information about the percentage of people responding to the various antigens. The available information is population specific. For Multitest, polycentric studies performed in various European countries on apparently healthy individuals permitted the definition of an average score value of 15 mm in women and 20 mm in men [42]. Analogous investigations on American population groups gave mean values of 19 mm in women and 23 mm in men [43]. In a study performed on 768 healthy Italian individuals, Dionigi (1986, unpublished data) reported a mean score of 15.7 ± 9.2 mm for both sexes combined, 18 ± 9.9 mm ($n = 377$) for men and 13.4 ± 9 mm ($n = 391$) for women. The number of positive reactions was 3.4 ± 1.5 mm ($n = 767$) for both sexes combined, 3.8 ± 1.5 mm ($n = 377$) for men and 3.0 ± 1.4 mm ($n = 390$) for women.

On 46 individuals aged 60 years and over we obtained a mean score of 9.7 ± 7.9 mm, a number of positive antigens of 2.4 ± 1.4, and a mean antigenic diameter of 3.9 ± 1.5 (Sarchielli (1987) unpublished data).

9.3.6 Interpretation

The immune response is very complex and not all of its components participate in the response evoked by the injection of anamnestic antigens. It is therefore not correct to consider the cutaneous test an efficient method that alone permits evaluation of adequate immunity, even cell-mediated, of an individual. For this reason the skin tests could be considered a simple one-time image of some aspects of the immune response. A relatively crude and complex test such as the DCH is not subject to subtle immunological interpretations, but if used carefully and accurately it certainly has considerable clinical importance in the identification of patients at high risk of developing complications.

Many clinical situations are characterized by a reduction of DCH: severe or recurrent infections (e.g. miliary tuberculosis, measles), Hodgkin's disease, sarcoidosis, certain kinds of malignancies (in these cases diminished reactions may be associated with poor diagnosis), and abuse of some drugs (corticosteroids and other immunosuppressors). Even clinically healthy volunteers show major differences in their ability to induce and express delayed hypersensitivity responses. The factors that should be taken into account are genetic influence, sex, and age. Whereas cell-mediated immunity can be demonstrated soon after birth, the specific response to selected antigens (e.g. PPD) develops later. Vaccinations with attenuated live viruses (measles for instance) often suppress the DCH.

Some individuals who do not respond to an intermediate strength of an antigen, may do so to a higher strength. People respond more efficiently to the antigens to which they are commonly exposed and therefore the selection of such appropriate antigens could be useful.

As in any other test a variety of variables can affect DCH. Some of these factors are biological, whereas others are of a technical nature. Among these latter we include the choice of antigens, their quality and purity, storage, inappropriate administration, degradation (heat exposure), and absorption of antigens on the walls of the containers. An inappropriate dilution should be taken into account, particularly for the conventional method. Use of Multitest has been proposed as an attempt to eliminate or reduce some of these variables.

Certain skin conditions may not allow the development of a positive reaction (e.g. skin atrophy, contact dermatitis, atopic diseases). Moreover, there may coexist a defect of the non-specific inflammatory response (differential diagnosis using sodium benzyl sulphide that gives positive reactions in 90% of individuals with an efficient non-specific inflammatory response). Furthermore the patients may not have been exposed to the skin test antigens; this is particularly relevant to children. Subcutaneous rather than intradermal injection of antigens results in rapid removal before a reaction is apparent. The presence of oedema of the skin sometimes gives negative reactions due to an increased lymphatic clearance of the antigen.

9.4 COMPLEMENT C3 AND FACTOR B

9.4.1 Purpose and scope

The complement system includes many serum proteins which interact among themselves and function as regulators, initiators, and effectors of cell lysis and inflammation. There are two major pathways of complement activation. The major serum antibody components IgA and IgG activate the classic pathway. Endotoxins, certain drugs, and IgA immunoglobulins activate the alternative pathway. These two pathways intersect at a common reaction point, C3, giving the final reaction sequence.

The classic C pathway can be divided into recognition (C1q, C1r, C1s), activation (C4, C2, C3), and attack (C5, C6, C7, C8, C9) portions respective to their function in cytolysis.

The alternative or properdin pathway consists of another four proteins: an

most probably points to a defective population of helper T cells, which have been shown to be particularly sensitive to nutritional manipulation [67]. In addition, the specific memory and suppressor cells may be significantly reduced. Optimum IgA production depends upon both cell-mediated and humoral immunity. Its thymus dependence may explain in part its reduction in PEM secondary to impairment of the cell-mediated immunity [68]. Other possible mechanisms involved in the impairment of the secretory immune response are the decreased synthesis of the secretory component, an essential constituent of the secretory IgA molecule, due to atrophied mucosal epithelium, and the decreased number of mucosal plasma cells producing IgA. Often the defect involves only the secretory antibody response whereas serum antibody response is normal, or a decreased synthesis by a reduced number of IgA-bearing cells of the submucous membrane. The finding of normal or even increased levels of secretory IgA in children with PEM and infection may be attributed to the latter [69].

The impact of specific nutrient deficiency on secretory immune response has not been studied adequately. Both iron and vitamin A deficiencies are associated with reduced sIgA levels and antibody responses to viral vaccines [9]. There is no information on the quality of secretory IgA antibodies. In the serum, antibody affinity is reduced.

9.5.2 Principle of the method

Determination of the concentration of secretory IgA (tear, saliva) is carried out by the radial immunodiffusion method (RID) [50, 59, 68–70].

9.5.3 Procedure

For preparation of the sample we refer to the recommendation of Urbaniak *et al.* [71]. For the procedure we refer to the method reported in the manufacturer's Instructions, e.g. for LC-Partigen IgA that of the Behring Institute.

9.5.4 Performance characteristics

(a) Range of linearity

See the manufacturer's Instructions, e.g. LC-Partigen IgA, Behring Institute. (Assay range: 0.5–7.9 IU/ml using the protein standard serum LC–V – 1:8, 1:4, 1:2 dilutions – or 0.8–13.3 mg/dl using the standard human serum stabilized – 1:200, 1:50, 1:25 dilutions.)

> *Note 2.*
> 1 mg of IgA is equivalent to 59.5 IU of IgA.

(b) Reproducibility

The intraobserver coefficient of reproducibility, calculated in 46 apparently healthy individuals (22 females and 24 males) between 20 and 40 years of age, for secretory IgA determination performed in duplicate, was 0.97 with a SEM of $\pm$ 1.30 mg/dl ($\bar{x} = 19.7 \pm 8.5$).

9.5.5 Reference values

In Table 9.1 we report the quartile distributions of the values obtained in two groups of 46 young persons and 46 elderly persons from the Perugia area.

Table 9.1 Means, SD, quartile distribution of salivary IgA (mg/dl) of two groups of 46 young persons and 46 apparently healthy elderly persons from the Perugia area

| | Aged 20–40 years | | Aged > 60 years | |
	Women n = 22	Men n = 24	Women n = 31	Men n = 15
Percentiles				
Min	7.5	9.1	6.2	6.3
25	10.0	23.3	7.0	8.2
50	16.0	18.5	7.6	15.6
75	21.4	23.3	13.6	23.1
Max	38.7	46.2	26.9	30.5
Mean	16.2	19.3	8.6	14.7
SD	7.8	9.0	6.6	10.2

9.6 T-LYMPHOCYTE AND SUBSET PERCENTAGE

9.6.1 Purpose and scope

T lymphocytes mediate a complex range of functions. They may be classified into subpopulations on the basis of cell surface markers and biological functions. In particular two specific subpopulations of T lymphocytes have been investigated *in vitro*: the helper/induced subpopulation and the cytotoxic/suppressor subpopulation [72].

The identification and enumeration of T cells and their subpopulations by monoclonal antibodies appears to be a useful tool for the detection and grading of impairment of cell-mediated immunity in nutritional deficiency disorders and also in the monitoring of nutritional therapeutic intervention [73].

Clinical human or experimental animal PEM is accompanied by a reduction of T cell number, which may be due to reduced clonal proliferation or a consequence of thymic atrophy and the reduction of thymic hormone levels [74, 75]. The availability of monoclonal antibodies reactive against surface antigens of lymphocytes revealing antigenically and functionally distinct subsets of T cells allowed the observation of a marked reduction of inducer $CD4^+$ cells and a moderate reduction of suppressor $CD8^+$ cells, thus resulting in a very sigificantly lower $CD4^+/CD8^+$ ratio.

The changes were reversed by nutritional supplementation given for a period of at least 4–8 weeks. The inducer/suppressor ratio was lower before nutritional therapy was started and rose thereafter [8].

Protein deprivation is characterized by a defective function of T helper cell populations, which may reflect the thymic dependency of antibody response, particularly secondary.

Populations of antigen-specific T suppressor cells are also deficient in the condition which compromises immunoregulation in nutritional deficiency [76].

Zinc-deficient animals and humans (acrodermatitis enteropathica) present a loss of T cells and a proportional increase in the number of cells bearing Fc receptors. Fraker suggested, on the basis of animal studies, that the immune defect in zinc deprivation predominantly affects T helper cell function. A progressive appearance of autologous rosette-forming cells, a property of a specific subset of immature T cells, occurs also in zinc-deprived animals.

The transfer of thymocytes from immunologically competent to zinc-deprived mice restored the antibody response (T helper dependent) to sheep red blood cells (SRBC) immunization [77–79].

The number of circulating T cells has also been reported to be slightly reduced with iron deficiency, in particular reduced T helper activity that can contribute to the impaired immunocompetence associated with an increased risk of infection [35, 36]. Laboratory animals deprived of copper and selenium exhibit changes in T cell number and function. Studies using moderate supplements of vitamins A, B_6 and E have shown an increase in the number of T cells [80–82].

9.6.2 Principle of the methods

In the past the E^+ rosette method was available for estimating T lymphocytes. Those that have surface receptors for sheep red cells are believed to be thymus-dependent (T cells). Lymphocytes with these receptors will bind to a cluster of SRBC, forming an erythrocyte rosette. The treatment of sheep red cells with 2 amino-ethylisothiouronium-hydrobromide (AET) stabilizes the bond, giving more reproducible results [83].

For the estimation of T lymphocytes and subpopulations [84], a range of mouse monoclonal anti-human T cell antibodies are commercially available, the most popular being the OKT series (Ortho), the LEU series (Becton Dickinson), and the LYT series (New England Nuclear).

The classic method is based on indirect immunofluorescence. These cells become coated with monoclonal antibodies and can be visualized and enumerated by staining with fluorescein-labelled goat anti-mouse immuno-globulins. Flow cytometric analysis is now available for the enumeration of the T cells and subsets. Lymphocyte fluorescence is analysed using a Coulter flow cytometer with the laser light tuned to 488 nm [85].

9.6.3 Procedure

For the E^+ rosette technique, T cell and subset enumeration, we refer to the methods as reported by Urbaniak *et al.* [86]. For the cytofluorometric procedure, we refer to the instructions of the flow cytometer (e.g. Coulter Epics V Instrument, Coulter Electronics, Hialeah, FL, or System 50H Cytofluorograph Cell Sorter).

All results are expressed as percentage of positive cells.

9.6.4 Performance characteristics

See information from the above-named manufacturers.

Reproducibility

The reproducibility of T lymphocyte quantitation by the E^+ rosettes technique by one observer calculated by us on 46 apparently healthy individuals (22 females and 24 males) between 20 and 40 years of age, is 0.98 with a SEM of 1.52 ($\bar{x} = 71.3 \pm 3.8$).

The intrameasurer reliability calculated by us on the same individuals for the T lymphocyte and subset percentage quantitation by indirect immunofluorescence is very high, with a coefficient ranging from 0.97 to 0.98 (CD3$^+$: 0.971, $\bar{x} = 69.0 \pm 5.7$; CD8$^+$: 0.978, $\bar{x} = 28.3 \pm 3.3$; CD4$^+$: 0.981, $\bar{x} = 40.7 \pm 5.0$) and a standard error of measurement from 1.39 to 1.61 (CD3$^+$: 1.57, CD8$^+$: 1.61 and CD4$^+$: 1.39).

9.7 LYMPHOCYTE PROLIFERATION RESPONSE

9.7.1 Purpose and scope

Lymphocyte function can be assessed quantitatively *in vitro* by stimulation with lectins and other substances that result in increased synthesis of DNA. This can be measured best by incorporation of radioactive DNA precursors into the cells.

The stimulating substances can be grouped as follows:

1. Polyclonal mitogens, e.g. phytohaemagglutinin (PHA), concanavalin A (Con A), pokeweed mitogen (PWM), OKT3 antibody, lipopolysaccharide, anti-immunoglobulin antibodies, protein A of *Staphylococcus aureus*, EB virus, Klebsiella;
2. Specific antigens, e.g. purified protein derivative (PPD) of *Mycobacterium tuberculosis*, candidin, streptokinase, streptodornase;
3. Allogeneic lymphocytes in mixed lymphocyte reaction (MLR) [87, 88].

Measurement of lymphocyte transformation is useful for diagnosis of primary or secondary immunodeficiencies and for monitoring various therapies for the successful functional recovery of the immune system.

Measurement of lymphocyte transformation to specific antigens can be useful in determining the sensitization to a particular antigen (better if coupled with delayed cutaneous hypersensitivity *in vivo* and stimulation of lymphokine release in specific tests *in vitro*). The pattern of responsiveness to various antigens can also be informative in identifying specific defects of cell-mediated immunity (CMI).

Autologous or heterologous sera may be used for maximal lymphocyte transformation and cell viability.

Sometimes autologous sera can have an inhibitory property, as has been shown for sera of kwashiorkor patients. This can explain the lack of correlation that sometimes occurs between *in vivo* and *in vitro* tests of CMI.

Peripheral blood blastization lymphocyte response is influenced by nutritional status [89]. The response to mitogens specific for T cells, e.g. concanavalin A and phytohaemagglutinin, has in fact been demonstrated to be reduced in PEM. Many factors can influence mitogen responsiveness: dose and source of the mitogen, culture conditions, incubation time, and type of serum utilized.

Chandra attributed decreased transformation in PEM to a decreased number of T cells capable of response (independently of the above-mentioned interfering variables). Nutritional supplementation causes full recovery of T cell responsiveness [90]. Factors inhibiting the cell-mediated response *in vitro* have also been revealed. Experiments in which autologous serum was obtained from PEM patients were not able to promote an optimal proliferation response of T cells.

The presence of immunosuppressive substances of embryonal origin (e.g. alpha-fetoprotein) can also be involved [91, 92, 93].

In starved individuals a decreased synthesis of DNA following stimulation with PHA and PPD can be observed, but not after incubation with Con A [94]. Indeed Golla *et al.* [32] found that patients with anorexia nervosa showed an enhanced response to T cell mitogens Con A and PHA and to the B cell mitogen PWM. These enhanced responses declined with appropriate nutritional repletion. On the other hand, obese patients presented a reduced lymphocyte blastization in response to PHA [17]. These results in obese subjects can in part be explained by a concurrent presence of iron or zinc deficiency.

Because zinc can play an important role in immune responses mediated by T and B cells, it obviously has a remarkable effect on lymphocyte responsiveness. The specific population that is particularly sensitive to zinc deficiency is the T helper population. Zinc supplementation can reverse the *in vitro* T and B cell responsiveness impairment [95]. Manganese can interact with Con A, of which it is an integral part, but the biological significance of this interaction is not clear and further studies are necessary to identify their nature [96]. Copper and selenium deficiency also appear to influence T cell mitogenic response but existing studies have been performed only on experimental animals.

Iron deficiency anaemia is also characterized by an impairment of T cell proliferation, which can be corrected by iron supplementation [35]. A marked reduction in the level of response to T cell mitogen phytohaemagglutinin and B cell mitogen LPS was observed in vitamin A deficiency [97].

Retinoic acid, which is added to cultures of human lymphocytes, enhances T cell response to mitogen PHA. In contrast, response to Con A and PWM is not affected.

Vitamin E stimulates Con A and PHA response (at low levels of mitogens) even in the absence of Ia+ adherent cells. Moreover, the mixed lymphocyte culture is enhanced [98]. Vitamin E also stimulates LPS response, but not in athymic animals, suggesting the importance of thymic factors for vitamin E lymphocyte stimulation.

Among water-soluble vitamins, vitamin B_6 in particular impairs the *in vitro* ^{3}H uridine incorporation after mitogenic stimulation, affecting DNA and protein lymphocyte synthesis [99]. Lymphocyte transformation responses to mitogen phytohaemagglutinin in patients with pernicious anaemia were significantly depressed [100].

9.7.2 Principle of the method

Stimulation with PHA, Con A, PWM mitogens, or other stimulators at different concentrations is carried out on cell cultures in triplicate, using flat-bottom microwell plates. For evaluation of proliferation, radioactive tracer 5-(^{125}I) iododeoxyuridine- or (^{3}H)-deoxythymidine is used. Results are expressed as net c.p.m. of the tracer uptake or as mitotic index (ratio between the response c.p.m. to a mitogen at a certain concentration and the basal count, without mitogen) [101–103].

9.7.3   Procedure

For lymphocyte response to PHA, Con A, and PWM, we refer to the procedure reported by Urbaniak *et al.* [103].

9.7.4   Performance characteristics

(a) General considerations

Human lymphocyte transformation has a marked variability. This has been demonstrated in normal human volunteers by many authors, even with the quantitation of the tracer in dose-response curves. Variability can be the result of *in vivo* and *in vitro* transient events. Viral infections and sometimes immunization responses can depress lymphocyte responses. Lymphocytes can be damaged during preparation by excessive mechanical manipulation. If the recovery level is 80% there is an increased variability of the relative number of T and B cells in the separated cell suspension.

This variability may also be due to different ratios of lymphocytes to monocytes. Both high and low concentrations of lymphocytes may be associated with a decreased lymphocyte transformation responsiveness.

Various studies reported a great variation in the response of both young and older adults, but particularly in young people [104, 105].

A reduced number of mitogen-responsive cells in the elderly, and failure of these cells to undergo clonal expansion have been reported, and a decrease in the production and responsiveness to IL2 could produce a 'ceiling' on the lymphocyte functions and result in a decreased variability of mitogen-induced, dose-dependent lymphocyte responsiveness.

(b) Reproducibility

Variability data can be found in the study reported by Robert [104]. In 46 clinically healthy young individuals (20–40 years of age) from the Perugia area we found the following standard errors of measurement: PHA (12.5 µg/ml) 643.9 c.p.m. (mean = 29724 ± SD 5766); Con A (2 µg/ml) 364.59 c.p.m. (mean = 19656 ± SD 3759); PWM (10 µg/ml) 368.79 c.p.m. (mean = 20559 ± SD 3144).

(c) Reference values

Each laboratory should calculate reference values from healthy individuals. For evaluating an individual for primary or acquired immunodeficiency, it may be necessary to compare the results with those of an age-matched healthy control tested at the same time.

REFERENCES

1. Chandra, R.K. (1981) Immunocompetence as a functional index of nutritional status. *Br. Med. Bull.*, **37**, 89–94.
2. Puri, S. and Chandra, P.K. (1985) Nutritional regulation of host resistance and predictive value of immunologic tests in assessment of outcome. *Ped. Clin. North Am.*, **32**(2), 499–515.
3. Cunningham-Rundles, S. (1982) Effects of nutritional status on immunological function. *Am. J. Clin. Nutr.*, **35**, 1202–10.

4. Gershwin, M.E., Beach, R.S. and Hurley, L.S. (1985) *Nutrition and immunity*, Academic Press, Orlando (Florida).

5. Chandra, R.K. (1980) Cell-mediated immunity in nutritional imbalance. *Fed. Proc.*, **39**, 3088–92.

6. MacMurray, D.N. (1984) Cell-mediated immunity in nutritional deficiency. *Prog. Food Nutr. Sci.*, **8**, 193–228.

7. Sirisinha, S., Suskind, R.M., Edelman, R. *et al.* (1973) Complement and C3-proactivator levels in children with protein–calorie malnutrition and effect of dietary treatment. *Lancet*, **i**, 1016–20.

8. Chandra, R.K., Gupta, S. and Singh, H. (1982) Inducer and suppressor T cell subsets in protein–energy malnutrition: Analysis by monoclonal antibodies. *Nutr. Res.*, **2**, 21–6.

9. Chandra, R.K. (1975) Reduced secretory antibody response to live attenuated measles and polio vaccines in malnourished children. *Br. Med. J.*, **2**, 583–5.

10. Seth, V. and Chandra, R.K. (1972) Opsonic activity, phagocytosis and bactericidal capacity of polymorphs in undernutrition. *Arch. Dis. Child.*, **47**, 282–4.

11. Panush, R.S. and Delafuente, J.C. (1985) Vitamins and immunocompetence. *World Rev. Nutr. Diet.*, **45**, 97–132.

12. Chandra, R.K. and Dayton, D. (1982) Trace element regulation of immunity and infection. *Nutr. Res.*, **2**, 721–33.

13. Chandra, S. and Chandra, R.K. (1985) Nutritional regulation of the immune responses: Basic considerations and practical applications. *J. Burn Care Rehab.*, **6**, 174–8.

14. Neuvonen, P.T. and Salo, M. (1984) Effects of short-term starvation on the immune response. *Nutr. Res.*, **4**, 771–6.

15. Mann, G.V. (1976) The influence of obesity on health. *N. Engl. J. Med.*, **291**, 178–83.

16. Chandra, R.K. (1981) Immune response in overnutrition. *Cancer Res.*, **411**, 3795–6.

17. Chandra, R.K. and Kutty, K.M. (1980) Immunocompetence in obesity. *Acta Pediatr. Scand.*, **69**, 25–30.

18. Makinodan, T. and Kay, M.M.B. (1980) Age influence on the immune system. *Adv. Immunol.*, **29**, 287–330.

19. Chandra, R.K. (1985) *Nutrition, Immunity and Illness in the Elderly*, Pergamon Press, New York.

20. Chandra, R.K. (in press) Nutritional regulation of immunity and infection in the elderly, in *Nutrition of the Elderly* (ed. A. Horowitz), Oxford University Press, Oxford.

21. Agarwal, S., Shukla, H.S., Verma, M. *et al.* (1982) Investigation of lymphocyte subpopulations and hypersensitivity skin tests during the menstrual cycle and pregnancy. *Ann. Chir. Gynaecol.*, **71**(2), 117–21.

22. Chandra, R.K. (1975) Fetal malnutrition and post-natal immunocompetence. *Am. J. Dis. Child.*, **129**, 450–5.

23. Neumann, C.G., Shilem, E.R., Zahradnick, J. *et al.* (1984) Immune function in intrauterine growth retardation. *Nutr. Res.*, **4**, 399–419.

24. Chandra, R.K. and Matsumura, T. (1980) Development aspects of cell-mediated immunity and findings in low birth weight infants. *Indian J. Pediatr.*, **47**, 25–31.

25. Carandente, F., Angeli, A., DeVecchi, A. *et al.* (1988) Multifrequency rhythms of immunological functions. *Chronobiologia*, **15**, 7–23.

26. Smythe, P.M., Schonland, M., Brerenton-Stiles, G.G. *et al.* (1971) Thymolymphatic deficiency and depression of cell-mediated immunity in protein–calorie malnutrition. *Lancet*, **ii**, 939–44.

27. Alleyne, G.A.O., Hay, R.W., Picon, D.I. *et al.* (1977) *Protein Energy Malnutrition*, Arnold, London.

28. Keusch, G.T. (1981) Host defense mechanisms in protein–energy malnutrition. *Adv. Exp. Med. Biol.*, **135**, 183–209.

29. Dionigi, P., Dionigi, R. and Nazari, S. (1986) Multicentric trial on nutritional assessment methods, in *Nutritional Status Assessment Methodology for Individuals and Population Groups* (ed. F. Fidanza), Group of European Nutritionists, Perugia, pp. 339–47.

30. Bowers, T.K. and Eckert, E. (1978) Leukopenia in anorexia nervosa. *Arch. Intern. Med.*, **138**, 1520–3.

31. Chandra, R.K., Baker, M. and Kumar, V. (1985) Body composition, albumin levels and delayed cutaneous cell-mediated immunity. *Nutr. Res.*, **5**, 679–84.

32. Golla, J.A., Larson, L.A., Anderson, C.F. *et al.* (1981) An immunological assessment of patients with anorexia nervosa. *Am. J. Clin. Nutr.*, **34**, 2756–62.

33. Armstrong-Esther, C.A., Lacy, J.H., Crisp, A.H. and Bryant, T.M. (1978) An investigation of the immune response of patients suffering from anorexia nervosa. *Postgrad. Med. J.*, **54**, 395–9.

34. Chandra, R.K. (1980) Acrodermatitis enteropathica: zinc levels and cell mediated immunity. *Pediatrics*, **66**, 789–91.

35. Bhaskaram, P., Prascad, J.S. and Krishnamachari, K.A.V.R. (1977) Anaemia and immune response. *Lancet*, **i**, 1000.

36. Joynson, D.H.M., Walker, D.M., Jacobs, A. and Dolly, A.E. (1972) Defect of cell-mediated immunity in patient with iron deficiency anaemia. *Lancet*, **ii**, 1058–9.

37. Frazer, I.H., Collins, E.J., Fox, J.S. *et al.* (1985) Assessment of delayed-type hypersensitivity in man: A comparison of the 'Multitest' and conventional intradermal injection of six antigens. *Clin. Immunol. Immunopathol.*, **35**, 182–90.

38. Urbaniak, S.J., McCann, M.C., White, A.G. *et al.* (1986) Tests of immune function, in *Handbook of Experimental Immunology. 4. Applications of Immunological Method in Biomedical Sciences* (eds D.M. Weir *et al.*), Blackwell Scientific Publications, Oxford, pp. 126.10–11.

39. WHO Scientific Group. (1978) *Immunodeficiency*. WHO, Geneva, Techn. Rep. Series No. 630.

40. Kniker, W.T., Anderson, C.T. and Roumiantzeff, M. (1979) The Multitest system. A standardized approach to evaluation of delayed cutaneous hypersensitivity and cell-mediated immunity. *Ann. Allergy*, **43**, 73–9.

41. Catalona, W.J., Taylor, P.T., Rabson, A.S. and Chretien, P.B. (1972) A method for dinitrochlorobenzene contact sensitization. A clinicopathological study. *N. Engl. J. Med.*, **286**, 399–402.

42. Biron, G., Rouminatzeff, M., Ajjan, N. *et al.* (1981) Etude sur une population française de référence de l'hypersensibilité cutanée retardée par le dispositif Multitest IMC. *Ann. Anesth. Franc.*, **3**, 270–8.

43. Kniker, W.T., Anderson, C.T. and Rouminatzeff, M. (1984) Multitest CMI for standardized measurement of delayed cutaneous hypersensitivity and cell-mediated immunity. Normal values and proposed scoring system for healthy adults in the USA. *Ann. Allergy*, **52(2)**, 75–82.

44. Spitzer, R.E. (1977) The complement system. *Pediatr. Clin. North Am.*, **24(2)**, 341–64.

45. Chandra, R.K. (1975) Serum complement and immunoconglutinin in malnutrition. *Arch. Dis. Child.*, **50**, 225–9.

46. Olusi, S.O., McFarlane, H., Ade-Serrano, M. *et al.* (1976) Complement components in children with protein calorie malnutrition. *Trop. Geogr. Med.*, **28**, 323–8.

47. Haller, L., Zubler, R.H. and Lambert, P.H. (1978) Plasma levels of complement

components and complement haemolytic activity in protein–energy malnutrition. *Clin. Exp. Immunol.*, **34**, 248–52.

48. Jagadeesan, V. and Reddy, V. (1979) Serum complement levels in malnourished children. *Indian J. Med. Res.*, **70**, 745–9.
49. Kielmann, A.A. and Curcio, L.M. (1979) Complement C3, nutrition and infection. *Bull. WHO*, **57(1)**, 113–21.
50. Chandra, R.K. (1980) *Immunology of Nutritional Disorders*, Edward Arnold, London.
51. Kumar, R. (1986) Discriminant function of complement C3, serum albumin and anthropometric measurements in identifying malnutrition. *Nutr. Res.*, **6**, 1147–60.
52. Palmblad, J., Cantell, K., Holm, G. *et al.* (1977) Acute energy deprivation in man: Effect on serum immunoglobulins antibody response, complement factors C3 and C4, acute phase reactants and interferon-producing capacity of blood lymphocytes. *Clin. Exp. Immunol.*, **30**, 50–6.
53. Kim, Y. and Michael, A.F. (1975) Hypocomplementemia in anorexia nervosa. *J. Pediatr.*, **87**, 538–42.
54. Palmblad, J. (1979) Plasma levels of complement factors 3 and 4, orosomucoid and opsonic function in anorexia nervosa. *Acta Paediatr. Scand.*, **68**, 617–21.
55. Chandra, R.K. and Saraya, A.K. (1975) Impaired immunocompetence associated with iron deficiency. *J. Pediatr.*, **86**, 899–902.
56. Montgomery, D.W., Don, L., Zukoski, C.F. and Chvapil, M. (1974) The effect of zinc and other metals on complement hemolysis of sheep red blood cells in vitro. *Proc. Soc. Exp. Biol. Med.*, **145**, 263–7.
57. Yamamoto, K. and Takahashi, M. (1975) Inhibition of the terminal stage of complement-mediated lysis (reactive lysis) by zinc and copper ions. *Int. Arch. Allergy Appl. Immunol.*, **48**, 653–63.
58. Amivaian, K., McKinney, J.A. and Tuchna, L. (1974) Effect of zinc and cadmium on guinea-pig complement. *Immunology*, **26**, 1135–44.
59. Mancini, G., Carbonara, A.O. and Haremaus, J.F. (1965) Immunochemical quantitation of antigens by single radial immuno-diffusion. *Immunochemistry*, **2**, 235–54.
60. Fahey, J.L. and McKelvey, E.M. (1965) Quantitative determination of serum immunoglobulins in antibody agar plates. *J. Immunol.*, **94**, 84–90.
61. Buffone, G.J. (1980) Immunonephelometric and turbidometric measurement of specific plasma proteins, in *Manual of Clinical Immunology*, 2nd edn (eds N.R. Rose and H. Friedman), American Society for Microbiology, Washington (DC).
62. Blanchard, G.C. and Gardner, R. (1982) Two nephelometric methods compared with a radial immunodiffusion method for measurement of IgG, IgA and IgM. *Clin. Biochem.*, **198**, 132–7.
63. Larson, C., Orenstein, P. and Ritchie, R. (1970) An automated method for quantitation of protein in body fluids. *Adv. Automat. Anal.*, **1**, 9–13.
64. Beckman Instructions (1983) Beckman Instruments Inc., Fullerton, California.
65. McMurray, D.N., Rey, H., Casazza, L.J. and Watson R.R. (1977) Effect of moderate malnutrition on concentrations of immunoglobulins and enzymes in tears and saliva of young Columbian children. *Am. J. Clin. Nutr.*, **30**, 1944–8.
66. Watson, R.R., Reyes, M.A. and McMurray, D.N. (1978) Influence of malnutrition on the concentration of IgA, lysozyme, amylase and aminopeptidase in children's tears. *Proc. Soc. Exp. Biol. Med.*, **157**, 215–9.
67. Chandra, R.K. (1980) Mucosal immunity in nutritional deficiency, in *Mucosal Post Defenses in Health and Disease* (eds P.L. Ogra and J. Bienenstock), Ross Laboratories, Columbus (Ohio).
68. Guy-Grand, D., Griscelli, C. and Vassalli, P. (1975) Peyer's patches, gut IgA

plasma cells and thymus function: Study in nude mice bearing thymic grafts. *J. Immunol.*, **115**, 361–4.

69. Bell, R.G., Turner, R.J., Gracey, M. *et al.* (1976) Serum and small intestinal immunoglobulin levels in undernourished children. *Am. J. Clin. Nutr.*, **29**, 392–7.

70. Becker, W. (1980) Die Standardizerung immunochemischer Plasmaprotein best-immungen. *Laboratoriumblätter*, **30**, 26–33.

71. Urbaniak, S.J., McCann, M.C., White, A.G. *et al.* (1986) Test of immune function, in *Handbook of Experimental Immunology. 4. Applications of Immunological Method in Biomedical Sciences* (eds D.M. Weir *et al.*), Blackwell Scientific Publications, Oxford, pp. 126.16.

72. Kung, P.C., Goldstein, G., Reinherz, E.L. and Schlossman, S.F. (1979) Mono-clonal antibodies defining distinctive human T cell surface antigens. *Science*, **206**, 347–9.

73. Reinherz, E.L. and Schlossman, S.F. (1980) Regulation of immune response: inducer and suppressor T lymphocyte subsets in human beings. *N. Engl. J. Med.*, **303**, 317–73.

74. Chandra, R.K. (1974) Rosette-forming T lymphocytes and cell-mediated immunity in malnutrition. *Br. Med. J.*, **3**, 608–9.

75. Ferguson, A.C., Lawlor, G.J., Neuman, C.G. *et al.* (1974) Decreased rosette-forming lymphocytes in malnutrition and intrauterine growth retardation. *J. Pediatr.*, **85**, 714–24.

76. Price, P. and Bell, R.G. (1977) Factors determining the effects of chronic protein-deficiency on antibody responses to sheep red blood cells and *Brucella abortus* vaccine in mice. *Aust. J. Exp. Biol. Med. Sci.*, **55**, 59–78.

77. Nash, L., Iwata, T., Fernandes, G. *et al.* (1979) Effect of zinc deficiency on autologous rosette forming cells. *Cell Immunol.*, **48**, 238–43.

78. Fernandes, G., Nair, M., Onoe, K. *et al.* (1979) Impairment of cell-mediated immunity functions by dietary zinc deficiency in mice. *Proc. Natl. Acad. Sci. (USA)*, **76**, 457–61.

79. Fraker, P.J., De Pasquali-Jardieu, P., Zwickle, C.M. and Luecke, R.W. (1978) Regeneration of T cell helper function in zinc-deficient adult mice. *Proc. Natl. Acad. Sci. (USA)*, **75**, 5660–4.

80. Malkovsky, M., Edwards, A.J., Hunt, R. *et al.* (1983) T cell-mediated enhancement of host-versus-graft reactivity in mice fed a diet enriched in vitamin A acetate. *Nature*, **302**, 338–42.

81. Lim, T.S., Putt, N., Safransky, D. *et al.* (1981) Effect of vitamin E on cell-mediated immune responses and serum corticosterone in young and maturing mice. *Immunology*, **44**, 289–93.

82. Williams, E.A.J., Gross, R.L. and Newberne, P.M. (1975) Effect of folate deficiency on the cell-mediated immune response in rats. *Nutr. Rep. Int.*, **12**, 137–48.

83. Kaplan, E. and Clark, C. (1974) Improved rosetting assay for detecting T lymphocytes. *J. Immunol. Methods*, **5**, 131–6.

84. Bach, M.A. and Bach, J.F. (1981) The use of monoclonal anti T cell antibodies to study T cell imbalances in human disease. *Clin. Exp. Immunol.*, **45**, 449–56.

85. Dean, P.N. and Pinkel, D. (1978) High resolution dual laser flow cytometer. *J. Histochem. Cytochem.*, **26**, 622–9.

86. Urbaniak, S.J., McCann, M.C., White, A.C. *et al.* (1986) Tests of immune functions, in *Handbook of Experimental Immunology. 4. Applications of Immunological Method in Biomedical Sciences* (eds D.M. Weir *et al.*), Blackwell Scientific Publications, Oxford, pp. 126.5–6.

87. Oppenheim, J.J. and Schecter, B. (1980) Lymphocyte transformation, in *Manual of*

Clinical Immunology (eds N.R. Rose and H. Friedman), American Society for Microbiology, Washington (DC), pp. 233–41.

88. Van Wauve, J.P., DeMey, J.R. and Goossens, J.G. (1980) OKT$_3$: a monoclonal anti-human lymphocyte antibody with potent mitogenic properties. *J. Immunol.*, **124**, 2708–13.

89. Chandra, R.K. (1972) Immunocompetence in undernutrition. *J. Pediatr.*, **81**, 1194–200.

90. Sellmeyer, E., Bhettay, E., Truswell, A.S. *et al.* (1972) Lymphocyte transformation in malnourished children. *Arch. Dis. Child.*, **47**, 429–35.

91. Salimonu, L.S., Johnson, A.O.K., Williams, A.I.O. *et al.* (1982) The occurrence and properties of E rosette inhibitory substance in the sera of malnourished children. *Clin. Exp. Immunol.*, **47**, 626–34.

92. Beatty, D.W. and Dowdle, E.B. (1979) Deficiency in kwashiorkor serum of factors required for optimal lymphocyte transformation *in vitro*. *Clin. Exp. Immunol.*, **35**, 433–8.

93. Chandra, R.K. and Bhujwala, R.A. (1977) Elevated serum fetoprotein and impaired immune response in malnutrition. *Int. Arch. Allergy Appl. Immunol.*, **53**, 180–5.

94. Holm, G. and Palmblad, J. (1976) Acute energy deprivation in man: effect on cell-mediated immunological reactions. *Clin. Exp. Immunol.*, **26**, 207–14.

95. Rao, K.M.K., Schwartz, S.A. and Goods, R.A. (1979) Age-dependent effect of zinc on the transformation response of human lymphocytes to mitogens. *Cell Immunol.*, **42**, 270–8.

96. Brown, R.D., Brewer, C.F. and Koenig, S.H. (1977) Conformation states of concanavalin A: Kinetics of transitions induced by interaction with Mn^{2+} and Ca^{2+} ions. *Biochemistry*, **6**, 3883–8.

97. Chandra, R.K. and Au, B. (1981) Single nutrient deficiency and cell-mediated immune responses. III. Vitamin A. *Nutr. Res.*, **1**, 81–3.

98. Corwin, L.M. and Gordon, R.K. (1982) Vitamin E and immune regulation. *Ann. N.Y. Acad. Sci.*, **393**, 437–51.

99. Robson, L.C. and Schwarz, M.R. (1975) Vitamin B$_6$ deficiency and the lymphoid system. Effects on cellular immunology and *in vitro* incorporation of ^{3}H uridine by small lymphocytes. *Cell Immunol.*, **16**, 135–44.

100. MacCuish, A.C., Urbaniak, S.J., Goldstone, A.H. and Irvine, W.J. (1974) PHA responsiveness and subpopulations of circulating lymphocytes in pernicious anemia. *Blood*, **44**, 849–55.

101. Vyes, G., States, D.A. and Breeher, G. (1974) *Laboratory Diagnosis of Immunological Disorders*, Grune and Stratton, New York, pp. 87–95.

102. Pryjma, J., Munoz, J. Galbraith, R.M. *et al.* (1980) Induction and suppression of immunoglobulin synthesis in cultures of human lymphocytes: effect of pokeweed mitogen and *Staphylococcus aureus*. *J. Immunol.*, **124**, 656–61.

103. Urbaniak, S.J., McCann, M.C., White, A.G. *et al.* (1986) Tests of immune function, in *Handbook of Experimental Immunology. 4. Applications of Immunological Methods in Biomedical Sciences* (eds D.M. Weir *et al.*), Blackwell Scientific Publications, Oxford, pp. 126.6–9

104. Robert, N.J. (1978) Variability of results of lymphocyte transformation. Assays in normal human volunteers. *Am. J. Clin. Pathol.*, **73(2)**, 160–4.

105. Hicks, M.J., James, J.F., Thies, A.C. *et al.* (1983) Age-related changes in mitogen-induced lymphocyte function from birth to old age. *Am. J. Clin. Pathol.*, **80(2)**, 159–63.

10 Clinical nutriture methodology

F. Fidanza and S.B. Heymsfield

At a late stage in the natural history of malnutrition physical signs and symptoms are present. To assess these signs and symptoms various forms are available. We have found that the most convenient and practical are those used for the Ten-State Nutrition Survey 1968–1970 [1] and reported in Fig. 10.1 and 10.2. These forms can be considered an improvement on those included in the Manual for Nutrition Surveys of Interdepartmental Committee on Nutrition for National Defense [2].

The description of the signs and symptoms can be found in the WHO Report of Expert Committee on Medical Assessment of Nutritional Status [3]. This Committee has classified these signs into the following three groups: (1) signs known to be of value in nutrition surveys; (2) signs that need further investigation; and (3) some signs not related to nutrition. More recently they have been examined critically in the Proceedings of the Conference on Nutritional Assessment [4]. For practical purposes they have been collected in Table 10.1 [5]. In addition a very useful colour atlas of most of them is available [6].

A more comprehensive form has been used in the Health and Nutrition Examination surveys in the USA, but this form is rather long and time-consuming. It can be obtained on request from National Center for Health Statistics, US Department of Health, Education and Welfare, Public Health Service, Center Building, 3700 East–West Highway, Hyattsville, Maryland 20782, USA.

If other clinical signs and symptoms have also to be assessed, the forms included in specialized publications such as WHO Monograph Series No 56 *Cardiovascular Survey Methods* [7], can be used. Some workers, however, do not like forms for clinical signs and symptoms assessment. In these cases the evaluation of their prevalence or incidence will be rather difficult and not valid, because they are based on subjective impressions. As in other cases it is very important to have standard forms.

Naturally at individual clinical levels the situation will be rather different. But this is not the case here.

Table 10.1 Signs of clinical deficiency states*

Clinical finding	Consider deficiency	Comment
Hair		
Easily pluckable, sparse	Protein, biotin	Loss of scalp and body hair may also occur
Straight, dull	Protein	Hair should be fine and silky
Flag sign	Protein	Reddening of normally black scalp; occurs in black-skinned children, possibly due to abnormal sebaceous gland activity
Coiled, corkscrew-like	Vitamin A, C	Due to follicular change; due to a keratinization disturbance and possibly abnormal sebaceous gland activity
Skin		
Xerosis	Essential fatty acid	Dryness of skin
Petechiae	Vitamin A, vitamin C	Pin-headed size haemorrhages
Pigmentation Desquamation	Niacin	Sign of pellagra distributed symmetrically in sun-exposed areas; also seen in haemochromatosis, an iron storage disease
Follicular keratosis	Vitamin A, possibly essential fatty acid	Keratin plugs in follicles, sandpaper feel of skin
'Flaky-paint' dermatitis	Protein	
Subcutaneous fat loss, fine wrinkling	Protein–energy	Minimal fat reserves; low values for anthropometric indices
Poor tissue turgor	Water	
Oedema	Protein, thiamin, vitamin E (in premature infants)	Seen in protein–energy malnutrition with hypoalbuminaemia and in wet beriberi due to thiamin deficiency
Purpura (subcutaneous skin haemorrhage)	Vitamin C, vitamin K	
Perifollicular haemorrhage	Vitamin C	
Pallor	Folacin, iron, B_{12}, copper, biotin	
Excessive hair growth	Protein–energy	Like fetal lanugo; noticeable in girls with anorexia nervosa; may be heat-retaining mechanism
Tendency toward excessive bruising (ecchymoses)	Vitamin C, vitamin K	Due to increased fragility of capillary walls
Pressure sores	Protein–energy	Common in pressure and bony points
Seborrheic dermatitis	Essential fatty acid, pyridoxine, zinc, biotin, riboflavin in infants	Also seen in acrodermatitis enteropathica due to a defect in zinc absorption
Poor wound healing	Protein–energy, zinc, and possibly essential fatty acids	Scrotal or vulvar in riboflavin deficiency; naso–labial in pyridoxine deficiency
Dermatitis	Biotin, possibly manganese	
Dry scaling	Non-specific	
Thickening of skin	Essential fatty acid	
Eyes		
Dull, dry (xerosis)	Vitamin A	Can lead to xerophthalmia in severe deficiency

Table 10.1 Continued

Clinical finding	Consider deficiency	Comment
conjunctiva		
Blepharitis	B-complex	Angular in riboflavin deficiency
Ophthalmoplegia	Thiamin	Wernicke's syndrome; prompt treatment necessary
Keratomalacia	Vitamin A	Softening of cornea
Bitot's spot	Vitamin A	Early evidence of deficiency
Corneal vascularization	Riboflavin	
Photophobia	Zinc	
Lips and Oral Structures		
Angular fissures, scars, or stomatitis	B-complex, iron, protein, riboflavin	Also seen with ill-fitting dentures
Cheilosis	B_6, niacin, riboflavin, protein	Seen especially at corners of mouth
Ageusia, dysgeusia	Zinc	Also associated with altered sense of smell
Swollen, spongy, bleeding gums	Ascorbic acid	If not edentulous
Tongue		
Magenta tongue	Riboflavin	Controversial; magenta colour may also be due to poor general nutrition
Fissuring, raw	Niacin	
Glossitis	Pyridoxine, folacin, iron, B_{12}	Due to inadequate repair of epithelial tissues
Large size, swollen	Iodine, niacin	In niacin deficiency the tongue can be deeply fissured and infected
Fiery red tongue	Folacin, B_{12}	Seen if anaemia is not pronounced
Pale	Iron, B_{12}	Seen in severe cases
Atrophic lingual papillae	Riboflavin, niacin, iron	
Teeth		
Higher frequency of tooth decay	Fluorine	May also be due to poor dental care
Loss of dental fillings, dental caries	Vitamin C	Scurvy
Glands		
Parotid enlargement	Protein	Rare, seen in alcoholic patients
'Sicca' syndrome	Ascorbic acid	Includes changes in salivary and tear glands
Thyroid enlargement	Iodine	Seen in inland areas where deficiency has not been corrected by iodination of table salt. Rarely due to a goitrogenic agent such as cabbage or brussels sprouts
Hypogonadism, delayed puberty	Zinc	
Nails		
Spoon-shaped nails (koilonychia)	Chromium, iron	Rare in the U.S.
Brittle, ridged, lined nails	Non-specific	May be protein undernutrition

Table 10.1 Continued

Clinical finding	Consider deficiency	Comment
Heart		
Tachycardia, cardiomegaly, congestive heart failure	Thiamin	'Wet' beriberi associated with high output congestive heart failure
Decreased cardiac function	Phosphorus	
Cardiac arrhythmias	Magnesium, potassium	
Cardiomyopathy	Selenium	Referred to as Keshan disease in the Orient. Occurrence in the U.S. with parenteral nutrition
Small heart, decreased output, bradycardia	Protein–energy	Prone to congestive heart failure during refeeding
Sudden failure, death	Ascorbic acid, thiamin	In ascorbic acid deficiency death may be due to small haemorrhages in the myocardium
Abdomen		
Hepatomegaly (fatty liver)	Protein	Also commonly seen in alcoholics
Wasting	Energy	Found in marasmus
Enlarged spleen	Iron	Found in 15 to 25% subjects with a significant degree of iron-deficiency anaemia
Bones and Joints		
Epiphyseal thickening, deformities	Vitamin D	Rickets in children
Bone pain	Calcium, vitamin D, phosphorus, vitamin C	(Adult) – osteomalacia due to repeated pregnancies with poor Ca^{2+} intake, little sun, light steatorrhoea (Child) – superiosteal haemorrhage in scurvy
Muscles, Extremities		
Wasting	Protein–energy	Evident in temporal area, dorsum of hand between thumb and index fingers, calf muscles
Pain in calves, weak thighs	Thiamin	
Oedema	Protein, thiamin	
Muscular twitching	Pyridoxine	
Muscular pains	Biotin, selenium	
Muscular weakness	Sodium, potassium	
Muscle cramps	Sodium, chloride	
Neurological		
Ophthalmoplegia, foot-drop	Thiamin	Wernicke's encephalopathy
Disorientation	Thiamin, sodium, water	Korsakoff's psychosis; confabulation occurs in thiamin-deficient alcoholics
Decreased position, vibratory sense, ataxia, optic neuritis	B_{12}	Subacute combined cord degeneration

Table 10.1 Continued

Clinical finding	Consider deficiency	Comment
Weakness, paraesthesia of legs	Thiamin, pyridoxine, pantothenic acid, B_{12}	Nutritional polyneuropathy, especially with alcoholism; 'burning foot' syndrome with pantothenic acid deficiency
Hyporeflexia	Thiamin	
Mental disorders	Niacin, magnesium, B_{12},	In untreated B_{12} deficiency mental disorders may progress to severe psychosis
Convulsions	Pyridoxine, calcium, thiamin (infants), magnesium, phosphorus	
Depression, lethargy	Biotin, folacin, vitamin C	
Sleep disturbances, impaired co-ordination	Pantothenic acid	
Non-ketonic hyperosmolar syndrome	Sodium	Due to large glucose infusions that result in an osmotic diuresis; occurs in TPN patients
Aphonia	Thiamin	Infants
Hyperaesthesia	Biotin	
Peripheral neuropathy	Pyridoxine	
Other		
Diarrhoea	Niacin, folacin, B_{12}	
Delayed wound healing and tissue repair	Vitamin C, zinc, protein–energy	
Anaemia, pallor	Vitamin E, pyridoxine, B_{12}, iron, folacin, biotin, copper	
Anorexia	B_{12}, chloride, sodium, thiamin, vitamin C	
Nausea	Biotin, pantothenic acid	
Fatigue, lassitude, apathy	Energy, biotin, pantothenic acid, magnesium, phosphorus,iron, potassium, vitamin C, (infants), sodium	
Growth retardation	Protein–energy, magnesium, zinc, vitamin D, calcium	
Constipation	Thiamin	Gastrointestinal atony
Headache	Pantothenic acid	
Glucose intolerance	Chromium	
Bleeding diathesis	Vitamin K	

* This table was compiled from numerous sources (from [5], with permission).

NATIONAL NUTRITION SURVEY
PEDIATRIC CLINICAL EXAMINATION
(Children under 6 years of age)

A. Identification code

State (1–2)   County (3–5)   E.D. (6–7)

Household No. (8–9)   Family (10)   Line No. (11–12)

Dietary (13)   Date of Birth (14–19)
                  Month   Day   Year   Sex (20)

B. Name *(First, middle, last)*

C. GENERAL EXAMINATION—Code: 0–Negative; 1–Positive; unless other positive codes are designated; 8–Not applicable

Examination		Doubt-ful	Col. No.	Code	Examination		Doubt-ful	Col. No.	Code
1. HAIR	a. Dry staring		(21)		6. TONGUE	a. Filiform papillary atrophy 1—Mild 2—Moderate 3—Severe		(39)	
All Neg.	b. Dyspigmented		(22)			b. Fungiform papillary hypertrophy or hyperemia 1—Mild 2—Moderate 3—Severe		(4()	
	c. Easily Pluckable		(23)						
	d. Abnormal texture or loss of curl		(24)		All Neg.				
2. EYES	a. Circumcorneal injection, bilateral		(25)			c. Geographic		(41)	
	b. Conjunctival injection, bilateral		(26)			d. Fissures		(42)	
	c. Xerosis conjunctivae		(27)			e. Serrations or swellings		(43)	
All Neg.	d. Bitot's spots		(28)			f. Red edges		(44)	
	e. Keratomalacia		(29)			g. Scarlet Beefy (Glossitis)		(45)	
	f. Xerophthalmia		(30)			h. Magenta		(46)	
3. LIPS	a. 1—Angular lesions 2—Angular scars 3—Both		(31)		7. FACE AND NECK	a. Nasalabial Seborrhea		(47)	
All Neg.					All Neg.	b. Parotids visibly enlarged		(48)	
	b. Cheilosis		(32)			c. Thyroid enlarged 0, 1, 2, 3		(49)	
4. TEETH	a. Visible caries 4+		(33)		8. FINGERS AND NAILS Neg.	1—Clubbed 2—Spooned 3—Ridged 4—Combinations		(50)	
All Neg.	b. 1—Debris 2—Calculus, 3—Both		(34)						
	c. Fluorosis		(35)		9. SKIN	a. Follicular Hyperkeratosis, Arms		(51)	
5. GUMS	a. Marginal redness or swelling 1—Local 2—Diffuse		(36)		All Neg.	b. Follicular Hyperkeratosis, Back		(52)	
All Neg.	b. Swollen red papillae, 1—Local 2—Diffuse		(37)			c. Dry or scaling (Xerosis)		(53)	
	c. Bleeding gums 1—Local 2—Diffuse		(38)			d. Hyperpigmentation, Face and hands		(54)	
						e. Thickened Pressure Points		(55)	

Fig. 10.1 Form for children under 6 years of age, from [1] with permission.

C. GENERAL EXAMINATION—Continued

	Examination	Doubt-ful	Col. No.	Code		Examination	Doubt-ful	Col. No.	Code
9. SKIN *(Continued)*	d. Hyperpigmentation face or hands		(24)		**11. LOWER EXTREM-ITIES**	a. Calf tenderness		(32)	
	e. Thickened pressure points, not elbow or knee		(25)						
	f. Perifolliculosis		(26)			b. Pretibial edema, bilateral		(33)	
All Neg. ☐	g. Purpura or petechiae		(27)		**All Neg.** ☐	c. Absent knee jerk, bilateral		(34)	
	h. Crackled skin *(mosaic)*		(28)			d. Absent ankle jerk, bilateral		(35)	
	i. Loss of elasticity		(29)			e. Absent vibratory sense, ankle		(36)	
	j. Pellagrous dermatitis *(comments)*		(30)						
10. ABDO-MEN Neg. ☐	a. Hepatomegaly		(31)		**12. SCRO-TUM Neg.** ☐	a. Scrotal dermatitis (8 — Not applicable)		(37)	

13. Pulse *(code direct)* (38–40) ☐☐☐	14. Blood pressure *(code direct)* (mm Hg)	Systolic (41–43) ☐☐☐	Diastolic (44–46) ☐☐☐

D. Date of examination (69–74) Month ☐☐ Day ☐☐ Year ☐☐	E. Completion code 0 — Completed 3 — Informant incapable 1 — Refusal 4 — Other 2 — Not available (75) ☐
F. Examiner's name Code No. (76–77) ☐☐	G. Card number 2 (78–80) 0 5 2

H. Comments

**NATIONAL NUTRITION SURVEY
GENERAL CLINICAL EXAMINATION**
(Adults and children 6 years of age and over)

A. Identification code

State (1–2)   County (3–5)   E.D. (6–7)

Household No. (8–9)   Family (10)   Line No. (11–12)

Date of birth (14–19)

Dietary (13)   Month   Day   Year   Sex (20)

B. Name

C. GENERAL EXAMINATION—Code: 0—Negative; 1—Positive, unless other positive codes are designated; 8—Not appl.

Examination		Doubt-ful	Col. No.	Code	Examination		Doubt-ful	Col. No.	Code
1. HAIR Neg.	a. Dry, staring		(21)		**6. TONGUE** All Neg.	a. Filiform papillary atrophy 1—Mild 2—Moderate 3—Severe		(39)	
2. EYES All Neg.	a. Thickened opaque bulbar conjunctivae		(22)			b. Fungiform papillary hypertrophy 1—Mild 2—Moderate 3—Severe		(40)	
	b. Angular lesions of eyelids		(23)						
	c. Circumcorneal injection, bilateral		(24)			c. Geographic		(41)	
	d. Conjunctival injection, bilateral		(25)			d. Fissures		(42)	
	e. Xerosis conjunctivae		(26)			e. Serrations or swellings		(43)	
	f. Bitot's spots		(27)			f. Red edges		(44)	
	g. Xerophthalmia		(28)			g. Scarlet beefy (*Glossitis*)		(45)	
3. LIPS All Neg.	a. 1—Angular lesions 2—Angular scars 3—Both		(29)			h. Magenta		(46)	
	b. Cheilosis		(30)		**7. FACE AND NECK** All Neg.	a. Malar pigmentation		(47)	
4. TEETH All Neg.	a. 1—Edent. 3—Both 2—Plates 8—Has teeth		(31)			b. Nasolabial seborrhea		(48)	
	b. Visible caries, 4+		(32)			c. Parotids visibly enlarged		(49)	
	c. 1—Debris 2—Calculus 3—Both		(33)			d. Thyroid enlarged 0, 1, 2, 3		(50)	
	d. Fluorosis		(34)		**8. FINGERS AND NAILS** Neg.	1—Clubbed 2—Spooned 3—Ridged 4—Combinations		(51)	
5. GUMS All Neg.	a. Atrophy, recession, inflammation 1—Local 2—Diffuse		(35)						

END CARD NUMBER 1   (78–80) 0 | 5 | 1

START CARD NO. 2 (Repeat Cols. 1–20 from card 1)

5. GUMS (cont.)	b. Marginal redness or swelling 1—Local 2—Diffuse		(36)		**9. SKIN** All Neg.	a. Follicular hyperkeratosis, arms		(21)	
	c. Swollen red papillae 1—Local 2—Diffuse		(37)			b. Follicular hyperkeratosis, back		(22)	
	d. Bleeding gums 1—Local 2—Diffuse		(38)			c. Dry or scaling (*Xerosis*)		(23)	

Fig. 10.2   Form for adults and children 6 years of age and over, from [1] with permission.

C. GENERAL EXAMINATION—continued

	Examination	Doubt-ful	Col. No.	Code		Examination	Doubt-ful	Col. No.	Code
10. ABDO-MEN All Neg.	a. Pot belly		(56)		**12. SKEL-ETAL** (Con-tinued) All Neg.	c. Epiphyseal Enlargement, wrists		(61)	
	b. Hepatomegaly		(57)			d. Bossing of skull		(62)	
11. LOWER EXTREM-ITIES Neg.	a. Pretibial Edema-Bilateral		(58)			e. Winged scapula		(63)	
12. SKEL-ETAL All Neg.	a. Beading of ribs		(59)		**13. IM-PRES-SIONS** All Neg.	1—Skinny 2—Fat 3—Neither		(64)	
	b. Bowed legs		(60)			1—Apathetic 2—Irritable 3—Both		(65)	

D. Date of Examination (69-74)

Month	Day	Year

E. Completion code

0—Completed   2—Not available   (75)
1—Refusal   3—Informant incapable
4—Other

F. Examiner's name (76-77)

Code No.

G. Card number (78-80)

0	3	1

Comments:

REFERENCES

1. *Ten-State Nutrition Survey 1968–1970* (1972) U.S. Department of Health, Education and Welfare. Center for Disease Control, DHEW Publication (HSM) 72–8130.
2. ICNND (1963) *Manual for Nutrition Surveys.* Interdepartmental Committee on Nutrition for National Defense, Bethesda.
3. WHO (1963) *Expert Committee on Medical Assessment of Nutritional Status – Report.* Techn. Rep. Series No. 258. WHO, Geneva.
4. Christakis, G. (ed.) (1973) Nutritional assessment in health programs. *Am. J. Public Health*, **63** (Suppl. November).
5. Heymsfield, S.B. and Williams, P.J. (1988) Nutritional assessment by clinical and biochemical methods, in *Modern Nutrition in Health and Disease*, 7th edn, (eds M.E., Shils and V.R. Young), Lea and Febiger, Philadelphia, pp. 817–60.
6. McLaren, D.S. (1981) *A Colour Atlas of Nutritional Disorders.* Wolfe Medical Publications, London.
7. Rose, G.A., Blackburn, H., Gillum, R.F. and Prineas, R.J. (1982) *Cardiovascular Survey Methods*, 2nd edn, WHO, Geneva.

11 Psychometrics and nutrition

K.J. Connolly

11.1 Purpose and scope

The term psychometrics has a variety of meanings. Collectively it deals with the branches of psychology concerned with measurement and more specifically with the measurement of mental function. Etymologically psychometry means measuring the mind, though in contemporary psychology it has come to be linked with psychological testing. Measurement in the physical sciences generally seems nowadays a fairly straightforward business. With some exceptions units of measurement have been agreed and the actual physical measurements are quite precise; rarely is the measurement of variables such as length, volume, and mass the subject of controversy. In some branches of the life sciences and particularly in the social sciences the position is rather different. Here the problem is not simply the precision with which measurements can be made, but often with the constructs themselves. Intelligence, for example, does not have a universally agreed definition but it is a concept we cannot easily do without.

Psychological tests, in the usually understood sense, represent one approach to measuring behaviour and mental function. Many hundreds of tests have been devised to assess different functions for different purposes in different populations. In addition to psychometric tests there are other approaches to describing and measuring psychological functions. For example, experimental methods are likely to be more reliable and penetrating when it comes to dealing with motor skills and the methods of direct observation are probably more useful when it comes to dealing with some aspects of social behaviour than are psychometric tests. This essay, however, focuses on psychological testing as this is generally understood; the basic features of psychological measurement are outlined and attention is drawn to some of the constraints. Examples of the principal types of tests and measures devised for a variety of purposes are given.

Psychological functions tend to be complex, in part this complexity is because they are affected by a wide range of variables. Almost any given end state, by which I mean the set of psychological characteristics displayed by an individual, can be produced by a variety of means. For example, we know from clinical investigations that mental subnormality may be produced by both biological and experiential factors. Intelligence is affected by, amongst other things, genetic, environmental and cultural agents. From this interconnecting network of variables, teasing out effects that can be attributed to a single variable, or even a class of variables, is extremely difficult. Moreover the various contributing factors act not only independently but also synergistically.

From clinical observations on chronically undernourished children it is known that there are correlated psychological effects, but it is difficult to tie these directly to malnutrition. Children suffering severe or even mild malnutrition are also likely to have different social and psychological experiences, so what causes what is extremely difficult to establish. Malnourished infants have been reported to show impaired attentional processes, reduced social responsiveness, heightened irritability, low activity, diminished affect, and so on. Depending on their nature, timing, duration, and severity nutritional factors can affect psychological functions in a number of ways. The effects of malnutrition on behaviour may be direct, via some physiological route such as affecting brain growth, or indirect through the organism's experience of and interaction with its environment, or by various kinds of covariation between these. Nutritional variables may have general or specific effects, they may alter the course of development and their effects may be reversible or irreversible.

The interaction of psychosocial factors with nutritional deficits has been demonstrated in an intervention study by Super *et al.* [1], and Barrett and Frank [2] provide a wide-ranging summary and critique of problems associated with investigating the effects of protein–energy malnutrition on behaviour and psychological function. The greater part of the published research on nutrition and psychological function is concerned with the consequences of severe protein–energy malnutrition, and the effects of nutritional supplementation on development and recovery [3, 4]. There is some work on the effects of specific nutritional deficits, for example, iron deficiency [5] and iodine deficiency [6, 7]. However there is little systematically developed theory to guide the search for links between nutrition and psychological function. The 'needle in the haystack' metaphor has some force.

11.2 Fundamentals of psychological testing

A standardized test offers a set of tasks presented under specified conditions and designed to assess some aspect of a person's knowledge, performance, ability, skill, personality or behaviour. It provides a scale on which individuals can be ranked on a given dimension, in some cases in relation to other individuals, in other cases in relation to a specified criterion. These are norm-referenced and criterion-referenced tests respectively.

To be useful any measuring device needs to be valid and reliable. Validity and reliability are inherent properties of tests, though of course they vary widely. In its simplest sense validity has to do with the property of truth, and is concerned with whether the test measures what it claims to measure. Reliability refers to the reproducibility of scores on a test, and also to the internal consistency of components of a test score. A test of course is unlikely to be valid if it is unreliable. All tests are samples, samples of behaviour or of mental functions, and they are used for a variety of purposes, but essentially they should provide measures typical of the individual's capacities and performance in specified circumstances.

(a) Reliability

There are two distinct meanings of the term reliability; the first relates to the reproducibility of results over time, the second to the internal consistency of the test. The usual way in which the reproducibility of results is assessed is by examining the agreement between results obtained on different occasions. This is known as test–retest reliability. If a test is reliable in terms of the reproducibility of results, then correlations between scores obtained from an individual on different occasions should approach 1. With some psychological tests this is the case, but with others test–retest reliability drops to around 0.3. It is possible to overestimate reliability if the interval between test and retest is too short. It is important also to appreciate that reliability is not simply a property of a test, it can be interpreted only as applying to the population from which the estimates were obtained. A test highly reliable among university students might be much less reliable among psychiatric patients.

Two other factors that affect test–retest reliability are the scoring procedure involved and the lability of the variable under investigation. If the scoring system is objective, that is, where the response can be clearly and simply scored as correct or incorrect, then there is less variability than arises in cases where the examiner has to exercise judgement about the response. Where the scoring system is not simple and objective, the examiner introduces variability. Some variables are naturally labile and subject to considerable variation, for example measures of anxiety. In such cases low test–retest correlations may not reflect the accuracy of a measure, but real changes in the level of the variable that have occurred in the intervening interval.

If a 50 cm ruler is broken in half, measurements made with either half will be identical; the ruler is internally consistent. If we split a psychological test in half we would not get perfectly correlated scores. Various methods are available to assess the internal consistency of tests. A common method is the split-half reliability, where scores on the first half of the test are correlated with scores on the second half. The higher the correlation the greater the internal consistency. Many tests use items arranged in order of increasing difficulty and for these a split-half method is inappropriate. This difficulty can be overcome by an odd–even split, where scores from even-numbered items are compared with scores from odd-numbered items. Since reliability is related to length of a sequence split-half methods tend to underestimate the reliability of the whole test. Procedures exist to correct such effects.

(b) Validity

Validity is concerned with what a test measures and how well it does so. The meaning of the term is quite straightforward but it is difficult to assess. The validity of a test cannot be reported in general terms: a test does not have a high or low validity in the abstract; it is valid for a purpose. Various methods have been devised to investigate validity, which has in fact become a term with a number of different meanings. Generally, to demonstrate that a test is valid it is necessary to set up criteria against which it can be judged. If good criteria can be established it is comparatively easy to demonstrate the validity or otherwise of a test. In the case of an intelligence test three kinds of criteria might be employed to investigate its validity; (a) correlations with scores from established tests of intelligence, (b) a demonstration that some groups score more highly than others, say research scientists or industrialists compared with factory operatives or shopkeepers, (c) by following up a group of individuals to whom the test was administered and examining the prediction that those scoring highly on the test would also do better in terms of other measures such as examination results, occupational status, income, responsibility in the community, etc. Positive results on each of these would lend support to the validity of the new test, but none is definitive. There is no single preferred means of establishing validity and in the absence of a widely accepted criterion validity should be considered in relation to a range of criteria. The overall outcome from these is the best indicator.

The validity of a test needs to be considered in relation to specified purposes, be it diagnosis or selection. Different kinds of validity are emphasized in investigations having different purposes. The principal kinds are as follows.

Face validity. This is inherently subjective but important. It refers not to what a test actually measures but to what it seems to measure. In testing adults, and also children though in a slightly different way, it is essential that the test has face validity. It must seem to the person being examined that the test is reasonable and sensible. If the test seems absurd or silly then a subject is likely either to refuse to be tested or not to take it seriously. The consequences with regard to the results are obvious, they could not be relied upon as a proper sample of the individual's capabilities.

Content validity. This is an estimate based on a detailed examination of the content of test items. Content validity applies where the subject matter is fixed and specific, it is most obviously applicable to tests of attainment and ability. A test purporting to measure the English vocabulary of children would obviously involve knowledge of the meaning of English words. Test items must constitute a sample of common nouns, verbs, etc. in a proportion similar to that found in the language. If the items concern word meaning and the words involved are an appropriate sample, then the test is self-evidently valid.

Concurrent validity. This refers to the relationship between scores on a test and established criterion scores. For example, a way of evaluating the validity of a test for clerical skills would be to see how the scores on the test correlate with known clerical skills of a group of individuals where performance was assessed in actual office conditions.

Construct validity. This refers to procedures for evaluating validity based on the degree to which the test item captures the hypothetical quality it was designed to measure. Thus if a test purports to measure intelligence it is necessary to ask what constructs (qualities or traits) actually characterize intelligence; and, do the test items actually tap such constructs? The initial stages of test construction are usually concerned with construct validity.

Predictive validity. This relates to evidence from the predictive power of the test, that is its correlation with a criterion subject to the test. Predictive validity provides good support for a psychological test.

(c) Standardization and norms

The standardization of a test consists in establishing firstly uniform conditions under which it is administered, and secondly specified ways of evaluating the responses made by subjects. Any test, irrespective of whether it is psychological or biochemical, requires specified standard conditions for its administration; this is nothing more than prescribing controlled conditions under which scientific observations are made. Only when conditions are standardized can differences be attributed to the individual; without these variable error is introduced and the test reliability is reduced.

In addition to establishing uniform procedures, standardization also involves establishing norms. Without norms it is impossible to evaluate an individual's performance on many tests. Norms are sets of scores on a test from various defined groups with which it is possible to compare an individual's performance. Norms are fundamental to establishing psychological facts; with good norms we can discover the developmental course of any psychological characteristic. A norm is a value, or range of values, that is representative of a group on a specified test. It provides a basis against which the performance of an individual can be assessed. A psychological test norm represents the test performance of a standardization sample. Norms are thus empirically established by determining how a representative group of persons performs on a specified test. An individual's score may then be compared to the scores from the standardization sample to determine how it relates to the distribution. Various transformations and scaling procedures are often employed in constructing standardized norms.

The construction of adequate norms for a test depends on sampling, not only on the size of the sample but on its containing a representative subset of individuals with respect to any variables that are of importance. Which variables will be of importance is an empirical question, though on the basis of accumulated experience we know something of the major variables that need to be included in the standardization of a test. They include the following: social class, urban or rural residence, occupational status, ethnic grouping, age, sex, and so forth. A normal adult sample would have to reflect the population in respect of these factors. In addition the size of the sample must be adequate. In the case of a variable known to change with age, and where such changes are important, there must be sufficiently homogeneous age groups to enable satisfactory comparisons to be made. For example in measuring infant vocabulary, change is so rapid during the second and third years that standardization groups need to be taken at three-month intervals. Generally rates of change slow with advancing age, which allows longer sample intervals to be used.

11.3 Types of psychological test

Psychological tests and scales can be classified in various ways. They may be grouped according to the function which they are designed to measure, for example intelligence, personality, specific abilities and aptitudes, etc. Another classification is in terms of the purpose for which the instrument is designed. For example as a screening test, as a selection device, as a diagnostic instrument, or as a means of evaluating the effectiveness of a therapeutic or educational intervention. There are a very large number of psychological scales, tests, and inventories. They are classified and catalogued in various handbooks the most extensive of which is the *Mental Measurements Yearbook* series [8].

Intelligence is difficult to define, but the various meanings of the concept are linked to fundamental cognitive processes. It is generally regarded as the ability to profit from experience, which implies the capacity to behave adaptively and function successfully within particular environmental contexts. A valid intelligence test, therefore, is one that predicts adaptive and successful functioning within specified environments. The principal use of intelligence tests has been as a predictor of scholastic success, and from this it follows that 'adaptive and successful' behaviours have been those such as reasoning, the ability to abstract, learning, and particular kinds of problem solving.

Various models of intelligence have been proposed [9, 10] and though this is not the place to discuss them, one distinction that will probably be helpful is that proposed by Cattell [11] between fluid and crystallized intelligence. Fluid intelligence is that which is assessed by those components of a test that are based on the ability to solve novel problems. It is in fact abstract intelligence and can be roughly equated with innate reasoning ability. Crystallized intelligence on the other hand is assessed by tests based on factual knowledge and the ability to utilize this knowledge. It is a concrete capacity and reflects the knowledge an individual gains from living within any culture. A good education serves to increase crystallized intelligence. Intelligence or general ability is essential for all cognitive activity involving any degree of problem solving; whether it is made up of one, a few, or many factors is not generally agreed.

There are tests designed to be administered to individuals and others designed to be administered to groups. Some tests attempt to examine fluid intelligence free from the trappings of a specified culture (culture-free tests), though whether this is possible, and if so to what extent is the subject of controversy. Some tests have been extremely well standardized and for specified populations excellent norms are available. A further distinction can be made between verbal tests or verbal items within tests which rely upon language and ability with language, and non-verbal or performance items that make minimal use of verbal materials. Tests of general intelligence have both verbal and performance sub-tests.

Stanford–Binet Scales. These are made up of an essentially atheoretical set of tasks involving verbal ability, perceptual skills, short-term memory, and eye–hand co-ordination. The test was designed for the American culture and language and is based on the Binet–Simon scale of 1911. The emphasis on verbal items has restricted the overall applicability of the test even within the USA. Criticisms have also been made of the standardization procedure. It is a time-consuming test. For further information see Terman and Merrill [12].

Wechsler Intelligence Scales. These comprise a series of verbal sub-tests (vocabulary, information or general knowledge, arithmetic, comprehension, similarities, digit-span or forward and reverse immediate memory span), and a series of performance sub-tests (block design or constructing patterns of different degrees of complexity, arranging sequences of pictures, object assembly – a jigsaw like task, mazes, a coding test, a picture completion task). The first three sub-tests in the verbal scale are very dependent on education and therefore measure crystallized intelligence. The performance tests measure fluid intelligence to a greater degree. Although they are novel to many subjects they are nonetheless firmly grounded in the familiar material culture of the developed industrialized countries – pictures, symbols, patterns, paper and pencil activities. The sub-tests are timed. A total IQ score can be obtained, as can verbal and performance IQs; a profile of the sub-test scores is also produced. The sub-test profile is sometimes used in neuropsychological diagnosis. Verbal and performance IQs have good reliability and the full-scale IQ has a test–retest reliability of about 0.9. The test is administered to individuals and takes about one hour; for further information see Wechsler [13]. Wechsler scales and norms are available over the age range 2.5 years to adult.

British Ability Scales. These were developed specifically for use in Britain and have British norms. These scales take account of some of the shortcomings of the Wechsler scales and also incorporate items that assess development in terms of Piaget's theory of cognitive growth. The scales are primarily intended for the age-group 5–12 years, though it can be extended upwards and downwards. The test provides six sub-scores corresponding to Thurstone's Primary Mental Abilities (reasoning, verbal ability, spatial ability, numerical ability, memory, fluency where creativity items are used) and a general ability score. Further details are given in the test manual [14].

Group intelligence tests. A good number of these are available, though many are very similar. They are designed principally as instruments for mass testing. They have certain obvious advantages in that many individuals can be tested simultaneously, the examiner's role is simplified and minimized, scoring is usually more objective (that is to say that there is less room for interpretation by the examiner). The tests usually have well-established norms because of the comparative ease of taking large samples. Group tests also have certain limitations, the most important of which is that nothing whatever is known of the subject's state. Group tests do not involve the examiner in gaining the subject's rapport, ensuring co-operation, and maintaining interest. Individuals who are unaccustomed to testing may be more handicapped on group tests than they are on individual tests; group tests are thus less satisfactory for use with young children or with persons from another culture or even sub-culture. Many of the available group tests are very dependent on verbal ability.

Performance tests. Measures such as the Wechsler scales require that the subject comprehend written and spoken instructions, in fact they rely to a great extent on verbal ability. An individual who is deaf, culturally disadvantaged, from another culture, or simply very young cannot be tested satisfactorily using the general tests referred to above. In such a performance test the subject does not necessarily have to read, speak, write, or understand spoken language, since the instructions can be mimed or demonstrated. A variety of performance tests have been devised, their value and quality is variable. Among the best known are:

1. *Kohs Block Design Test.* This involves constructing patterns of different degrees of difficulty from a set of coloured blocks. For details see Kohs [15].
2. *Porteus Maze Test.* This is a paper and pencil test which involves solving maze puzzles of varying degrees of difficulty. See Porteus [16, 17].
3. *Knox Cube Test.* This is essentially a test of immediate memory for a series of movements. See Knox [18].
4. *Raven's Progressive Matrices.* The test is made up of a set of matrices each with a section cut out. The subject must choose, from a set of 6–8 possibilities, which section matches that which has been cut out, in order to complete the overall pattern. Items of the test become progressively more difficult. The test has been extensively used and there are well-established British norms [19].
5. *Goodenough–Harris Drawing Test.* This requires the subject to draw a man, a woman, and him or herself. A detailed scoring system and North American norms are available [20]. It may be given as an individual or as a group test. There is no time limit, which for many purposes is an advantage. The test presumes a familiarity with pictures and pencil and paper.

(b) Personality and temperament

Although commonly used terms, personality and temperament are difficult to define and the meaning given to them depends in part on the theoretical bias of the user. In general the terms refer to basic elements of behavioural functioning, elements which within an individual show substantial consistency over time. There is now an enormous amount of evidence demonstrating individual differences in behaviour from birth throughout life. Many of these characteristics are constitutional in that they reflect some intrinsic aspect of personal functioning, though their origins may be experiential rather than genetic.

It has been argued that a person's behaviour is largely determined by the situation in which it occurs. While there is no doubt about the importance of situations, the significance of personality is shown by the great variation in individual responses to any one situation. The 'fuzziness' surrounding the concept of personality certainly makes for difficulties but it does not remove the utility of the notion. It is concerned with individual differences in patterns of reactivity and self-regulation, with a broad array of behavioural styles, some of which may be discernible in infancy, whereas others do not become clear until later. The cause of these relatively stable patterns no doubt varies but is likely to include genetic, physiological, experiential, and environmental factors. For some the terms personality and temperament are used interchangeably whereas others use personality only in referring to adults and temperament only for children. This is not the place to discuss such differences though it is perhaps worth mentioning that dimensions along which temperament is thought to vary include; physique, activity, sociability, emotionality, and cognition. Personality is seen by some of the principal contemporary theorists in terms of a collection of traits. These traits have been derived empirically by factor analysis.

Since it is well known that situational variables exert an important effect on a person's behaviour, it follows that if we wish to make general statements about characteristic styles of response it is necessary to sample behaviour over a wide range of situations, and over a reasonably long time-scale. This makes for some practical difficulties. The direct observation of behaviour in a variety of situations by the examiner is impracticable, so other methods of obtaining information are necessary. In the case of children parental questionnaires have been used. Parents are seen as a source of information because of their extensive direct experience of the child over a number of situations and a considerable period of time. There are obviously limitations (parents do not see their children in some situations) and there is a danger of systematic bias. Another source is information from the individual directly in the form of answers to specially constructed questionnaires.

The 16 Personality Factor Test. This test was developed by Cattell and Eber [21]. There are two parallel forms each of 187 items. The items comprise a series of statements with three possible answers to each, and the subjects are asked to choose one, avoiding the middle option as far as possible. An example would be; I prefer people who are (a) reserved, (b) in between, (c) make friends quickly. Subjects are asked to respond quickly, giving the answer that comes to mind first. This is because on careful examination many of the questions are ambiguous and what is sought is an individual's 'basic' response. The items relate to dimensions such as sociability, energy, nervousness, independence, feelings of guilt, moodiness. As the name of the test implies there are 16 factors which Cattell argues make up human personality.

Eysenck Personality Questionnaire. Eysenck considers personality to be composed of two basic variables, extraversion and neuroticism. These dimensions were arrived at by factor analysis. The E scale measures extraversion, which has to do with an individual's being outward looking, noisy, cheerful, impulsive and the like. The N scale measures neuroticism and is concerned with the individual's tendency to worry and be anxious, moody, and irritable. The EPQ is a refinement of the Eysenck Personality Inventory, to which was added a new P scale which refers to psychoticism, a factor defining a particular abnormal group [22]. There are also scales for children. The E and N factors are for the most part identical with Cattell's second-order factors labelled extraversion and anxiety.

Minnesota Multiphasic Personality Inventory. This consists of some 567 items to which the subject must answer true or false. Items are built in which detect deception on the part of the subject. The various items in the scale, which takes a long time to complete, were selected for their capacity to discriminate between individuals falling into psychiatric categories such as schizophrenia and depression, and normal individuals. The test was devised almost 50 years ago and has been the subject of extensive research, its usefulness is confined very largely to a clinical context.

Projective techniques. This means simply a procedure for discovering a person's characteristic modes of behaviour, motivations, and dynamic traits.

The idea is that the individual will, if provided with the right eliciting stimuli, reveal his or her enduring personality characteristics. The notion is simple and probably basically sound, but the scoring and interpretation of this kind of material presents great difficulties. Test–retest reliability tends to be low and validity is difficult to demonstrate. Probably the best known projective test is the Rorschach, a series of ten symmetrical inkblots which the subject has to describe. The Thematic Apperception test presents a series of rather indistinct pictures and again the subject must describe was is going on in these pictures. It is presumed that such tasks elicit from the subject characteristic responses that reflect enduring personality features. These tests may be useful for clinical purposes but their utility in research is very limited.

Temperament questionnaires for infants and children. From a longitudinal study carried out in New York Thomas *et al.* [23, 24] identified nine temperament variables. These were; activity level, rhythmicity, approach–withdrawal, adaptability, intensity of reaction, threshold of responsiveness, quality of mood, distractability, and attention span and persistence.

Persson-Blennow and McNeil [25, 26] devised parental questionnaires, based on the Thomas *et al.* variables, to assess temperament in infancy, specifically at 6, 12, and 24 months. The questionnaires consist of multiple-choice questions based on situations represented in the Thomas *et al.* work. The degree of overlap between the 6- and 12-month and the 12- and 24-month sets was about 75% and 70% respectively. The questionnaires were standardized on 147 Swedish infants at all three ages. The questionnaires consist of between 50 and 55 questions and take approximately 15 minutes to administer. The general level of test–retest reliability in the two-year sample is from 0.56 to 0.84 with a mean of 0.65 [27].

Bates [28] has recently reviewed concepts and measures of temperament in childhood.

(c) Motor performance

The ability to make accurate controlled movements is important for everyday life in all cultures. Walking, speaking, and using simple manual tools are commonplace examples of skilled motor action. Motor skills are learned and the quality of behaviour depends on factors such as the amount and kind of practice, and an individual's motivation. The range of individual variation in motor performance is very great and cannot be explained simply in terms of factors such as differential practice. There appears to be extensive variability in some set of underlying abilities, and the assessment of motor performance entails measuring these abilities. The nature of these capacities and particularly their organization change in important ways during development so that the predictive utility of measurements made in infancy will be limited. A similar limitation applies to the specificity of skills; a high level of performance on one is no guarantee of a similar high level of performance on another. Because of the great flexibility evident in skilled motor action, correlations between tasks are for the most part low. However, if some fundamental component of skilled motor action is impaired, or limited (such as precision in timing) then the effects of this may be evident in many tasks.

The idea of a general all-encompassing motor ability, analogous with the general factor in intelligence, is not supported by empirical studies; for the most part high inter-task correlations have not been found. Motor skills have complex and variable structures and different tasks are likely to require different combinations of underlying abilities. Although motor skills are highly specific, some proportion of the observed variance is associated with factors such as speed, steadiness, spatial precision, and strength. Individuals may have a relatively high capability on one factor while being low on another. The blend most appropriate for one task will not be that specially suited to another, so quite marked variability will be observed.

The assessment of motor performance is complex, partly because of the great range of factors that contribute, but especially because of the paucity of adequate theory with which to guide the process. Many variables can and do affect the development of motor performance; moreover, motivation will certainly differentially affect the individual's performance on given tasks at given times. The approach to assessing motor performance through abilities has been subject to criticism on several grounds; the range of subjects employed has been severely limited (largely young men), the structure of the underlying abilities may change over the lifespan, etc.

In infants and young children the assessment of motor development is based largely on the time at which different behaviours appear during development and the typical patterns of change. Various scales of motor development, and tests of motor impairment and general motor proficiency have been devised. There are a large number of tests available most of them being of doubtful value [29]. The analysis of skilled motor performance undertaken by experimental psychologists provides another approach to measurement and assessment. Here a more adequate theoretical base has been developed and methods of measuring performance speed, accuracy, timing, information processing capacity, etc. have all been devised [29, 30].

(d) Developmental schedules   The assessment of psychological development and competence in infancy poses special problems. Because of the infant's linguistic limitations control of the testing situation by verbal instructions is not possible; moreover the infant cannot be relied upon to co-operate with the examiner's efforts. These difficulties coupled with the rapid changes that occur in infancy and the quite marked individual differences that exist present special problems. Developmental schedules are based on the pattern and timing of behaviour development, which appears generally typical of the species, at least so far as this can be judged from any one culture. These schedules are firmly based therefore in a normative view of development and are concerned less with the processes of developmental change than with the product of development and the timing of events.

Gesell's Developmental Schedule. Initially published in 1925, the scale consisted of 144 items grouped into four sets, beginning at the age of four months and extending up to six years. The four general fields of development were: (a) motor behaviour including postural control, locomotion, prehension, drawing, and hand control (items in this set are designed to assess co-ordination and motor capacity); (b) language behaviour, assessed by means of vocabulary, word comprehension, and conversation; (c) adaptive behaviour, comprising eye–hand coordination, object recovery, comprehension, discriminative performance, etc. (items in this set are designed to assess the child's responsiveness to environmental change); (d) personal and social behaviour including reactions to persons, personal habits, initiative and independence, play responses, etc.

Each of the infant schedules contains on average 32 items, some of which appear in more than one schedule. The make-up of the scales is varied; motor items comprise 45% of the four-month schedule and language items only 3%. By 24 months motor items are down to 11% and language up to 21%. Attempts to estimate the predictive validity of the scale by correlating scores with intelligence test scores have produced varying results. A major revision and updating of the scales has been published which provides more adequate norms [31]. The revision also divides the motor behaviour category into gross and fine motor behaviour. The scales are not measures of intelligence, rather they provide a picture of overall development in early childhood. They may be helpful in detecting quite large disturbances in development but more minor variations may well be of no biological or predictive significance.

Bayley's Infant Scales. These scales were designed to provide a measure of the developmental progress of infants from 2 to 30 months which would be of use for clinical and research purposes [32]. An overall mental development index is obtained from the combined scores of the mental and motor scales. The mental scale contains 163 items which include shape discrimination, imitation, comprehension, problem solving, and manipulation of objects. The 81 items making up the motor scale include activities such as sitting, standing, walking and grasping. Additionally there is also an infant behaviour record used to evaluate the child's co-operativeness, endurance, emotional tone, and other factors likely to influence performance on the test. Norms are provided at half-month intervals from two to five months and at monthly intervals from 6 to 30 months. The test was standardized on a carefully drawn sample of 1262 American infants. Split-half reliabilities average at 0.86. Inter-observer agreement is generally high at 89% and 93% respectively on the mental and motor scales at eight months. Good correlations with the Standford–Binet test at 36 months have been reported [33].

The Bayley scale is not only the most thoroughly developed of the infant assessment instruments, it is also the most widely used. Francis-Williams and Yule [34] found British infants to be broadly comparable to the USA norms. In a sample of Indian infants Phatak [35] found them to be advanced on the US norms during the first 6–9 months, though during the latter part of the second year their scores were lower than the USA norms. Solomons and Solomons [36] used the motor scale in a study of Yucatecan infants and found variations from the USA norms; in some instances these children were advanced but in others delayed. There is evidence of cultural differences in the rate and pattern of early motor development and some indication of acceleration in traditionally reared infants. Comparisons with American norms are therefore likely to be misleading.

The Denver Developmental Screening Test. As the name implies the test is designed to detect developmental delay in preschool children, it is not a diagnostic instrument. The test comprises four scales; gross motor, fine motor and adaptive, language, and personal/social [37]. Items are arranged in order of appearance and the age at which 50% of the children pass is given. The test was standardized on 1036 US children aged two weeks to six years four months. Mean inter-observer agreement is reported as 96% and the test–retest reliability of items ranged from 0.66 to 0.93 [38].

Scores were found to correlate with scores from the Stanford–Binet and Bayley scales between 0.86 and 0.97. The relative ease with which an examiner can learn to administer and interpret the test, along with high inter-observer agreement, makes it a most useful screening device for preschool children.

(e) Cognitive psychology and neuropsychological evaluation

Cognitive psychology is concerned with how people mentally represent and process information. It includes processes such as perception, learning, memory, reasoning, problem solving, decision making, etc., functions that are, in fact, related to performance on general intelligence tests. Neuropsychology links these complex psychological functions to systems within the brain and is particularly concerned with the behavioural, that is functional, expression of brain disease and brain damage. Many of the component abilities tapped by tests such as the Wechsler scales can be explored in greater depth and with greater precision if experimental tasks are employed. For example, different aspects or types of memory may be investigated directly, or the difficulty of certain mental operations can be assessed by the time required to carry them out. Procedures of this kind are not usually norm referenced; they are used in experimental investigations and sometimes in criterion-referenced diagnostic tests.

Neuropsychological tests are used to identify deficits in particular psychological functions and to relate these to pathology of the brain. They are primarily diagnostic tests and are used to detect deficits in functions such as attention, concentration, scanning, the mental rotation of objects, etc. Various batteries of tests have been compiled the purpose of which is to aid the understanding of organic disability. These batteries provide a standard procedure for collecting data on a broad sample of behaviour and they measure major intellectual functions across auditory, visual, verbal and non-symbolic modalities. Memory tests need to examine encoding, retention, retrieval, recognition, etc. in order more exactly to identify the form that a memory deficit may take.

Halstead–Reitan Battery. This set of tests has gradually grown from the original collection employed by Halstead [39] and has been extended by Reitan [40].

The tests include a category test that requires the subject to discover the principles by which collections of objects are grouped, a tactual performance test – the Seguin Formboard, a rhythm test requiring the subject to discriminate between like and unlike pairs of musical beats, a finger tapping test which is sensitive to cortical lesions, and a time–sense test involving visual reaction time and the ability to estimate a just elapsed time-span.

A. Smith's neuropsychological battery. The tests making up this battery were chosen to provide a balanced examination of intellectual function. The battery comprises six standard tests with the Wechsler Adult Intelligence Scale – WAIS (or in the case of children the Wechsler Intelligence Scale for Children – WISC), the Hooper [41] Visual Organisation Test (pictures of cut-up objects which the subject is asked to identify), Raven's Matrices, the Benton Visual Retention Test (a visual memory test) [42], the Purdue Pegboard (a test of manual dexterity), the Symbol Digital Modalities Test (where symbols have to be matched to digits), the Peabody Picture Vocabulary Test (pictures of objects must be named), colour naming, identifying body parts, tactile inattention, and memory. Details of the battery are given in Smith [43]. There are no norms for the battery as a whole but each of the component tests has demonstrated sensitivity to a well-defined modality or functional impairment. The whole battery takes about three hours to administer.

Various other test batteries have been compiled such as that developed by Luria [44]. In addition some tests are essentially screening tests for brain damage. Most of the neuropsychological tests in use are designed to detect severe focal lesions; they are, in the hands of a skilled examiner, sensitive and frequently they detect early signs of a deteriorating condition in the CNS.

11.4 Cross-cultural assessment

The fundamental difficulty in cross-cultural assessment is that a test valid in one culture is not necessarily valid in another. Some of the reasons for this are common to all kinds of test but the problems are most acute in measuring what are commonly called higher cognitive functions. Where groups do not share a common language, similar social conventions and norms, patterns of child rearing, and a broadly similar material culture, then it is inevitable that comparisons will be difficult. Culture-free tests do not exist (except perhaps at a psychophysiological and sensory level). The manner in which an individual thinks is strongly influenced by linguistic structure, by semantic categories, and by the way in which the world is perceived and interpreted. Even at the level of motor skills the material culture exerts its effects. Although language is the most powerful cultural instrument, simply changing a test from verbal to non-verbal (say a pictorial form) does not alter the difference in the conceptual approach it will invoke in the subject. Moreover many societies will be quite unfamiliar with pictures and diagrams. At the perceptual level the way in which the environment is perceived is influenced not only by the visual habits built up in response to the physical features of the childhood environment but also by patterns of conformity demanded by a particular society and the way in which the conformity is maintained.

In an attempt to find a common medium through which mental functioning can be validly examined across cultures, the idea of 'culture-fair' tests has been introduced. Culture-fair means that the more obviously culture-bound features of a test are avoided. Thus, for example, an emphasis on speed of performance (which is quite foreign to many cultures) and a reliance on pictures to present objects or situations (in many cultures the conventions of pictorial representation are not understood) would be avoided. Fundamental issues such as the way in which reality is perceived, the way in which problems are understood, and differences in style of thought are not affected by such relatively minor adjustments.

While comparisons between cultures are very difficult, and their validity remains doubtful, it is possible to use culture-fair tests to measure individual differences within a cultural group. As long as it is appreciated that what these tests measure may be far from identical in different groups, then they can be useful tools. Although culture produces very basic differences in the style of psychological functioning, there are some common features between individuals across cultures. For example, memory is a capacity possessed not only by the urban European but also the villager in a remote region of the Papua New Guinea Highlands. To be sure the culture will affect the ways in which memory is organized, used, and accessed but it may nevertheless, by using means appropriate for a specific culture, be possible to make valid comparisons. One promising possibility for the cross-cultural study of the processes of cognitive development and intellectual functioning stems from Piaget's theory, and this has been linked with the investigation of malnutrition [45, 46]. Problems associated with mental testing in pre-literate societies have been discussed in some detail by Ord [47]. Ord's own work has been largely with Melanesians and the various cultures in Papua New Guinea, though work in other regions is also reviewed. Cross-cultural factors in human assessment are discussed in considerable detail in a volume edited by Irvine and Berry [48].

REFERENCES

1. Super, C.M., Clement, J., Vuori, L. *et al.* (1981) Infant and caretaker behavior as mediators of nutritional and social intervention in the barrios of Bogota, in *Culture and Early Interactions* (eds T.M. Field, A.M. Sostek, P. Vletze and P.H. Leiderman), Erlbaum, Hillsdale NJ.
2. Barret, D.E. and Frank, D.A. (1987) *The Effects of Undernutrition on Children's Behavior*, Gordon and Breach, New York.
3. Stock, M.B. and Smythe, P.M. (1976) 15 year developmental study on effects of severe under-nutrition during infancy on subsequent physical growth and intellectual functioning. *Arch. Dis. Child.*, **51**, 327–31.
4. Joos, S.K. and Pollitt, E. (1984) Effects of supplementation on behavioral development in children up to the age of two years: A comparison of four studies, in *Malnutrition and Behavior: Critical Assessment of Key Issues* (eds J. Brozek and B. Schurch), Nestlè Foundation, Lausanne.
5. Pollitt, E., Soemantri, A.G., Yunis, F. and Scrimshaw, N.S. (1985) Cognitive effects of iron deficiency anaemia. *Lancet*, **i**, 58.
6. Pharoah, P.O.D., Connolly, K.J., Ekins, R.P. and Harding A.G. (1984) Maternal thyroid hormone levels in pregnancy and the subsequent cognitive and motor performance of the children. *Clin. Endocrinol.*, **21**, 265–70.
7. Pharoah, P.O.D. and Connolly, K.J. (1987) A controlled trial of iodinated oil for the prevention of endemic cretinism: A long term follow-up. *Int. J. Epidemiol.*, **16**, 68–73.
8. Buros, O.K. (1978) *The Eighth Mental Measurements Yearbook.* 2 volumes. The Gryphon Press, Highland Park, New York.
9. Sternberg, R.J. (ed.) (1982) *Handbook of Human Intelligence*, Cambridge University Press, Cambridge.
10. Wolman, B.B. (1985) *Handbook of Intelligence*, Wiley, New York.
11. Cattell, R.B. (1971) *Abilities: Their Structure, Growth and Action*, Houghton–Mifflin, Boston.
12. Terman, L.M. and Merrill, M.A. (1937) *Stanford–Binet Intelligence Scale*, G.G. Harrap, London.

13. Wechsler, D. (1958) *The Measurement and Appraisal of Adult Intelligence*, Williams and Wilkins, Baltimore.
14. Elliott, C.D., Murray, D.J. and Pearson, L.S. (1978) *British Ability Scales*, National Foundation for Educational Research, Windsor.
15. Kohs, S.C. (1923) *Intelligence Measurement: A Psychological and Statistical Study based upon the Block-design Tests*, Macmillan, New York.
16. Porteus, S.D. (1952) *The Porteus Maze Test Manual*, Harrap, London.
17. Porteus, S.S. (1965) *Porteus Maze Test: Fifty Years Application*, Pacific Books, Palo Alto.
18. Knox, H.A.A. (1914) A scale based on the work at Ellis Island for estimating mental defect. *JAMA*, **62**, 741–7.
19. Raven, J.C. (1965) *Progressive Matrices*, H.K. Lewis, London.
20. Harris, D.B. (1963) *Children's Drawings as Measures of Intellectual Maturity*, Harcourt Brace Jovanovich, New York.
21. Cattell, R.B. and Eber, H.W. (1963) *Handbook for the Sixteen Personality Factor Questionnaire*, IPAT, Champaign (Illinois).
22. Eysenck, H.J. and Eysenck, S.B.G. (1975) *The EPQ*, University of London Press, London.
23. Thomas, A., Birch, H.G., Chess, S. *et al.* (1963) *Behavioral Individuality in Early Childhood*, New York University Press, New York.
24. Thomas, A., Chess, S. and Birch, H.G. (1968) *Temperament and Behavior Disorders in Children*, New York University Press, New York.
25. Persson-Blennow, I. and McNeil, T.F. (1979) A questionnaire for measurement of temperament in six-month-old infants: Development and standardization. *J. Child Psychol. Psychiat.*, **20**, 1–13.
26. Persson-Blennow, I. and McNeil, T.F. (1980) Questionnaire for measurement of temperament in one- and two-year-old children. Development and standardization. *J. Child Psychol. Psychiat.*, **21**, 37–46.
27. Persson-Blennow, I. and McNeil, T.F. (1982) Research note: new data on test–retest reliability for three temperament scales. *J. Child Psychol. Psychiat.*, **23**, 181–4.
28. Bates, J.E. (1989) Concepts and measures of temperament, in *Temperament in Childhood* (eds G.A. Kohnstamm, J.E. Bates and M.K. Rothbart), Wiley, Chichester.
29. Connolly, K.J. (1984) The assessment of motor performance in children, in *Malnutrition and Behavior: Critical Assessment of Key Issues* (eds J. Brozek and B. Schurch), Nestlè Foundation, Lausanne.
30. Brozek, J. (1984) The assessment of motor functions in adults, in *Malnutrition and Behavior: Critical Assessment of Key Issues* (eds J. Brozek and B. Schurch), Nestlè Foundation, Lausanne.
31. Knoblock, H. and Pasamanick, B. (1974) *Gesell and Amatruda's Developmental Diagnosis: The Evaluation and Management of Normal and Abnormal Neuropsychologic Development in Infancy and Early Childhood*, 3rd edn, Harper and Row, New York.
32. Bayley, N. (1969) *Bayley Scales of Infant Development*, Psychological Corporation, New York.
33. Ramey, C.T., Campbell, F.A. and Nicholson, J.E. (1973) The predictive power of the Bayley scales of infant development and the Stanford–Binet intelligence test in a relatively constant environment. *Child Dev.*, **44**, 790–5.
34. Francis-Williams, J. and Yule, W. (1967) The Bayley scales of motor and mental development: An exploratory study with an English sample. *Dev. Med. Child Neurol.*, **9**, 391–401.
35. Phatak, P. (1970) Motor growth patterns of Indian babies and some related factors. *Indian Pediatr.*, **7**, 619–24.

36. Solomons, G. and Solomons, H.C. (1975) Motor development of Yucatecan infants. *Dev. Med. Child Neurol.,* **17,** 41–6.
37. Frankenburg, W.K. and Dodds, J.B. (1967) The Denver Developmental Screening Test. *J. Pediatr.,* **71,** 181–91.
38. Frankenburg, W.K., Camp, B.W., Van Natta, P.A. and Demersseman, J.A. (1971) Reliability and stability of Denver Developmental Screening Test. *Child Dev.,* **42,** 1315–25.
39. Halstead, W.C. (1947) *Brain and intelligence,* Chicago University Press, Chicago.
40. Reitan, R.M. and Davison, L.A. (1977) *Clinical Neuropsychology: Current Status and Applications,* Winston/Wiley, New York.
41. Hooper, H.E. (1958) *The Hooper Visual Organisation Test Manual,* Western Psychological Services, Los Angeles.
42. Benton, A.L. (1974) *The Revised Visual Retention Test,* 4th edn, Psychological Corporation, New York.
43. Smith, A. (1975) Neuropsychological testing in neurological disorders, in *Advances in Neurology* (ed. W.J. Friedlander), Raven Press, New York.
44. Christensen, A.L. (1975) *Luria's Neuropsychological Investigation,* Muntesgaard, Copenhagen.
45. Dasen, P.R. (1977) Cross-cultural cognitive development: The cultural aspects of Piaget's theory. *Ann. N.Y. Acad. Sci.,* **285,** 332–7.
46. Dasen, P.R. (1984) Cross-cultural uses of Piagetian methodology, in *Malnutrition and Behavior: Critical Assessment of Key Issues* (eds J. Brozek and B. Schurch), Nestlè Foundation, Lausanne.
47. Ord, I.G. (1971) *Mental Tests for Pre-Literates,* Ginn, London.
48. Irvine, S.M. and Berry, J.W. (1983) *Human Assessment and Cultural Factors,* Plenum Press, New York.

Index

Abdomen
  skinfold 33
Absorptiometry photon dual *see* Dual
    photon absorptiometry
Activation neutron analysis *see* Neutron
    activation analysis
Advanced methods
  body composition 83–96
Albumin
  plasma 170–3
Alkaline phosphatase *see* Phosphatase
    alkaline
Anthropometer 4
Anthropometic measurements 1–62
  introduction 1
Apparatus
  body density 65
  body weight 8
  calorimetry, indirect 121
  crown-rump length 4
  skeletal diameters 41
  skinfold thickness 30
  stature 4
  supine length 4
Arachidonic acid
  cascade 153–9
Area
  fat 16
  muscle 16
Arm
  circumference 18
  span 5
Aspartate transaminase 266
  interpretation 270
  performance characteristics 269
  procedure 268
  reference values 270

Benn
  index 12
Biacromial
  breadth 41

Biceps
  skinfold 31
Bicondylar humerus
  breadth 42
Biiliac
  breadth 41
Bioimpedence analysis 87
  evaluation 92
  interpretation 95
  procedure 89
Biotin 296–304
  plasma-urine 300
    interpretation 304
    performance characteristics 303
    procedure 302
    reference values 304
  whole blood 296
    interpretation 300
    performance characteristics 299
    procedure 298
    reference values 300
Bistyloid
  breadth 42
Bitrochanteric
  breadth 41
Bodily mass
  index 12
Body
  cell mass 72
  composition 63–99
    introduction 63
  density *see* Densitometry
  fat 73
  mass *see* Body weight
    index 12–6
  weight 6
    apparatus 8
    interpretation 11
    performance characteristics 10
    procedure 9
    reference values 11
Breadth

biacromial 41
bicondylar humerus 42
biiliac 41
bistyloid 42
bitrochanteric 41

Caeruloplasmin, serum 396
  interpretation 398
  performance characteristics 398
  procedure 397
  reference values 398
Calcium 342–50
  ionized 345
    interpretation 346
    performance characteristics 346
    procedure 346
    reference values 346
  metacarpal indices 346–8
  serum osteocalcin 349–50
  total, serum-plasma 344
    interpretation 345
    performance characteristics 345
    procedure 344
    reference values 345
  urine hydroxyproline 348–9
Calf
  circumference 18
Calorimetry, indirect 119
  apparatus 121
  performance characteristics 127
  procedure 122
Carbohydrate
  tolerance test XV
Cardiorespiratory efficiency 102
  interpretation 105
  performance characteristics 104
  procedure 103
  reference values 105
β-Carotene 200
  performance characteristics 202
  procedure 201
  reference values 203
Chest
  circumference 23
    performance characteristics 24
    procedure 24
    reference values 24
Child
  growth 9–10
Children
  height data 44–53
  weight data 44–53

Cholesterol, serum 140
  procedure 142
Chromium 408
  interpretation 410
  procedure 409
  reference values 410
Circumferences
  arm 18
  calf 18
  chest 23
  forearm 18
  head 23
  hip 27
  thigh 18, 27
  waist 27
Clinical nutriture 447–56
  forms 452–5
  signs of deficiency 448–51
Cobalamin(s) *see* Vitamin B_{12}
Cognitive psychology
  psychological tests 469
Complement C3 432
  performance characteristics 434
  procedure 434
  reference values 434
Computerized axial tomography 83
  evaluation 90
  interpretation 95
  procedure 88
Conductivity, electrical total body *see*
    Total body electrical conductivity
Copper 395–401
  caeruloplasmin, serum 396–8
  plasma-serum 395–6
    by AAS 395
      interpretation 395
      performance characteristics 395
      procedure 395
      reference values 395
    by colorimetry 396
  superoxide dismutase 398
    interpretation 401
    performance characteristics 400
    procedure 400
    reference values 401
Counting whole-body *see* Whole-body
    counting
Creatinine, urine 173
  interpretation 175
  performance characteristics 175
  procedure 174
  reference values 175

Cross cultural assessment
  psychological tests 470
Crown-rump
  length 4–5

Delayed cutaneous hypersensitivity 429
  interpretation 431
  performance characteristics 431
  procedure 431
  reference values 431
Densitometry 64
  apparatus 65
  interpretation 70
  performance characteristics 68
  procedure 66
  reference values 70
Developmental schedules
  psychological tests 467
Diameters, skeletal 40
  apparatus 41
  interpretation 43
  performance characteristics 42
  procedure 41
  reference values 43
Dilutometry 71
  exchangeable potassium 77
  total body potassium 79
  total body water 74
Douglas bag
  technique 122
Dual photon absorptiometry 86
  evaluation 91
  interpretation 95
  procedure 89

Energy
  balance 113–30
    introduction 113
  expenditure 117
  intake 115
Equations
  fat mass 34, 65
  per cent fat 34, 65

Factor B 432
  performance characteristics 434
  procedure 434
  reference values 434
Fat
  area 16
    interpretation 21
    performance characteristics 19

    procedure 18
    reference values 21
  mass 64
    equation 34, 65
    percent 34, 65
Fat-free
  extracellular solids 72
  mass 64
Fatty acids, essential 131
  interpretation 137
  performance characteristics 134
  procedure 133
  reference values 137
Ferritin, serum 360–2
  procedure 362
Fibronectin
  plasma 170–3
Fitness, physical 101–12
Flavin adenine dinucleotide (FAD) 251
  interpretation 256
  performance characteristics 254
  procedure 253
  reference values 255
Folic acid (5-Me-THF) 283
  interpretation 287
  performance characteristics 286
  procedure 285
  reference values 287
Forearm
  circumference 18

Glutathione
  peroxidase 406
    interpretation 408
    performance characteristics 408
    procedure 407
    reference values 408
  reductase 244–51
    macromethod 244
      interpretation 247
      performance characteristics 247
      procedure 246
      reference values 247
    micromethod 248
      interpretation 251
      performance characteristics 251
      procedure 249
      reference values 251

Haematocrit 374
  procedure 375
Haemoglobin 372

procedure 374
HDL-cholesterol 148–53
 procedure 149–52
Head
 circumference 23
  performance characteristics 24
  procedure 24
  reference values 24
Height *see* Stature
Height
 for age 6
  calculation 9
  interpretation 12
 data, children 44–53
 sitting 2, 4, 6
  reference values 6
Hip
 circumference 27
Hydroxyproline, urine 348
 interpretation 349
 performance characteristics 349
 procedure 348
 reference values 349
Hypersensitivity cutaneous delayed *see*
  Delayed cutaneous
  hypersensitivity

IgA, secretory 434
 performance characteristics 435
 procedure 435
 reference values 435
IGF-1 *see* Insulin-like growth factor-1
Immunocompetence 425–45
 introduction 425
 malnutrition 426
Index
 Benn 12
 body mass 12
 bodily mass 12
 obesity 13
 ponderal 12
 power family 13
 Quetelet 12
 Rohrer 12
Indices, metacarpal *see* Metacarpal indices
Indirect calorimetry *see* Calorimetry,
  indirect
Insulin-like growth factor-1, 178
 interpretation 180
 performance characteristics 180
 procedure 179
 reference values 180

Intelligence
 psychological tests 462
Interpretation
 albumin 172
 aspartate transaminase 270
 biotin
  plasma-urine 304
  whole blood 300
 body
  density 70
  weight 11
 caeruloplasmin, serum 398
 calcium
  ionized 346
  total serum-plasma 345
 cardiorespiratory efficiency 105
 chromium 410
 copper 395
 creatinine, urine 175
 diameters, skeletal 43
 fat area 21
 fatty acids, essential 137
 fibronectin 172
 flavin adenin dinucleotide (FAD) 256
 folic acid (5-Me-THF) 287
 glutathione
  peroxidase 408
  reductase 247, 251
 height
  for age 12
  sitting 11
 hydroxyproline, urine 349
 IGF-1 180
 length, supine 6
 manganese 412
 metacarpal indices 348
 3-methyl-histidine 177
 muscle area 21
 niacin
  metabolites, urine 266
  whole blood 263
 osteocalcin 350
 pantothenic acid 309
 phosphatase, alkaline 395
 phylloquinone 220
 plasma transport proteins 172
 potassium 342
  exchangeable 79
  total body 83
 pyridoxal 5'-phosphate (PLP)
  plasma 280
  whole blood 276

selenium
  by AAS 403
  by fluorometry 406
skinfold thickness 39
sodium 337
stature 6
superoxide dismutase 401
thiamine
    transketolase 232, 235
    whole blood 241
trans-vitamin K_1 227
vitamin A (retinol) 195, 200
vitamin B_{12} 295
vitamin C
    buffy coat layer 315
    plasma 315, 319
    whole blood 319
vitamin D (25-OHD) 209
vitamin E 213
waist/hip ratio 28
weight
    for height 11
    height ratios 15
zinc
    leukocytes 390
    plasma-serum 386
Infants
  body weight 15
Iron 355-85
  deficiency 376–85
    criteria 382–3
    indicators 376–81
  ferritin, serum 360–2
  haematocrit 374–5
  haemoglobin 372–4
  protoporphyrin, erythrocyte 369–72
  serum 362–7
    procedure 367
Iron binding capacity 367–9
  procedure 369

Jump standing broad *see* Standing broad
  jump

Kofranyi-Mickaelis
  technique 123

Length
  crown-rump 4–5
  supine 3
    apparatus 4
    interpretation 6

performance characteristics 5
  procedure 4
  reference values 6
Lipid pattern 131–63
Lipids, plasma 139
  cholesterol 140
  lipoproteins 144
  triglycerides 142
Lipoproteins, plasma 144
  HDL-cholesterol 148
  procedure 147
Lymphocyte
  count 428–9
    performance characteristics 429
    procedure 429
  proliferation response 438–40
    performance characteristics 440
    procedure 440
  T 436–8
    performance characteristics 437
    procedure 437

Magnesium 353–5
  serum 353
    by AAS 353–4
    by colorimetry 354–5
  urine, by AAS 353
    procedure 354
    reference values 354
Manganese 410
  interpretation 412
  performance characteristics 411
  procedure 411
  reference values 412
Mass
  body 6
  fat 73
  fat free 74
Medial calf
  skinfold 33
Metacarpal indices 346
  interpretation 348
  performance characteristics 347
  procedure 346
  reference values 347
3-methyl-histidine 175
  interpretation 177
  performance characteristics 176
  procedure 176
  reference values 177
Midaxillary
  skinfold 33

Mineral nutriture 332–412
  introduction 332
Motor performance 108
  performance characteristics 111
  procedure 109
    pull-ups 109
    shuttle run 110
    sit-ups 110
    soft ball throw distance 111
    standing broad jump 110
    50-yard dash 110
    600-yard run walk 111
  psychological tests 466
  reference values 111
Muscle
  area 16
    interpretation 21
    performance characteristics 19
    procedure 18
    reference values 21
  strength 106
    performance characteristics 107
    procedure 107
    reference values 107

Neuropsychological evaluation
  psychological tests 469
Neutron activation analysis 84
  evaluation 91
  interpretation 95
  procedure 89
Niacin 258–66
  metabolites, urine 263
    interpretation 266
    performance characteristics 265
    procedure 265
  whole blood 258
    interpretation 263
    performance characteristics 262
    procedure 261
    reference values 262
Nomogram
  body mass index 14
Nuclear magnetic resonance 84
  evaluation 90
  interpretation 95
  procedure 89

Obesity
  index 13
25-OHD *see* Vitamin D
Osteocalcin, serum 349

interpretation 350
performance characteristics 350
procedure 350
reference values 350

Pantothenic acid 304–9
  interpretation 309
  performance characteristics 308
  procedure 307
  reference values 309
Percent, fat 34, 65
Performance characteristics
  albumin 171–2
  aspartate transaminase 269
  biotin
    plasma-urine 303
    whole blood 299
  body weight 10
  caeruloplasmin, serum 398
  calcium
    ionized 346
    total, serum-plasma 345
  calorimetry, indirect 127
  cardiorespiratory efficiency 104
  β-carotene 202
  complement C3 434
  copper 395
  creatinine, urine 175
  delayed cutaneous hypersensitivity 431
  densitometry 68
  diameters, skeletal 42
  factor B 434
  fat area 19
  fatty acids, essential 134
  fibronectin 171–2
  flavin adenin dinucleotide (FAD) 254
  folic acid (5-Me-THF) 286
  glutathione
    peroxidase 408
    reductase 247, 251
  head circumference 24
  hydroxyproline, urine 349
  IgA secretory 435
  IGF-1 180
  lymphocyte
    count 429
    proliferation response 440
    T 437
  magnesium 355
  manganese 411
  metacarpal indices 347
3-methyl-histidine 176

motor performance 111
muscle
   area 19
   strength 107
niacin
   metabolites, urine 265
   whole blood 262
osteocalcin 350
pantothenic acid 308
phosphatase, alkaline 394
phosphorus 353
phylloquinone 218
potassium 342
   exchangeable 78
   total body 79
proteins, plasma transport 171–2
pyridoxal 5′-phosphate (PLP)
   plasma 279
   whole blood 274
4-pyridoxic acid, urine 282
riboflavin, urine 257
selenium 403, 405
skeletal diameters 65–66
skinfold thickness 33
stature 5
superoxide dismutase 400
supine length 5
thiamin
   urine 243
   whole blood 239
transketolase 231, 235
trans-vitamin K_1 225
vitamin A 194, 198
vitamin B_{12} 294
vitamin C
   buffy coat layer 314
   plasma 314, 318
   whole blood 318
vitamin D (25-OHD) 208
vitamin E 212
waist/hip ratio 27
water
   total body 76
weight/height ratios 14
zinc
   hair 392
   leukocytes 390
   plasma-serum 386
   plasma-urine 387
Personality
   psychological tests 464
Phosphatase, alkaline 392

interpretation 395
   performance characteristics 394
   procedure 394
   reference values 395
Phosphorus 350
   performance characteristics 353
   procedure 352
   reference values 353
Phylloquinone (vitamin K_1) 214
   interpretation 220
   performance characteristics 218
   procedure 217
   reference values 219
Plasma transport proteins 170–3
PLP *see* Pyridoxal 5′-phosphate
Ponderal index 12
Potassium 340–2
   exchangeable 77
      interpretation 79
      performance characteristics 78
      procedure 77
      reference values 79
   total body 79, 340
      interpretation 83
      performance characteristics 79
      procedure 79
      reference values 82
Procedure
   albumin 171
   arm
      circumference 18
      span 5
   aspartate transaminase 268
   biotin
      plasma-urine 302
      whole blood 298
   body weight 9
   caeruloplasmin, serum 397
   calcium
      ionized 346
      total, serum-plasma 344
   calf circumference 18
   calorimetry, indirect 122
   cardiorespiratory efficiency 103
   β-carotene 201
   chest circumference 24
   cholesterol 142
   chromium 409
   complement C3 434
   copper 395
   creatinine, urine 174
   crown-rump length 5

delayed cutaneous hypersensitivity 431
factor B 434
fatty acids, essential 133
ferritin, serum 362
fibronectin 171
flavin adenin dinucleotide (FAD) 253
folic acid (5-Me-THF) 285
forearm circumference 18
glutathione
    peroxidase 407
    reductase 246, 249
haematocrit 375
haemoglobin 374
HDL-cholesterol 149, 152
head circumference 24
hip circumference 27
hydroxiproline, urine 348
IgA secretory 435
IGF-1 179
infant body weight 9
iron, serum 367
iron binding capacity 369
lymphocyte
    count 429
    proliferation response 440
    T 437
magnesium 354
manganese 411
metacarpal indices 346
3-methyl-histidine 176
motor performance 109
muscle
    area 18
    strength 107
niacin
    metabolites, urine 265
    whole blood 261
osteocalcin 350
pantothenic acid 307
phosphatase, alkaline 394
phosphorus 352
phylloquinone 217
plasma transport proteins 171
potassium 341
    exchangeable 77
    total body 79
protoporphyrin 371
pyridoxal 5'-phosphate (PLP)
    plasma 278
    whole blood 273
4-pyridoxic acid, urine 282
riboflavin, urine 257

selenium 402, 405
skinfold thickness 31
sodium 337
stature 4-5
superoxide dismutase 400
supine length 4
thiamin
    urine 242
    whole blood 238
thigh
    circumference 18, 27
lymphocyte T percentage 437
transketolase 230, 234
trans-vitamin K_1 223
triglycerides 144
vitamin A 193, 197
vitamin B_{12} 293
vitamin C
    buffy coat layer 312
    plasma 312, 317
    whole blood 317
vitamin D (25-OHD) 206
vitamin E 211
waist circumference 27
water, total body 75
weight/height ratios 13
zinc
    hair 392
    leukocytes 389
    plasma-serum 386
    plasma-urine 387
Protein
    nutriture 165–84
        introduction 165
    plasma 169–73
        interpretation 172
        performance characteristics 171
        procedure 171
        reference values 172
Protoporphyrin, erythrocyte
    procedures 371
Psychological
    testing 458–61
    tests 461–70
Psychometric and nutrition 457–73
Pull-ups 109
Pyridoxal 5'-phosphate (PLP) 271–6
    plasma 276
        interpretation 280
        performance characteristics 279
        procedure 278
        reference values 280

whole blood, by HPLC 271
   interpretation 276
   performance characteristics 274
   procedure 273
   reference values 275
4-pyridoxic acid, urine 280
  performance characteristics 282
  procedure 282
  reference values 282

Quetelet index 12

Ratio
  waist/hip 24
  waist/thigh 24
  weight/height 6, 8, 12
Reference values
  albumin 172
  aspartate transaminase 270
  biotin
    plasma-urine 304
    whole blood 300
  body
    density 70
    weight 11
  caeruloplasmin 398
  calcium
    ionized 346
    total, serum-plasma 345
  cardiorespiratory efficiency 105
  β-carotene 203
  chest circumference 24
  child growth 11
  chromium 410
  complement C3 434
  copper 395
  creatinine, urine 175
  delayed cutaneous hypersensitivity 431
  diometers, skeletal 43
  factor B 434
  fat area 21
  fibronectin 172
  flavin adenin dinucleotide (FAD) 255
  folic acid (5-Me-THF) 287
  glutathione
    peroxidase 408
    reductase 247, 251
  head circumference 24
  height, sitting 6
  hydroxyproline, urine 349
  IgA secretory 435
  IGF-1 180

length, supine 6
magnesium, serum-urine 354
manganese 412
metacarpal indices 347
3-methyl-histidine 177
motor performance 111
muscle
  area 21
  strength 107
niacin, whole blood 262
osteocalcin 350
pantothenic acid 309
phosphatase, alkaline 395
phosphorus 353
phylloquinone 219
potassium 342
  exchangeable 79
  total body 82
protein plasma 172
pyridoxal 5'-phosphate
  plasma 280
  whole blood 275
4-pyridoxic acid 282
riboflavin, urine 258
selenium, whole blood
  by AAS 403
  by fluorometry 406
skinfold thickness 38
superoxide dismutase 401
thiamin
  urine 243
  whole blood 240
transketolase 232, 235
trans-vitamin K_1 226
vitamin A 194, 199
vitamin B_{12} 295
vitamin C
  buffy coat layer 314
  plasma 314, 319
  whole blood 319
vitamin D (25-OHD) 208
vitamin E 212
water, total body 77
weight/height ratios 15
zinc
  hair 392
  leukocytes 390
  plasma-serum 386
  plasma-urine 387
Resonance magnetic, nuclear *see* Nuclear
  magnetic resonance
Retinol *see* vitamin A

Riboflavin 244–58
  erythrocyte
    glutathione reductase 244–51
  whole blood
    FAD 251–6
  urine 256
    performance characteristics 257
    procedure 257
    reference values 258
Rohrer index 12

Score Z 10
Secretory, IgA *see* IgA Secretory
Segment lengths 5
Selenium 401–8
  by AAS 402
    interpretation 403
    performance characteristics 403
    procedure 402
    reference values 403
  by fluorometry 404
    interpretation 406
    performance characteristics 405
    procedure 405
    reference values 406
  glutathione peroxidase 406–8
Shuttle run 110
Siri's equation 65
Sit-ups 110
Skinfold
  thickness 29
    apparatus 30
    interpretation 39
    performance characteristics 33
    procedure 31
      sites 31–3
    reference values 38
Sodium 335
  interpretation 337
  procedure 337
Soft-ball throw 111
Somatomedin C *see* IGF-1
Stadiometer 4
Standardization of methods XV
Standing broad jump 110
Stature (standing height) 3
  apparatus 4
  interpretation 6
  performance characteristics 5
  procedure 4
  reference values 6
Subscapular

skinfold 32
Superoxide dismutase 398
  interpretation 401
  performance characteristics 400
  procedure 400
  reference values 401
Suprailiac
  skinfold 32

Temperament
  psychological tests 464
Testing, psychological *see* Psychological
    testing
Tests, psychological *see* Psychological tests
Thiamin 228–43
  erythrocyte
    transketolase 228-35
  urine 241
    performance characteristics 243
    procedure 242
    reference values 243
  whole blood, total 235
    interpretation 241
    performance characteristics 239
    procedure 238
    reference values 240
Thigh
  circumference 18, 27
  skinfold 33
T-lymphocyte *see* Lymphocyte T
α-tocopherol *see* vitamin E
Tomography, computerized axial *see*
    Computerized axial tomography
Total body electrical conductivity 87
  evaluation 92
  interpretation 96
  procedure 89
Trace elements nutriture 332–423
Transport proteins 170–3
Trans-vitamin K_1 220
  interpretation 227
  performance characteristics 225
  procedure 223
  reference values 226
Transketolase, erythrocyte 228–35
  macromethod 228
    interpretation 232
    performance characteristics 231
    procedure 230
    reference values 232
  micromethod 233
    interpretation 235

performance characteristics 235
  procedure 234
  reference values 235
Triceps
  skinfold 31
Triglycerides, serum 142
  procedure 144

Vitamin A (retinol) 191–200
  macromethod 191
    interpretation 195
    performance characteristics 194
    procedure 193
    reference values 194
  micromethod 195
    interpretation 200
    performance characteristics 198
    procedure 197
    reference values 199
Vitamin B_6 266–83
  erythrocyte
    aspartate transaminase 266–71
  plasma
    pyridoxal 5′-phosphate (PLP) 276–80
  whole blood
    pyridoxal 5′-phosphate (PLP) 271–6
  urine
    4-piridoxic acid 280–3
Vitamin B_{12} 290
  interpretation 295
  performance characteristics 294
  procedure 293
  reference values 295
Vitamin C 309–19
  buffy coat layer 309
    interpretation 315
    performance characteristics 314
    procedure 312
    reference values 314
  plasma, macromethod 309
    interpretation 315
    performance characteristics 314
    procedure 312
    reference values 314
  plasma, micromethod 315
    interpretation 319
    performance characteristics 318
    procedure 317
    reference values 319
  whole blood 315
    interpretation 319

performance characteristics 318
  procedure 317
  reference values 319
Vitamin D (25-OHD) 203
  interpretation 209
  performance characteristics 208
  procedure 206
  reference values 208
Vitamin E (α-tocopherol) 209
  interpretation 213
  performance characteristics 212
  procedure 211
  reference values 212
Vitamin K_1 *see* Phylloquinone and Trans-vitamin K_1
Vitamin nutriture 186–330
  introduction 187

Waist circumference 27
Waist/hip ratio 24
  interpretation 28
  performance characteristics 27
  procedure 27
Waist-thigh ratio 24
  interpretation 28
  performance characteristics 27
  procedure 27
Water
  extracellular 73
  intracellular 73
  total body 74
    interpretation 77
    performance characteristics 76
    procedure 75
    reference values 77
Weight
  body *see* Body weight
  data, children 44–53
  underwater 64, 67
Weight for
  age 7
    interpretation 11
  height 9–10
    procedure 9
  length 9–10
    procedure 9
Weight/height ratios 12
  interpretation 15
  performance characteristics 14
  procedure 13
  reference values 15
Whole-body counting 79, 84

interpretation 83, 95
evaluation 91
procedure 79, 89
Working capacity 101–12
introduction 101

50-yard dash 110
600-yard walk 111

Zinc 385–95
hair 391
performance characteristics 392
procedure 392
reference values 392
leukocytes 388
interpretation 390

performance characteristics 390
procedure 389
reference values 390
phosphatase, alkaline 392–5
plasma-serum 385–8
by AAS 385
interpretation 386
performance characteristics 386
procedure 386
reference values 386
by alternative method 387–8
plasma-urine 386
performance characteristics 387
procedure 387
reference values 387
Z-score 10